Gastrointestinal Motility

CONFERENCE DATA

This volume contains the Proceedings of the 9th International Symposium on Gastrointestinal Motility held in Aix-en-Provence, France, September 12–16, 1983.

International steering committee
J. H. Szurszewski (Chairman), (USA)
T. Burks (USA)
C. Roman (France)
M. Wienbeck (FRG)
D. Wingate (Great Britain)

Local organizing committee
(Marseille)
J. Gonella
N. Mei
J. P. Miolan
C. Roman
J. Salducci
Mrs. E. Dussauze
Miss A. M. Lajard

Local planning committee
L. Bueno, Toulouse
J. P. Delmont, Nice
J. Frexinos, Toulouse
J. Gonella, Marseille
R. Lambert, Lyon
N. Mei, Marseille
P. Meunier, Lyon
J. P. Miolan, Marseille
C. Roman, Marseille
J. Salducci, Marseille

SPONSORS

GASTROINTESTINAL MOTILITY

EDITED BY

Claude ROMAN Dr. Sc.

Professor of Physiology,
Department of Physiology and
Neurophysiology L.A. CNRS 205,
Faculty of Sciences St Jérôme,
University AIX-MARSEILLE III,
13397 MARSEILLE CEDEX 13

Proceedings of the 9th International Symposium
on Gastrointestinal Motility held in Aix-en-Provence, France,
September 12–16, 1983

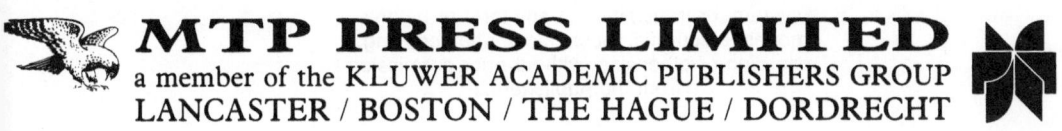

MTP PRESS LIMITED
a member of the KLUWER ACADEMIC PUBLISHERS GROUP
LANCASTER / BOSTON / THE HAGUE / DORDRECHT

Published in the UK and Europe by
MTP Press Limited
Falcon House
Lancaster, England

British Library Cataloguing in Publication Data

International Symposium on Gastrointestinal
Motility *(9th: 1983: Aix-en-Provence)*
Gastrointestinal motility
1. Gastrointestinal motility
I. Title   II. Roman, Claude
612'.32   QP145

ISBN 978-94-010-9354-5   ISBN 978-94-010-9352-1 (eBook)
DOI 10.1007/978-94-010-9352-1

Published in the USA by
MTP Press
A division of Kluwer Boston Inc
190 Old Derby Street
Hingham, MA 02043, USA

Library of Congress Cataloging in Publication Data

International Symposium on Gastrointestinal Motility
(9th: 1983: Aix-en-Provence, France)
Gastrointestinal motility.

"Proceedings of the 9th International Symposium on
Gastrointestinal Motility held in Aix-en-Provence,
France, September 12–16, 1983."
Includes bibliographies and index.
1. Gastrointestinal system—Motility—Congresses.
2. Gastrointestinal system—Motility—Disorders—Congresses.
I. Roman, Claude, 1938–   II. Title.
[DNLM: 1. Gastrointestinal motility—Congress.
W3 IN918L 9th 1983g/WI 102 1603 1983g]
QP145.I53   1983   599'.0132   83-24921

ISBN 978-94-010-9354-5

Butler & Tanner Limited, Frome and London

Preface

This volume reviews the most recent knowledge in the field of gastrointestinal motility in health and disease. The topics addressed include basic as well as clinical data concerning the motor functions of the entire gut: the lower oesophageal sphincter and the gastro-oesophageal reflux; the gastric emptying and the role of the pylorus; the motility of the biliary tract and its disorders; the cyclic motor activity of the gut and intestinal transit; the colonic and ano-rectal motility. There are also important contributions in physiology and pharmacology relating to the neurohumoral regulation of the gut, and the function of digestive smooth muscle. Several papers explore the nature of the linkage between brain and gut, a link which has long been deduced by clinicians but not, until recently, systematically explored by scientists. The individual papers, selected from a large number of submissions, have been subject to 'peer-review' by an international committee which includes both clinicians and basic scientists. Therefore this book should serve as an up to date source of information for researchers concerned with basic sciences as well as for clinicians in gastroenterology, medicine and surgery.

C. Roman

This volume is dedicated to the memory of two
friends and colleagues:

Professor Dr J. HELLEMANS
Professor Dr H. MONGES

Acknowledgments

This was the 9th of this series of symposia held alternatively in Europe and North America, and the first to be held in France. I had a great deal of advice and help from the international steering committee and from the French planning committee. Their membership is listed elsewhere in this volume. These committees helped particularly in abstract review, fund-raising and publicity.

Many crucial responsibilities were assumed by my associates and colleagues here at the University of Aix-Marseille. Mrs. E. Dussauze and Miss A. M. Lajard worked very hard for months and were secretaries, hostesses and general organizers. Drs. J. Gonella, J. P. Miolan, N. Mei and J. Salducci gave invaluable assistance in program planning and greatly contributed to the success of the meeting. Mrs. Dany (Office du ·Tourisme of Aix-en-Provence) arranged the accommodation and the social program. I want also to mention the contributions of two other collaborators who acted as projectionists and general assistants: D. Catalin and P. Rega. I am very grateful to the authors for their cooperation in submitting their camera-ready papers in time, and to MTP Press (England) for publishing the proceedings so soon after the symposium. Last but not least, the financial assistance of many firms and agencies (listed elsewhere in this volume) was both generous and greatly appreciated.

List of Participants

Dr A. ABITA
Laboratoire Janssen Le Brun
Département Expérimental
4 rue Dumont d'Urville
75116 Paris
France

Dr L. M. A. AKKERMANS
Academic Hospital Utrecht
Department of Surgery
Catharijnesingel 101
NL-3500 CG Utrecht
The Netherlands

Dr R. S. ALPHIN (A. H. ROBINS)
1211 Sherwood Avenue
Richmond, VA 23229
USA

Dr M. AL-SAFFAR
Department of Pharmacology
Karolinska Institutet
Box 60 400
S-104 01 Stockholm
Sweden

Dr F. ANGEL
Department of Physiology and Biophysics
Mayo Clinic and Foundation
Rochester, MN 55905
USA

Dr E. ATANASSOVA
Institute of Physiology
Bulgarian Academy of Sciences
PO BOX 131
1113 Sofia
Bulgaria

Dr F. BALDI
Cattedra di Clinica Medica III
Policlinico S. Orsola
Via Massarenti 9
I-40138 Bologna
Italy

Dr D. L. BARENDS
Janssen Pharmaceutical
Chapel Street
Marlow
Bucks. S47 1ET
England

Dr P. BASS
Department of Pharmacology
University of Wisconsin
425 N. Charter
Madison, WI 53706
USA

Dr BAUER
Federal Republic of Germany

Dr G. BAZZOCHI
Istituto di Clinica Medica e
  Gastroenterologia
Policlinico S. Orsola
Via Massarenti 9
I-40138 Bologna
Italy

Dr J. BEHAR
Department of Gastroenterology
Rhode Island Hospital
593 Eddy Street, APC 421
Providence, RI 02902
USA

Dr A. BENNANI
Avicenne Hospital
Gastroenterology Department
Rabbat
Morocco

Dr W. E. BERQUIST
Division of Gastroenterology and
  Clinical Nutrition
UCLA Hospitals and Clinics
University of California
Los Angeles, CA 90024
USA

Dr P. BIANCANI
Division of Gastroenterology
Department of Medicine
Rhode Island Hospital
593 Eddy Street
Providence, RI 02902
USA

Dr A. L. BLUM
Division of Gastroenterology
Department of Internal Medicine
Triemli Hospital
CH-8063 Zurich
Switzerland

Dr G. BONORA
Istituto di Clinica Medica e
  Gastroenterologia
Policlinico S. Orsola
Via Massarenti 9
I-40138 Bologna
Italy

Dr A. BORTOFF
Department of Physiology
Upstate University of NY
Syracuse, NY 13210
USA

Dr M. BORTOLOTTI
Istituto di Clinica Medica I e
  Gastroenterologia
Università di Bologna
Policlinico S. Orsola
I-40138 Bologna
Italy

Dr M. BOUVIER
Institut Neurophysiologie,
  Psychophysiologie CNRS
Département de Neurophysiologie
  Végétative
31 chemin Joseph Aiguier
F-13277 Marseille Cédex 9
France

Dr K. L. BOWES
Division of General Surgery
University of Alberta
Edmonton, Alberta T6G 2G3
Canada

Dr L. BUENO
Station Pharmacologie-Toxicologie INRA
180 chemin de Tournefeuille
31300 Toulouse
France

Dr S. BUHOT
4 rue Rollin
75005 Paris
France

Dr T. F. BURKS
Department of Pharmacology
University of Arizona
Health Science Center
Tucson, AZ 85724
USA

Dr G. CARGILL
6–8 rue Général Camou
75007 Paris
France

Dr CASPI
Laboratoire Théraplix
46–58 rue Albert
75640 Paris Cédex 13
France

Dr O. CASTELL
Gastroenterology Section
Department of Medicine
Bowman-Gray School of Medicine
Winston Salem, NC 27103
USA

Dr B. CATCHPOLE
Department of Surgery
University of Western Australia
Queen Elizabeth II Medical Center
Nedlands, Western Australia 6009
Australia

Dr M. M. CHAMBERS
Department of Surgery
University of Alberta
Edmonton, Alberta T6G 2G7
Canada

Dr W. Y. CHEY
The Genesee Hospital
224 Alexander Street
Rochester, NY 14607
USA

Dr J. CHRISTENSEN
Division of Gastroenterology-Hepatology
Department of Internal Medicine
University of Iowa Hospital and Clinic
Iowa City, IA 52242
USA

Dr A. S. CLANACHAN
Department of Pharmacology
University of Alberta
Edmonton, Alberta T6G 2H7
Canada

Dr S. M. COLLINS
Gastroenterology
Department of Internal Medicine
McMaster University
1200 Main Street West
Hamilton, Ontario L8N 3Z5
Canada

Dr P. I. COLLMAN
Department of Physiology
The University
Sheffield S10 2TN
England

Dr M. COOK
Department of Pharmacology
University of Western Ontario
London, Ontario N6A 5C1
Canada

Dr E. CORAZZIARI
Cattedra di Gastroenterologia
Clinica Medica II
Policlino Umberto 1
I-00161 Roma
Italy

Dr D. COUTURIER
Service d'Hépato-Gastroentérologie
Hôpital Cochin
27 rue du Faubourg St. Jacques
F-75674 Paris Cédex 14
France

Dr COVILLE
Laboratoire Théraplix
46–52 rue Albert
75640 Paris
France

Dr F. CRENNER
Department of Bioengineering
INSERM Unit 61
Avenue Molière
F-67200 Strasbourg
France

Dr R. F. CROCHELT
843B. S. American Street
Philadelphia, PA 19147
USA

Dr J. C. CUBER
Laboratoire de Physiologie
  de la Nutrition
INRA CNRZ
78350 Jouy en Josas
France

Dr E. E. DANIEL
McMaster University
Department of Neurosciences
Faculty of Health Sciences
1200 Main Street West
Hamilton, Ontario L8N 3ZS
Canada

Dr E. DANQUECHIN-DORVAL
Department of Medicine
USUHS
Bethesda, MD 20814
USA

Dr J. DAVISON
Department of Medical Physiology
University of Calgary
Calgary, Alberta T2N 1N4
Canada

Dr L. DEBSKI
Department of Surgery
University of Alberta
Edmonton, Alberta T6G 2G3
Canada

Dr D. J. DE CARLE
Department of Medicine
University of New South Wales
St George Hospital
Kogarah, New South Wales 2217
Australia

Dr M. DELILLE
Laboratoire Théraplix
46–52 rue Albert
F-75640 Paris Cédex 13
France

Dr N. E. DIAMANT
Toronto Western Hospital
Department of Medicine and Clinical
  Science
399 Bathurst Street
Toronto, Ontario M5S 2T8
Canada

Dr DIEGMAN
Krankenhaus Schwabing
Koelner Platz 1
D-8000 München 40
Federal Republic of Germany

Dr M. T. DROY
Institut IPSEN
30 rue Cambrone
75015 Paris
France

Dr A. DUBOIS
Digestive Disease Division
Department of Internal Medicine
Uniformed Services School of Medicine
4301 Jones Bridge Road
Bethesda, MD 20814
USA

Dr DUCROT
Janssen Le Brun
24 rue Hamelin
75116 Paris
France

Dr N. G. DURDLE
Department of Electrical Engineering
University of Alberta
Edmonton, Alberta T6G 2G7
Canada

Dr D. A. V. EDWARDS
Department of Clinical Research
University College Hospital
  Medical School
University Street
London WC1E 6GG
England

Dr H. J. EHRLEIN
Institute of Zoophysiology
University of Hohenheim
D-7000 Stuttgart 70
Federal Republic of Germany

Dr L. ELOUAER-BLANC
Service d'Hépato-Gastroentérologie
Hôpital Cochin
27 rue du Faubourg, St. Jacques
F-75674 Paris Cédex 14
France

Dr J. ERCKENBRECHT
University Hospitals
Department of Medicine D
Moorenstrasse 5
D-4000 Düsseldorf
Federal Republic of Germany

Dr D. F. EVANS
Department of Surgery, Floor E
University Hospital
Nottingham NG7 2UH
England

Dr W. EWART
The London Hospital Medical College
London E1 2AD
England

Dr I. EYRE-BROOK
Department of Surgery
Royal Hallamshire Hospital
Glossop Road
Sheffield S10 2JF
England

Dr M. FALEMPIN
Université des Sciences et Techniques Lille I
Laboratoire de Neurophysiologie
  Végétative SN4
59655 Villeneuve d'Ascq Cédex
France

Dr G. FELDER
INSERM U 61
3 avenue Molière
67200 Strasbourg
France

Dr T. FENTON
Queen Mary Hospital
Carshalton
Surrey
England

Dr F. FERRARINI
Via Tito Speri 30
46100 Mantova
Italy

Dr J. FIORAMONTI
Physio-pathologie Digestive
Ecole Nationale Vétérinaire
23 chemin des Capelles
F-31076 Toulouse Cédex
France

Dr G. FOSTER
Department of Surgery, Floor E
University Hospital
Nottingham NG7 2UH
England

Dr D. A. FOX
University of Wisconsin
425 N. Charter St.
Madison, WI 53705
USA

Dr J. E. T. FOX
School of Nursing
McMaster University
Hamilton, Ontario L8N 3Z5
Canada

Dr J. FREXINOS
Département Gastroentérologie
C.H.U. Rangueil
F-31954 Toulouse Cédex
France

Dr J. FURNESS
Medical School, Flinders University of
  South Australia
Bedford Park
South Australia 5042
Australia

Dr L. GARNIER
CNRS INP 1
B.P. 91
13277 Marseille Cédex 9
France

Dr R. J. GILBERT
Gastroenterology Division
Beth Israel Hospital
330 Brooklin Avenue
Boston, MA 02215
USA

Dr R. GILL
Department of Surgery
University of Alberta
Edmonton, Alberta T6G 2G3
Canada

Dr J. J. GLEYSTEEN
Department of Surgery
Veterans Administration Medical Center
5700 West National Avenue
Wisconsin 53193
USA

Dr K. GOLENHOFEN
Department of Physiology
University of Marburg
Deutschhausstrasse 2
D-3550 Marburg/Lahn
Federal Republic of Germany

Dr J. GONELLA
Institut Neurophysiologie, Psychophysiologie
  CNRS
Département de Neurophysiologie Végétative
31 chemin Joseph Aiguier
F-13277 Marseille Cédex 9
France

Dr R. K. GOYAL
Department of Medicine
Beth Israel Hospital
330 Brooklin Avenue
Boston, MA 02215
USA

Dr J. F. GRENIER
INSERM Unit 61
Avenue Molière
F-67200 Strasbourg
France

Dr J. C. GRIMAUD
Département de Gastroentérologie
Hôpital Nord
13326 Marseille Cédex 3
France

Dr D. GRUNDY
Department of Physiology
University of Sheffield
Sheffield S10 2TN
England

Dr S. GUSTAVSSON
Department of Surgery
University Hospital
S-750 14 Uppsala
Sweden

Dr F. HALTER
Gastrointestinal Unit
Inselspital
3010 Berne
Switzerland

Dr M. HELLSTRÖM
Department of Pharmacology
Karolinska Institutet
Box 60400
S-104 01 Stockholm 60
Sweden

Dr J. HELM
Section of Gastroenterology
Medical College of Wisconsin
Milwaukee, WI 53226
USA

Dr C. HILLEMEIER
Pediatric Gastroenterology
Rhode Island Hospital
Brown University Medical Center
Providence, RI 02902
USA

Dr G. HOLLE
Lindenstrasse 7
D-8000 München 90
Federal Republic of Germany

Dr R. H. HOLLOWAY
Department of Gastroenterology
Department of Internal Medicine
Yale University School of Medicine
New Haven, CT 06510
USA

Dr A. H. HOLSCHER
Ismaninger Strasse 22
Chirurgische Klinik Medicine
Isar der TU
D-8000 München 80
Federal Republic of Germany

Dr C. HONDE
Station de Pharmacologie INRA
180 chemin de Tournefeuille
31300 Toulouse
France

Dr J. HOSTEIN
AZ St. Rafael
3000 Leuven
Belgium

Dr J. D. HUIZINGA
Department of Physiology
University of Toronto
Toronto, Ontario M5S 1AS
Canada

Dr M. R. E. HUTTON
Gastrointestinal Science Research Unit
26 Ashfield Street
Whitechapel
London E1
England

Dr Z. ITOH
Department of Surgery
Gunma University School of Medicine
Maebashi Gunma 371
Japan

Dr L. P. JAGER
C.D.I.
Postbus 65
NL-0200 AB Lelystad
The Netherlands

Dr J. JANSSENS
Department of Gastroenterology
AZ St. Rafael
University of Leuven
B-3000 Leuven
Belgium

Dr A. JEAN
Département de Physiologie et
  Neurophysiologie
Faculté St. Jérôme
13397 Marseille Cédex 13
France

Dr R. JIAN
Hôpital Saint-Lazare
107 bis, rue du Faubourg St. Denis
75010 Paris
France

Dr A. G. JOHNSON
University Surgical Unit, Floor K
Royal Hallamshire Hospital
Sheffield S10 2JF
England

Dr J. L. JUNIEN
Laboratoire Jouveinal
1 rue des Moissons
Sofilic 423
94263 Fresnes Cédex
France

Dr M. KARAUS
University Hospital
Department of Internal Medicine
Moorenstrasse 5
D-4000 Düsseldorf
Federal Republic of Germany

Dr K. A. KELLY
Department of Surgery
Mayo Medical School
Rochester, MN 55905
USA

Dr Y. J. KINGMA
Department of Electrical Engineering
University of Alberta
Edmonton, Alberta T6G 2G7
Canada

Dr R. KINSMAN
Department of Physiology
University of Sheffield
Sheffield S10 2TN
England

Dr P. KITABGI
Centre de Biochimie
Université de Nice
06000 Nice
France

Dr K. L. KOCH
Gastroenterology Division
The Milton S. Hershey Medical Center
The Pennsylvania State University
PO Box 850
Hershey, PA 17033
USA

Dr S. J. KONTUREK
Institute of Physiology
Medical Academy
31–531 Krakow
Poland

Dr K. KRAGLUND
Department of Gastrointestinal Surgery
Aarhus University Hospital
DK-8000 Aarhus C
Denmark

Dr S. KRISHNAMURTHY
University of Washington
Department of Medicine
Division of Gastroenterology
Seattle Public Hospital
PO Box 3145
Seattle, WA 98114
USA

Miss A. M. LAJARD
Département de Neurophysiologie
Faculté des Sciences St. Jérôme
Rue H. Poincaré
13397 Marseille Cédex 13
France

Dr G. LAKE BAKAAR
Janssen Pharmaceutical
Chapel Street
Marlow
Bucks. SL7 1ET
England

Dr G. A. LANFRANCHI
Istituto di Clinica Medica e
  Gastroenterologia
Policlinico S. Orsola
Via Massarenti 9
I-40138 Bologna
Italy

Dr I. M. LANG
Surgical Research
Gastrointestinal Motility
Department of Surgery
Medical College of Wisconsin
Milwaukee, WI 53226
USA

Dr P. LEDERER
Medizinische Universitätsklinik
Krantenhausstrasse 12
PO Box 3560
D-8520 Erlangen
Federal Republic of Germany

Dr K. Y. LEE
The Genesee Hospital
224 Alexander Street
Rochester, NY 14607
USA

Dr S. P. LIM
Department of Pharmacology
University of Glasgow
Glasgow G12 8QQ
Scotland

Dr J. F. LONG
Janssen Pharmaceutica Inc.
40 Kingsbridge Road
Piscataway, NJ 08854
USA

Dr F. D. LOO
Department of Medicine
Gastroenterology Section
Froedtert Memorial Lutheran Hospital
9200 W. Wisconsin Avenue
Milwaukee, WI 53226
USA

Dr F. E. LUDTKE
Klinik für Allgemeinchirurgie
Robert Koch Strasse 40
D-3400 Göttingen
Federal Republic of Germany

Dr T. MARUYAMA
Department of Applied Physiology
Tohoku University School of Medicine
Sendai 980
Japan

Dr L. MARZIO
Unita Locale
Socio Sanitaria 04
I-66100 Chieti
Italy

Dr S. MATTIOLI
Clinica Chirurgica II
Università di Bologna
Via Massarenti 9
I-40138 Bologna
Italy

Dr N. MEI
Institut Neurophysiologie, Psychophysiologie
  CNRS
Département de Neurophysiologie Végétative
31 chemin Joseph Aiguier
F-13277 Marseille Cédex 9
France

Dr E. H. METMAN
Service de Gastroentérologie
CHR Trousseau
37044 Tours Cédex
France

Dr P. MEUNIER
Laboratoire d'Exploitation Fonctionelle
Manométrique
Hôpital Debrousse
69322 Lyon Cédex 05
France

Dr J. P. MIOLAN
Département de Neurophysiologie
Faculté des Sciences St. Jérôme
Avenue Henri Poincaré
F-13397 Marseille Cédex 13
France

Dr I. MORRIS
Department of Surgery
University of Liverpool
Royal Liverpool Hospital
Prescott Street
Liverpool L7 8XP
England

Dr T. C. MUIR
Department of Pharmacology
University of Glasgow
Glasgow G12 8QQ
Scotland

Dr B. NAUDY
Département de Médecine Interne
Centre Hospitalier
84120 Pertuis
France

Dr J. P. NIEL
Département de Physiologie et
  Neurophysiologie
Faculté St. Jérôme
Rue Henri Poincaré
13397 Marseille Cédex 13
France

Dr S. NIKOLIC
Wüstener Strasse 3
4902 Bad Salzuflen
Federal Republic of Germany

Dr O. OLERUP
Department of Pharmacology
Karolinska Institutet
Box 60 400
S-104 01 Stockholm
Sweden

Dr K. ONO
2nd Department of Surgery
Hirosaki University
School of Medicine
5-Zaifu Sho Hirosaki-shi
Aomori 036
Japan

Dr H. S. ORMSBEE III
Department of Pharmacology
Smith, Kline and French Laboratory
1500 Spring Garden Street
Philadelphia, PA 19101
USA

Dr A. OUYANG
Gastrointestinal Section
Hospital of University of Pennsylvania
3600 Spruce Street
Philadelphia, PA 19104
USA

Dr N. PANDOLFO
Patologia Chirurgica II
Università di Genova
Via Benedetto XV
Genova
Italy

Dr X. PASCAUD
Laboratoires Jouveinal
1 rue des Moissons
94263 Fresnes Cédex
France

Dr S. A. PEDERSEN
Department of Gastrointestinal Surgery
Arhus University Hospital
DK-8000 Arhus C
Denmark

Dr T. L. PEETERS
Division of Gastroenterology
Gasthuisberg O & N
University of Leuven
B-3000 Leuven
Belgium

Dr S. R. PEIKIN
Division of Gastroenterology
Jefferson Medical College
1025 Walnut Street
Philadelphia, PA 19107
USA

Dr M. PESCATORI
Clinica Chirurgica
Università Cattolica
Via della Pineta Sacchetti 644
I-00168 Roma
Italy

Dr I. PFEUFFER-FRIEDERICH
Division of Neuropharmacology
University of Mainz
D-6500 Mainz
Federal Republic of Germany

Dr S. F. PHILLIPS
Division of Gastroenterology
Department of Internal Medicine
Mayo Clinic
Rochester, MN 55905
USA

Dr M. A. PILOT
Surgical Unit
London Hospital
Whitechapel
London E1
England

Dr D. PLANCHE
Département d'Hépato-gastro-entérologie
Hôpital Nord
Chemin Bourelly
13015 Marseille
France

Dr C. E. POPE II
Gastroenterology Service
Veterans Administration Hospital
4435 Beacon Avenue South
Seattle, WA 98108
USA

Dr F. PORRECA
College of Medicine
Department of Pharmacology
University of Arizona Health Sciences
 Center
Tucson, AZ 85724
USA

Dr E. M. QUIGLEY
Hope Hospital
Eccles Old Road
Salford M6 84D
England

Dr V. RAYNER
Physiology Department
Rowett Research Institute
Aberdeen AB2 9SB
Scotland

Dr N. W. READ
Clinical Research Unit
Royal Hallamshire Hospital
Sheffield S10 2TN
England

Dr P. REGA
Département de Neurophysiologie
Faculté des Sciences St. Jérôme
Avenue Henri Poincaré
13397 Marseille Cédex 13
France

Dr S. REISER
Chirurgie Klinik
Klinikum M. Cl. Isar
Ismaningerstrasse 22
D-8000 München 80
Federal Republic of Germany

Dr J. C. REYNOLDS
Gastroenterology
Department of Medicine
University of Pennsylvania
Philadelphia, PA 19104
USA

Dr A. REYNTJENS
Janssen Pharmaceutica
Turnhoutseweg 30
B-2340 Beerse
Belgium

Dr J. E. RICHTER
Gastroenterology Division
Department of Medicine
Bowman-Gray School of Medicine
Winston Salem, NC 27103
USA

Dr C. ROMAN
Département de Physiologie et
    Neurophysiologie
Faculté des Sciences et Techniques
Avenue Henri Poincaré
F-13397 Marseille Cédex 13
France

Dr C. ROZE
Faculté de Médicine
X. Bichat
INSERM, U 239
F-75018 Paris
France

Dr Y. RUCKEBUSCH
Laboratoire de Physio-Pathologie Digestive
Ecole Nationale Vétérinaire
23 chemin des Capelles
F-31076 Toulouse
France

Dr J. SALDUCCI
Département de Gastroentérologie
Hôpital Nord
F-13326 Marseille Cédex 15
France

Dr K. M. SANDERS
School of Medicine
Department of Physiology
University of Nevada
Reno, NV 89557
USA

Dr S. K. SARNA
Department of Surgery
Milwaukee County Medical Complex
Milwaukee, WI 53226
USA

Dr M. SATO
2nd Department of Surgery
Hirosaki University
School of Medicine
5-Zaifu-sho Hirosaki-shi
Aomori 036
Japan

Dr C. SCARPIGNATO
Institute of Pharmacology
University of Parma
43100 Parma
Italy

Dr J. C. SCHANG
Département de Chirurgie
Centre Hospitalier Universitaire
Sherbrooke J1H 5N4
Quebec
Canada

Dr SCHATZE
Institut IPSEN
30 rue Cambrone
75015 Paris
France

Dr M. SCHEMANN
Institut für Zoophysiologie
Universität Hohenheim
D-7000 Stuttgart 70
Federal Republic of Germany

Dr U. SCHEURER
Gastrointestinal Unit
University Hospital
Inselspital
CH-3010 Berne
Switzerland

Dr E. SCHIPPERS
AZ St. Rafael
Kapucinjnenvoer 33
B-3000 Leuven
Belgium

Dr C. SCHNEIDER
Psychophysiology Unit
Psychiatric & 1st Surgical Clinic
A-1097 Vienna
Austria

Dr M. D. SCHUFFLER
Department of Medicine
Division of Gastroenterology
Seattle Public Health Hospital
PO Box 3145
Seattle, WA 98114
USA

Dr K. SCHULZE-DELRIEU
Division of Gastroenterology-Hepatology
Department of Internal Medicine
University of Iowa Hospital and Clinic
Iowa City, IA 52242
USA

Dr J. A. J. SCHUURKES
Department of Pharmacology
Janssen Pharmaceutica
B-2340 Beerse
Belgium

Dr G. W. SCOTT
Department of Surgery
University of Alberta
Edmonton, Alberta T6G 2N8
Canada

Dr R. B. SCOTT
Division of Gastroenterology
Department of Pediatrics
Alberta Children's Hospital and University of
   Calgary
Calgary, Alberta T2T 5C7
Canada

Dr S. SHIRAZI
Department of Surgery
University of Iowa Hospital and Clinics
Iowa City, IA 52242
USA

Dr L. F. SILLIN
Department of Surgery
Upstate Medical Center
750 E Adams Street
Syracuse, NY 13210
USA

Dr J. SIMON
Rhône Poulenc
Direction des Recherches Thérapeutiques
18 avenue d'Alsace
92400 Courbevoie
France

Dr R. W. SJOGREN
Department of Gastroenterology
Division of Medicine
Walter Reed Army Institute of Research
Washington, DC 20012
USA

Dr J. P. M. SMOUT
Department of Gastroenterology
University Hospital Utrecht
PO Box 16250
NL-3500 CG Utrecht
Netherlands

Dr G. SOLDANI
Farmacologica Veterinaria
Viale delle Piagge 2
56100 Pisa
Italy

Dr G. STACHER
Psychophysiology Unit
Psychiatric and 1st Surgical Clinic
A-1090 Wien
Austria

Dr E. STAHLE
Department of Surgery
University Hospital
75185 Uppsala
Sweden

Dr R. W. SUMMERS
Division of Gastroenterology-Hepatology
Department of Internal Medicine
University of Iowa Hospital and Clinics
Iowa City, IA 52242
USA

Dr T. SUZUKI
Gastroenterology Laboratory
Department of Surgery
Gunma University School of Medicine
Maebashi 371
Japan

Dr J. H. SZURSZEWSKI
Department of Physiology and Biophysics
Mayo Medical School
Rochester, MN 55905
USA

Dr I. TAKAHASHI
Department of Radiology
Milwaukee County Medical Complex
Milwaukee, WI 53226
USA

Dr B. TAYLOR
Welsh National School of Medicine
Heath Park
Cardiff CF4 4XN
Wales

Dr M. TEBLICK
Janssen Pharmaceutica
Turnhoutseweg 30
B-2340 Beerse
Belgium

Dr D. THIERMAN
Laboratoire Jouveinal
1 rue des Moissons
Sofilic 423
94263 Fresnes Cédex
France

Dr K. THOR
Department of Pharmacology
Karolinska Institutet
S-104 01 Stockholm
Sweden

Dr P. THOR
Institute of Physiology
Medical Academy
31–531 Krakow
Poland

Dr L. TIBBLING
ENT Department
University Hospital
S. 581 8S
Linkoping
Sweden

Dr S. TOYAMA
2nd Department of Surgery
Hirosaki University
School of Medicine
5 Zaifu-sho Hirosaki-shi
Aomori 036
Japan

Dr L. THUNEBERG
Anatomy Department C
University of Copenhagen
Blegdamsvej 3C
DK-2200 Copenhagen N
Denmark

Dr R. VALORI
Gastrointestinal Science Research Unit
London Hospital Medical College
London E1 2AD
England

Dr E. J. VAN DER SCHEE
Department of Medical Technology
Medical Faculty
Erasmus University
NL-3000 DR Rotterdam
Netherlands

Dr J. M. VAN NUETEN
Department of Pharmacology
Janssen Pharmaceutica
B-2340 Beerse
Belgium

Dr G. VANTRAPPEN
Department of Internal Medicine
AZ St. Rafael
University Hospital Leuven
B-3000 Leuven
Belgium

Dr M. VERLINDEN
Janssen Pharmaceutica
Turnhoutseweg 30
B-2340 Beerse
Belgium

Dr H. F. WEISER
Department of Surgery
Technical University of Munich
Ismaningerstrasse 80
D-8000 München 80
Federal Republic of Germany

Dr M. WIENBECK
University Hospital
Department of Medicine D
Moorenstrasse 5
D-4000 Düsseldorf 1
Federal Republic of Germany

Dr D. WINGATE
Department of Gastroenterology
London Hospital Medical College
Whitechapel
London E1 2AD
England

Dr E. R. WOZNIAK
Institute of Child Health
Department of Child Health
30 Guildford Street
London WC1
England

Dr ZARA
GI Science Research Unit
The London Hospital
26 Ashfield Street
Whitechapel
London E1
England

Contents

SECTION 2   GASTRIC MOTILITY AND EMPTYING

SECTION 6   SMOOTH MUSCLE, NERVOUS AND HORMONAL CONTROL

Section 1
Oesophagus, Lower Oesophageal Sphincter

1

Effects of Vagal Deafferentation on Oesophageal Motility in the Conscious Sheep

M. FALEMPIN and J. P. ROUSSEAU

INTRODUCTION

The pharyngeal and oesophageal stages of swallowing depend on a central
pattern generator. This theory has come from the early observation of
MOSSO (1876) that primary peristalsis could jump a gap produced by
oesophageal transection in dog. More recent studies of the effects of
oesophageal transection (CARVETH, SCHLEGEL, CODE and ELLIS, 1962) and
demonstration that sequential efferent signals proceed to all oesophageal muscles (ROMAN, 1966 ; ROMAN and TIEFFENBACH, 1972) support this
theory that mammalian nervous control of peristalsis is governed by a
central pattern generator. However, the decrease in the number of peristaltic waves observed following deviation of the bolus (JANSSENS,
1978) suggests that control of oesophageal peristalsis depends on peripheral feedback. Direct evidence for oesophageal afferents has come
from neural recordings. The passage of a peristaltic wave and distension of the oesophagus elicited discharges in sensory fibres (ANDREW,
1946 ; MEI, 1970 ; FALEMPIN, MEI and ROUSSEAU, 1978 ; FALEMPIN and
ROUSSEAU, 1983). In spite of the evidence that swallowing depends on a
central pattern generator, peripheral inputs to the medullary centres
seem to modify the central neural program. So the contribution of afferents in the control of the swallowing centre could be evaluated if
the contingent of sensory fibres alone was cut in both vagus nerves.
The surgical isolation of the vagal sensory fibres is actually possible
at the level of the nodose ganglion in sheep. However as cutting both

ganglia, leaving the bundles of motor fibres intact, is followed by death of the sheep in most cases, section of one vagus nerve was associated in the present work with division of the nodose ganglion of the contralateral nerve to test the effects of vagal deafferentation on electromyographic oesophageal activity and transit of a bolus.

METHODS

Vagal deafferentation was performed in 12 sheep 5-6 months old. The right vagus nerve was severed first either in its lower cervical part (n = 2) or in its thoracic part (n = 10), then the left nodose ganglion. The entire thoracic oesophagus or its distal part was thus free of its sensory innervation.

Preparation of the animals consisted of the following steps, during which sheep were anaesthetized with halothane/oxygene anasthesia after induction with a mixture of pentobarbitone sodium (200 mg) and thiopentone sodium (0.5 g) in 25 ml saline I.V :

i) siting of electrodes in the oesophageal wall at cervical and thoracic levels (upper, lower cervical and mid thoracic oesophagus)

ii) section of the right vagus nerve

iii) siting of a steal wire around the surgically isolated left nodose ganglion, which could subsequently be divided in conscious sheep by to-and-fro movements of the wire.

Oesophageal balloons, filled with 20 ml of air, were connected to pressure transducers (TELCO, France) to record the intra-oesophageal pressure. E.m.g. activity and pressure were displayed on a Beckman chartpaper recorder. After each step of the preparation recordings were made in conscious animals.

RESULTS

<u>In normal sheep</u>, the inflation of a balloon in the pharyngeal cavity led to primary peristalsis. Bursts of e.m.g activity occurred successively in the upper and lower parts of the cervical oesophagus, then in the thoracic oesophagus just preceding the characteristic peak of oesophageal pressure indicating the passage of the balloon into the stomach. Swallowing of the balloon was successful within 2-2.3 seconds at every attempt.

<u>After cutting the vagus nerve</u>, the balloon was propelled as in normal sheep in 431 of the 481 attempts. Failure of transit of the balloon occurred in the range of 4-16 % of the attempts in different animals. In these attempts, the balloon stopped in the lower cervical attempts, the balloon stopped in the lower cervical oesophagus, in those animals in which the right vagus nerve was cut in the neck. The presence of the balloon there led to a series of secondary peristaltic waves propagating along the remainder of the oesophagus, as is suggested by successive recordings of bursts in the lower cervical oesophagus, then in the mid-thoracic oesophagus. When the balloon was stopped in sheep in which the vagus nerve has been cut in the thorax local reflux contractions were elicited in the thoracic oesophagus. In every case when the balloon failed to be normally propelled into the stomach, the motor reflex responses of the oesophagus contributed to push it down into the stomach within less than one minute.

<u>The effect of the subsequent division of the left ganglion</u> was drastic: the balloon failed to be moved downwards in each of the 317 attempts of swallowing. It was constantly stopped at the beginning of the deafferented part of the oesophagus (the entire thoracic oesophagus or its last 10-15 cm). It finally passed down through the cardia within 5-8 minutes as a result of several spontaneous swallows of saliva. The presence of the balloon in the deafferented oesophagus failed to elicit the reflex responses that had been observed in the unilaterally vagotomized sheep just before the division of the contralateral nodose ganglion was performed. In addition, a decrease was observed in the amplitude and the duration of the e.m.g. bursts recorded in the deafferented oesophagus during swallowing of the balloon and of saliva.

DISCUSSION

The surgical isolation of the vagal sensory fibres and their section
at the level of the nodose ganglion have been performed previously in
the cat (MEI and DUSSARDIER, 1966) and in the guinea-pig (RECH, 1966),
but the effects of vagal deafferentation on gastric motility were
studied first in sheep (FALEMPIN and ROUSSEAU, 1979) and in the pig
(DARCY, FALEMPIN, LAPLACE and ROUSSEAU, 1979).

As cutting both ganglia was usually followed by death of the animals,
section of one vagus nerve was associated with division of the contralateral nodose ganglion. Thus oesophageal motility and transit had
to be compared in ipsilaterally vagotomized sheep, before and after
the section of the contralateral nodose ganglion to assess the role
of oesophageal afferents.

Evidence of deafferentation of the entire thoracic oesophagus or of
its last 10-15 cm has come from the failure of inflated balloons to
elicit local reflex contractions or secondary peristalsis during distension of the presumed deafferented part of the oesophagus, in contrast to what was observed in the vagotomized sheep before ganglionec-
tomy.

The large increase in the rate of failure of oesophageal transit from
10 % in vagotomized animals to 100 % after section of the nodose vagal afferents in achieving the successful swallowing of a bolus.

These results confirm the evidence of facilitation of the activity
both in oesophageal motoneurones (ROMAN, 1966 ; ROMAN and TIEFFENBACH,
1972) and in medullary interneurones (JEAN, 1972, 1978) obtained by
afferent stimulation. Thus the central pattern generator is constantly
modified by sensory feedback to adjust the intensity and velocity of
peristalsis according to the oesophageal content.

The swallowing of saliva was apparently not disturbed in deafferented
sheep, but diminution of the amplitude of the bursts recorded in the
deafferented part of the oesophagus was regularly observed. As saliva
is unlikely to distend the oesophagus, the vagal input when saliva is
swallowed could only consist of afferents stimulated by the oesophageal contractions. This is consistent with evidence of oesophageal
receptors which are only stimulated by primary peristalsis during
swallowing in conscious sheep (FALEMPIN and ROUSSEAU, in press).

ACKNOWLEGMENTS

It is a pleasure to thank Miss G.M. O'Brien for help with the English.

REFERENCES

1. Andrew, B.L. (1956). The nervous control of cervical oesophagus of the rat. *J. Physiol.* (*London*). 134, 729-740.

2. Carveth, S.W., Schlegel, J.F., Code, C.F. and Ellis, F.H. (1962). Esophageal motility after vagotomy, phrenicotomy, myotomy and myosnectomy in dogs. *Surg. Gynacol. Obstrt.*, 114, 31-42.

3. Darcy, B., Falempin, M., Laplace, J.P. and Rousseau, J.P. (1979). Importance de la voie vagale sensitive : recherche d'une technique de déafferentation sélective chez le Porc et le Mouton. *Ann. Biol. anim., Bioch., Biophys.*, 19, 881-888.

4. Falempin, M., Mei, N. and Rousseau, J.P. (1978). Vagal mechanoreceptors of the inferior thoracic oesophagus, the lower oesophageal sphincter, and the stomach in sheep. *Pflügers Arch.*, 373, 25-30.

5. Falempin, M. and Rousseau, J.P. (1979). Vagal digestive deafferentation in sheep. *Ann. Rech. Vet.*, 10, 186-188.

6. Falempin, M. and Rousseau, J.P. (1983). Reinnervation of skeletal muscles by vagal sensory fibres in the sheep, cat and rabbit. *J. Physiol.* (*London*)., 335, 467-479.

7. Falempin, M. and Rousseau, J.P. (1983). Activity of lingual, laryngeal and oesophageal receptors in conscious sheep. In press.

8. Janssen, J. (eds) (1978). The peristaltic mechanism of the oesophagus. Acco, Lewen, cited by Roman, C. and Gonella, J. in *Physiology of*

the gastrointestinal tract (1981). L.R. Johson Ed. Raven Press, New-York, p. 297.

9. Jean, A. (1972). Localisation et activité des neurones déglutiteurs bulbaires. *J. Physiol. (Paris).*,64, 227-268.

10. Jean, A. (1978). Contrôle bulbaire de la déglutition et de la motricité oesophagienne. Thèse. Doct. es-Sciences Marseille.

11. Mei, N. and Dussardier, M. (1966). Etude des lésions pulmonaires produites par la section des fibres sensitives vagales. *J. Physiol. (Paris).*, 58, 427-431.

12. Mei, N. (1970). Mécanorécepteurs digestifs chez le chat. *Exp. Brain. Res.* 11, 502-514.

13. Mosso, A. (1876). Ueber die Bewegungen der Speiseröhre. *Untersuch. Z. Natur.*, 11, 327-349.

14. Rech, R.H. (1966). The fiber component of the midcervical vagus nerve implicated in vagotomy inducted lung edema. *Exper. Neurol.*, 14, 475-483.

15. Roman, C. (1966). Contrôle nerveux du péristaltisme oesophagien. *J. Physiol. (Paris).*, 58, 79-108.

16. Roman, C. and Tieffenbach, L. (1972). Enregistrement de l'activité unitaire des fibres motrices vagales destinées à l'oesophage de babouin. *J. Physiol. (Paris).*, 64, 479-506.

2

Electrophysiological and Pharmacological Characterization of the NANC Nerve Mediated Inhibition of the Circular Muscle Layer of the Opossum Esophagus

L. P. JAGER, J. JURY and E. E. DANIEL

ABSTRACT

Field stimulation of strips from the circular muscle of the esophagus of the North American opossum induced a transient nerve mediated hyperpolarization of the smooth muscle cell membrane (IJP), followed by an "off" depolarization, usually accompanied by spike activity and muscle contraction. Optimum stimulus parameters were 0.1 to 0.2 ms pulse duration and 20 pps for 0.3 s. Tetrodotoxin and scorpion venom abolished responses at these parameters.

These responses were unaffected by atropine, guanethidine or indomethacin in effective doses. ATP, ADP, AMP and adenosine had no consistent effects on membrane potential or on the IJP in concentrations up to 10^{-4} M. VIP from 10^{-8} M upward caused enhanced "off" depolarization and initiated spontaneous activity.

Manipulation of external potassium ion concentration and of membrane potential effected the IJP amplitude consistent with its origin from increased conductance towards potassium ions. Double sucrose gap studies showed that during the IJP the membrane resistance decreased. A conditioning hyperpolarization of more than about 40 mV reversed the IJP. This reversal potential of the IJP was dependent on the potassium concentation of the super fusion medium. Thus the IJP seems to be due to a selective increase in the permeability of the smooth muscle cell membrane towards potassium ions.

Apamine up to 10^{-5} M did not affect the membrane potential or the IJP. Tetra-ethylammonium (TEA) $1 - 3 \times 10^{-2}$ M induced a depolarization of muscle cell membrane and increased the membrane resistance and increased the IJP. These results suggest that the potassium channels of the smooth muscle cell membrane in this preparation are apamine-insensitive and probably voltage-regulated.

However, the potassium channels opened by the inhibitory neurotransmitter are qualitatively different from those functioning at rest. Like TEA, quinine (10^{-3} M) induced a depolarization at rest, but unlike TEA it did block the IJP. This effect may be due to an interference of quinine with the conductance change underlying the IJP or with the impulse propagation by the intramural nerves.

The pharmacological properties of the potassium channels in the opossum esophagus employed by the inhibitory transmitter are unlike those of other smooth muscle preparations of the gastrointestinal tract.

INTRODUCTION

Field stimulation of most circular smooth muscle preparations and some longitudinal muscle preparations from the alimentary canal can induce responses which are mediated via intrinsic non-adrenergic non-cholinergic (NANC) nerves. Among these the inhibitory response of the guinea pig's taenia caecum has been studied extensively to establish the existence of intramural NANC nerves (2, 3) to investigate the mechanisms of action of the endogenous neurotransmitters on the smooth muscle cell membrane (1, 14) and to test hypotheses concerning the identity of the neurotransmitters (1, 14, 17, 19).

The purinergic nerve hypothesis put forward by Burnstock and his co-workers (5) that purines (esp.: ATP) may be the mediator still is a central working hypothesis. The main obstacle in testing the purinergic nerve hypothesis is the lack of a selective receptor antagonist which only interferes postsynaptically with the NANC nerve mediated response (6, 15, 16, 18, 23, 25).

In recent years the peptidergic hypothesis emerged, (see: 13), in which the vasoactive intestinal peptide (VIP) is regarded as the most likely candidate for the neurotransmitter of NANC nerves (11, 12, 24), but the data presented so far are indirect and unsupported by electrophysiological evidence.

The electrophysiological characteristics of NANC-nerve mediated responses (21) in the North American opossum were studied to assess whether purines or VIP can account for the observed effects of endogenous mediator(s). The esophagus of the North American opossum is a useful model for electrophysiological anlysis of NANC nerves and their mediator(s): the circular muscle of the oppossum esophageal body might represent a nearly pure NANC nerve—muscle preparation. It meets the requirements for the use of the sucrose gap technique. The opossum esophagus resembles the human esophagus with regard to anatomical characteristics. Furthermore, the NANC-nerves are probably evolutionairy old attributes of the vertebrate alimentary canal. As the NANC nerves reported so far might all belong to a single class of nerves, observations of a NANC-nerve mediated response in a 'living fossil' as a marsupial might produce a basically similar but less complicated picture than that of eutheria.

MATERIALS and METHODS

The materials and methods used have been described extensively (9), for the single sucrose gap. The double sucrose gap used was similar to that described earlier (17) and employed in experimental circumstances identical to those of the single sucrose gap.

RESULTS

General

Field stimulation with a single pulse evoked a transient hyperpolarization of the smooth muscle cell membrane, followed by a small, but longer lasting depolarization. The amplitude of the hyperpolarization evoked by an optimal dimensioned single pulse (0.1 − 0.2 ms) was doubled by field stimulation with a train (0.3 s) of the same pulses (20 − 30 pps). As a rule the depolarizations following hyperpolarizations evoked by a pulse train were accompanied by muscle action potentials and a transient increase in tension. (Fig. 1). A similar configuration of junction potentials was obtained with intracellular recording and the membrane potential at rest was found to be about 50 mV.

With prolonged trains of stimuli the initial hyperpolarization (IJP) decreased in time, but the membrane remained hyperpolarized during stimulation. Only after

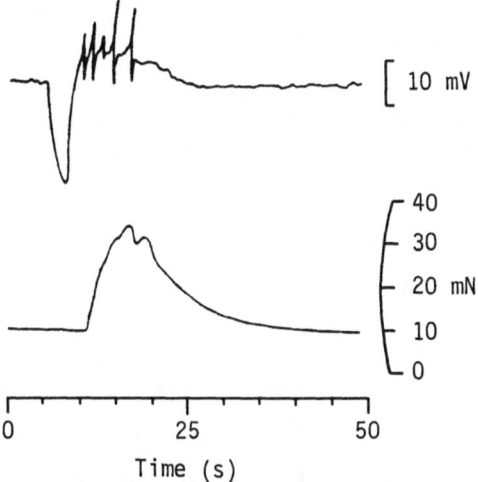

Figure 1: The IJP induced by field stimulation with a train of pulses (train duration 0.3 s, pulse rate 30 pps, pulse width 0.1 ms, supramaximal voltage) and the 'off' or 'rebound' depolarization and contraction following it. Single sucrose gap recording obtained using Krebs solution at 27°C. (From ref. 9 with permission).

cessation of the stimulus the depolarizing phase developed and is therefore referred to as the "off" response.

The optimal pulse width observed for field stimulation suggests that the membrane response observed is evoked via stimulation of intramural neurones. This suggestion was corroborated by the inhibition of the response by TTX (Fig. 2). Furthermore, scorpion venom blocked irreversibly the responses evoked by field stimulation.

To ascertain that the IJP is mediated by nonadrenergic, non-cholinergic nerves the effects of selective antagonists and inhibitors were investigated. No significant effect on the IJP by atropine, guanethidine, propranolol, phentolamine and indomethacin became apparent.

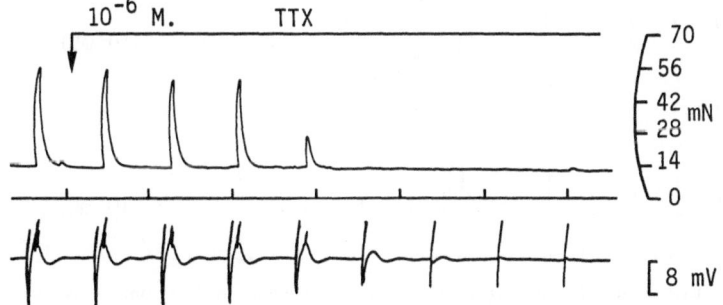

Fig. 2. Blockade by tetrodotoxin of the IJP evoked in cells of the circular smooth muscle layer of the opossum esophagus by field stimulation (0.3 s, 30 pps, 0.1 ms, supramaximal pulse amplitude). Time marker: 1 min. Sucrose gap recording at 27 ± 1°C using Krebs solution to superfuse the preparation.

IJP and putative transmitters.

ATP, ADP or AMP in high concentrations usually induced a transientdepolariza-
tion of the cell membrane, but in general no distinct effect on the membrane potential at rest was observed. Consequently a transient increase in the contractile force
which lasted for a few minutes was observed. Superfusion with adenosine and its
2-chloroderivative did not induce measurable effects on the membrane potential or on
the contractility of this smooth muscle-preparation at rest.

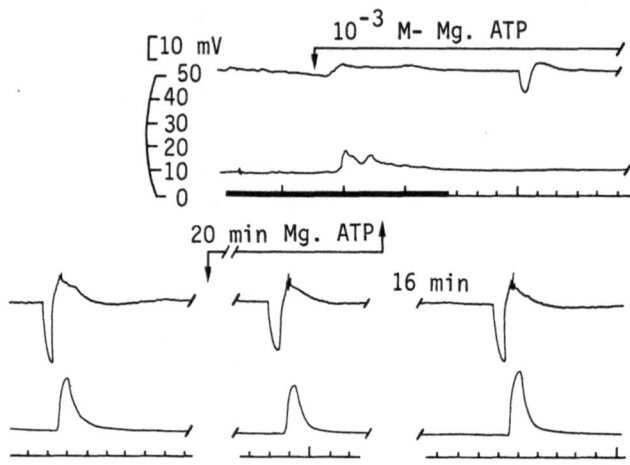

Fig. 3. Effects of ATP (10^{-3} M) on the cell membrane potential at rest and
on the responses evoked by field stimulation of the circular smooth muscle layer of
the opossum esophagus. Sucrose-gap recordings using different paper speeds at 27 ±
1° C. (Time marker: 1 min (large), 5 s (small)). The upper set of traces was made
after the first and before the second set of the lower traces. Stimulus parameters: 0.3
s, 30 p.p.s., 0.1 ms, supramaximal amplitude. (From ref. 9 with permission).

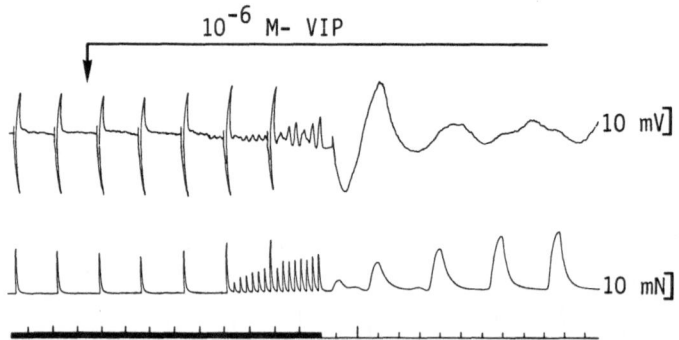

Fig. 4. Effects of VIP (10^{-6} M) on the smooth muscle and on the responses evoked
by field stimulation (0.01 t.p.s., 0.3 s, 50 p.p.s., 0.1 ms, pulse height supramaximal)
in the circular muscle of the opossum esophagus. Responses were obtained in the
presence of antagonists, using two paper speeds and at 27 ± 1° C. Timer markers: 1
min (large), 5 s (small). (From ref 9, with permission).

Adenosine and adenosine nucleotides in various concentrations were also found to be without effect on the responses following stimulation of the NANC nerves. (Fig. 3). ATP at high concentrations only induced a transient decrease in the amplitude of IJP and of the rebound contraction. In the presence of ATP these responses recovered to control values within 20 minutes. Adenosine and its chloride analog however depressed more persistently the amplitude of the IJP.

As shown in Fig. 4 VIP induced repetitive contractions and depolarizations in this preparation under the circumstances used (26). Even in the lowest concentration studied (10^{-8} M) this cyclic response was observed albeit the amplitudes were smaller and the delay between start of the superfusion and the first response was considerably longer. At higher concentrations the amplitude of the responses increased but remained cyclic (tonic contractions and depolarizations were not observed), and the response started almost instantaneously. The responses elicited by stimulation of the intramural NANC nerves, remained essentially unchanged in the presence of VIP, although transient inhibitions of the VIP induced contractions were observed.

Mechanisms underlying the IJP.

Experiments in which the effect of varying the ionic composition of the superfusion medium on the IJP was studied revealed that IJP-amplitude depended on the extracellular potassium ion concentration (9). The suggestion that the IJP might be due to an increase in the permeability of the smooth muscle cell membrane towards potassium ions was corroborated by the following observations (20) with the double sucrose gap. (i). During the IJP the membrane resistance, as reflected in the amplitude of electrotonic potentials evoked with constant current pulses, decreased to about half its resting value (fig. 5) (ii). The amplitude of the IJP was decreased by increasing conditioning hyperpolarizations of the smooth muscle cell membrane and showed a reversal potential at about 40 mV more negative than the resting membrane potential

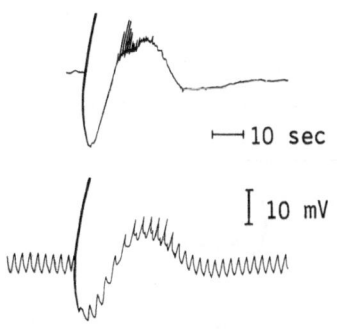

⊢——⊣ 10 sec

⌶ 10 mV

Fig. 5. Electrotonic potentials and the IJP recorded simultaneously with double sucrose-gap method. The IJP produced by field stimulation (0.1 s, 30 pps, 1.0 s, supramaximal voltage) is shown in the upper trace. Decrease of the amplitude of the electrotonic potentials (pulse rate: 0.5 pps; intensity: 10^{-6} A) evoked during the IJP is demonstrated in the lower trace.

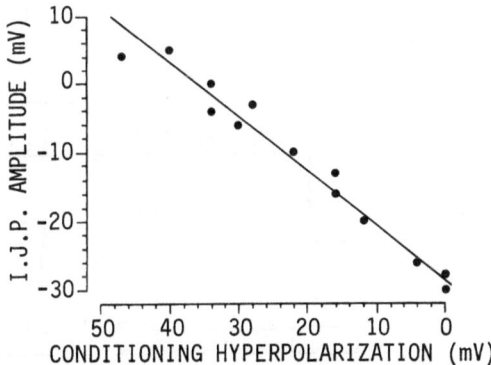

Fig. 6. Relationship between the IJP amplitude and the conditioning hyperpolarization during wich the NANC-nerve mediated response was evoked. Note that the IJP reverses at hyperpolarizations of about 40 mV.

(Fig. 6). (iii). This reversal potential changed with the potassium ion concentration in the medium in a manner predicted by the Nernst-Goldman equations.

Pharmacology of Potassium Conductance.

Agents which supposedly block voltage-dependent potassium conductance channels in cell membranes, induced a depolarization of the smooth muscle cell membrane and (TEA) a marked increase in membrane resistance (Fig. 7). Apamin (5, 22), which interferes with the calcium-dependent potassium channels, was without effect in this preparation (9). Quinidine, which has a questionable selectivity, depolarized the smooth muscle cells and increased the membrane resistance. Thus in our experimental circumstances the contribution of the potassium conductance to the resting membrane potential is largely covered by voltage dependent potassium channels (20). However, none of the potassium-channels drugs available had any effect on the IJP. If the drug tested depolarized the smooth muscle cell membrane a concomittant increase in IJP-amplitude was observed.

Morphology of NANC innervation.

The suggestion from the electrophysiological observations that the circular smooth muscle coat of the body from the opossum esophagus is innervated by only one type of nerves was born out by electromicroscopic studies. Only one type of nerve profiles was observed, characterized by varicosities containing mostly small agranular and occasionally also large granular vesicles (10).

A striking feature was that the varicosities were close to the interstitial cell of Cajal and not to smooth muscle cells. The interstitial cells of Cajal were found in gap junction contact with each other and with smooth muscle cells. Furthermore, the

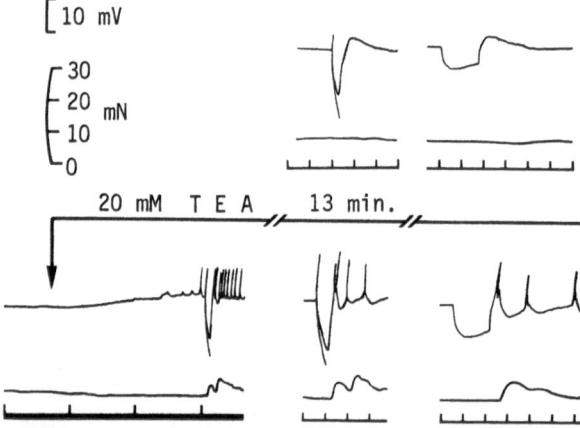

Fig. 7. The effect of tetraethylammonium on the membrane potential, membrane resistance and the IJP. The upper set of traces show the control responses: IJP evoked by field stimulation and electrotonic potential evoked by a long lasting current pulse. The lower set of traces show the depolarization induced by TEA, the lack of effect on the IJP and the increased electrotonic potential, reflecting a larger membrane resistance. Note the mechanical activity in the presence of TEA. Time markers: 1 min (large) and 5 s (small), three different paper speeds.

smooth muscle cells are in extensively gap junction contact with each other, which might be expected from the fact that the sucrose gap technique could be used with this preparation.

DISCUSSION

As is often the case more questions are raised than answered by our observations. To start with the latter: (i) The IJP, observed in smooth muscle cells of the opossum esophagus body circular muscle, evoked by stimulation of intramural NANC nerves is not mimicked by the putative neurotransmitters ATP, ADP, AMP, adenosine and VIP. (ii) The IJP is brought about by a selective increase in the permeability towards potassium ions, mediated via the endogenously released NANC transmitter. (iii) This marsupial smooth muscle-nerve preparation is relatively simple in the sense that only one nerve-mediated response and only one type of nerve profiles were observed. However, the question is raised whether the identity of action criterium for putative neurotransmitters can be invoked when it seems likely that the nerve mediated response is mediated via the interstitial cells of Cajal.

Our earlier suggestion that in this preparation, as in guinea pig taenia caecum, the IJP and the 'off'-response might be mediated via different cotransmitters can reflect that the IJP is mediated via actions of the NANC-neurotransmitter on interstitial cells of Cajal and the 'off'-response via actions on the smooth muscle cells (10). Comparing the NANC nerve mediated IJP in the circular smooth of the opossum esophageal body with that in the longitudinal smooth muscle of the guinea pig taenia caecum reveals besides strong similarities intriguing differences. Although both seem to be due to a selective increase in membrane permeabilities towards potassium ions, this increase is inhibited by apamine in guinea pig where as this bee venom was ineffective in opossum as were other potassium channel blockers. In guinea-pig the nerve profile ascribed to NANC-nerves is varicosities with large opaque vesicles (5) while in opossum the NANC-nerves are characterized as having varicosities with mostly agranular small vesicles. As earlier attempts to identify the NANC-nerves in mammalian intestinal preparations failed to confirm the 'large opaque vesicle profile' (7, 8) the current observations seem to indicate the NANC-nerve profile resembles the 'cholinergic nerve profile'. This providing that there does exist a single, homogenous type of intramural NANC nerves in the entodermal organs throughout the vertebrate realm.

REFERENCES

1. Bennet, M.R., Burnstock, G. & Holman, M.E. (1963). *The effect of potassium and chloride ions on the inhibitory potential recorded in the guinea pig taenia coli.* J. Physiol. **169**, 33-34P.
2. Bennet, M.R. Burnstock, G. & Holman, M. E. (1966). *Transmission from intramural inhibitory nerves to the smooth muscle of the guinea-pig taenia coli.* J. Physiol. **182**, 541-558.
3. Bülbring, E. & Tomita, T. (1967). *Properties of the inhibitory potential of smooth muscle as observed in the response to field stimulation of the guinea-pig taenia coli.* J. Physiol. **189**, 299-315.
4. Burgess, G.M., Claret, M. & Jenkinson, D.H. (1981). *Effects of quinine and apamine on the calcium-dependent potassium permeability of mammalian hepatocytes and red cells.* J. Physiol. **317**, 67-90.
5. Burnstock, G. (1972). *Purinergic Nerves.* Pharmacol. Rev. **24**, 509-581.
6. Choo, L.K. (1981). *The effect of reactive blue, an antagonist of ATP, on the isolated urinary bladders of guinea-pig and rat.* J. Pharm. Pharmacol. **33**, 248-250.

7. Daniel, E.E. (1979). *The distribution of non-adrenergic inhibitory nerves in the intestine. Their structural identification, and the role of prostaglandins in their function.* In: *Physiological and Regulatory Functions of Adenosine and Adenine Nucleotides,* Eds.: H.P. Bear, & G.I. Drummond, New York, Raven Press, pp. 61-68.

8. Daniel, E.E., Taylor, G.S., Daniel, V.P. & Holman, M.E. (1977). *Can non-adrenergic inhibitory varicosities be identified structurally.* Can. J. Physiol. Pharmacol. **55**, 243-250.

9. Daniel, E.E., Helmy-Elkholy, A., Jager, L.P., Kannan, M.S. (1983). *Neither a purine nor VIP is the mediator of inhibitory nerves of opossum oesophageal smooth muscle,* J. Physiol. **336**, 243-260.

10. Daniel, E.E., Jager, L.P., Jury, J., Helmy-Elkholy, A., Kannan, M.S. & Posey-Daniel, V (1983). *The mediators and mechanisms causing the non-adrenergic non-cholinergic nerve responses in opossum esophagus. Role of interstitial cells of Cajal.* Biomed. Res. (in press).

11. Fahrenkrug, J. (1979). *Vasoactive Polypeptide: Measurement, distribution and putative neurotransmitter function.* Digestion **19**, 149-169.

12. Goyal, R.K., Rattan, S. & Said, S.I. (1980). *VIP as a possible neurotransmitter of non-cholinergic inhibitory neurones.* Nature **288**, 378-380.

13. Hakanson, R., Leander, S., Sundler, F. & Uddman, R. (1981). *P-type nerves: Purinergic or Peptidergic?* In: *Cellular Basis of Chemical Messengers in the Digestive System,* UCLA Forum in Med. Sc. 23, New York, Academic Press, pp. 169-200.

14. Den Hertog, A. and Jager, L.P. (1975). *Ion fluxes during the inhibitory junction potential in the guinea-pig taenia coli.* J. Physiol. **250**, 681-691.

15. Hooper, M., Spedding, M., Sweetman, A.J. & Weetman, D.F. (1979). *Effects of 2-2'-Pyridylisatogen on responses to adenosine 5'-triphosphate in isolated smooth muscle preparations.* In: *Physiological and Regulatory Functions of Adenosine and Adenine Nucleotides,* Eds.: H.P. Baer & G.I. Drummond, New York, Raven Press, pp. 85-93.

16. Huizinga, J.D. & Den Hertog, A. (1980). *Inhibition of fundic strips from guinea-pig stomach: the effect of theophylline on responses to adenosine, ATP and intramural nerve stimulation.* Eur. J. Pharmacol. **63**, 259-265.

17. Jager, L.P. (1974). *The effect of catecholamines and ATP and the smooth muscle membrane of the guinea pig taenia coli.* Eur. J. Pharmacol. **25**, 372-382.

18. Jager, L.P. (1976). *Effects of dipyridamole on the smooth muscle cells of the guinea-pig's taenia coli.* Arch. Int. Pharmacodyn. Ther. **221**, 40-53.

19. Jager, L.P. & Schevers, J.A.M. (1980). *A comparison of effects evoked in guinea-pig taenia ceacum by purine nucleotides and by "purinergic" nerve stimulation.* J. Physiol. **299**, 75-83.

20. Jury, J., Jager, L.P. & Daniel, E.E. (1984). *NANC-nerve mediated inhibition of the N-American opossum esophageal smooth muscle is potassium dependent.* Can. J. Physiol. Pharmacol. (submitted).

21. Lund, G.F. & Christensen, J. (1969). *Electrical stimulation of esophageal smooth muscle and effects of antagonists.* Am. J. Physiol. **214**: 1369-1374.

22. Maas, A.J.J. (1981). *The effect of apamin on responses evoked by field stimulation in guinea-pig taenia caeci.* Eur. J. Pharmacol. **73**: 1-9.

23. Maas, A.J.J. & Den Hertog, A. (1979). *The effect of apamin on the smooth muscle cells of the guinea-pig taenica coli.* Eur. J. Pharmacol. **58**: 151-156.

24. Matsuzaki, Y., Hamasaki, Y. & Said, S.I. (1980). *Vasoactive intestinal peptide: a possible transmitter of non-adrenergic relaxation of guinea pig airways.* Sciences **210**: 1252-1253.

25. Muller, M.J. & Baer, H.P. (1980). *Apamin, a non-specific antagonist of smooth muscle relaxants.* Naunyn-Schmiedeberg's Arch. Pharmacol. **311**: 105-107.

26. Rattan, S., Grady, M. & Goyal, R.K. (1982). *Vasoactive intestinal peptide causes peristaltic contraction in the esophageal body.* Life Sc. **30**, 1557-1563.

Acknowledgements

This study was supported by grants from the MRC of Canada to L.P.J., E.E.D. & Dr. J.E.T. Fox. We are indebted to Mrs. and Mr. Propsma for their help in the preparation of the manuscript.

3

The Edrophonium Response: Use in Diagnosis and Possible Understanding of Mechanisms of Esophageal Chest Pain

J. E. RICHTER, W. C. WU, J. N. BLACKWELL, D. N. JOHNS, B. T. HACKSHAW and D. O. CASTELL

A frustrating problem in evaluating patients with suspected esopha-geal chest pain has been a general inability to clearly implicate the esophagus. Most patients report they have intermittent episodes of chest pain and are rarely obliging enough to experience the pain during the manometric study. A definite statement can only be made when the patient has a typical attack of chest pain during the manometric exami-nation. If a characteristic pattern appears (i.e., diffuse spasm) or the intensity of the pain can be predicted from the manometric record-ing (i.e., excessive high amplitude peristalsis), then a clear-cut case can be made for an esophageal origin of the chest pain especially if coronary artery disease has been excluded. Unfortunately, in our experiences and others, spontaneous pain with manometric correlation occurs in less than 20% of patients studied. Therefore, a variety of techniques have been suggested to provide an esophageal "stress test." These have included ice water swallows (1), intraesophageal acid per-fusion (2), and injections of bethanechol (3), edrophonium (4), penta-gastrin (5), and ergonovine (6). Recent studies from our laboratory have suggested that edrophonium is the best tolerated and most effec-tive provocative test for esophageal chest pains (7). These findings are supported by another study in which patients responding to ergo-novine with chest pain and manometry abnormalities were generally found to have a similar response with edrophonium (4).

The purpose of this study was to expand our experience with edrophonium as an esophageal stress test and hopefully better understand the mechanism by which edrophonium provokes esophageal pain. We therefore studied prospectively a consecutive series of patients with chest pain and normal coronary arteriograms. By comparison with age matched controls, we have attempted to correlate the manometric changes associated with the patients' chest pain in order to get a better insight into the pathogenesis of esophageal chest pain.

PATIENTS AND METHODS

Patients

Thirty eight consecutive patients with chest pain and recent normal coronary arteriography (no lesion obstructing the lumen of a coronary artery by greater than 25%) were entered into this prospective manometric study. This group included 19 men and 19 women with a mean age of 54 years. The control group consisted of 25 healthy subjects (10 men, 15 women, mean age 55 years) who had undergone similar manometry studies.

Methods

Esophageal manometric studies were performed using a round 8 lumen polyvinyl catheter (diameter 4.5mm; internal diameters 0.8mm; Arndorfer Specialties, Inc. Greendale, Wisconsin, USA). The distal four openings are located 1cm apart at 90° angles while the four proximal openings are spaced at 5cm intervals. Each lumen was continuously perfused with distilled water at a rate of 0.5ml/min using a low compliance pneumohydraulic capillary infusion system (Arndorfer Specialties, Inc.). The catheter was connected to external transducers (Beckman, Model 4-327-C, Norcross, Georgia, USA) with output to a Beckman recorder (Model R-612). This manometric system has a pressure rise rate of 400mmHg/sec.

All subjects were studied in the supine position after an overnight fast. All medications known to effect esophageal contractions or modulate esophageal pain were held for forty-eight hours. The catheter was introduced through the nose into the stomach. After the lower esophageal sphincter was measured, the four proximal openings were positioned in the body of the esophagus 2,7,12 and 17cm above the sphincter. Esophageal contractions were recorded from these openings in response to 5ml H_2O given at 30 sec intervals. The basal study consisted of ten consecutive esophageal contractions analyzed for mean amplitude and duration. Wave amplitude, in millimeters of mercury, was measured from the onset of the major upstroke to the end of wave. Following completion of the basal study, a single blinded edrophonium provocative study was performed. Each patient received edrophonium chloride (Tensilon) 80mcg/kg IV bolus. Immediately after this injection, ten esophageal contractions induced by 5cc H_2O were recorded and the patient asked about chest pain and the similarities of symptoms to their chronic pain syndrome. A positive test was defined as the replication of the patient's chest pain by edrophonium with or without an associated new abnormality of esophageal motility not present on the baseline tracing. Patients were also observed for unpleasant or dangerous side effects. Atropine was available if an untoward response to edrophonium should occur. The ten esophageal contractions after edrophonium were analyzed similar to the basal study. Note was also made of simultaneous contractions and repetitive waves characterized by three or more pressure peaks occurring in succession following a single swallow.

Statistical Analysis

To compensate for variable individual basal pressures, percent changes in amplitude and duration were calculated and compared between basal studies and after edrophonium. Because of the short duration of action of edrophonium, a separate analysis was made of the first five and second five esophageal contractions after the drug. Statistical studies were performed using the student t test for paired and unpaired samples as appropriate. All values are presented as mean ± SE.

RESULTS

Edrophonium provoked chest pain in 10/38 patients (26%) who had recently had normal coronary arteriography. In all cases, the drug induced chest pain was similar to the chronic pains for which the patients had sought medical attention. None of the 25 age-matched control subjects experienced chest pain after edrophonium. All esophageal contractions induced by wet swallows after edrophonium were peristaltic, although repetitive waves were frequent. Simultaneous contractions were not observed. Patients tolerated edrophonium well and no important side effects were noted.

In all groups, increases in distal amplitude and duration of esophageal contractions were significant and consistent with the expected pharmacologic response to edrophonium (Tables 1 and 2).

Table 1.   Distal Esophageal Amplitude (mmHg, $\bar{x}$ ± SE)

	Basal	Edrophonium (1st 5)	Edrophonium (2nd 5)
Controls	133±9	159 ± 12*	154 ± 13*
-CAD, -E	131±10	150 ± 12*	137 ± 10**
-CAD, +E	136±12	191 ± 16*	180 ± 21*

*p < 0.01 compared to basal; **p < 0.05 compared to basal

Table 2.   Distal Esophageal Duration (sec, $\bar{x}$ ± SE)

	Basal	Edrophonium (1st 5)	Edrophonium (2nd 5)
Controls	4.7±0.2	7.3 ± 0.5*	6.6 ± 0.3*
-CAD, -E	4.4±0.2	6.9 ± 0.4*	6.2 ± 0.4*
-CAD, +E	4.7±0.3	9.9 ± 1.0*	7.5 ± 1.1*

*p < 0.01 compared to basal

The most striking responses in both amplitude and duration usually occurred within the first 5 esophageal contractions, but the last 5 contractions were also significantly greater than the basal values. Distal
esophageal amplitude increased from 133±9mmHg ($\bar{x}$±SE) to 159±12mmHg
(p < 0.01) after edrophonium in the control subjects; 131±10mmHg to
150±12mmHg (p < 0.01) in the patients with normal coronary arteriograms
and negative edrophonium test (-CAD, -E); and 136±12mmHg to 191±16mmHg
(p < 0.01) in the patients with normal coronary arteriograms and a
positive edrophonium test (-CAD, +E).   Likewise, distal esophageal duration increased from 4.7±0.2 sec to 7.3±0.5 sec (p < 0.01) after edrophonium in the control subjects; 4.4±0.2 sec to 6.9±0.4 sec (p < 0.01)
in the patients with the negative edrophonium test; and 4.7±0.3 to 9.9±
1.0 sec (p < 0.01) in the patients with a positive edrophonium test. As
shown in Table 3, when the three groups were compared the magnitude of
responses as expressed by percentage change was significantly greater
for both amplitude and duration in the group with a positive edrophonium test.

Table 3.   The Magnitude of Response to Edrophonium ($\bar{x}$ ± SE)

	Controls	-CAD,-E	-CAD,+E
△ Amp	21 ± 5%	22 ± 8%	46 ± 9%*,**
△ Dur	53 ± 9%	59 ± 8%	93 ± 16%[+]

*   p < 0.01 compared to controls

** p < 0.05 compared to -CAD, -E

[+] p < 0.02 compared to controls and -CAD, -E

Overall the edrophonium positive group increased their distal amplitude by 46 ± 9% and distal duration by 93 ± 16% in the first 5 contractions after edrophonium as compared to 21 ± 5% and 53 ± 9% respectively for control subjects and 22 ± 8% and 59 ± 8% respectively for the patients with a negative edrophonium test. Among individual patients, however, overlap was observed between the individual mean amplitudes and/or duration of esophageal contractions after edrophonium and the production of esophageal chest pain.

DISCUSSION

This study extends our previous clinical experience with edrophonium and confirms it is a useful and safe "stress test" for implicating the esophagus as the cause of non-cardiac chest pain. Ten of thirty-eight patients (26%) had replication of their non-cardiac chest pain after edrophonium. This is slightly higher than our previous report in which 6 of 34 (18%) patients had a positive edrophonium response (7). However in this earlier report which did not have control subjects, a positive response required both chest pain and a change in the baseline manometry. Our current study with age-matched control subjects suggests that individual manometric responses usually reflect the pharmacologic action of edrophonium in which case the replication of chest pain becomes the decisive factor. Using this new definition, 10 of 34 (29%) patients would have had a positive edrophonium test in our earlier study. The safety of edrophonium as a provocative test has been substantiated by the lack of any important adverse affects in over 75 patients ranging in age from 20 to 72 years.

This study suggests that esophageal chest pain is related to increased amplitude and/or prolonged duration of esophageal contractions. Since all contractions were peristaltic, simultaneous contractions were not the cause of the chest pains observed in our patients. These observations support the theory that esophageal pain may result from myoischemia, occurring as a result of intramural tension produced by high amplitude prolonged contractions, inhibiting blood flow in the muscles for a critical period of time (3). Simultaneous contractions may certainly inhibit bolus transport and cause dysphagia (8), but their relationship to non-cardiac chest pain is probably more dependent on the amplitude and/or duration of the esophageal contraction.

The observed overlap in individual pressure responses (both absolute

amplitude/duration and percentage change) after edrophonium and the
production of chest pain raises many unanswered questions. Our studies
suggest that pressure changes alone are not sufficient to consistently
elicit esophageal pain and other variables must be considered. Possibly
patients have individual pain thresholds or varying critical times in
esophageal blood flow where changes in esophageal pressures are more
likely to bring out pain. Certainly this study and others (9,10) would
confirm that no single manometric factor can universally account for
esophageal chest pain. One author has even gone as far as to recently
suggest that esophageal chest pain may not result from changes in
esophageal motility or pressures (10). We do not believe this is the
case and suggest the edrophonium "stress test" gives us some insight
into the etiology of esophageal chest pain. Further understanding a-
waits the development of new technology which will permit ambulatory
long-term monitoring of esophageal pressures under more physiologic
conditions.

REFERENCES

1. Meyer GW, Castell DO. Human esophageal response during chest pain
induced by swallowing cold liquids. JAMA 1981;246:2057-59.
2. Siegel CI, Hendrix TR. Esophageal motor abnormalities induced by
acid infusion in patients with heartburn. J Clin Invest 1963;42:686-95.
3. Mellow M. Symptomatic diffuse esophageal spasm: manometric follow-
up and response to cholinergic stimulation and cholinesterase inhibition. Gastroenterology 1981;81:10-14.
5. Wexler RM, Kay MD. Pentagastrin in diffuse esophageal spasm.
Gut 1981;22:213-16.
6. Alban Davis H, Kay MD, Rhodes J, Dart AM, Henderson AH. Diagnosis
of esophageal spasm by ergometrive provocation. Gut 1982;23:89-97.
7. Benjamin SB, Richter JE, Cordova CM, Knuff TE, Castell DO. Prospective manometric evaluation with pharmacologic provocation of patients with suspected esophageal motility dysfunction. Gastroenterology
1981;84:893-901.
8. Richter JE, Blackwell JN, Wu WC, Cowan RJ, Johns DN, Castell DO.
Assessment of liquid bolus transit by simultaneous radionuclide transit
and esophageal manometry. Gastroenterology 1983;84:128.
9. Mellow MH. Esophageal motility during food ingestion: a physiologic
test of esophageal motor function. Gastroenterology 1983;85:570-7.

4

The Diabetic Esophagus – Revisited

F. D. LOO, W. J. DODDS, R. C. ARNDORFER, K. H. SOERGEL,
W. J. HOGAN and J. F. HELM

Diabetic patients with overt neuropathy exhibit asymptomatic abnormalities of esophageal motor function. Previously reported abnormal findings include frequent non-peristaltic contractions, delayed clearance and decreased lower esophageal sphincter (LES) pressure. We have noted an esophageal manometric aberration in diabetic patients with neuropathy that has not been described previously. Fourteen insulin-dependent diabetics (age 21-64 yrs) with peripheral and autonomic neuropathy were investigated. None had esophageal symptoms, but 6 complained of vomiting, 5 had diarrhea and 3 had both. Gastric emptying of a radiolabelled solid meal was abnormal in 11 of 14. Small bowel manometric findings were abnormal in the 5 patients with diarrhea. Control subjects included 6 diabetic patients without neuropathy (16-64 yrs), 100 consecutive non-diabetic patients evaluated for suspected esophageal disease and 30 healthy volunteers (18-32 yrs). We used a multilumen manometric tube that featured an orifice for measuring gastric pressure, a sleeve device for measuring LES pressure and 6 orifices spaced at 3-cm intervals for recording pressure activity in the esophageal body. Each lumen was perfused with distilled water (0.5 ml/min) by a minimally compliant hydraulic system. Three rapid pull-throughs across the LES were performed using the 4 recording sites above the sleeve. The sleeve was then positioned straddling the LES. Esophageal responses were recorded for 10 wet swallows (5 ml H_2O), at intervals of 30 seconds, under basal conditions, after amyl nitrite, edrophonium (80 ug/kg IV) and atropine (3 ug/kg IV). Results: Resting LESP (22.5 ± 6 SD mm/Hg) and LES relaxation were normal. The incidence

23

of complete primary peristalsis was normal (>80%) in 12 patients. Two patients had 50-80% failed swallows. Thirteen patients exhibited a singular manometric aberration of multiphasic peristaltic pressure waves in the smooth-muscle esophagus. These complexes usually had a "rabbit-ear", double-peaked profile, but in some cases had several peaks. Peak amplitudes ranged from 40-200 mmHg. Propagation measured from onset of the multiphasic pressure complex or from the initial pressure peak was normal. Concurrent fluroscopic and manometric monitoring demonstrated that the multiphasic wave complexes stripped barium from the smooth-muscle esophageal segment in a normal fashion. The second wave of the multiphasic wave complex was simultaneous at two or more sites in 34%, appeared retrograde in 4% and was antigrade in 62%. Edrophonium (80 ug/kg IV) increased the number and amplitude of the phasic waves, whereas atropine (3 ug/kg IV) reduced the number and amplitude, often to a single-peaked peristaltic complex. Only 2 subjects in the control groups demonstrated multiphasic peristaltic pressure complexes phenomenon. We conclude: 1) Most of our diabetics with neuropathy (13/14) had multiphasic esophageal peristaltic pressure complexes with normal bolus transport. 2) Although the underlying cause of this aberration remains to be determined, increased cholinergic sensitivity appears to play a role.

5

Abnormalities of Esophageal Motor Function in Diabetic Patients

E. H. METMAN, B. PANTIN, P. LE MARCHAND, E. DANQUECHIN DORVAL and J. BERTRAND

Occurence of a peripheral neuropathy (PN) increase the frequency of abnormal esophageal motility in diabetic patients (DP) (1) (2) but results concerning LES function are either incomplete (1) or contradictory (2) (3) (4).

The aims of the study were to establish the frequency of esophageal and LES abnormalities in DP with and without PN compared to an healthy control group.

MATERIAL AND METHODS

Eighty-two DP (age 28 - 87) were studied ; 38 were insulin-dependent, 42 had a PN.

Fifty-seven healthy subjects (age I6 - 84) composed the control group (C).

Esophageal recording were performed using a strain-gauge probe GAELTEC.

Recording involved :

1 - LES basal pressure and relaxation. LES basal pressure was considered as the end expiratory pressure recorded both in thoracic and abdominal areas.

2 - Esophageal waves. Amplitude, duration and velocity of peristalsis and frequency of abnormal waves in response to dry swallow, were calculated.

RESULTS

A - <u>WHEN COMPARING DP TO CONTROL GROUP</u>

   - no difference were found in amplitude or duration of peristalsis .

   - In contrast

    * LES resting pressure was decreased in its thoracic
area (P < 0.0I).

    * Abnormal relaxation occurred in 32.9 % in DP versus
I0.4 % in C (P < 0.0I).

    * Velocity of peristalsis was decreased in the lower
third of the esophagus (P < 0.0I).

    * Abnormal waves were more frequent (Fig. 1).

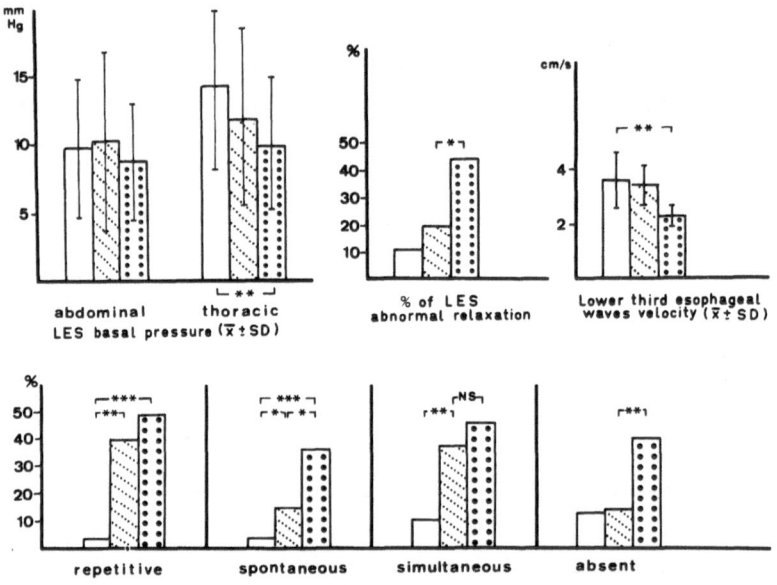

Figure 1 - Comparison of LES basal pressure, LES abnormal relaxation,
   peristalsis velocity and frequency of abnormal waves in
   controls, diabetic patients (DP) without peripheral neuropathy (PN) and DP with PN.

B - <u>AMONG DP</u>

      - Incidence of PN increased frequency of abnormal waves (I9 out of 40 DP without PN, versus 29 out of 42 DP with PN), decreased velocity of peristalsis and increased incomplete relaxation of the LES (Fig. 1).

      - In contrast no difference was found due to duration of diabetic state or to insulin-dependence.

DISCUSSION

      In DP, decreased velocity of peritalsis, incomplete relaxation of LES, and high frequency of abnormal motor activity of esophagus suggest a dysfunction of the autonomous nervous system. Absence of variation in the amplitude of waves accounts for the integrity of the smooth muscle (5).

      In our study repetitive and simultaneous waves are significantly more frequent in DP with or without PN than in controls.

      In contrast decrease velocity of peristalsis, spontaneous contractions and absence of contractions after swallow are significantly enhanced by the presence of PN suggesting a more advanced visceral neuropathy.

      We have found dysfunction of LES in DP ; this suggests an abnormal neurologic control of LES.

      LES dysfunction and/or abnormal peristalsis are not found in all DP with PN : this agrees with a report (6) who show with radionuclide transit studies that esophageal dysfunction is better correlated with clinical gastroenteropathy than with PN.

CONCLUSION

      Asymptomatic dysfunction of autonomous nervous system of the esophagus is frequent in DP and frequency increases with presence of PN ; this affects both esophagus motility and LES function. However 3I % DP with PN had no esophageal dysfunction suggesting that visceral neuropathy may occur later than PN.

REFERENCES

(1) - HOLLIS J.B., BASTELL D.O., BRADDOM R.L.
      Esophageal function in diabetes mellitus and its relation to
      peripheral neuropathy.
      Gastroenterology I977, 73, I098-II02

(2) - HEITMANN P., STÖSS U., GOTTESBÜREN H., MARTINI G.A.
      Strörungen der Speiseröhrenfunction bei Diabetikern
      Dtsch. Med. Wschr. I973, 98, II5I-II55

(3) - LOO F.D., DODDS W.J., ARNDORFER R.C., SOERGEL K.H., HOGAN W.J.,
      HELM J.H.
      The diabetic esophagus-revisited.
      Gastroenterology, I983, 84, 1233 (abstr.).

(4) - LEVINE R.A.
      Diabetic esophageal dysmotility unassociated with peripheral
      neuropathy.
      Dig. Dis. Sc. I980, 25, 7I5 (abstr.)

(5) - HOLLIS J.B., CASTELL D.O.
      Comparison of esophageal function abnormalities in diabetes and
      aging.
      V° Int. Symposium on Gastro-intestinal motility
      Vantrappen Ed. Typoff-Press, I975, 406-4I0

(6) - RUSSELL C.O.J., GANNAN R., COATSWORTH J., NEILSEN R., ALLEN F.,
      HILL L.D., POPE C.E.
      Relationship among esophageal dysfunction, diabetic gastroente-
      ropathy and peripheral neuropathy.
      Dig. Dis. Sc. I983, 28, 289-293

6

In Vitro Study of the Effects of Leu-Enkephalin and Related Drugs on the Vagally Induced Responses of the Cat Lower Esophageal Sphincter

A. JEAN, J. P. MIOLAN and C. ROMAN

INTRODUCTION

The lower esophageal sphincter (LES) has a double extrinsic innervation (parasympathetic and sympathetic). The parasympathetic pathway running in the vagus nerves is composed of cholinergic preganglionic fibers connected either with excitatory cholinergic intramural neurons or with inhibitory non-adrenergic non-cholinergic neurons (1, 2). In physiological conditions the inhibitory vagal pathway is involved in the LES opening during swallowing and secondary esophageal peristalsis ; the excitatory vagal pathway probably participates in the closure observed afterwards and in the maintenance and reflex modulation of resting tone (2, 3).

Recent data have evidenced the existence of enkephalin intramural neurons in LES, specially in man and cat (4). Moreover, several opiate receptors have been identified in the LES of the opossum (5). Thus, endogenous opiates and opiate receptors are likely to be involved in the physiological regulation of LES function, as also suggested by conflicting results observed in man (6, 7).

The aim of this work was to investigate the role of opiate receptors in LES motility by studying the effects of opiate-related drugs (Leucine enkephalin and morphine) and that of a therapeutic agent (Trimebutine maleate) on the excitatory and inhibitory responses of LES muscle elicited by electrical stimulation of vagal preganglionic fibers.

METHODS

Adult cats were used for this study ; the animals were fasted
24 h before the experiments. After a brief induction with halothane
(halothane 2 %, air 98 %), cats were anaesthetized with sodium thiopentone injected intravenously (thiopentone 10 % in 0.9 % Na Cl solution).
The approach to the lower esophageal sphincter was carried out on the
left side after resection of the last ribs. The distal part of the
esophagus was excised with the attached vagus nerves. Then, the organ
was opened by a longitudinal section on the right border and the mucosa
was removed. The preparation was placed in an organ bath perfused with
a saline solution of the following composition (mmol) : NaCl 133, KCl
4.7, $CaCl_2$ 1.9, $MgCl_2$ 0.49, NaH_2PO_4 1.0 and glucose 7.8. The solution
was bubbled with 95 % O_2 and 5 % CO_2 gas mixture and maintained at a
temperature of 30°C.

The nerves were stimulated at 30 sec. intervals (2-6 pulses,
1-2 msec, 20 Hz, 10-20 V) with an appropriate device. Monopolar electromyographic (EMG) responses of the LES muscle were recorded with extracellular pressure electrodes placed on the serosa or directly on the
circular muscle (8).

Statistical analysis was performed using Student's test for
paired samples. When the value of P was greater than 0.05, the difference was considered as non-significant. The mean values are given with
standard deviation.

The following drugs were used : Leucine enkephalin (Leu-Enk ;
Serva), naloxone hydrochloride (Mallet S.A. Chemical), morphine hydrochloride (Coop. Pharmaceutique Française), atropine sulfate (Merck),
trimebutine maleate (Jouveinal).

RESULTS

1. Effects of stimulation of vagal efferent fibers
As previously demonstrated by Gonella et al. (1), stimulation
of preganglionic vagal fibers with short trains of pulses (2-6) induced
either excitatory or inhibitory responses at the LES level. The exci-

tatory responses consisted of slow depolarizations (excitatory junction potentials, EJPs) which often gave rise to a burst of spikes inducing a contraction of the muscle. These excitatory responses were suppressed by atropine and also hexamethonium indicating that the excitatory pathway is entirely cholinergic. The inhibitory responses corresponded to slow hyperpolarizations (inhibitory junction potentials, IJPs) of smooth muscle fibers. The IJPs remained after atropine treatment. As they were not affected by antiadrenergic drugs but suppressed by hexamethonium (1), it was concluded that the inhibitory pathway involves a cholinergic preganglionic fiber and a non-adrenergic non-cholinergic postganglionic neuron (2).

2. Effects of drugs on the EMG responses

2.1 Excitatory responses

Perfusion of the organ bath with Leu-Enk (10^{-6} M ; n = 7) in normal saline solution resulted within 2-3 min in a powerful decrease of the excitatory responses. When the responses showed a burst of spike potentials superimposed on EJP, the application of the drug produced a reduction in the number of spikes and even a suppression of the spike burst which is always accompanied by a decrease of the amplitude of EJP (Fig. 1). The mean decrease of the amplitude of EJPs was 68 % $\pm$ 4.8 significantly different from control at $P \leqslant 0.001$ (Fig. 3). After removing the drug from the perfusing saline solution, the response returned to normal within 5-6 min. This inhibitory effect of Leu-Enk was markedly decreased when naloxone ($1-5.10^{-6}$ M ; n = 2) was added in the saline solution.

Preliminary results obtained with morphine ($1-6.10^{-6}$ M ; n = 3) indicated that this drug did not produce appreciable changes in the excitatory responses. Only a slight decrease of the excitatory responses was hardly observed.

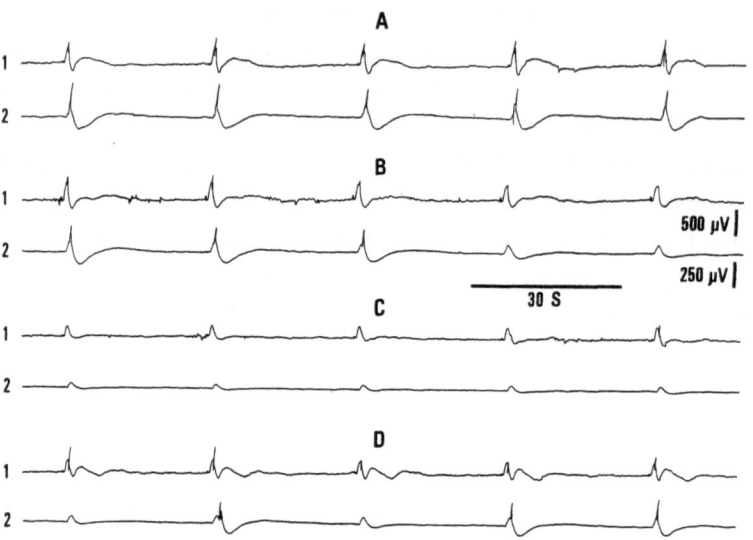

Fig. 1 : Action of Leu-enkephalin on EJPs and superimposed spikes
recorded on the LES after vagal stimulation.
(A) control
(B) 2-3 min after perfusion with Leu-Enk (10^{-6} M)
(C) and (D) 2 and 5 min respectively, after removing the drug
from the organ bath. Stimulation of vagus nerve (4 pulses ;
1 msec, 20 Hz, 10 V) evokes EJPs and spike bursts recorded
on two sites of the LES (1 and 2). Notice the powerful inhibitory effect of Leu-Enk on the excitatory responses causing
first the suppression of spike bursts, then a marked decrease
of the amplitude of EJPs.

The application of the therapeutic agent, Trimebutine maleate
($2-5.10^{-5}$ M ; n = 8), produced effects rather similar to those of Leu-
Enk. This drug caused within 2-4 min a suppression of spike bursts,
followed by a decrease of the amplitude of EJPs (Fig. 2A). The mean
decrease of the amplitude of EJPs was 26 % $\pm$ 12, significantly different from control at $P \leqslant 0.01$ (Fig. 3). After the bath was rinsed with
fresh saline solution, the response returned to normal within 4-6 min.
Naloxone ($1-5.10^{-6}$ M ; n = 3) added in the saline solution antagonized
the inhibitory effect of Trimebutine maleate (Fig. 2B).

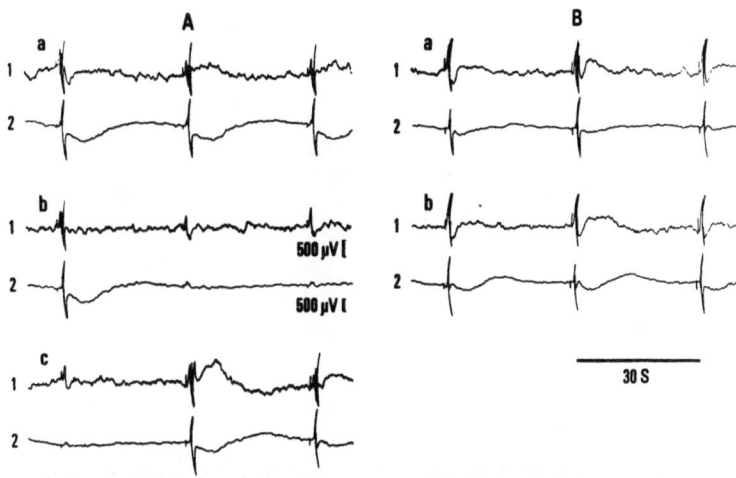

Fig. 2 : Action of Trimebutine maleate on vagal excitatory responses
A. (a) control : stimulation of vagus nerve (4-5 pulses ;
2 msec ; 20 Hz ; 12 V) evokes EJPs with superimposed spikes.
Records (1 and 2) are obtained from two sites of the LES.
     (b) 3 min after perfusion with Trimebutine maleate (4.10^{-5}
M).
     (c) 4 min after removing the drug from the organ bath. Note
the inhibitory effect of the drug which causes the suppression
of spike bursts.
B. Naloxone (5.10^{-6} M) is added in the physiological solution.
     (a) control
     (b) 3 min after perfusion with Trimebutine maleate. Notice
that the inhibitory effect of the drug is antagonized by the
opiate antagonist, Naloxone.

2.2 Inhibitory responses

In order to record IJPs without EJPs the experiments were performed under atropine (10^{-6} M). The application of either Leu-Enk
(n = 5) or morphine (n = 3) in doses similar to those previously found
to be effective on EJPs did not produce any significant modification
of the amplitude of IJPs (Fig. 3). Similarly, perfusion with Trimebutine maleate ($2-5.10^{-5}$ M ; n = 5) resulted in non-significant changes
in the amplitude of IJPs (Fig. 3).

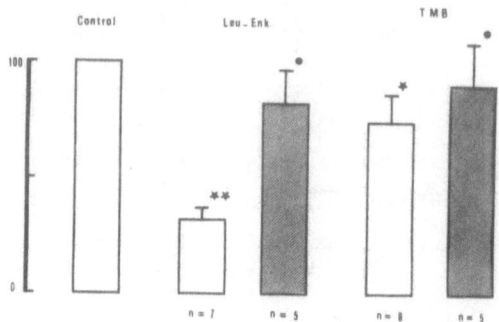

Fig. 3 : Modification of EJP and IJP amplitude by Leu-Enk and
Trimebutine maleate(TMB)
The mean control amplitude (left column) was taken as 100 %.
The open columns represent the effect of drugs on EJPs and
the shaded that on IJPs. The vertical line on the top of each
column is standard deviation. Results significantly different
from control (t test for paired samples) are indicated by
(✱✱) P ≤ 0.001, (✱) P ≤ 0.01 ; columns with dots (●) correspond to non-significant variations. n indicates the number of
tests.

DISCUSSION

The present results demonstrate that enkephalins are involved
in the regulation of LES motility through opiate receptors. The action
of Leu-Enk can result from an activation of receptors which might be
localized either in the myenteric plexus or on the LES muscle itself,
as suggested by recent results obtained in opossum (5). As Leu-Enk can
modulate (decrease) only the EJPs and the superimposed spikes whereas
the IJPs remain unaffected, it may be assumed that the opiate receptors
are likely located on the neural pathway (preganglionic or postganglionic fibers), since any modification of the muscular membrane potential
should have changed both excitatory and inhibitory vagal responses.
Thus, the powerful inhibitory effect of the drug on EJPs probably results from a blockade of the excitatory cholinergic pathway. Opiates
may act on preganglionic nerve endings or intramural cholinergic neu-

rons. Such conclusions are in agreement with results of Furness et al. (9) and Morita and North (10), showing that enkephalins acted by preventing the release of acetylcholine from enteric neurons.

In addition, our results indicate that Trimebutine maleate produces effects similar to those of Leu-Enk, although less powerful. This drug acts also on opiate receptors since the effects were antagonized by the specific opiate antagonist, naloxone. Trimebutine maleate may act through the same receptor as Leu-Enk or may excite endogenous opiate containing neurons which are present in the myenteric plexus of the cat LES (4).

CONCLUSION

Our results suggest that peripheral opiate receptors are able to modulate the activity of the excitatory (cholinergic) vagal pathway to the cat LES, but not that of the inhibitory vagal pathway. Thus, in physiological conditions the opiates might be involved, at the peripheral level, in the maintenance and reflex modulation of LES resting tone, whereas the relaxation of the sphincter would result from a central nervous mechanism unaffected at least by peripheral opiate receptors.

This work was supported by a grant from Jouveinal Labs. We appreciated the kind wellcome of J. Gonella and M. Bouvier in their laboratory for some experiments. The technical help of A.M. Lajard and D. Catalin is also gratefully acknowledged.

REFERENCES

1. Gonella, J., Niel, J.P. and Roman, C. (1977). Vagal control of lower oesophageal sphincter motility in the cat. J. Physiol. (London), 273, 647-664.

2. Roman, C. and Gonella, J. (1981). Extrinsic control of digestive tract motility. In : Johnson, L.R. (ed). Physiology of the gastrointestinal tract. pp. 289-333. (New York : Raven Press).

3. Goyal, R.K. and Cobb, B.W. (1981). Motility of the pharynx, esophagus and esophageal sphincters. In : Johnson, L.R. (ed). Physiology of the gastrointestinal tract. pp. 359-391. (New York : Raven Press).

4. Uddman, R., Alumets, J., Hakanson, R., Sundler, F. and Walles, B. (1980). Peptidergic (Enkephalin) innervation of the mammalian esophagus. Gastroenterol., 78, 732-737.

5. Rattan, S. and Goyal, R.K. (1983). Identification and localization of opioid receptors in the opossum lower esophageal sphincter. J. Pharmacol. exp. therap., 224, 391-397.

6. Hall, A.W., Moossa, A.R., Clark, J., Cooley, G.R. and Skinner, D.B. (1975). The effects of premedication drugs on the lower oesophageal high pressure zone and reflux status of Rhesus monkeys and man. Gut, 16, 347-352.

7. Howard, J.M., Belsheim, M.R. and Sullivan, S.N. (1982). Enkephalin inhibits relaxation of the lower oesophageal sphincter. Brit. med. j., 285, 1605-1606.

8. Gonella, J. (1972). Modifications of electrical activity of the rabbit duodenum longitudinal muscle after contractions of the circular muscle. Am. J. Dig. Dis., 17, 327-332.

9. Furness, J.B., Costa, M., Franco, R. and Llewellyn-Smith, I.J. (1980). Neuronal peptides in the intestine : distribution and possible functions. In : Costa, M. and Trabucchi, M. (eds). Neural peptides and neuronal communication. pp. 601-617 (New York : Raven Press).

10. Morita, K. and North, R.A. (1981). Opiates and enkephalin reduce the excitability of neuronal processes. Neuroscience, 6, 1943-1951.

7

Relation between Lower Esophageal Sphincter Pressure and Plasma Concentration of Neurotensin (1–13) during Intravenous Infusion of Neurotensin (1–13) and (Gln⁴)-Neurotensin (1–13) in Man

K. THOR, E. THEODORSSON-NORHEIM and Å. RÖKAEUS

INTRODUCTION

Recent studies indicate that neurotensin, or a molecule with neurotensin homologies, may function as a hormone, which is released from the
small intestine after the ingestion of fat (1, 2) and, among other
things, may be involved in the postprandial regulation of gastrointestinal motility (3). Thus, upon intravenous infusion of (Glu^4)-neurotensin
(NT) or its analogue (Gln^4)-neurotensin (GNT) in man, the lower esophageal sphincter (LES) pressure is reduced (4, 5), the motility in the
duodenum is increased with a change in the pressure gradient between
antrum and duodenum (6), the migrating motor complexes (MMC) in the proximal small intestine is inhibited with a change from a fasting- to a
fed-type of motility (7) and with an increase in colonic motility (8).

In the previous studies on LES pressure neurotensin-like immunoreactivity was measured in plasma (p-NTLI). p-NTLI is due to several NT
sequences, some of which may be biologically inactive. Experiments in
rats on gastrointestinal motility have shown that only the whole neurotensin sequence NT(1-13) or GNT(1-13) is biologically active (9). Recently, we have shown that the concentration of immunoreactive molecules corresponding to NT(1-13) increases almost tenfold in unextracted
peripheral plasma in healthy subjects after ingestion of fat (10). The
question then arises whether the increase in the plasma concentration
of NT(1-13) after ingestion of fat is sufficient to cause changes in
LES pressure. The aim of the present investigation was to find out
whether plasma concentrations of NT(1-13) in the physiological range

can have any effect on the LES pressure. We also compared the effects
of NT and GNT, since in previous studies of LES pressure only GNT has
been used. In addition, we studied the effect of GNT on a pentagastrin-
induced increase in LES pressure and the importance of cholinergic innervation since studies in animals have shown that some of the effects
of GNT on gastrointestinal motility can be blocked by atropine (11,12).

MATERIAL AND METHODS

The studies were performed in 14 healthy male volunteers, median age
32 years (range 19-43). The experiments were carried out between 8 a.m.
and 10 a.m. after a fasting period of at least 11 h. LES pressure was
recorded with a continuous pullthrough method and calculated as described by Thor and Rökaeus (6).

Thirty min after the catheter had been introduced, indwelling cannulas were inserted into the antecubital vein of one arm for blood
sampling and into the other arm for intravenous infusion of NT or GNT.
Both peptides were infused at a rate of 12 pmol x kg^{-1} x min^{-1}; both
were obtained from Peninsula, Calif., USA. Blood samples were taken
and analyzed with chromatography and radioimmunoassay as described before (6, 13).

Atropine (1 mg) was administered as an intravenous bolus injection.
Pentagastrin (0.6 µg x kg^{-1}, Peptavlon, ICI) was administered by intravenous injections during 30 sec.

Statistical evaluation

Two-way analyses of variance and multiple comparisons with the Student's t-test were performed on a NORD-10 computer using the STATPAC
interactive computer program package (Systemgruppen, Karolinska Institutet). The results are reported as mean $\pm$ standard error of the mean
(M $\pm$ S.E.). P-values less than 0.05 were regarded as significant.

RESULTS

One min after the start of the infusion of NT(1-13) or GNT(1-13) during 5 min LES pressure was diminished by 43%, and did not decrease
further during the infusion period (n=3). After the end of the infusion, the LES pressure returned to control level (Fig. 1). The chromatographic pattern of p-NTLI was similar in all three subjects. The
mean concentration of NT(1-13) in plasma increased from a basal value

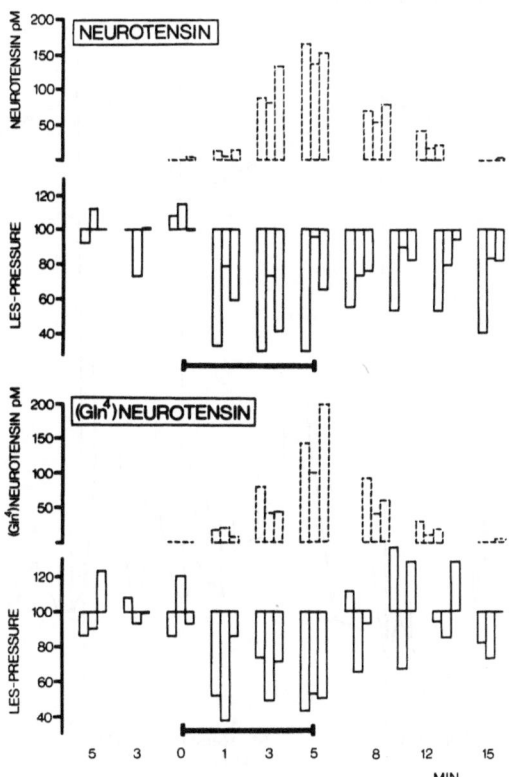

FIGURE 1 Relation between the concentration of the intact tridecapep-
tides and the LES pressure (per cent of resting level). The
concentrations of the intact peptides in pM and the LES
pressure expressed as percentage change from the mean resting
value are shown on the ordinate. The abscissa shows the time
scale. The horizontal bar indicates the infusion period.
(Reproduced from ref. 3).

of 1 pM to 14 pM at 1 min and to a maximal value of 156 pM at 5 min
(n=3). The mean concentration of GNT(1-13) increased from 1 pM to 16 pM
at 1 min and to a maximal value of 142 pM at 5 min (n=3). Ion-exchange
chromatography revealed that the principal metabolic product was probably NT(1-8) and GNT(1-8). Other N- or C-terminal fragments were not
detected. The plasma half-lives of NT(1-13) and GNT(1-13) were both
2.5 min. The half-lives of NT(1-8) and GNT(1-8) could not be estimated,
but apparently they are considerably longer than those of NT(1-13) and
GNT(1-13).

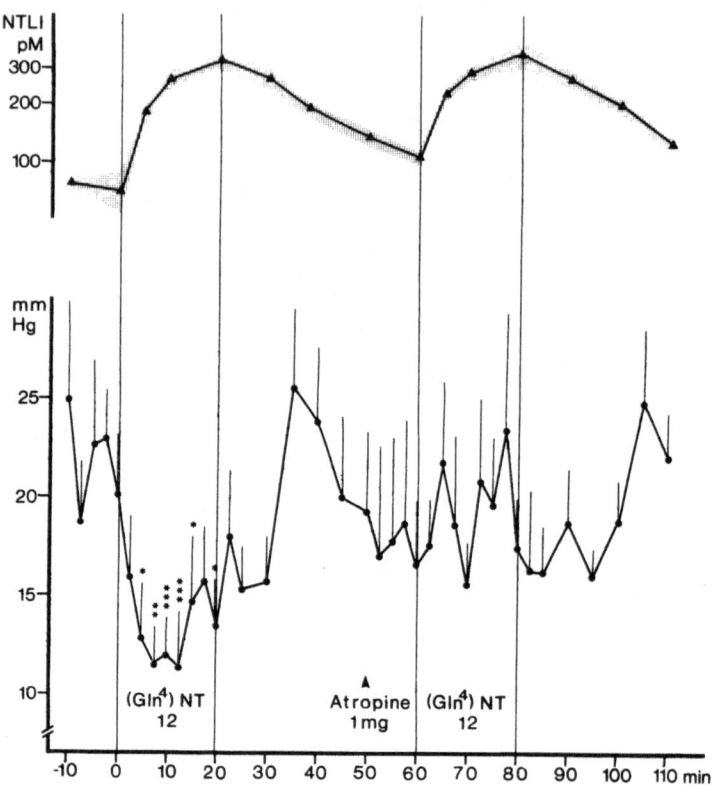

FIGURE 2   Changes in p-NTLI (pM) and LES pressure (mm Hg) following
intravenous infusion of (Gln^4)-neurotensin (12 pmol x kg^{-1} x
min^{-1}) during 20 min, before and after atropine injection.
Vertical lines indicate the infusion period. Shaded area and
vertical bars indicate means ± S.E. (n=7).
P<0.05*, P<0.01**, P<0.001***. (Reproduced from ref. 5).

Intravenous infusion (n=7) of GNT (12 pmol x kg^{-1} x min^{-1}) during
20 min significantly decreased the LES pressure from 21.8 ± 3.2 mm Hg
to 11.4 ± 2.8 mm Hg. During the postinfusion period there was a gradual
return of the pressure to preinfusion values (Fig. 2). The administration of atropine (1 mg) as a single intravenous bolus injection resulted in a 20 % fall in the mean basal pressure compared to preinfusion
values, but this change was not significant (P>0.05). After atropine,
the LES pressure response to GNT was abolished, but the increases in
p-NTLI in the two infusion periods were not significantly different
(Fig. 2).

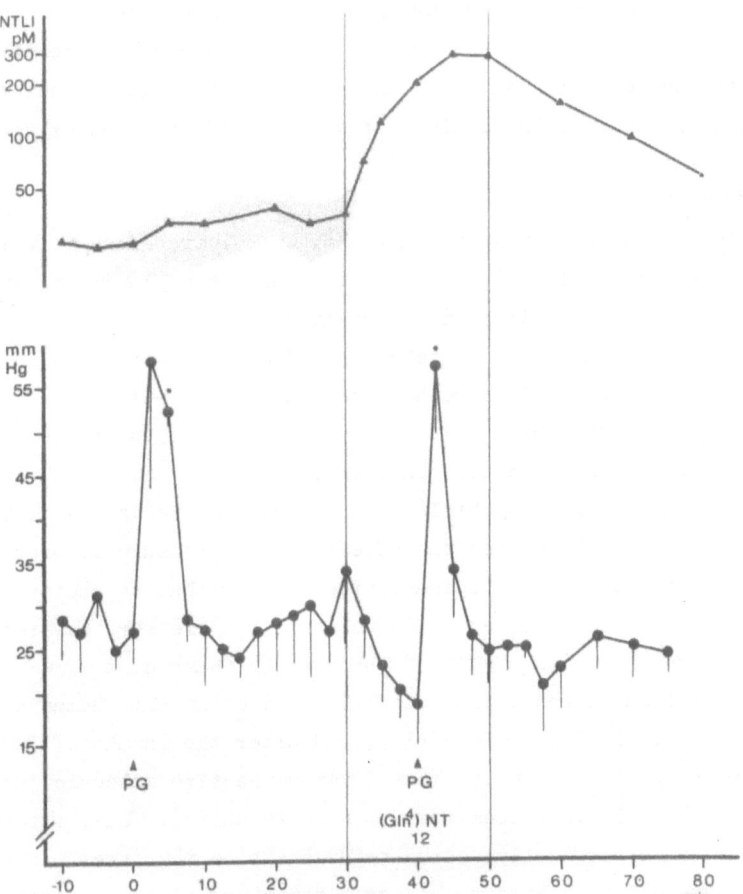

FIGURE 3   Changes in p-NTLI and LES pressure (mm Hg) in response to
intravenous bolus injection of pentagastrin (0.6 µg x kg^{-1})
alone and during an intravenous infusion of (Gln^4)-neuroten-
sin (12 pmol x kg^{-1} x min^{-1}) for 20 min. The shaded area and
the vertical bars indicate means ± S.E. (n=4). P<0.05 *.
(Reproduced from ref. 5).

Bolus injections (n=4) of pentagastrin (0.6 µg x kg^{-1}) increased
the LES pressure from 28.4 $\pm$ 3.9 to 52.3 $\pm$ 1.5 mm Hg at 2.5 min after
the injection (Fig. 3). Following the injection of pentagastrin, there
was a tendency for p-NTLI levels to rise, but this change was not
statistically significant (P>0.5). An intravenous infusion of GNT,
starting 10 min before the injection of pentagastrin, did not inhibit
the effect of pentagastrin. The concentration of p-NTLI increased from

27 ± 11 pM to 274 ± 19 pM during the infusion period.

All volunteers reported dryness of the mouth after the atropine injection and experienced flush and a "sinking" feeling after the pentagastrin injections, regardless of whether GNT was used or not.

DISCUSSION

The results of the present study show that intravenous infusion of GNT or NT at a dose of 12 pmol x kg^{-1} increased the plasma concentration of GNT(1-13) and NT(1-13) to about 15 pM at one min. At that time the LES pressure had been diminished by 43% of the resting value. These data indicate that the threshold plasma concentrations of NT(1-13) or GNT(1-13) for producing relaxation of LES were 15 pM or less. As mentioned in the introduction, shorter sequences of NT or GNT have not been found to exert any biological effects on the gastrointestinal tract in vivo. Therefore, the effect on LES pressure is probably due to actions of the intact tridecapeptide, rather than to shorter sequences such as NT(1-8) since, at 1 min when the LES pressure was reduced, the plasma concentration of NT(1-8) had hardly changed.

The plasma concentration of NT(1-13) increases in human subjects after the ingestion of food (14), and after the intake of 300 ml of cream the plasma concentration of immunoreactive molecules corresponding to NT(1-13) increases from 3 pM to 26 pM (6). Thus, after ingestion of fat the biologically active tridecapeptide may reach a concentration in plasma which is higher than that necessary to cause a reduction in LES pressure. This is strong evidence that the increase in the plasma concentration of NT(1-13) after a meal containing fat is sufficient for the NT(1-13) to exert hormonal actions.

It has been shown in man and animals that NT(1-13) brings about changes in gastrointestinal motility and secretion upon intravenous infusion of doses as low as 1.4-3 pmol x kg^{-1} x min^{-1} (9, 15, 16, 7). In view of the present findings, this dose range seems to result in concentrations of NT(1-13) found physiologically. The present data also indicate that NT(1-13) and GNT(1-13) have equal potencies in decreasing LES pressure in man.

Neurotensin does not reduce a pentagastrin-induced increase in LES pressure, which indicates that postprandially released neurotensin is probably not involved in the reduction of the pentagastrin-stimulated

LES pressure, while the inhibitory action of GNT on the LES pressure seems to involve a cholinergic nervous pathway, rather than being due to a direct myogenic action.

ACKNOWLEDGEMENTS

This study was most generously supported by Åhlén's Foundation and Tore Nilson's Foundation.

REFERENCES

1.   Rosell, S. and Rökaeus, Å. (1979). The effect of ingestion of amino acids, glucose and fat on circulating neurotensin-like immuno-reactivity (NTLI) in man. Acta Physiol. Scand., 107, 263-267

2.   Rosell, S. and Rökaeus, Å. (1981). Actions and possible hormonal functions of circulating neurotensin. Clin. Physiol., 1, 3-20

3.   Rosell, S., Al-Saffar, A. and Thor, K. (1983). The role of neuro-tensin in gut motility. Scand. J. Gastroent. In press.

4.   Rosell, S., Thor, K., Rökaeus, Å., Nyquist, O., Lewenhaupt, A., Kager, L. and Folkers, K. (1980). Plasma concentration of neurotensin-like immunoreactivity (NTLI) and lower esophageal sphincter (LES) pressure in man following infusion of (Gln^4)-neurotensin. Acta Physiol. Scand., 109, 369-375

5.   Thor, K. and Rökaeus, Å. (1983). Studies on the mechanisms by which (Gln^4)-neurotensin reduces lower esophageal sphincter (LES) pressure in man. Acta Physiol. Scand. In press.

6.   Thor, K. and Rökaeus, Å. (1983). Antroduodenal motor response induced by (Gln^4)-neurotensin in man. Acta Physiol. Scand. In press.

7.   Thor, K., Rosell, S., Rökaeus, Å. and Kager, L. (1982). (Gln^4)-neurotensin changes the motility pattern of the duodenum and proximal jejunum from a fasting-type to a fed-type. Gastroenterology, 83, 569-574.

8.   Thor, K. and Rosell, S. (1983). Neurotensin increases colonic motility. (Manuscript).

9.   Al-Saffar, A. and Rosell, S. (1981). Effects of neurotensin and neurotensin analogues on the migrating myoelectrical complexes in the small intestine of rats. Acta Physiol Scand., 112, 203-208

10. Theodorsson-Norheim, E. and Rosell, S. (1983). Chromatographic characterization of the increase in human plasma neurotensin-like immunoreactivity (p-NTLI) after fat ingestion. Regulatory Peptides, 6, 221-234

11. Hellström, P.M. and Rosell, S. (1982). The stimulatory effect of neurotensin on colonic motility is mediated via nervous pathways. In Annals of the New York Academy of Sciences. 400, 381-383

12. Al-Saffar, A. (1983). Analysis of the control of intestinal motility in fasted rats, with special reference to neurotensin. Acta Physiol. Scand. (Submitted).

13. Theodorsson-Norheim, E., Thor, K. and Rosell, S. (1983). Relation between lower esophageal sphincter (LES) pressure and the plasma concentration of neurotensin during intravenous infusion of neurotensin (1-13) and (Gln^4) neurotensin (1-13) in man. Acta Physiol. Scand. Suppl. 515, 29-35

14. Blackburn, A. and Bloom, S. (1979). A radioimmunoassay for neurotensin in human plasma. J. Endocrinol. 83, 175-181

15. Blackburn, A.M., Fletcher, D.R., Adrian, T.E. and Bloom, S.E. (1980). Neurotensin infusion in man: pharmacokinetics and effect on gastrointestinal and pituitary hormones. J. Clin. Endocrinol. Metab. 51, 1257-1261

16. Fletcher, D.R., Blackburn, A.M., Adrian, T.E., Chadwick, V.S. and Bloom, S.R. (1981). Effect of neurotensin on pancreatic function in man. Life Sci., 29, 2157-2161.

8

D-Pro^2, D-Trp^{7,9} Substance P: an Effective Antagonist of Exogenous and Endogenous Substance P

C. REYNOLDS, A. OUYANG and S. COHEN

INTRODUCTION

Substance P has been identified by immunohistochemical techniques throughout the gastrointestinal tract (1,2). The opposum lower eso- phageal sphincter contracts in the presence of substance P via direct and indirect mechanisms (3). The role of substance P as a neurotrans- mitter remains incompletely understood (4,5). The recent development of substance P antagonists (6) may provide a method to define the physiologic effects of substance P. We investigated D-Pro^2, D-Trp^{7,9} substance P on the feline lower esophageal sphincter response to exo- genous substance P and to distal esophageal acidification.

METHODS

The methods used in this study have been described in detail pre- viously (7). Studies were performed in fasted adult cats using keta- mine and chloralose anesthesia. Intraluminal pressures were recorded using a pneumohydraulically perfused catheter assembly fixed by a pinning technique in the position that recorded maximal LES pressure. The pin also secured a serosal Ag-AgCl bipolar electrode directly over the LES perfusion ports. Intraluminal pressures were also re- corded from 3.0 and 6.0 cm orad to the LES. Myoelectric activity was recorded from the gastric fundus 1 cm aborad to the LES, the antrum 1.0 and 2.0 cm orad to the pylorus and from the duodenum. Catheters were attached to pressure transducers (Statham Instruments).

Signals from the electrodes and transducers were amplified and graphed on a multichannel rectilinear recorder.

The following drugs were used: pentagastrin (Ayerst Laboratories, (0.5 µg/kg), phenylephrine HCL (Winthrop Laboratories, 25.0 µg/kg, tetrodotoxin (Sankyo Company, 2.5 µg/kg/bolus), substance P (Peninsula Laboratories) and D-Pro^2, D-Trp^{7,9} substance P (Peninsula Laboratories). All peptides were dissolved in a 0.1N acetic acid solution and handled in glassware treated with a silicone solution (Sigma Cote).

RESULTS

(a) Pharmacologic studies

The lower esophageal sphincter response to substance P is shown in Figure 1. Substance P 1.0 µg/kg gave a prompt, increase in LES pressure (32.1 + 7.1 mmHg) and spike activity (41.7 + 11.7 spikes/ 30 sec). Substance P gave a dose-dependent increase in LES pressure and spike activity. The threshold dose was 0.5 µg/kg i.v. The maximal dose was 10.0 µg/kg i.v.

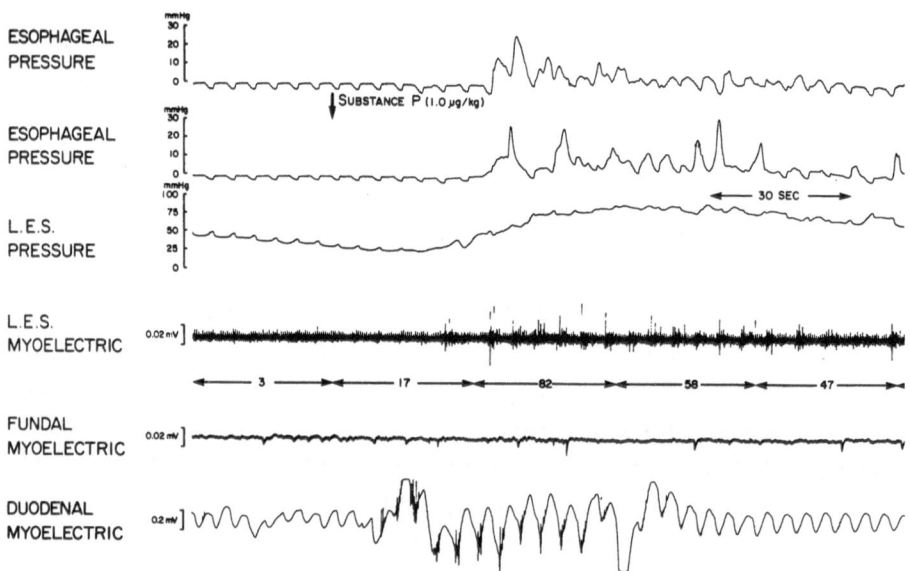

FIGURE 1

Desensitization of the LES response to substance P 1.0 μg/kg was established by repeated administration of a supra-maximal dose (100 μg/kg i.v.). Substance P tachyphylaxis abolished the LES response to exogenous substance P (1.0 μg/kg). This antagonism was specific, and had no effect on the LES response to the ED_{50} dose of phenylephrine or pentagastrin.

The substance P analogue D-Pro^2, D-Trp^{7,9} substance P gave a dose-dependent increase in LES pressure and spike activity that was less potent than the parent compound. The analogue gave 22.4% of the contractile response to substance P at 1.0 μg/kg i.v. and 47.8% of the response to the parent compound at supra-maximal doses (200.0 μg/kg). The inhibitory effect of D-Pro^2, D-Trp^{7,9} substance P on the LES response to 1.0 μg/kg is shown in Figure 2. Significant inhibition was achieved only when molar ratios exceeded 100:1.

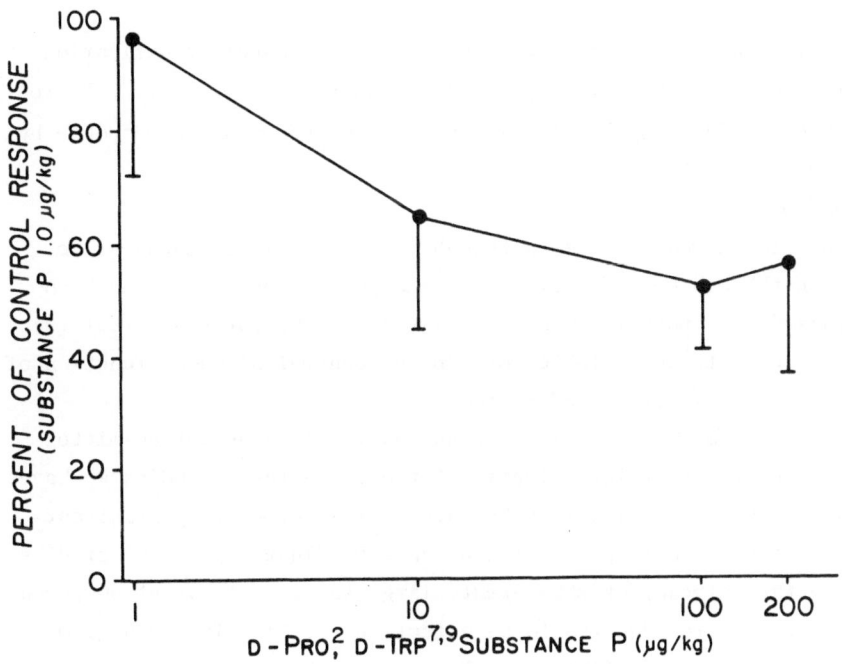

FIGURE 2

$D-Pro^2$, $D-Trp^{7,9}$ substance P (200.0 µg/kg i.v) inhibited the response to substance P by 48.7% of the control response. The substance
P analogue had no effect on the responses to the ED$_{50}$ doses of pentagastrin or phenylephrine.

(b) Physiologic studies

Acidification of the distal esophagus (3.0 ml, 0.1N HCl) produced a
prompt increase in lower esophageal sphincter pressure that presis-
ted for 3-4 minutes (8). The mean increases in LES pressure (27.1 $\pm$
4.9 mmHg) and spike activity (133.8 $\pm$ 22.6 spikes/min) were significantly greater than following saline (p<0.001). Acidification of the
fundus had no effect. In previous studies we showed that the LES
response to acid was abolished by neural blockade by tetrodotoxin or
intraluminal benzocaine (8). Antagonists to acetylcholine, phenylephrine, histamine, serotonin, opioid peptides or dopamine and bilateral cervical vagotomy had no effect on the increase in LES pressure (8).

The increase in LES pressure following esophageal acidification
was reduced by 81.5 $\pm$ 5.5% (p<0.05) by tachyphylaxis. $D-Pro^2$, $D-Trp^{7,9}$
substance P (200.0 µg/kg, i.v.) reduced the LES pressure response by
61.3 $\pm$ 19.3% (p<0.05).

DISCUSSION

The enteric nervous system is thought to play a major integrative
function through neural reflexes in the gut. Substance P has been
recognized as a putative neurotransmitter in the gut since 1931 (9).
Nevertheless its physiologic role in the control of motor function of
the gut is incompletely understood.

The development of a selective antagonist to a neurotransmitter
creates an important investigational tool. In these studies we have
shown that $D-Pro^2$, $D-Trp^{7,9}$ substance P is a selective partial antagonist of the LES response to substance P. In all previous studies
showing the efficacy of this agent, large antagonist/parent compound
molar ratios were required to be effective (6,10). The mechanism for
a partial antagonist effect is unknown. In these studies, larger
doses of the antagonist were not effective in producing a greater
inhibition beyond a molar ratio of 100 to 1. In these doses, the
contractile response of the LES to $D-Pro^2$, $D-Trp^{7,9}$ substance P approached that of the parent compound. This suggests that part of its

antagonist effect could be via desensitization. The binding properties of D-Pro^2, D-Trp^{7,9} substance P have not been compared to the
parent compound. Antagonism by competitive binding would not be
expected to produce a partial effect. Previous studies have shown
that substance P may act at the LES directly on smooth muscle as well
as via tetrodotoxin - sensitive mechanisms. It is possible that
D-Pro^2, D-Trp^{7,9} substance P inhibits either the direct or the
tetrodotoxin-sensitive pathways but not both. Further studies will
be necessary to establish its mechanism of action and to develop
antagonists with less agonist effects.

Esophageal acidification increases lower esophageal sphincter
pressure in healthy controls but not in patients with reflux esophagitis (11). These studies demonstrate that this response occurs
in an animal model via local neural pathway that involve substance
P as a transmitter. This suggests that substance P may be an important mediator of physiologic reflexes in the gut.

REFERENCES

1. Schultzberg, M., Hokfelt, T., Nilssen, G., Terenius, L., Rehfeld,
J.F., Brown, M., Elde, M., Goldstein, M., and Said, S. (1980).
Distribution of peptide and catecholamine-containing neurons in the
gastrointestinal tract of the rat and guinea-pig: immunohistochemical studies with antisera to substance P, vasoactive intestinal
polypeptide, enkephalins, somatostatin, gastrin/cholecystokinin,
neurotensin and dopamine β-hydroxylase. Neuroscience 5, 689-744.

2. Holzer, P., Bucsics, A., Saria, A., and Lembeck, F. (1982). A
study of concentrations of substance P and neurotensin in the gastrointestinal tract of various mammals. Neuroscience 7, 2919-2924.

3. Mukhopadhyay, A.K. (1978). Effect of substance P on the lower
esophageal sphincter of the opossum. Gastroenterology 75, 278-282.

4. Franco, R., Costa, M., and Furness, J.B. (1979). Evidence for
release of endogenous substance P from intestinal nerves. Naunyn-
Schneidenberg's Arch. of Pharmacol. 306, 195-201.

5. Morita, K., North, R.A., and Katayama, Y. (1980). Evidence that
substance P is a neurotransmitter in the myenteric plexus. Nature
287, 151-154.

6. Leander, S., Hakanson, R., Rosell, S., Folkers, K., Sundler, F., and Tornquist, K. (1981). A specific substance P antagonist blocks smooth muscle contractions induced by non-cholinergic, non-adrenergic nerve stimulation. Nature 294, 467-469.

7. Reynolds, J.C., Ouyang, A., and Cohen, S. (1982). Electrically-coupled intrinsic responses of feline lower esophageal sphincter. Am. J. Physiol. 243 (Gastrointest. Liver Physiol. 6):G415-G423.

8. Reynolds, J.C., Ouyang, A., and Cohen, S. (1983). Substance P: a neurotransmitter in these intrinsic neural pathways mediating the feline lower esophageal sphincter response to esophageal acidification. Gastroenterology 84,1285.

9. vonEuler, U.S., and Gaddum, J.H. (1931). An unidentified pressor substance in certain tissue extracts. J. Physiol. (Lond). 72, 74-87.

10. Domoto, T., Jury, J., Berezin, I., Fox, J.E.T. and Daniel, E.E. (1983). Does substance P co-mediate with acetylcholine in nerves of opossum esophageal muscularis mucosa? Am. J. Physiol. (Gastrointest. Liver Physiol 8):G19-G28.

11. Ahtaridis, G., Snape, W.J., Jr., and Cohen, S. (1981). Lower esophageal sphincter pressure on an index of gastroesophageal acid reflux. Dig. Dis. and Sci. 26, 993-998.

9

Relationship of Functional Changes to Structural Changes in Megaesophagus of Chagas' Disease

J. E. T. FOX, E. E. DANIEL, C. R. DeFARIA, J. M. REZENDEZ,
L. RASSI, J. DeREZENDEZ JR. and V. P. DANIEL

INTRODUCTION

The denervation of the intrinsic nerves of the esophagus (1) in Chagas' disease has been attributed to activated lymphocytes following trypanasoma crusi infection (2). deRezendez and co-workers have classified the severity of the disease radiologically (3) and manometrically (4) into four groups. Complete retention of contrast media, gross dilatation and elongation of the esophageal body with complete loss of motor activity on x-ray was described for group 4, with other groups being intermediate. By manometry increased lower esophageal sphincter pressure and length and 95% loss of sphincter relaxation with swallowing characterized group 3. Increased sensitivity to methacholine (5) also occurs in Chagasics (2). Extremes of temperature induced increased contractile disco-ordination in group 2 (6). Pentagastrin contractions were found to be less in Chagasic patients (7). Since deRezendez (unpublished studies) found the reduction in LES relaxation by glucagon related to the severity of the disease, the reduced pentagastrin response may reflect a loss of cholinergic nerves.

Our objectives were to study the functional behaviour of the circular muscle of the lower esophagus in vitro to nerve stimulation and to analogues of neurotransmitters and to compare these results to structural changes in the neuromuscular apparatus.

METHODS

Surgical specimens of LES were obtained from 5 (Chagas' serological
positive) Brazilian patients with second and third stage magaesophagus.
As "normal" controls, unaffected tissue was obtained following resection for carcinoma in two Canadian patients. In vitro responses of
circular muscle strips were recorded on a Sandborn Recorder in Brazil
and a Beckman Dynograph in Canada. Adjacent segments were fixed for
electron microscopy in glutaraldehyde in 2% cacodylate buffer for 2
hours at $20^{\circ}C$, stored in phosphate buffer at $4^{\circ}C$ and post fixed in
$0_2 0_4$. Sections were observed and the numbers and types of nerves and
gap junctions per 100 smooth muscle cells quantified (8). Statistical
evaluation utilized students' unpaired t-test.

RESULTS

Control tissues responded to field stimulation of 0.5 ms by relaxation
or an "off" contraction. Only one out of 17 Chagas' tissues responded
at 0.5 ms. At higher durations a tetrodotoxin-insensitive contraction
occurred most frequently suggesting a direct muscle response. Carbachol increased tone in all tissues. The ED_{50} for Chagasic tissue (2.4
$\pm$ 0.4 x $10^{-7}M$) was significantly less than that of normal tissue (20.0
$\pm$ 5.0 x $10^{-7}M$) suggesting denervation supersensitivity is measurable in
vitro as well. All tissues responded to 1 ug/ml isoproterenol by
relaxation of resting or carbachol-induced tone.

MORPHOLOGICAL EVALUATION

Control tissues were found to have 19.7 $\pm$ 3.1 nerves per 100 smooth
muscle cells located within the muscle bundles and in nerve bundles
outside the muscle bundles. Nerve varicosities contained large
granular vesicles, small granular vesicles and small agranular
vesicles (Figure 1, Table 1). Interstitial cells of Cajal were found
between the muscle bundles in close association with the nerves and
the smooth muscle cells. Gap junctions were found between the smooth
muscle cells (Table 2, Figure 2).

In the Chagasic tissues there were 5 times fewer nerves. The remaining nerves were frequently damaged. There were a similar number
of varicosities containing small granular vesicles as control but
fewer varicosities contained small agranular vesicles and none were
found with large granular vesicles (Figure 3). A similar number of
interstitial cells/100 cells were found but fewer found associated

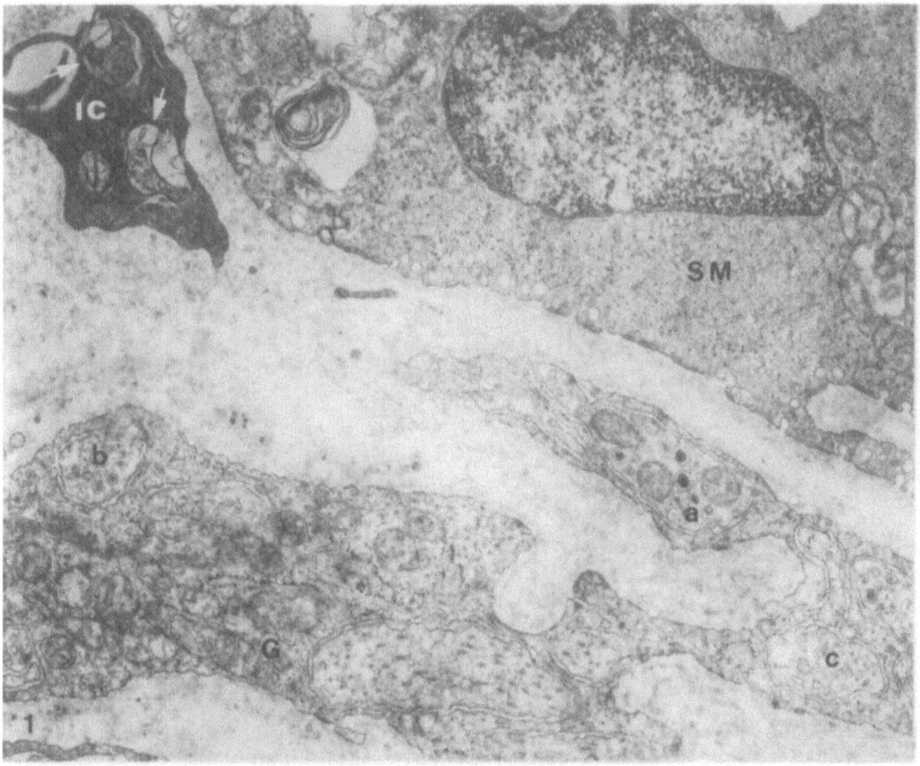

Nerve profiles and interstitial cell (IC) in muscle bundle of normal
esophagus. The nerve bundle contains one varicosity (a) with a predominance of large granular vesicles present in addition to mitochondria
and small granular vesicles; another varicosity (b) contains predominantly small granular vesicles, while one varicosity (c) may contain a
small agranular vesicle. Note the numerous neurotubules and neurofila-
ments, also glial filaments in the glial cell (G). The interstitial
cell apparently contains two damaged nerve profiles (small white
arrows). The smooth muscle cell (SM) appears normal as seen after
immersion fixation. Magnification = 25,200.

Gap junction (690 nm) in normal
esophagus. Note the typical
five-lined structure (no gap
noted in this case). Muscles
contained small and large filaments. Magnification = 80,000.

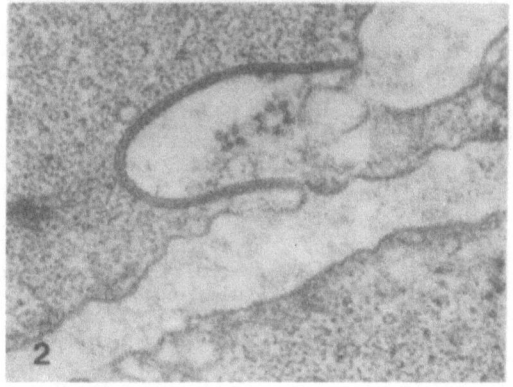

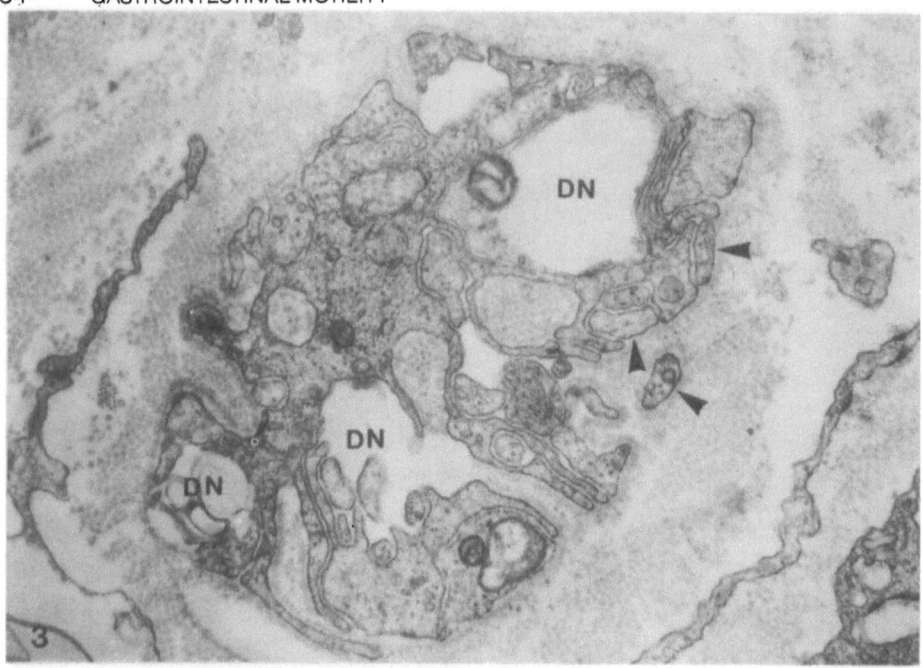

Nerve bundle in an esophagus of chagasic patient. Few nerves were
present inside muscle bundles and residual profiles were usually found
in small bundles outside the muscle as in this case. Note apparently
degenerating nerve profiles (DN), several small axons free of glial
cytoplasm which may be regenerating (arrowheads) and absence of any
varicosities with large granular vesicles. Magnification = 22,800.

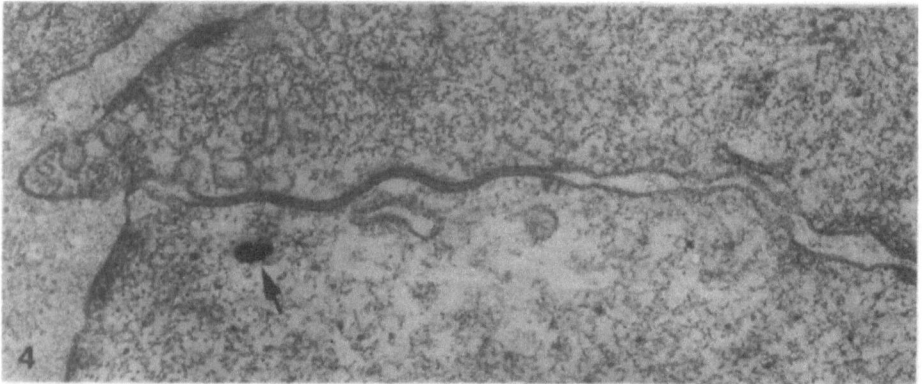

Gap junction (590 nm) in esophageal muscle from chagasic patient. Note
typical seven-lined structure (gap visible) and length of junction.
The smooth muscle is normal with thin and thick filaments, membrane
caveolae and other normal features. Magnification = 80,000.
Note dense intracellular body near gap junction (arrow).

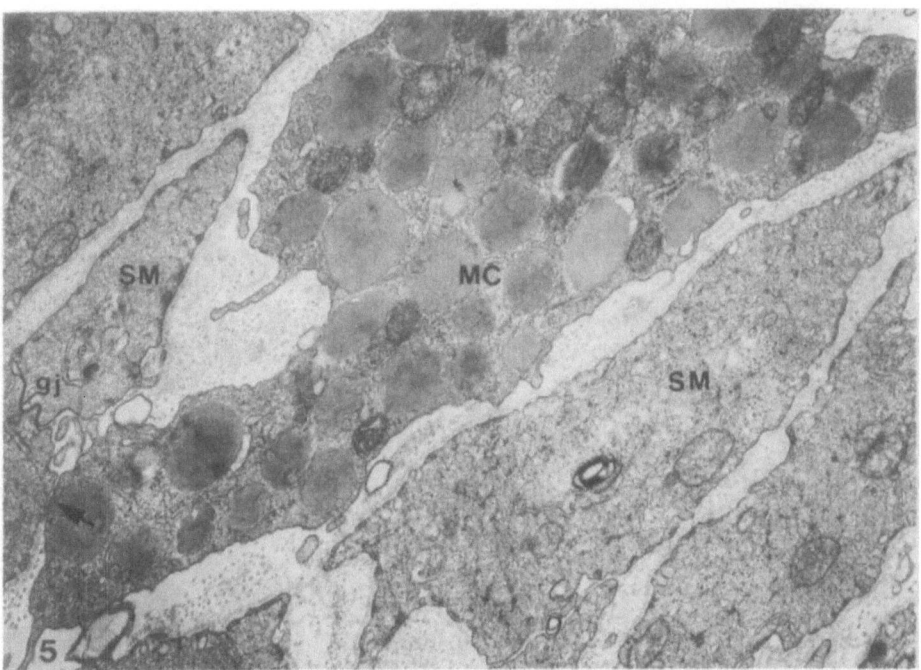

Mast cell like structure (MC) commonly seen in muscle bundles of esophagus from chagasic patients. Note close contact (arrow) between this
cell and a smooth muscle cell (SM) which is in gap junction contact(gj)
with another muscle cell. Magnification = 28,800.

TABLE I: Prominent Morphological Features of Esophageal
          Tissues Expressed per 100 Smooth Muscle Cells

	CONTROL	CHAGAS
# sections/# patients	8/2	39/5
# nerves	19.7 + 3.1	3.6 ± 1.0*
Nerve varicosities containing		
a) large granular vesicles	0.3 ± 0.2	0 ± 0
b) small granular vesicles	0.4 ± 0.2	0.3 ± 0.2
c) small agranular vesicles	3.1 + 1.1	0.2 ± 0.1
# of interstitial cells	0.7 ± 0.5	0.8 ± 0.3
a) associated with nerves	0.4 + 0.3	0.2 ± 0.1
b) not associated with nerves	0.4 + 0.2	0.7 ± 0.2
# of muscle cell nuclei	7.7 ± 1.3	7.4 ± 1.6

with nerves.

The smooth muscle cells appeared normal with similar numbers of nuclei visible. The major difference between the Chagasic tissues and controls was the four-fold increase in the number of gap junctions per 100 sm cells in the Chagasic tissues (2.1 $\pm$ 1.0, controls; 9.3 $\pm$ 1.1, Chagasics). These were only slightly longer (not significant) in the Chagasic tissues (156 $\pm$ 22 nm controls, 200 $\pm$ 12 nm Chagasics). Gap junctions associated with dense intracellular bodies were seen in four Chagasic patients' tissue (Fig. 4).

Most cell-like structures and platelets were found in the muscle cell bundles in only the Chagasic tissue (Fig. 5).

DISCUSSION

The normal innervated LES in vitro relaxes to field stimulation of nerves and β-agonists and contracts to cholinergic agonists (9). By electron microscopy nerve varicosities containing several types of granules are found both within and without the muscle bundles. Interstitial cells of Cajal are also found associated with the nerves in the muscle bundle. Gap junction contacts occur between cells.

In Chagas' disease the smooth muscle cells appear relatively normal but denervation of both the submucous and the myenteric plexus occurs (1). The achalasia of Chagas' disease with the increased sphincter pressure, the lack of LES relaxation and the increased sensitivity to cholinergic agonists is similar to that described for achalasia in the Northern Hemisphere (5, 10).

Our functional studies demonstrate the almost complete loss of nerves stimulated response which correlates well with our finding of reduced number and damaged nerves by microscopy. Thus systemic administration of a nerve stimulant would evoke a response which would reflect the amount of denervation such as that seen with glucagon or pentagastrin (7). Our finding of increased sensitivity to carbachol in vitro reflects the increased sensitivity to mecholyl found in vivo and can probably be classed as "denervation supersensitivity". The exact mechanism of this is unknown. Increased numbers of end organ receptors has been proposed (11). This has not been tested in Chagas' disease.

We present in our study a possible alternative mechanism for increased sensitivity, that of increased coupling and hence the area of low resistance pathways between cells, less stimulation should be required to produce a contractile response.

Thus the increased coupling may be a compensatory mechanism for denervation and the presence of nerves may reduce the number of gap junctions. Thus there may be factors released from nerves in smooth muscle which prevent the tight coupling of the muscles. Loss of nerves would then facilitate coupling.

ACKNOWLEDGEMENTS

Supported by the Medical Research Council of Canada. Dr. J.E.T. Fox is a MRC Scholar. The authors wish to thank R. Vonau for secretarial assistance and I. Berezin for assistance with microscopy pictures.

REFERENCES

1. Koberle, F. and Nador, E. (1955). Etiologia et patagenia do megaesofago no Brasil. Rev. Paul Med. 47: 643-661.

2. Teixeira, M.L., Rezendi Filho, J., Figueredo, F. and Teixeira, A.R.L. (1980). Chagas' disease: Selective affinity and cytotoxicity of trypanosome Cruzi-immune lymphocytes to parasympathetic gaglion cells. Mem. Inst. Oswaldo Cruz. 75: 33-45, 1980.

3. deRezendez, S.M. (1963). The endemic South American magaesophagus. Clinical aspects of endemic megaesopagus. In Ingelfinger, R.J. and Siffert, G., 2nd World Congress of Gastroenterology 1962 Vol. pp. 69-74 (N.Y. S. Kager).

4. dePaula-Costa, M.D. and deRezendez, J.M. (1978). Pressao basal do esofago no megaesofago Chagasico. Rev. Ass. Med. Brazil. 24: 269-727.

5. Kramer, P. and Ingelfinger, F.J. (1951). Esophageal sensitivity to mecholyl in Cardiospasm Gastroenterol 19: 242-253.

6. deRezendes, J.M.N., Montalvao, F. and Centeno, A.J. (1981). Efeito da temperatura dos ingesta sobre a motiladade esofaginana no megaesofago Chagasico. Estudo manometrico Arq. Gastroent. S. Paulo 18: 8-13.

7. Padovan, W. Godoy, R.A., Dantas, R.O., Menghelli, U.S., Oliveira, R.B. and Troncon, L.E.A. (1980). Lower oesophageal sphincter response to pentagastrin in Chagasic patients with magaoesophageal and megacolon. Gut 21: 85-90.

8. Jones, T.R., Kannon, M.S. and Daniel, E.E. (1980). Ultrastructural study of guinea pig tracheal smooth muscle and its innerovation. Can. J. Physiol. Pharmacol. 58: 974-983.

9. Marshall, R.W., McKirdy, H.C. and Duthie, H.C. (1982). Possible identification of sphincteric muscle from human lower oesophagus with observations on the effects of drugs and electrical field stimulation. In Wienbeck, M. (ed.) Motility of the Digestive Tract, pp. 333-338, (NY: Raven Press).

10. Cohen, S. and Lipshultz, W. (1971). Lower esophogeal dysfunction in achalasia. Gastroenterology, 61: 814-825.

11. Carrier, O. and Shibata, S. (1977). Supersensitivity, In Carrier, O. and Shibata, S. (eds.). Factors influencing vascular reactivity, pp. 255-267 (Tokyo, Igaku-Shoin).

10

Developmental Characteristics of the Kitten Lower Esophageal Sphincter

C. HILLEMEIER and P. BIANCANI

Gastroesophageal reflux is a common finding during infancy. In the cat, in vivo LES pressure increases with age from 9.5 ± 2.4 mmHg at 3 days to 21.5 ± 2.9 mmHg at 6 weeks to $43 + 4.5$ mmHg in the adult cat. In order to examine the genesis of this reduced pressure in the kitten, we determined the mechanical characteristics and responses to muscarinic stimulation of both the kitten and adult LES. Circumferentially oriented rings of the LES exhibited increased in vitro active force in response to + induced depolarization with advancing age (Figure 1). Normalizing active forces for the different amount of muscle present in the various age groups yields greater stresses in the kitten (Figure 2), suggesting that reduced LES pressures are not due to reduced contractility in the kitten. According to Laplace's law, pressure equals the product of the stress and the ratio of the circular muscle thickness to its inner radius ratio[1]. In the kitten thickness/radius ratio is such that despite higher stresses generated, lower pressures are developed.

The in vitro kitten LES contracts significantly less with low concentrations of bethanechol. The kitten LES responds with relaxation to low concentrations of nicotine while the adult LES contracts. However, after incubation in atropine the adult LES shows a dose-response curve to nicotine similar to that of the kitten. This suggest that at low-dosed nicotine stimulation in the adult activates excitatory cholinergic pathways not yet present in the kitten.

59

We conclude: (1) the muscle of the LES in our infant model has increased contractility but is at a mechanical disadvantage in generating LES pressure; (2) the kitten is less responsive to muscarinic stimulation than the adult.

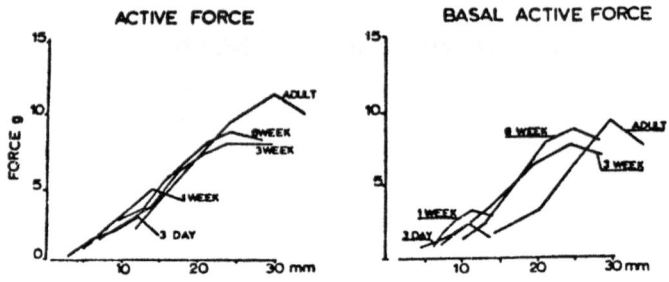

Figure 1

On the left are the active force length relationships, and on the right the basal active force length relationships. They show increasing force generated with age.

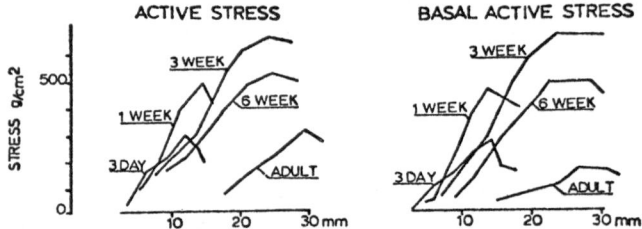

Figure 2

The active stress (Total active force/area of circular smooth muscle) length relationships at the LES (left panel). Basal active stresses at the LES (right panel). They shown infant LES is capable of generating greater stress than in the adult.

REFERENCE

1. Biancani, P., Zabinski, M.P., Behar, J. (1975). Pressure tension and force of closure of the human lower esophageal sphincter. J. Clin. Inv., 56:476-483

11

Variability of Pressure and Myoelectrical Activity Recorded from the Lower Esophageal Sphincter of Fasted Conscious Opossums

I. TAKAHASHI, E. BLANK, R. H. HOLLOWAY, W. J. DODDS, J. DENT, S. SARNA and W. J. HOGAN

The opossum has served as an important model for studies of lower esophageal sphincter (LES) function. Previous investigations, however, have been confined to studies in anesthetized animals. Our aim in this study was to record LES pressure and electrical activity concurrently from conscious opossums. In four animals, we performed a cervical esophagostomy and implanted bipolar electrodes on the abdominal esophagus, LES, gastric antrum and duodenum. Beginning several weeks after surgery, 15 to 20 recording sessions, each lasting 4-6 hr, were obtained in each animal. Intraluminal pressure from the gastric antrum, LES and esophageal body was recorded by a manometric assembly that incorporated a sleeve device, while myoelectric activity from comparable sites was recorded via the implanted electrodes. In fasted conscious animals, interdigestive migratory myoelectric complexes (MMC's) were readily recorded from the stomach and duodenum. These MMC's had a cycle length of 86 ± 2.9 (SE) min. The LES exhibited cyclic changes in its intraluminal pressure and myoelectrical activity that occurred in synchrony with the gastric MMC cycle. Basal LES pressure (24.1 ± 2.1 mmHg) was lowest during phase I of the gastric MMC cycle and reached a maximal value (29.5 ± 1.4 mmHg) during phase III of the gastric MMC. Phasic LES contractions began to appear during phase II of the gastric MMC, became pronounced during phase III and disappeared during phase I. These phasic contractions occurred at a rate of 1.1 ± 0.3 (SE) per min and had maximal amplitudes of 40-80 mmHg. During phase I of the gastric MMC, the LES exhibited irregular spikes of low magnitude (0.1 mV) that occurred at an average rate of 21 ± 2 per min. During the phasic LES contractions that occurred during phases II and III of the gastric MMC, the LES electrical spikes grouped into clusters of increased spike rate (31 ± 3 per min) and magnitude (0.8 mV). Each cluster of spikes corresponded to a phasic LES contraction. The phasic LES pressure and electrical activity associated with the MMC cycle was abolished by anesthesia, feeding or atropine. We conclude: 1) in conscious opossums, the LES exhibits cyclic changes of contractile and electrical activity that occur in synchrony with the gastric MMC, and 2) these variations in LES pressure and electrical activity do not occur during anesthesia.

12

Reflux Characteristics in Health and Disease

A. H. HÖLSCHER and H. F. WEISER

Via the development of a solid state pH-metry with little discomfort to patients it has become possible to quantitatively assess the gastroesophageal reflux (GER) in health and disease under almost physiological conditions. Based on initial studies of healthy subjects we have attempted to establish the borderline between physiological and pathological reflux (9).

According to this a gastroesophageal reflux can be interpreted as physiologic under the condition that
- the pH of the regurgitated fluids is more than 4 and less than 7
- the total reflux duration amounts to less than 7 % in 24 hours and
- a day-time reflux during the prandial and postprandial period respectively
- a reflux during the first half of the night is demonstrable.

This definition agrees with statements of other authors (1, 7, 8), who reported that a pH-value of <4 with a duration of 6 - 7 % of the entire measurement period has a good selectivity between physiological and pathological reflux. We were able to confirm the significance of the fasting reflux as well as the reflux during the second half of the night (deep sleep phase) for the development of reflux esophagitis (2, 3).

The question of our studies now was:
which pH-metrical differences can be found comparing healthy subjects to patients with slight respectively severe
stages of reflux disease?

Patients and methods:

We examined 31 healthy subjects and 77 patients with reflux
suspicious symptoms. According to manometric and endoscopic
findings the patients were differentiated into two groups
(Table 1).

Table 1. Subject characterization of the examined groups.

	n	♂:♀	Mean age (years)	Mano- metry	Endo- scopy	Classifi- cation
Control group	31	16:15	28	LES* suffi- ciency	no esopha- gitis	no reflux disease
Group I	30	14:16	49.7	comp. LES insuff.	esopha- gitis I - II	slight reflux disease
Group II	47	28:19	51.7	decomp. LES insuff.	esopha- gitis III-IV	severe reflux disease

* Lower Esophageal Sphincter

The classification of the endoscopic findings was done with
help of Savary and Miller's grading system (4). The uncom-
plicated endobrachyesophagus is, in our opinion, not a com-
plication of reflux disease but a stage of the healing process of reflux esophagitis and as a modification was therefore not classified as stage IV. Moreover, classification
into stages I, II, III, IV respectively was assigned depending on the oral findings of the endobrachyesophagus (11).

In the course of the consecutively conducted manometry the
sufficiency of the lower esophageal sphincter (LES) was
tested with the 3-point-manometry. The pentagastrin stimulated LES-pressure was checked with the rapid pull-through-
manometry (5, 6). A compensated LES-insufficiency was diag-

nosed under the condition that a positive common cavity phenomenon and a positive pentagastrin stimulation test was present; a decompensated LES-insufficiency was stated if a positive common cavity phenomenon but a negative pentagastrin stimulation test could be found (5).

The assessment of GER was conducted with the 24-hour-solid-state-pH-metry (Autronicord CM18pH) with combined miniature pH electrode (Ingold 440M4) (10). Following calculations were done: number of reflux episodes (n/h), mean reflux duration (min/h). The data showed a homogenous distribution, so that the statistical analysis was done by Student-t-test.

Results:
The typical decrease of the night-time reflux after sleeping in normals can not be found in patients with pathologi-

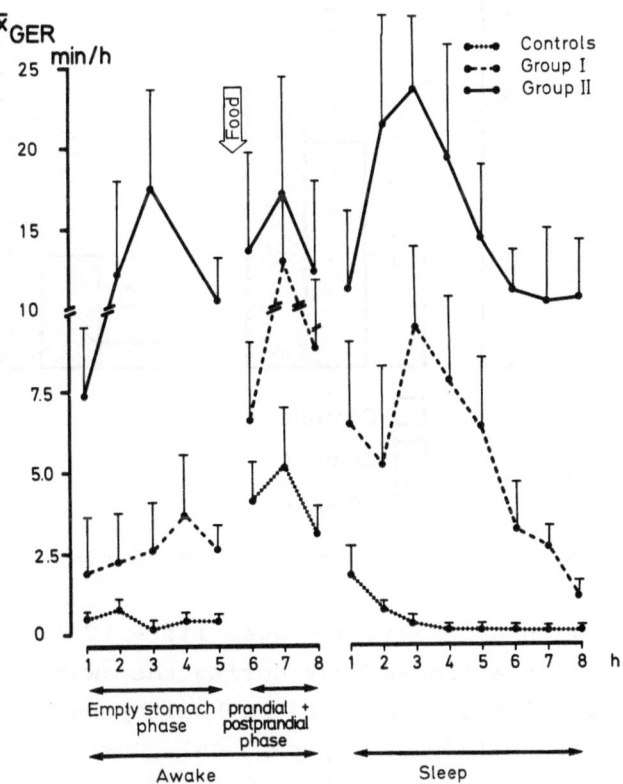

Fig. 1. Mean reflux duration (min/h) during the entire time of measurement.

cal GER. Patients with compensated LES-insufficiency (group I) have a continual but insufficient decrease of the GER during the second half of the night (Fig. 1). A persisting pathologic reflux is found in patients with decompensated LES-insufficiency (group II) during the second half of the night in comparison to healthy persons and to those of group I (p < 0.001, p < 0.01) (Fig. 1).

The number of reflux episodes/hour is significantly higher in patients with esophagitis stages I and II (group I) during the awake and sleep phase than it is in healthy subjects (p < 0.05, p < 0.01) (Fig. 2).

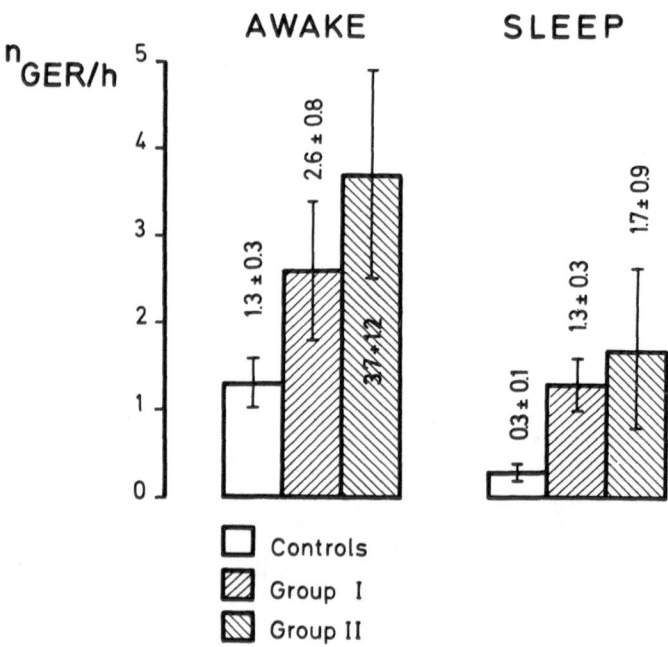

Fig. 2. Number of reflux episodes (n/h) during the awake and sleep phase.

In patients with esophagitis stages III - IV (group II) the number of reflux episodes/hour during the awake phase is significantly higher than it is in healthy persons and in patients of group I (p < 0.01, p < 0.05). During the sleep phase the patients of group II show a significant increase of reflux rate only in comparison to healthy subjects

(p < 0.01). There is an approximately identical reflux frequency in comparison to patients of group I (p > 0.05)(Fig.2)

The average reflux duration/hour is significantly increased
during the awake and sleep phase in patients of group I in
comparison to healthy subjects (p<0.01, p<0.01) (Fig. 3).

In patients of group II the average reflux duration/hour is
significantly higher during the awake and sleep phase than
in healthy subjects and in patients of group I (awake
phase: p < 0.01, p < 0.01, sleep phase: p < 0.001, p < 0.01)
(Fig. 3).

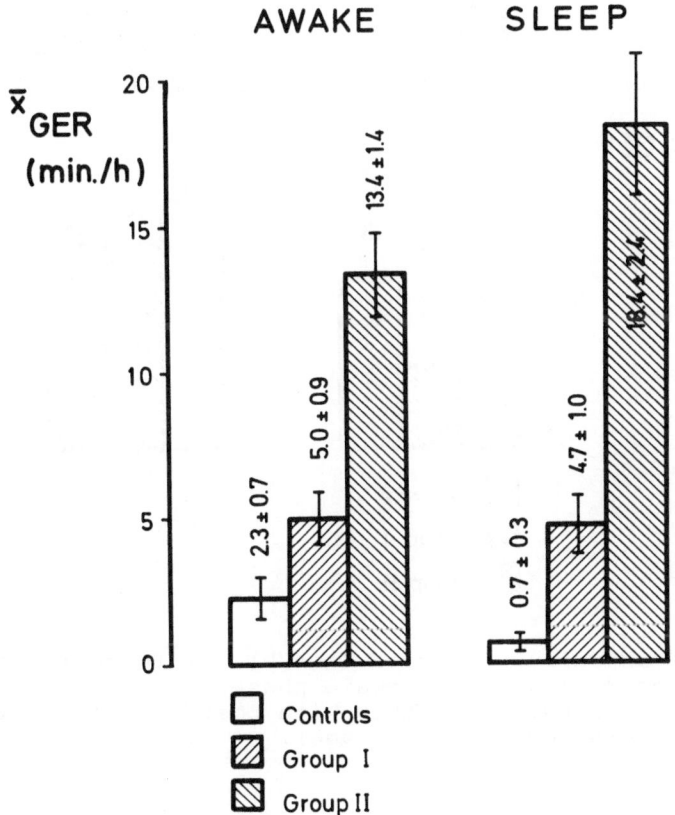

Fig. 3. Mean reflux duration (min/h) during the awake and
        the sleep phase.

After subtraction of the prandial and postprandial reflux
portion from the reflux of the awake phase, group II patients in contrast to healthy subjects and group I patients
show a significant shift in favour of the fasting reflux to
59.9 % of the measurement period ($p < 0.001$, $p < 0.01$)(Fig.4).

On the contrary patients of group I have in comparison to
normals only a slight decrease of the prandial and postprandial reflux   (71.3 % : 86.4 %) in favour of the
empty stomach reflux ($p > 0.05$) (Fig. 4).

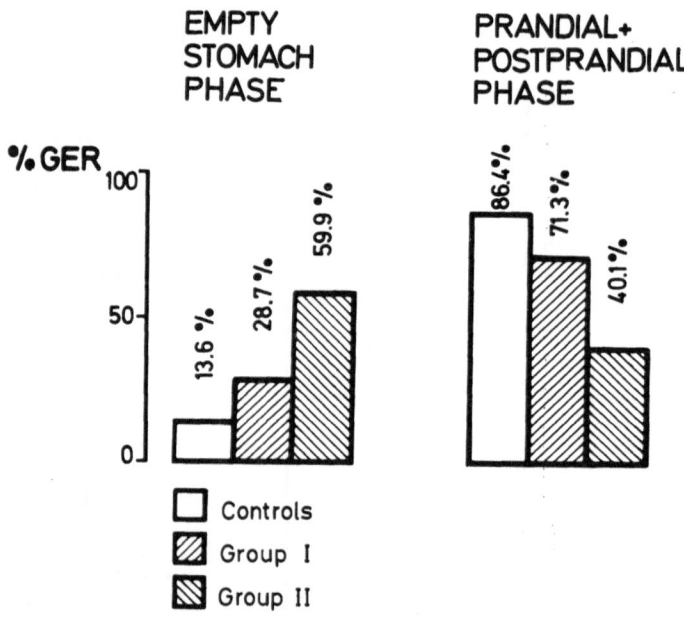

Fig. 4. Mean reflux duration (min/h). Differentiation of
        the reflux of the awake phase into fasting reflux
        and prandial together with postprandial reflux
        (expressed as percentage).

Conclusions:

1. Healthy subjects and patients with slight respectively
severe stages of reflux disease show significant differences of reflux frequency and reflux intensity in 24-hour-
pH-metry.

2. GER in normals occurs at day-time mainly postprandially and in the first half of the night. A slight reflux disease primarily has an increased night-time reflux, whereas in severe reflux disease also a clear shift of day-time reflux in favour of fasting reflux is found.

3. There is a good correlation between functional (manometrical, pH-metrical) and morphological findings in reflux disease.

References:

1. DeMeester, T.R., Johnson, L.F., Joseph, G.J., Toscano, M.S., Hall, A.W., Skinner, D.B. (1976). Patterns of gastroesophageal reflux in health and disease. Ann. Surg., 184, 459.
2. Dent, J., Dodds, W.J., Friedman, R.H., Sekiguchi, T., Hogan, W.J., Arndorfer, R.C., Petrie, D.J.(1980). Mechanism of gastroesophageal reflux in recumbent asymptomatic human subjects. J. clin. Invest., 65, 256.
3. Euler, A.R., Byrne, W.J.(1981). Twenty-four-hour esophageal intraluminal pH-probe testing. A comparative analysis. Gastroenterology, 80, 957
4. Savary, M. Miller, G. (1977). Der Ösophagus - Lehrbuch und endoskopischer Atlas. Gassman: Solothurn.
5. Siewert, J.R., Weiser, H.F., Jennewein, H.M., Waldeck, F. (1974). Clinical and manometric investigations of the lower esophageal sphincter and its reactivity to pentagastrin in patients with hiatus hernia.Digestion,10,287.
6. Siewert, J.R., Blum, A.L., Waldeck, F. (1976). Funktionsstörungen der Speiseröhre. Springer: Berlin - Heidelberg - New York.
7. Stanciu, C., Hoare, R.C., Bennett, J.R. (1977). Correlation between manometric and pH tests for gastro-esophageal reflux. Gut, 18, 536.
8. Wallin, L., Madsen, T. (1979). 12-hour simultaneous registration of acid reflux and peristaltic activity in the esophagus. A study in normal subjects. Scand. J. Gastroent., 14, 561.

9. Weiser, H.F., Pace, F., Lepsien, G., Müller-Lissner, S.A., Blum, A.L., Siewert, J.R. (1982). Gastroösophagealer Reflux - was ist physiologisch? Dtsch. med. Wschr., 107, 366.

10. Weiser, H.F. (1982). Reflux characteristics of healthy volunteers, examined by 24-hour-pH-recording. In: Wienbeck, M. (ed.). Motility of the Digestive Tract. (Raven Press: New York).

11. Weiser, H.F., Hölscher, A.H., Siewert, J.R. (1983). Gastroösophagealer Reflux: Besteht eine Korrelation zwischen Refluxausmaß und Refluxfolgen? Dtsch. med. Wschr., 108, 930 - 935.

Section 2
Gastric Motility
and Emptying

13

Effect of Dopamine or Dopamine Blocker on the Antral Motility in Isolated Perfused Rat Stomach

W. Y. CHEY, S. K. ODAIBO and K. Y. LEE

In isolated perfused rat stomach preparation, effects of dopamine; domperidone, a peripheral dopamine blocker; secretin; and cholecysto-kinin-octapeptide (CCK-OP) on the antral motility were studied. While the stomach was perfused with Krebs-Ringer (K-R) solution at a rate of 1.1 ml/min via celiac artery, motility was recorded through a open tip tube placed in the antrum which was connected to the Statham pressure transducer and Harvard peristaltic pump (0.03 ml/min). Gastric fluid was drained by a tube placed in the proximal duodenum. Peptides or drugs were infused through the celiac artery. Results: 1) Domperidone produced dose-dependent increases (r=0.68) in motility at doses of 0.08, 0.16, 0.32 and 0.64 μg, 2) Dopamine produced dose-dependent de-creases in motility (r=0.76) at dose of 0.13, 0.25 and 0.5 μg which were reversed by domperidone, 0.32 μg, 3) Secretin inhibited the motility in a dose-dependent manner (r=0.49) at doses of 62.5, 125 and 250 pg which were also reversed by domperidone, 0.64 μg, 4) CCK-OP produced inhibition of motility at dose of 40 ng (p<0.025) which was also reversed by domperidone, 0.32 μg. In conclusion, local dopamine receptors in the rat stomach have an inhibitory effect on antral motility, while a peripheral dopamine blocker, domperidone, exerts a gastrotonic effect on spontaneous and inhibited antral motility by either secretin or CCK-OP. Thus, local dopamine receptors in the stomach appear to play a significant role on regulation of antral motility in physiological state.

Effect of Dopamine or Dopamine Blocker on the
Antral Motility in Isolated Perfused Rat Stomach

14

Dual Effect of Substance P on Canine Antral Muscle

E. A. MAYER, S. KHAWAJA, J. ELASHOFF and J. H. WALSH

Substance P (SP) is widely distributed in neuronal structures of the mammalian gut. The peptide is known to have excitatory effects on various gastrointestinal tissues both in vivo and in vitro and this effect appears to be partially mediated by acetylcholine release from the myenteric plexus. In this study we sought (1) to describe the SP effect on the canine antral muscle in vitro and (2) to characterize its mechanism of action. Longitudinal (LAM) and circular (CAM) antral muscle strips from 30 mongrel dogs were studied using conventional organ bath techniques as previously described (Am. J. Physiol., 242: G141, 1982).

RESULTS

In both CAM and LAM, SP increased amplitude (A) and frequency (F) of spontaneously occurring contractions in a dose-dependent fashion with rapid development of tachyphylaxis. Dose-response curves for LAM and CAM were similar with threshold concentrations between 10^{-11}—10^{-10} and concentrations for maximal response around 10^{-6}M. Tetrodotoxin 3×10^{-6} M, atropine 3×10^{-6} M and hexamethonium 10^{-4} M partially inhibited the SP-induced A (but not F) response in LAM. In CAM both A and F response were resistant to tetrodotoxin whereas the calcium channel blocker diltiazem 10^{-5} M partially inhibited the A response. In contrast to previously reported data, somatostatin 14 10^{-6} M showed a small but significant inhibitory effect on

SP-induced A increase in LAM which was abolished by preincubation
with atropine.

CONCLUSION

These data suggest that the SP effect on frequency of spontaneously
occurring phasic contractions in LAM and CAM, as well as on frequency in LAM are myogenic, whereas the effect on amplitude in LAM
is partially mediated through release of Ach from pre-and-post-
ganglionic sites.   The cholinergic component is inhibited by high
concentrations of somatostatin.   The SP-induced amplitude response
in CAM, but not the frequency response is dependent on extracellular
calcium.   These findings of direct stimulation of CAM and additional
indirect cholinergic stimulation of LAM are similar to previously
reported effects of gastrin and bombesin on canine antral muscle and
may represent a general mechanism of action of various neuropeptides.

15

Regulation of Gastric Antral Slow Wave Frequency by Prostaglandins

K. M. SANDERS, A. J. BAUER and N. G. PUBLICOVER

INTRODUCTION

Metabolism of arachidonate results in the production of several prostaglandins (PGs) by gastric muscles (1-6). The physiological role of PGs in regulating electrical and mechanical behavior is not fully understood. In antral circular muscle, PGs decrease the force of contractions by decreasing maximum depolarization of the slow wave (7). Preliminary observations have suggested that endogenous PGs also regulate slow wave frequency (7). Experiments were conducted to examine the regulatory role of PGs in canine antral muscles. Data relating the motility effects of PGs to a case of human gastric psuedo-obstruction is included.

METHODS

Stomachs were removed from anesthetized dogs. A patch of antral muscle was dissected from the mucosa. Strips (2 x 8 mm) were cut parallel to the circular layer, and prepared as described previously (8). The strips were pinned to the floor of a recording chamber and perfused with Krebs solution (8). One end of the muscle strip was attached to a force transducer to record contractions of the circular muscle. The other end of the strip was secured to facilitate intracellular recordings. The muscles were spontaneously electrically and mechanically active. The muscles were stretched to optimal lengths.

Cells were impaled with microelectrodes having impedances of 20-40 M ohms. Membrane potential was measured and recorded by standard techniques (8). Contractile activity was amplified by a bridge circuit amplifier and recorded along with the electrical signals. In experiments where muscle strips were stimulated electrically, a partitioned chamber similar to that described by Abe and Tomita (9) was used. Drug solutions were prepared as described before (8).

77

RESULTS

Effects of Indomethacin (INDO) on Electrical and Mechanical Activities

Muscles of 5 dogs were studied to determine the effects of INDO on the amplitude and frequency of contractions. The muscles were equilibrated in Krebs solution and contractile activity was recorded. Then the muscles were treated with INDO, 10^{-5} M for 1 hour. During this time the frequency of contractions decreased by an average of 43 ± 9 % (Mean $\pm$ S.E.) and the amplitude of contractions increased 376 ± 58%. Data from a typical experiment are shown in Figure 1.

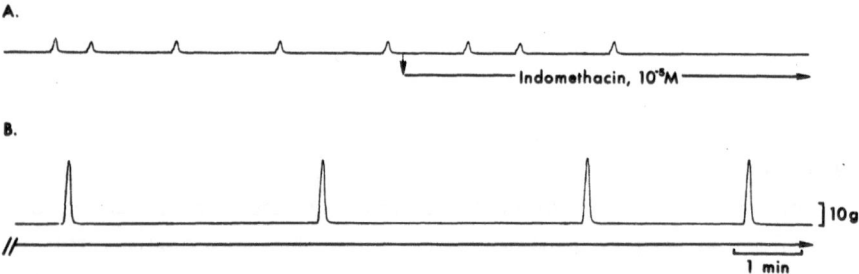

FIGURE 1   Effects of INDO on frequency and amplitude of contractions.

FIGURE 2   Effects of INDO on slow wave parameters. Each panel shows mechanical (upper trace, each panel) and electrical (lower trace, each panel) activities. Panel a shows activity recorded in Krebs solution. Panel b shows activity recorded from the same cell after 50 min of INDO, 10^{-5} M.

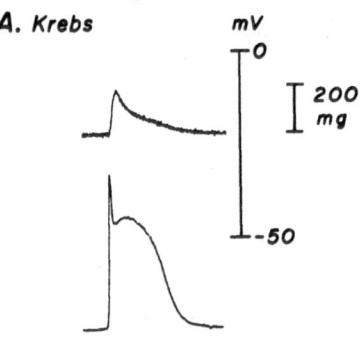

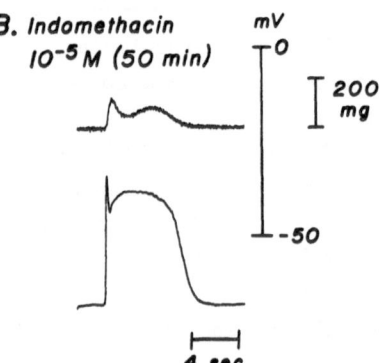

Intracellular recordings were made from muscles of 6 dogs to determine the effects of INDO on electrical activity. In these experiments, cells were impaled and after approximately 30 minutes of stable electrical activity, the muscles were treated with INDO, 10^{-5} M. There was no immediate effect, but after 40 minutes of INDO treatment several changes were noted: The membrane potentials depolarized from an average of 71 ± 1 mV to 68 ± 0.9 mV ($p < 0.05$); the duration of the plateau potential lengthened from an average of 5.4 ± 0.4 sec to 6.6 ± 0.3 sec ($p < 0.05$); and the maximum depolarizaton during the plateau phase of the slow wave increased from an average of 30 ± 0.2 mV to 34 ± 0.2 mV ($p < 0.005$). Figure 2 shows typical changes in the resting membrane potential and slow wave caused by INDO.

Effects of Exogenous PGE$_2$ on Contractile and Electrical Activities

Data above suggest that the dominant PG in antral circular muscle must: i) decrease slow waves and contractions; ii) increase slow wave frequency. PGE$_2$ is a potent inhibitory PG and probably one of the most abundantly produced PGs in antral circular muscles (6). Therefore, muscles were treated with exogenous PGE$_2$ to determine if this PG could reverse the effects of INDO.

In 6 muscles PGE$_2$, 10^{-8} M, reduced the plateau potential by an average of 3.9 ± 0.4 mV and shortened the duration by and average of 1 ± 0.2 sec. Associated with these changes was a 58% reduction in the

A.KRB

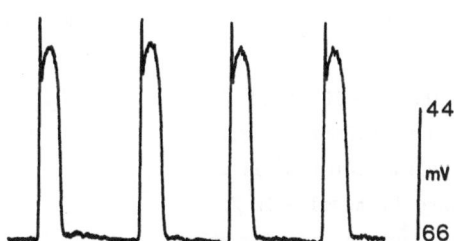

44

mV

66

FIGURE 3   Slow waves before (A) and in the presence (B) of PGE$_2$, 10^{-6} M.   PGE$_2$ increased the frequency of slow waves and decreased the amplitudes of the plateau phase of the slow waves.

B.PGE$_2$, 10^{-6}M

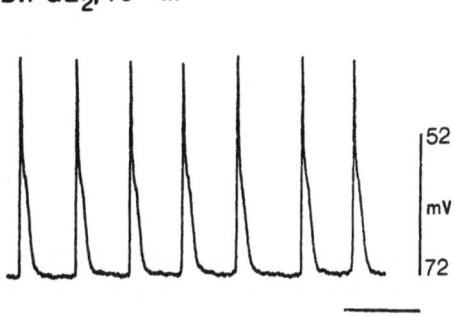

52

mV

72

20 sec

amplitude of the associated contractions. These changes were statistically significant (p < 0.025). The effects of PGE_2 were concentration dependent. At 10^{-6}M, PGE_2 drastically reduced the plateau depolarization and approximately doubled the frequency of slow waves (Figure 3).

Slow wave frequency appears to be determined by an absolute refractory period following each slow wave event. One of the ways in which PGE_2 could enhance slow wave frequency is to decrease this refractory period. To test this hypothesis 6 muscles were studied in the partitioned chamber (9), and slow waves were evoked at maximal frequency. The muscles could be driven at maximum frequencies ranging from 5–6 events/min. In other words, each slow wave was followed by an absolute refractory period of 7–15 sec. Then muscles were exposed to PGE_2, 10^{-6} M for several minutes. When muscles were paced in the presence of PGE_2, they could be driven at approximately twice the control rate (Figure 4). These data suggest that PGE_2 decreases the time required for the excitability mechanism to reset after each slow wave.

A.KRB

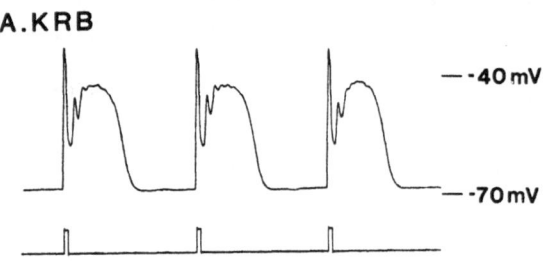

FIGURE 4 Effect of PGE_2 on the maximum frequency of pacing. Slow waves were evoked in muscles in Krebs solution (A) and in the presence of PGE_2, 10^{-6} M (b). PGE_2 increased the maximum rate of pacing.

B.PGE_2, 10^{-6} M

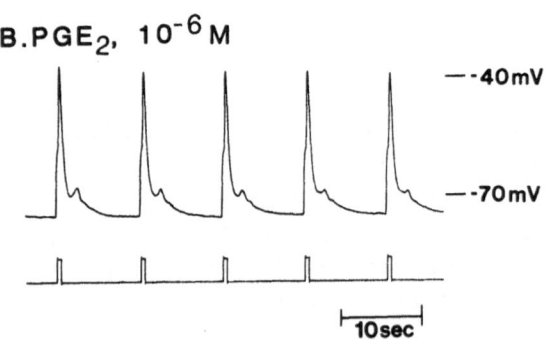

Frequency effects of pentagastrin dependent upon PG synthesis

Others have shown that gastrins increased antral slow wave frequency and the force contractions (10,11). We investigated the possibility that the frequency effect of pentagastrin might be related to the presence of PGs, because drugs which stimulate gastrointestinal muscles can increase PGE_2 synthesis (12,13). In these experiments muscles were first exposed to pentagastrin in Krebs solution and then they were treated with INDO, 10^{-5} M for 1 hr. After INDO, the muscles were re-exposed to pentagastrin. In Krebs solution, pentagastrin increased the frequency of the contractions and the force of the second phase of contraction (panel **a**, Figure 5). INDO increased the force effect of pentagastrin (averaged 750 $\pm$ 175 % in 4 muscles), but the frequency response was significantly decreased (panel **b**, Figure 5). The effects of pentagastrin on the amplitude and duration of slow waves were also enhanced by INDO (panels **c and d**, Figure 5).

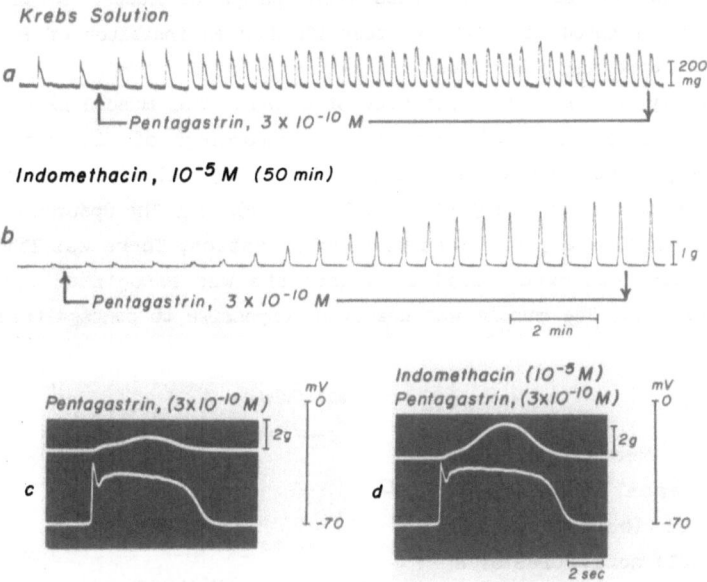

FIGURE 5   Responses to pentagastrin before and after INDO. INDO enhanced the force of contractions in response to pentagastrin, but blocked the frequency effect (panels a and b). INDO enhanced the mechanical (top trace, both panels) and intracellular electrical (bottom trace, both panels) responses to pentagastrin (panels c and d).

Pathological involvement of PGs in gastric motility

Data above demonstrate the involvement of PGs in the regulation of normal gastric muscle. It is possible that over-production of PGs could lead to serious motility disorders, such as gastric psuedo-obstruction. One such case has been studied and the results are summarized below.

A 26-year old, non-diabetic female with a history of gastric retention (14) underwent numerous studies including endoscopy, X-rays and evaluations of

esophageal motility. Impaired gastric emptying was the only abnormality
found. Clinical evaluation revealed that electrical slow wave frequency in
the antrum was abnormally high, 9–12 cycles/min, and antral contractions were
feeble. At the end of the clinical evaluation, a gastrojejunostomy was
performed to relieve her symptoms, and at the time of surgery a small sample
of antral muscle was removed after informed consent had been given.

This muscle was studied with techniques similar to those described above.
The fact that slow wave frequency was abnormally high and contractions were
weak suggested the possibility that antral muscle cells were exposed to an
over-abundance of PGE_2. To test this hypothesis, control mechanical and
electrical activities were recorded from strips of muscle <u>in vitro</u>. Then
muscles were treated with INDO to test whether an inhibitor of PG synthesis
could restore normal activities.

Normally the electrical activity of human antral muscle is very similar
to canine muscle (15). But intracellular recordings of electrical activity
from this patient revealed 4 striking differences: i) The spontaneous slow
wave frequency was between 9–12 (normal = 3/min). ii) The upstoke of the slow
wave was immediately followed by repolarization; There was little or no
plateau phase observed. iii) Each upstroke was associated with a weak
contraction. iv) The muscle was nearly unresponsive to pentagastrin, 10^{-9} M,

FIGURE 6 Mechanical (top
trace, each panel) and
electrical (bottom trace,
each panel) activities of a
muscle from a patient with
gastric psuedo-obstruction.
Panel a shows spontaneous
activity in Krebs solution.
Panel b shows changes that
occured when the muscle was
treated with INDO for 1 hour.
Panel c shows restoration of
abnormal activities when PGE_2
was given after INDO.

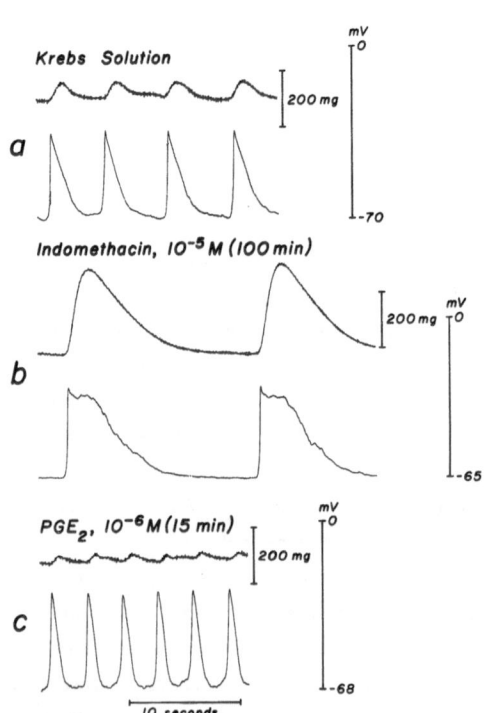

a concentration that causes large electrical and mechanical responses in normal human and canine muscles (10,11,15). These data are shown in panel **a** in Figures 6 and 7.

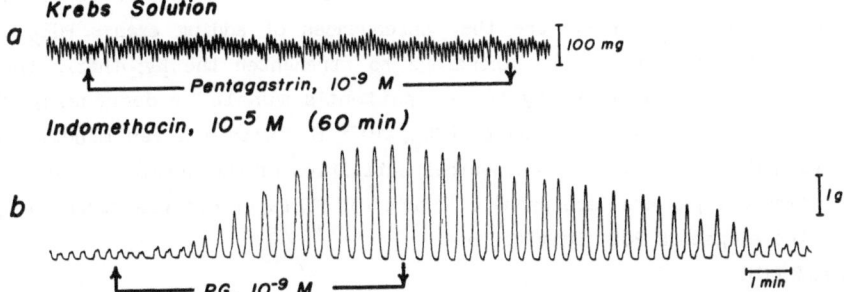

FIGURE 7 Mechanical responses to pentagastrin before (panel a) and after INDO (panel b). INDO enhanced the force response to pentagastrin, but did not restore the frequency response.

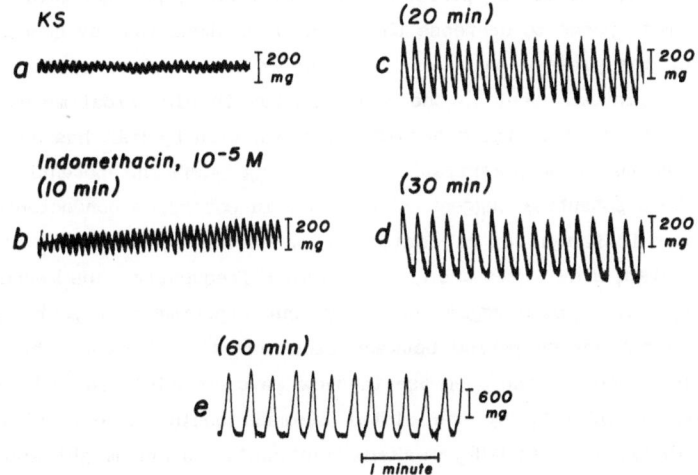

FIGURE 8 Effect of INDO on contractions of a muscle of a psuedo—obstruction patient. See text for details.

After control recordings were made, the muscle was treated with INDO. There was no response immediately, but within 1 hr INDO produced striking changes (Figure 8 and panel b Figure 6). INDO increased the force of contractions by at least 1000% and decreased the frequency to 3–4 cycles/min. INDO also affected the electrical activity; each upstoke was followed by a plateau depolarization. Then the muscles were re-exposed to pentagastrin, 10^{-9} M.

After INDO, pentagastrin increased the force of contractions, but **did not increase the frequency of contractions.** These data are consistent with the hypothesis that the abnormal activity of the antral muscle of this patient was a result of an over-abundance of a PG that inhibited contractile force and stimulated frequency. These are the consequences of adding excess PGE_2 to canine muscles (see Figure 3). Therefore to strenghten the hypothesis that INDO restored normal activity to the patient's muscle by decreasing PG synthesis, the muscle was exposed to PGE_2, 10^{-6} M. Within a few minutes of adding PGE_2 the electrical and mechanical activities of the muscle returned to the pathological pattern (see panel c Figure 6). This effect was reversed by washing the exogenous PGE_2 from the bath.

DISCUSSION

The data presented suggest that endogenous PGs have a 2-fold regulatory role in the gastric antrum: i) they have an inhibitory influence on the strength of contractions; and ii) they have an accelerating influence on the frequency of contractions. These 2 functions are manifest during basal, spontaneous activity, and during periods of stimulation by pentagastrin.

Endogenous PGs appear to decrease the force of contractions by decreasing the amplitude of the plateau phase of the slow wave. Previous studies have reported that the plateau event is the major factor in electrical-mechanical coupling in the antrum (16). The mechanism of inhibition by PGE_2 has not been investigated, but the hyperpolarization of resting membrane potential and decrease in plateau potential suggest an increase in potassium conductance.

The increase in frequency of contractions caused by PGE_2 also has an electrical mechanism; slow waves are generated more frequently. The mechanism of enhanced frequency is also vague currently, but experiments reported here suggest that the refractory period between slow waves is decreased by PGE_2. This might simply be due to the decrease in slow wave duration caused by PGE_2.

Over-production of PGE_2 by the distal stomach could cause significant motility disorders, because PGE_2 weakens contractions and might enhance frequency slow waves enough to drive the rest of the stomach from the antrum. Arrhythmias of this type have been reported in mammalian stomachs (17). In the antral arrhythmia reported here, the evidence supports the involvement of PGE_2. If other types of psuedo-obstruction are also associated with PG over-production, perhaps specific PG synthesis blockers will provide effective therapies for these syndromes.

ACKNOWLEDGEMENTS This study was supported by NIH grants AM 32176 and AA 05883. Dr. Sanders was supported by an NIH Research Career Development Award, AM01209. The clinical material was studied while Dr. Sanders was a post-doctoral fellow at the Mayo Medical School.

REFERENCES

1. Pace-Asciak, C.R. and Rangaraj, G. (1977). Distribution of prostaglandin biosynthetic pathways in several rat tissues. Formation of 6-keto-PGF$_{1a}$. Biochim. Biophys. Acta., 486, 579-582.

2. Bennett, A., Stamford, I.F. and Stockley, H.L. (1977). Estimation and characterization of prostaglandins in the human gastrointestinal tract. Br. J. Pharmacol., 61, 579-586.

3. Ali, M. and McDonald, J.W.D. (1980). Synthesis of thromboane B$_2$ and 6-keto-prostaglandin F$_{1a}$ by bovine gastric mucosal and muscle microsomes. Prostaglandins, 20, 245-254.

4. LeDuc, L.E. and Needleman, P. (1979). Regional localization of prostacyclin and thromboxane synthesis in dog stomach and intestinal tract. J. Pharmacol. Exp. Ther., 211, 181-188.

5. Bennett, A., Hensby, C.N., Sanger, G.J. and Stamford, I.F. (1981). Metabolites of arachidonic acid formed by human gastrointestinal tissues and their actions on the muscle layers. Br. J. Pharmacol., 74, 435-444.

6. Sanders, K.M. and Northrup, T.E. (1983). Prostaglandin synthesis by microsomes of circular and longitudinal gastrointestinal muscles. Am. J. Physiol., 244, G442-G448.

7. Sanders, K.M. and Szurszewski, J.H. (1981). Does endogenous prostaglandin affect gastric antral motility? Am. J. Physiol., 241, G191-G195.

8. Sanders, K.M. and Bauer, A.J. (1982). Ethyl alcohol interferes with excitation-contraction mechanisms of canine antral muscle. Am. J. Physiol., 242, G222-G230.

9. Abe, Y. and Tomita, T. (1968). Cable properties of smooth muscle. J. Physiol., 196, 87-100.

10. Szurszewski, J.H. (1975). Mechanism of action of pentagastrin and acetylcholine on the longitudinal muscle of the canine antrum. J. Physiol., 252, 335-361.

11. El-Sharkawy, T.Y. and Szurszewski, J.H. (1978). Modulation of canine antral circular smooth muscle by acetylcholine, noradrenaline and pentagastrin. J. Physiol., 279, 309-320.

12. Sanders, K.M. and Ross, G. (1978). Effects of endogenous prostaglandin E on intestinal motility. Am. J. Physiol., 234, 204-208.

13. Sanders, K.M. (1978). Endogenous prostaglandin E and contractile activity of isolated ileal smooth muscle. Am. J. Physiol., 234, E209-E212.

14. Sanders, K.M., Menguy, R., Chey, W., You, C., Lee, K., Morgan, K., Kreulen, D., Schmalz, P., Muir, T. and Szurszewski, J.H. (1979). One explanation for human antral tachygastria. Gastroenterology 76, 1234.

15. El-Sharkawy, T.Y., Morgan, K.G. and Szurszewski, J.H. (1978). Intracellular electrical activity of canine and human gastric smooth muscle. J. Physiol., 279, 291-307.

16. Morgan, K.G. and Szurszewski, J.H. (1979). Mechanisms of phasic and tonic actions of pentagastrin on canine gastric smooth muscle. J. Physiol., 301, 229-242.

17. Gullikson, G.W., Okuda, H., Shimizu, M. and Bass P. (1980). Electrical arrhythmias in gastric antrum of the dog. Am. J. Physiol., 239, G59-G68.

16

Mechanical Activity of Isolated Human Pyloric Muscle, in Comparison with Canine Pylorus

F. E. LÜDTKE, K. GOLENHOFEN and H. D. BECKER

INTRODUCTION

The role of the pylorus in the regulation of gastric emptying is still controversial. Some authors concluded that the pylorus only acts as the terminal part of the antrum (1-4), whereas other authors found evidence for a more specific function of the pylorus (5-10). We have observed in studies with isolated muscle preparations from canine pylorus that particularly the inner layer of the pyloric ring (inner pylorus) exhibits pronounced individual behaviour when compared with preparations from other regions of stomach and duodenum (11). In extension of these experiments we have now studied isolated muscle preparations from human pylorus.

METHODS

A total of 14 human stomachs were investigated. The specimens were removed during operations, predominantly from patients with gastric cancer. A segment extending about 3 cm above and below the pyloric ring was excised, opened along the lesser curvature, pinned to a dissection chamber, and the mucosa was removed. The thickened muscular ring, often referred to as "pyloric ring", or "pyloric sphincter", or "distal pyloric sphincter" (10) in the literature, is called the "pylorus" in this paper. Six circular strips were usually dissected from the "pyloric region": two from the inner layer of the pylorus (proximal and distal inner pylorus), two from the outer layer (proximal and distal outer pylorus), and two strips a few mm proximal and distal to the pylorus, respectively (prepyloric and postpyloric strip). In addition circular preparations from antrum (middle) and duodenum (3-4 cm distal to the pylorus), and sometimes a longitudinal strip from the fundus were excised (in situ length 20-25 mm, cross sectional area 1-2 mm^2). The strips were transferred to a conventional thermostatically controlled organ bath at $37^{\circ}C$. The standard saline solution contained: Na^+ 137, K^+ 5.5, Ca^{2+} 2.5, Mg^{2+} 1.2, Cl^- 124, HCO_3^- 25, $H_2PO_4^-$ 1.2, glucose 11.5 mmol/l; equilibrated with 95% O_2 and 5% CO_2, pH 7.4. The mechanical activity was in most cases recorded under auxotonic (near isotonic) conditions, with a preload of about 2 mN/mm^2. The changes were calculated as percentage of the resting length (% Δ l).The resting length was determined by complete suppression of the contractile processes (calcium removal or application of papaverine 10^{-3} mol/l). Isometric mechanical activity was calibrated in mN/mm^2. The following substances were used: acetylcholine (Lematte & Boinot), histamine (Merck), indomethacin (Sharp & Dohme), substance P (Beckmann), bombesin (Chemical Company, St. Louis), secretin (GIH Research Unit, Karolinska Institute, Stockholm), motilin and gastrointestinal inhibitory polypeptide (GIP) (Prof. John Brown, Vancouver), adrenaline and noradrenaline (Hoechst), bradykinin (Serva), prostaglandins E_1 and E_2 (Upjohn Comp.), vasoactive intestinal polypeptide (VIP) and cholecystokinin 33 (Prof. Mutt, Karolinska Institute, Stockholm).

RESULTS

Spontaneous activity

Fundus strips produced tonic, antrum and duodenum strips phasic activity. The phasic activity of human antrum strips was 3/min or slower, depending on their localisation. The maximum frequency of 3/min corresponds to the normal in situ-frequency of gastric peristalsis. The human duodenum strips showed phasic activity with a frequency around 12/min, corresponding to the segmentation rhythm in situ. In dogs, the maximum frequencies were higher, corresponding to the faster gastric peristalsis (4-5/min) and duodenal segmentation rhythm (18-20/min).

In pyloric preparations, the situation is quite complex. In canine inner pylorus strong phasic activity of minute-rhythm type was present in most cases, usually superimposed by a fast rhythm of duodenal type. The outer pyloric strips were not uniform. The proximal preparations were often antrum-like, the distal preparations often duodenum-like, and minute-rhythmical fluctuations as in the inner pylorus were sometimes also observed.

In man, most of the 37 inner pyloric strips exhibited spontaneous activity (80%). In 50% of all preparations, minute-rhythmical fluctuations were observed, as in the examples A, B, C and F of Fig. 1. In general, however, this

minute-rhythm was weaker than in canine pylorus. Some inner pyloric preparations showed regular phasic activity with a frequency of 3/min which is typical
for the gastric peristaltic pacemaker (E in Fig. 1). Other preparations showed
fast duodenum-like rhythmic activity as superimposed on the minute-rhythm in
F of Fig. 1. Even faster rhythms of around 20/min were also observed (B and C
in Fig. 1). Tonic elevations of the baseline were also abserved in some
preparations, usually superimposed by phasic fluctuations.

Indomethacin increased strongly the spontaneous activity in canine inner
pylorus but had no effect on human pyloric strips. This indicates that the
endogenous synthesis of an inhibitory prostaglandin is much weaker (probably
negligible) in human than in canine pyloric muscle.

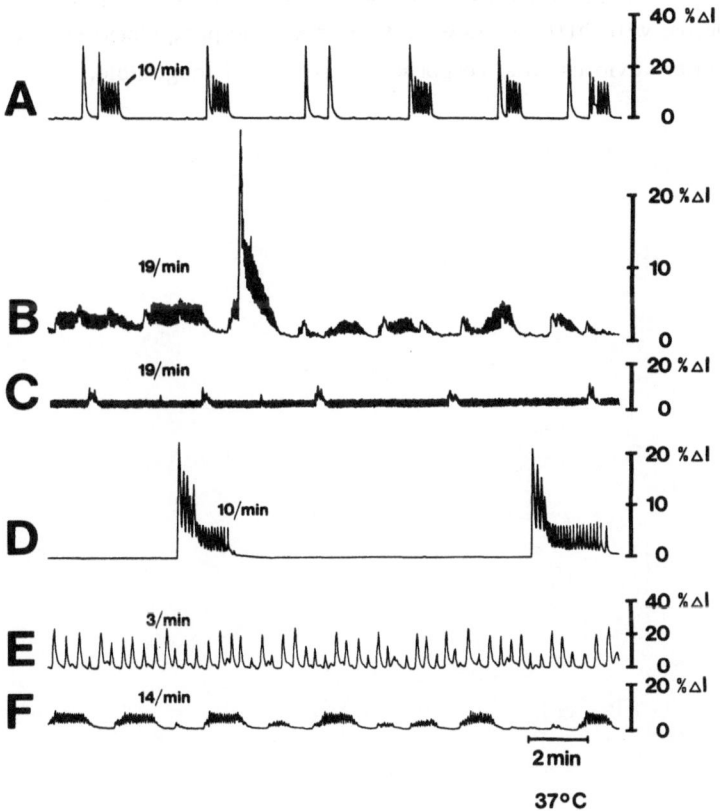

FIG. 1. Spontaneous mechanical activity of human inner pylorus. Examples from
six different human specimens. E and F from the same stomach, E
proximal, F distal inner pylorus.

Altogether, the spontaneous activity of human inner pylorus was much more variable than in canine pylorus. The spontaneous activity of the outer pyloric strips was qualitatively similar to that of the inner pylorus. The differentiation between inner and outer pylorus was in man not so marked as in dog.

Responses of pyloric muscle

Acetylcholine. Acetylcholine produced powerful activations in preparations of fundus, antrum, and duodenum, and often also in the outer pylorus. The excitatory responses of the inner pylorus to acetylcholine, however, were very weak or nearly absent (Fig. 2). These results with acetylcholine were similar in canine and human preparations.

Histamine. Histamine produced in canine preparations strong activation of the fundus. In the pyloric region, it stimulated selectively or preferentially the inner pylorus, with little or no effects on pre- and postpyloric strips, and even in the outer pylorus the responses were often negligible. The histamine

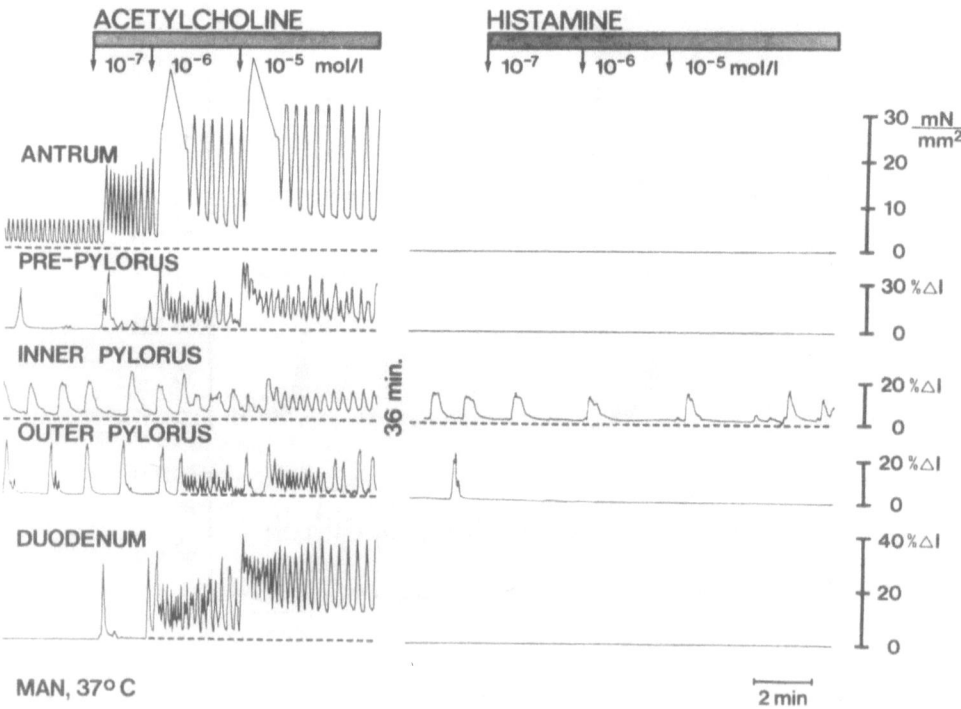

FIG. 2. Mechanical activity of 5 circular muscle strips from different regions of one and the same human stomach. Comparison of acetylcholine and histamine responses of the same strips. Isometric recording in the antrum, near-isotonic recording in the other strips.

responses of canine inner pylorus were often tonic in character, and the contractions reached near maximum values. Only few other substances are able to induce such strong contractions in the canine inner pylorus, e.g. substance P. In marked contrast to canine pylorus, however, no or only negligible excitatory effects of histamine could be observed in human pylorus (Fig. 2), independent of the degree of spontaneous activity.

Substance P. Marked excitatory responses to substance P were observed in all types of human preparations (Fig. 3). In antrum and pyloric preparations substance P increased the amplitude of the phasic contractions, without an increase of the baseline. In the pyloric strips, however, an increase of the baseline occurred in addition to the increase of amplitude. This tonic component of the substance P response was, however, in human pylorus less pronounced than in canine pylorus (12).

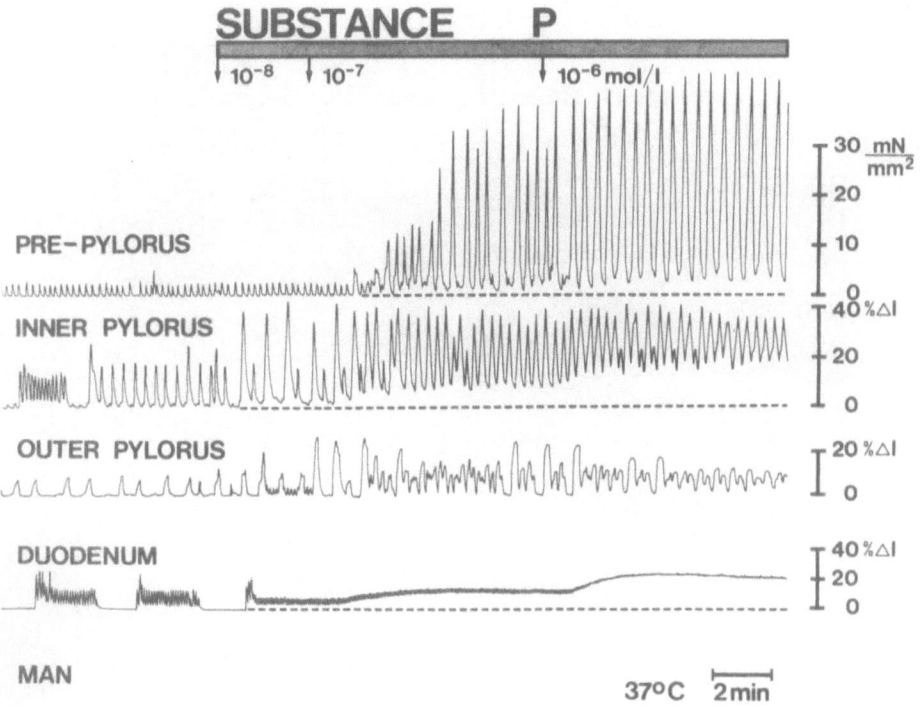

FIG. 3. Mechanical activity of four muscle strips from human pyloric region. All preparations from the same stomach. Spontaneous activity and substance P responses. Recording as in Fig. 2.

Bombesin. The most effective excitatory agent on human pylorus was bombesin. In antrum it increased the amplitude of the phasic contractions, and reduced its frequency at high concentrations (Fig. 4). In the human pylorus bombesin induced strong fluctuations of the minute-rhythm type on which faster contractions remained superimposed. A permanent elevation of the baseline was also often observed (not pronounced in the example of Fig. 4). The induction of minute-rhythm by bombesin is particularly clear in the duodenum of Fig. 4, where the spontaneous activity was near zero.

Other substances. Cholecystokinin, secretin, motilin and gastric inhibitory polypeptide (GIP) had no significant effects on human gastric muscle.

Inhibitory effects. Strong inhibitory responses were observed to application of adrenaline, noradrenaline, bradykinin, prostaglandins E_1 and E_2 and vasoactive intestinal polypeptide (VIP).

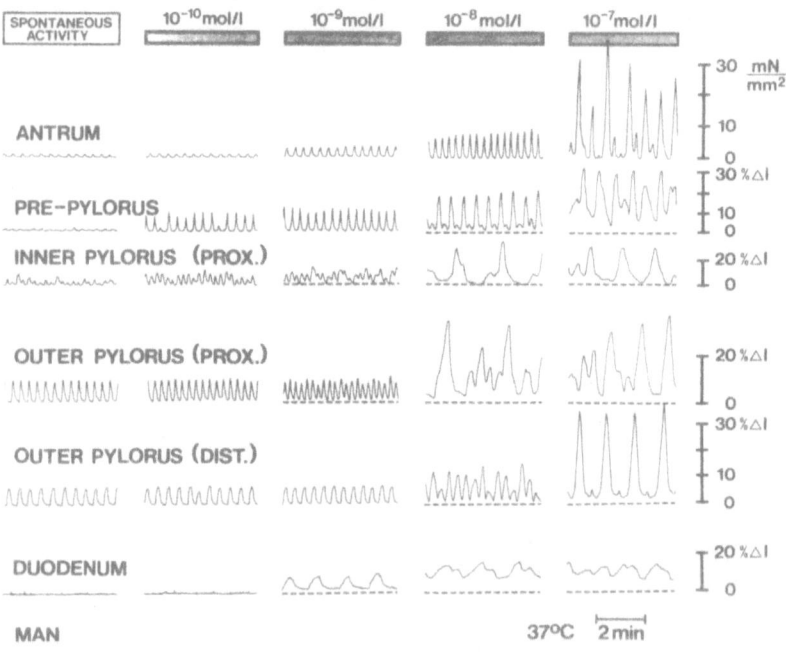

FIG. 4. Mechanical activity of six circular muscle strips from human pyloric region. All preparations from the same stomach. Spontaneous activity and bombesin responses. Recording as in Fig. 2.

DISCUSSION AND CONCLUSIONS

The present studies have demonstrated that marked differences exist in the basic properties of smooth muscle within the pyloric region, and in addition, species differences between man and dog were found. The most pronounced individual characteristics were observed in the inner pylorus. The spontaneous activity of the inner pylorus was qualitatively different from that of the neighbouring preparations: Strong phasic activity of the minute-rhythm type was present in most cases. In general, however, the minute-rhythm of human inner pylorus was much weaker than in canine pylorus. Compared with canine pylorus the spontaneous activity of human inner pylorus was more variable. The differentiation between inner and outer pylorus was in man not so marked as in dog.

Marked differences also exist in the responses of the inner pylorus, in comparison with preparations from antrum and duodenum. Acetylcholine as the classical excitatory agent for gastrointestinal muscle is in most cases nearly ineffective on inner pylorus, and only few other substances are able to induce strong contractions of the inner pylorus. On the other hand, many substances are very effective inhibitors of the inner pylorus.

Schulze-Delrieu and Shirazi (10) studied isolated preparations from human pylorus and concluded that "muscle from the human pylorus differs from muscle of the antrum and the duodenum by its high baseline tension, its prominent neurogenic relaxation response, and its poor spontaneous contractile activity." The latter statement about spontaneous activity is not in agreement with our observations, which seems to be partly due to differences in terminology. The "high baseline tension" is, in our opinion, an expression of tonic spontaneous contractile activity. The reason why the spontaneous activity was predominantly phasic in our studies and predominantly tonic in the observations of Schulze-Delrieu and Shirazi is not clear.

All these results indicate that the pylorus, particularly the inner layer of the pyloric ring (inner pylorus) may operate also in situ as a distinct organ, with specific control mechanisms.

REFERENCES

1. Thomas, J. E. (1957). Mechanics and regulation of gastric emptying. Physiol. Rev., 37, 453-474

2. Kelly, K. A. (1981). Motility of the stomach and gastroduodenal junction. In: Johnson, L. R. (ed). Physiology of the Gastrointestinal Tract. Vol. 1, pp. 393-410. (New York: Raven Press)

3. Pröve, J., and Ehrlein, H.-J. (1978). Studies on the mechanism of gastric emptying in dogs. Pflügers Arch., 377, Suppl., R27

4. Pröve, J., and Ehrlein, H.-J. (1982). Motor function of gastric antrum and pylorus for evacuation of low and high viscosity meals in dogs. Gut, 23, 150-156

5. Anuras, S., Cooke, A. R., and Christensen, J. (1974). An inhibitory innervation at the gastroduodenal junction. J.Clin.Invest., 54, 529-534

6. Fisher, R. S., Lipshutz, W., and Cohen, S. (1973). The hormonal regulation of pyloric sphincter function. J.Clin.Invest., 52, 1289-1296

7. Mir, S., Telford, G. L., Mason, G. R., and Ormsbee, H. S. (1979). Noncholinergic nonadrenergic inhibitory innervation of the canine pylorus. Gastroenterology, 76, 1443-1448

8. Munk, J. F., Gannaway, R. M., Hoare, M., and Johnson, A. G. (1978). Direct measurement of pyloric diameter and tone in man and their response to cholecystokinin. In: Duthie, H. L. (ed). Gastrointestinal Motility in Health and Disease. pp. 349-356. (Lancaster: MTP Press)

9. Phaosawasdi, K., and Fisher, R. S. (1982). Hormonal effects on the pylorus. Amer.J.Physiol., 243, G330-G335

10. Schulze-Delrieu, K., and Shirazi, S. S. (1983). Neuromuscular differentiation of the human pylorus. Gastroenterology, 84, 287-292

11. Golenhofen, K., Lüdtke, F. E., Milenov, K., and Siewert, R. (1980). Excitatory and inhibitory effects on canine pyloric musculature. In: Christensen, J. (ed). Gastrointestinal Motility. pp. 203-210. (New York: Raven Press)

12. Milenov, K., and Golenhofen, K. (1983). Differentiated contractile responses of gastric smooth muscle to substance P. Pflügers Arch., 397, 29-34

17

Stimulating Effects of Cisapride on Antroduodenal Motility in the Conscious Dog

J. A. J. SCHUURKES, L. M. A. AKKERMANS and J. M. VAN NUETEN

SUMMARY

The effects of cisapride on gastroduodenal motility and gastric emptying were studied in conscious dogs, implanted with strain gauge force transducers or gastric cannulas. In the digestive state, cisapride (1.25 mg/kg p.o.) doubled contractile amplitude, reduced (20 %) contractile frequencies of antrum and duodenum, and improved antroduodenal coordination (25 → 60 %). The minimal effective dose was 0.31 mg/kg p.o. Cisapride was significantly more effective than metoclopramide on all parameters tested. Isopropamide (0.04 mg/kg i.v.) abolished the motor-stimulating effects of cisapride. Cisapride accelerated the emptying of a liquid (gastric cannula dogs) and semi-solid and solid (Tc-99m tin colloid labelled) test meal. Minimal effective dose was 0.16 mg/kg i.v. In the interdigestive state, cisapride (0.63 mg/kg i.v.) induced contractions on antrum and duodenum as strong as but not similar to phase III contractions. Cisapride appears to be a potent stimulator of digestive and interdigestive gastroduodenal motility. It improves gastric emptying of liquid, semi-solid and solid test meals.

INTRODUCTION

Cisapride has been shown to exert motility stimulating effects on isolated gastrointestinal preparations (1) and to improve antroduodenal coordination in vitro (2) in the guinea pig.

The aim of this study was to quantify the effects of cisapride on antroduodenal motility and gastric emptying in the consciuos dog.

95

METHODS

Five beagle dogs were implanted with strain gauge force transducers
on antrum and duodenum, 4 and 8 cm from the pylorus respectively
(2). Half an hour after an interdigestive complex (IDC) had passed,
the dogs ate a test meal (5 g/kg), containing milk, rice and meat
(2). One hour later, either drug or solvent were administered
orally in 10 ml milk and the effects followed for 3 h. In the
interdigestive state, drugs were tested i.v. 15 minutes after the
end of an IDC. Mean amplitude, mean frequency (mean reciprocal
interval) and antroduodenal coordination ($\equiv$ the relative number of
antral cycles during which the sum of duodenal amplitudes in the
time interval between -1 and 5 seconds from the antral peak was more
than 90 % of the sum in the interval between -1 to 11 seconds) were
calculated. For statistical analysis the Wilcoxon Matched-Pairs
Sign-Ranks Test was used (3).

Gastric emptying of liquids was tested in 7 beagle dogs implanted
with gastric cannulas. After intragastric administration of the
test meal, the gastric volume was repeatedly determined by
drainage. In four beagle dogs gastric emptying of a semi-solid
(porridge) and solid (pancake) test meal labelled with Tc-99m tin
colloid was measured with a γ-camera. The test meals were
energetically equivalent and of similar composition (4, 5). Effects
on emptying were determined as effects on the lag phase (= time
between end of ingestion and first appearance of radioactivity in
the duodenum) and the percentage of the meal emptied in the first
hour after the end of the lag phase. Analysis of variance was used
to test differences in lag phase length; the Student-t-test was used
to test differences in emptying rate ($p < 0.05$). Cisapride was
administered 30 min before the meal.

RESULTS

Digestive motility

Cisapride enhanced digestive antroduodenal motor patterns within a
few minutes after oral administration. Antral frequencies were
easily recognizable in the duodenal signal (Fig. 1). Motor activity
could be abolished by isopropamide. Mean amplitude during the
interdigestive complex (IDC) for both antrum and duodenum was 65 %

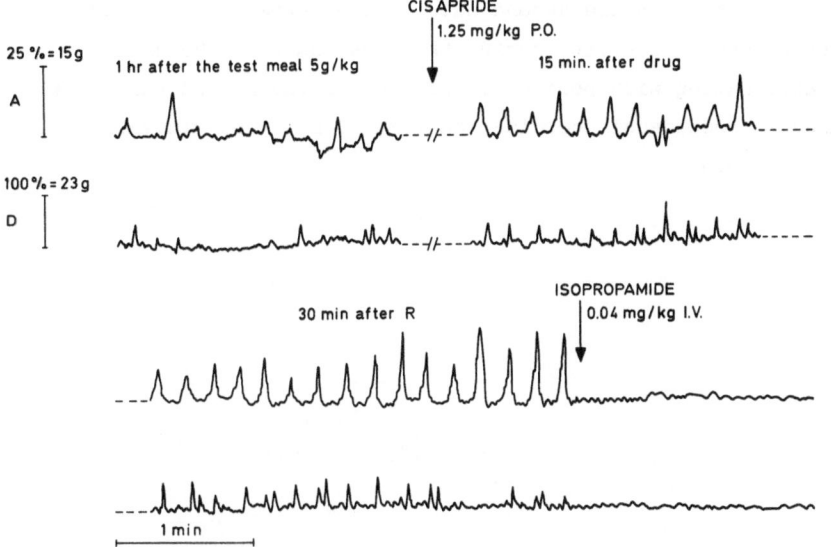

**FIGURE 1   Cisapride stimulates digestive motor patterns of antrum
(A) and duodenum (D) of the conscious dog.**

of the maximal amplitudes that occurred during the IDC.   After the
meal this value was only 23 % for antrum and duodenum.   Cisapride
enhanced the mean amplitude of both antrum and duodenum to
respectively 50 and 42 % of max IDC (Fig. 2 A).   Antral and duodenal
contractile frequencies were reduced by about 20 % (Fig. 2 B).
Antral frequency was reduced by a prolongation of the interval
between individual contractions that were continuously present (Fig.
3 A).   In contrast, duodenal frequency was reduced by disappearence

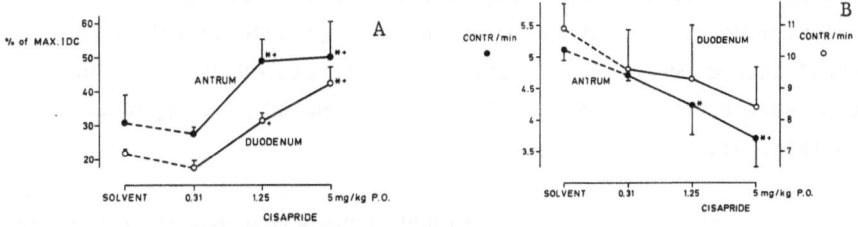

**FIGURE 2   Dose-response relation for cisapride (2 h after oral
administration to conscious dogs) on A. antral and
duodenal contractile amplitude, expressed as % of max
contractile amplitude during the interdigestive complex
and B. antral and duodenal contractile frequency
(reciprocal interval) ($\overline{m} \pm$ SEM, n = 5) different from
* solvent, + metoclopramide, p < 0.05.**

of waves occurring in the second half of the antral cycle, resulting
in short bursts of activity during the first half of the antral
cycle, alternating with periods of silence in the second half, i.e.
increased antroduodenal coordination (Fig. 3 B). The minimal

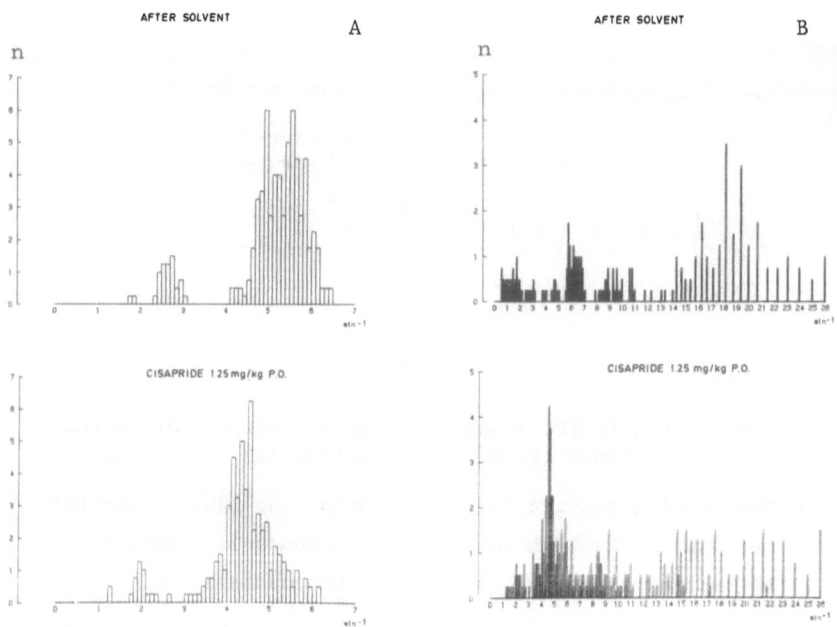

FIGURE 3   Frequency distribution of antral (A) and duodenal (B)
            frequencies (mean reciprocal interval), 120-135 min after
            oral administration of solvent or cisapride (n = 5).

effective dose to increase antroduodenal coordination was 0.31 mg/kg
p.o. (Fig. 4). In the dose range tested (up to 5 mg/kg p.o.)
metoclopramide did not affect contractile amplitude or frequency but
enhanced antroduodenal coordination; the effects of cisapride on
this parameter were significantly more pronounced at comparable
doses (Fig. 4).

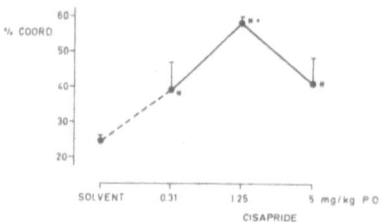

FIGURE 4 Dose-response relation for
         cisapride (2 h afteroral
         administration to
         conscious dogs) on
         antroduodenal coordination
         ($\overline{m} \pm$ SEM, n = 5) different
         from * solvent, +
         metoclopramide,p < 0.05.

Gastric emptying

Cisapride significantly accelerated the emptying of a liquid test
meal (Fig. 5). After 0.31 mg/kg i.v. the total emptying curve for
each of 7 dogs was below the emptying curve after solvent. Minimal
effective dose was 0.16 mg/kg i.v. The lag phase lengths after the
porridge and pancake meals (Fig. 6) were significantly reduced by
cisapride (0.16 mg/kg, i.v.) from 17.1 ± 2.1 to 9.9 ± 0.8 min ($\overline{m} \pm$
SEM) and from 31.9 ± 2.3 to 20.0 ± 1.5 min respectively. Cisapride
also significantly enhanced the emptying rate for both meals:
porridge 54.4 ± 0.2 to 80.0 ± 0.8 %/h, pancake 39.7 ± 0.3 %/h to
43.5 ± 0.4 %/h.

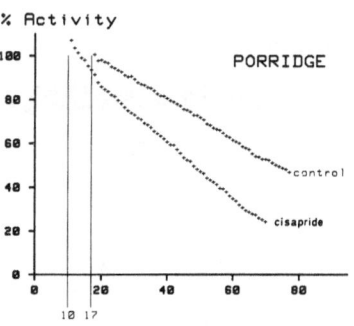

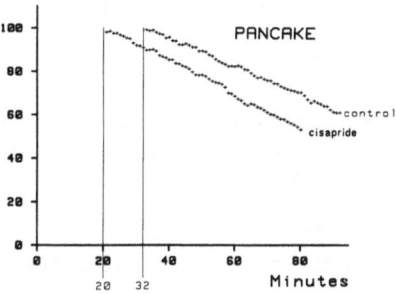

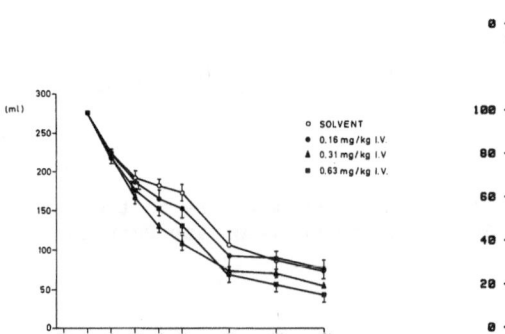

FIGURE 5 Effect of cisapride (R)
on gastric emptying of a
liquid test meal (250 ml
milk, 25 ml oleic acid
and 3 ml PEG 400) in the
conscious dog (gastric
cannula) ($\overline{m} \pm$ SEM, n = 7)

FIGURE 6 Effect of cisapride
(0.16 mg/kg, i.v.,
t –30 min) on gastric
emptying (lag phase
length and emptying
rate) of a semi-solid
(porridge) and solid
(pancake) test meal
(mean curves, 4 dogs,
5 replicas per dog).

Interdigestive motility

Cisapride (0.63 mg/kg i.v., 15 min after the IDC) induced
contractions on antrum and duodenum as strong as, but quite distinct
from phase III activity (Fig. 7). In 3 out of 5 dogs, it induced
coordinated antroduodenal patterns, characteristic for the digestive
state, but only exceptionally observed in phase II of the IDC. The
minimal effective dose for this effect was 0.16 mg/kg i.v.

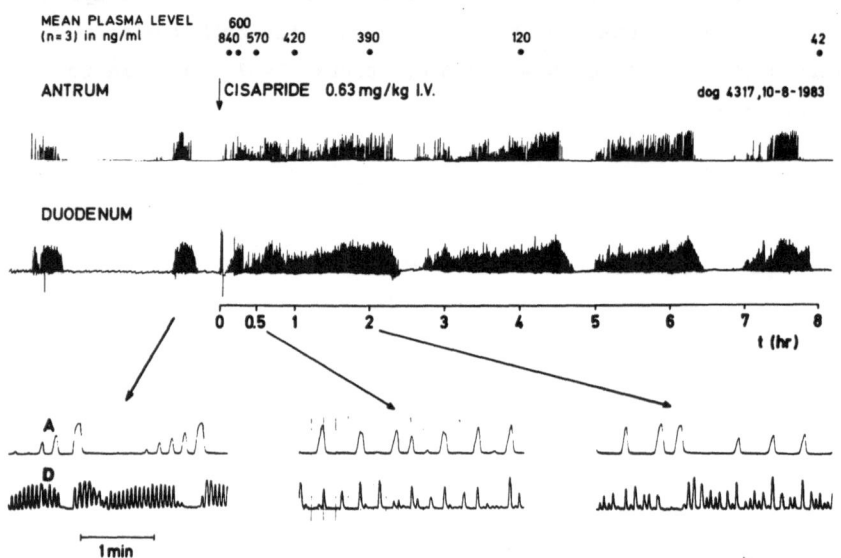

FIGURE 7   Effect of cisapride on interdigestive motility in the
           concious dog. Plasma levels by courtesy of Van Peer et
           al., 1982.

DISCUSSION

Oral administration of cisapride effectively enhances antral and
duodenal amplitude. On the antrum it reduces the frequency of
contractions by lengthening the time lag between pacesetter
potentials (unpublished), whereas the occurrence of duodenal
contractions becomes related to the antral waves, i.e. increased
antroduodenal coordination. Our in vivo results confirm recent in
vitro results with cisapride on antroduodenal coordination in the
guinea pig (2). In both studies cisapride appeared more potent than
metoclopramide, a difference also observed on other in vitro
preparations (1). The blockade of the effects of cisapride by the

anticholinergic isopropamide shows the cholinergic nature of upper gastrointestinal contractions and is in agreement with the hypothesis of facilitation of the release of acetylcholine as the mechanism of action of cisapride (1).

Possibly as a consequence of its motor stimulating properties, cisapride accelerates the emptying of liquid and solid test meals. Our study does not allow a conclusion whether the increased antral amplitude, the decreased frequency or the increased antroduodenal coordination, with stronger duodenal contractions associated with the antral waves, or yet another mechanism is responsible for the acceleration of gastric emptying. This effect on emptying was even seen after administration of a liquid test meal containing 25 ml oleic acid, known to inhibit gastric emptying, most likely via a maximal release of neurotensin (Rosell, personal communication).

In the interdigestive state, cisapride was able to induce a coordinated motor pattern with contractions similar in strength to phase III contractions. This coordinated pattern is dissimilar from phase III in its temporal distribution, and rarely observed during phase II of the interdigestive complex. Preliminary determinations on plasma levels of motilin, gastrin, cholecystokinin and pancreatic polypeptide in dogs and pigs do not implicate any of these gastrointestinal hormones in the action of cisapride (Itoh; Rose, personal communications).

In our study no side-effects were observed after oral administration of cisapride in doses up to 5 mg/kg. In one dog, i.v. injection of 0.63 mg/kg induced a short-lived salivation. Extensive tests on basal and submaximally stimulated (insulin and pentagastrin) gastric secretion revealed the absence of any secretory stimulant effects of cisapride (unpublished).

The pronounced stimulating properties of cisapride on antroduodenal motility as observed in this study in the conscious dog, together with its effects on lower oesophageal sphincter pressure (6) and colonic motility (1, 6), support its use as a gastrokinetic in motor dysfunctions [e.g. gastroesophageal reflux, gastroparesis and colonic atony (6)] of the gastrointestinal tract.

ACKNOWLEDGEMENT

The authors are indebted to Messrs. F. Mast, J.G.M.G. Eelen and E.C. Cruysberghs for skilfull technical assistance; to Mr. H. Vanhove for linguistic corrections and to Mrs. L. Geentjens for preparing the manuscript.

REFERENCES

1. Van Nueten, J.M., Van Daele, P.G.H., Reyntjens, A.J., Janssen, P.A.J. and Schuurkes, J.A.J. (1983). Gastrointestinal motility stimulating properties of cisapride, a non-antidopaminergic, non-cholinergic compound. This book, chapter   , pp.

2. Schuurkes, J.A.J. and Van Nueten, J.M. (1983). Control of gastroduodenal coordination: dopaminergic and cholinergic pathways. Scand. J. Gastroenterol. (Suppl. 2nd Int. Symp. Duodenogastric Reflux, Brunnen, June 1983), in press

3. Siegel, S. (1956). Nonparametric Statistics, pp. 75-83 (McGraw Hill, New York)

4. Jacobs, F., Akkermans, L.M.A., Hong Yoe, O. and Wittebol, P. (1981). Effects of domperidone on gastric emptying of semi-solid and solid food. In: Towse, G. (ed). Progress with Domperidone, a Gastrokinetic and Anti-Emetic Agent. pp. 11-20. (The Royal Society of Medicine, ICSS No. 36)

5. Jacobs, F., Akkermans, L.M.A., Hong You, O., Hoekstra, A. and Wittebol, P. (1982). A radioisotope method to quantify the function of fundus, antrum, and their contractile activity in gastric emptying of a semi-solid and solid meal. In: Wienbeck, M. (ed). Motility of the Digestive Tract. pp. 233-240. (Raven Press, N.Y.)

6. Reyntjens, A.J., Verlinden, M.H.J.J., Schuurkes, J.A.J., Van Nueten, J.M. and Janssen, P.A.J. (1983). New approach to gastro-intestinal motor dysfunction: non-antidopaminergic, non-cholinergic selective stimulation with cisapride. Submitted for publication.

18

Changes in the Innervation of the Fundus after Subtotal Gastrectomy

E. ATANASSOVA, O. BAYGUINOV and I. LOLOVA

INTRODUCTION

Our earlier studies show the changes of the nervous transmission from mainly inhibitory of the fundic smooth muscle cells to mainly excitatory of the gastric remnant after subtotal gastrectomy (Bayguinov, Atanassova 1981). It is of interest to know the dynamics of these changes and of the morphological changes in the intrinsic nervous system after surgery.

METHODS

Microelectrode studies were carried out on strips, 8 x 2 mm, from the smooth muscle wall of the dog fundus and gastric remnant in the course of 15 days, 1, 2, 5 and 7 months after subtotal gastrectomy. The electrical activi ty of single smooth muscle cells was led off by glass microelectrodes with a resistance of 20 to 50 Mohms, filled with 2,5 M KCL. The postsynaptic responses of the smooth muscle cells to transmural electrical stimulation were investigated. Single or rhythmic stimulation (2, 5, 8, 10 and 15 imp/s) of 0.2-0.5-1ms duration was applied. The excitatory and inhibitory responses were expressed as percentage of the total number of smooth muscle cells investigated from 3 dogs for each term.

For the morphological studies were tasted 6 experimental

and 6 control dogs. Tissue blocks of the whole thickness
of the gastric muscle coat of the proximal, middle and
distal part of the gastric remnant have been taken along
the great and small curvature. To demonstrate the acetyl-
cholineserase (AChE) was used the Baker's fixative. AChE
was examined by the Karnovsky-ROOts method and a selective
inhibitor of the nonspecific cholinesterase was iso-OMPA.

RESULTS

In response to transmural stimulation the fundic smooth
muscle cells of an intact stomach respond mainly with
hyperpolarization and relaxation of the strip – 40% and
only in 23% the response was excitatory (Bayguinov,
Atanassova 1981)

This character of the postsynaptic potentials changed
in the different periods after subtotal gastrectomy. As
early as the 15th day after surgery there was an increase
of the biphasic responses (depolarization, followed by
hyperpolarization and vice versa): 7.1% compared with 3.3%
under normal conditions (Fig. 1). The inhibitory responses

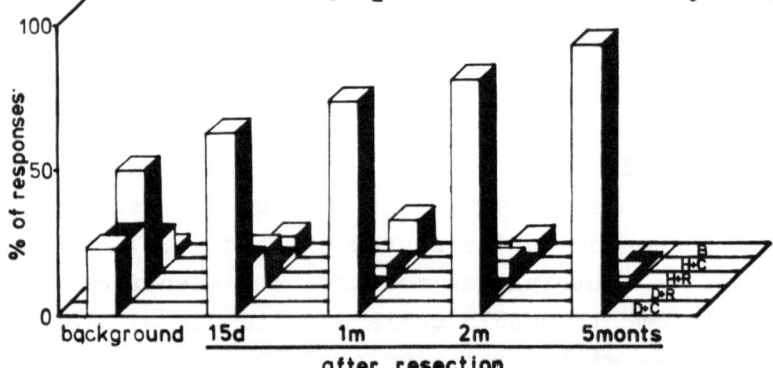

Fig. 1. Dynamics of the changes in the nerve transmission
in the gastric remnant after subtotal gastrectomy
D+C – depolarization and contraction of the smooth
muscle strip; D+R – depolarization and relaxation; H+R –
hyperpolarization and relaxation; H+C– hyperpolarization
and contraction; B – biphasic responses

were reduced almost by half (hyperpolarization and relaxation 13.1%). The percentage of the smooth muscle cells
which responded with depolarization and contraction

increased to 62%. Considerable increase of the excitatory
responses was observed at the end of the first month:
74.1%. In this period the biphasic responses still more
increased: 12.9% and the inhibitory responses were much
decreased: 7.5%. At the end of the second month responses
to single stimulation were frequently observed: inhibitory
junction potentials (Fig. 2 a) or depolarization preceding
contraction of the smooth muscle strip (Fig. 2 b). In some

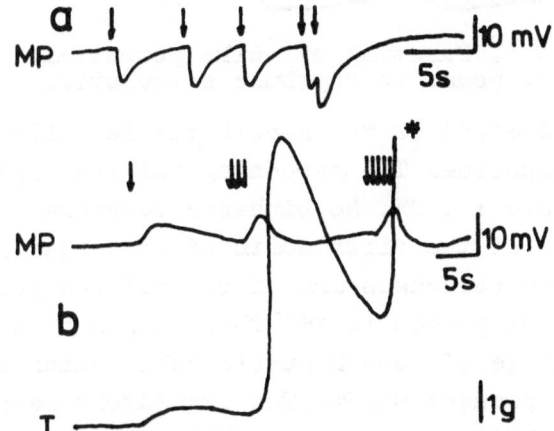

Fig. 2 Inhibitory (a) and excitatory
(b) junction potentials in response to
single transmural stimulations
MP - electrical activity; T - tension;
arrows - single electrical impulses

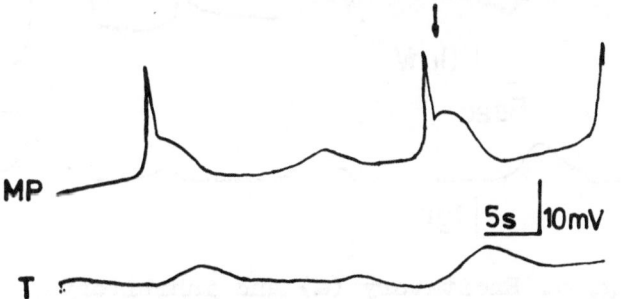

Fig. 3. Increase of the plateau level
in response to single stimulation

cases
single stimulation caused an increase of the plateau level
of the already formed plateau potential(Fig. 3). Rhythmic

stimulation evoked spike potentials on the plateau (Fig. 4)

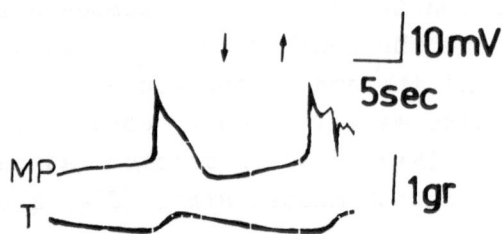

Fig. 4. Bursting of spike potentials
in response to rhythmic stimulation

In this period 81.4% of the smooth muscle cells exhibited
excitatory responses. The percentage of the biphsic responses decreased : 6.2%. No biphasic responses were elicited at the end of the fifth month after surgery. Instead
of the biphasic responses and of the reduced percentage
of inhibitory responses (4.1%) there was a high increase
of the percentage of smooth muscle cells which exhibited
excitatory responses: 93.5%. The excitatory responses to
rhythmic stimulation was occasionally manifested not only

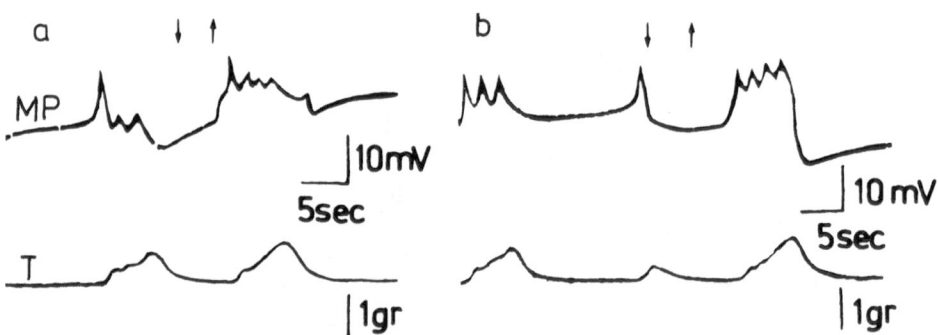

Fig. 5. Excitatory (a) and inhibitory
(b) responses to rhythmic stimulation

by depolarization but also by an increase in the number of
spike potentials on the plateau of the slow potential
(Fig. 5 a). The inhibitory responses was expressed by
abolition of the plateau and leading to a decrease of
the strip contraction (Fig. 5 b). The rebound excitation

was manifested by an increase of the number of spike potentials on the plateau. In some cases the transmural stimulation led to an increase of the of the followed potentials or to a delay of the appearance of the next potential.

Atropin $(10^{-6}M)$ added to the nutrient medium blocked the
larger part of the excitatory responses and led to hyperpolarization and relaxation of the muscle strip to transmural stimulation. Addition of adrenergic antagonists to
the bath suggests the participation of non-adrenergic
inhibitory systems in some of the inhibitory responses.

Comparative studies of the antrum muscle have shown
that 90% of the smooth muscle cells exhibit excitatory
postsynaptic responses as the majority of them are cholinergic (Dobreva, Bayguinov, Atanassova 1982).

The morphologic investigations showed at the first week
following subtotal gastrectomy the myenteric ganglia and
the connecting strands in the experimental dog (Fig. 6 a)
appearing larger in comparison to the control dog(Fig.6 b).
due to the number of glial cells. AChE activity was reduced and the neurons showed prominent chromatolysis. AChE
positive nerve fibers and terminals in the neuropil were
less numerous. At the second week the density of the myenteric ganglia decreased in the experimental dog. AChE
activity was higher in some of the neurons than in the
neurons of the control dog. In the neurons exhibiting axon
reaction the enzyme activity was less decreased than the
first week. The AChE positive nerve fibers and terminals
were scarce in the neuropil and some of them coarser. The
nerve bundles and fibers within the muscle coat were reduced as compared to the control animals. In the first month
the myenteric ganglia had the same density as in the
control dog. The ganglia of the experimental animal were
characterized by their variable size. AChE activity was
much higher in the neurons of the experimental animal
(Fig. 7 a) as compared to the control dog (Fig. 7 b). The
changes in the neuropil persisted as in the earlrer time
intervals though the enzyme activity increased. There was

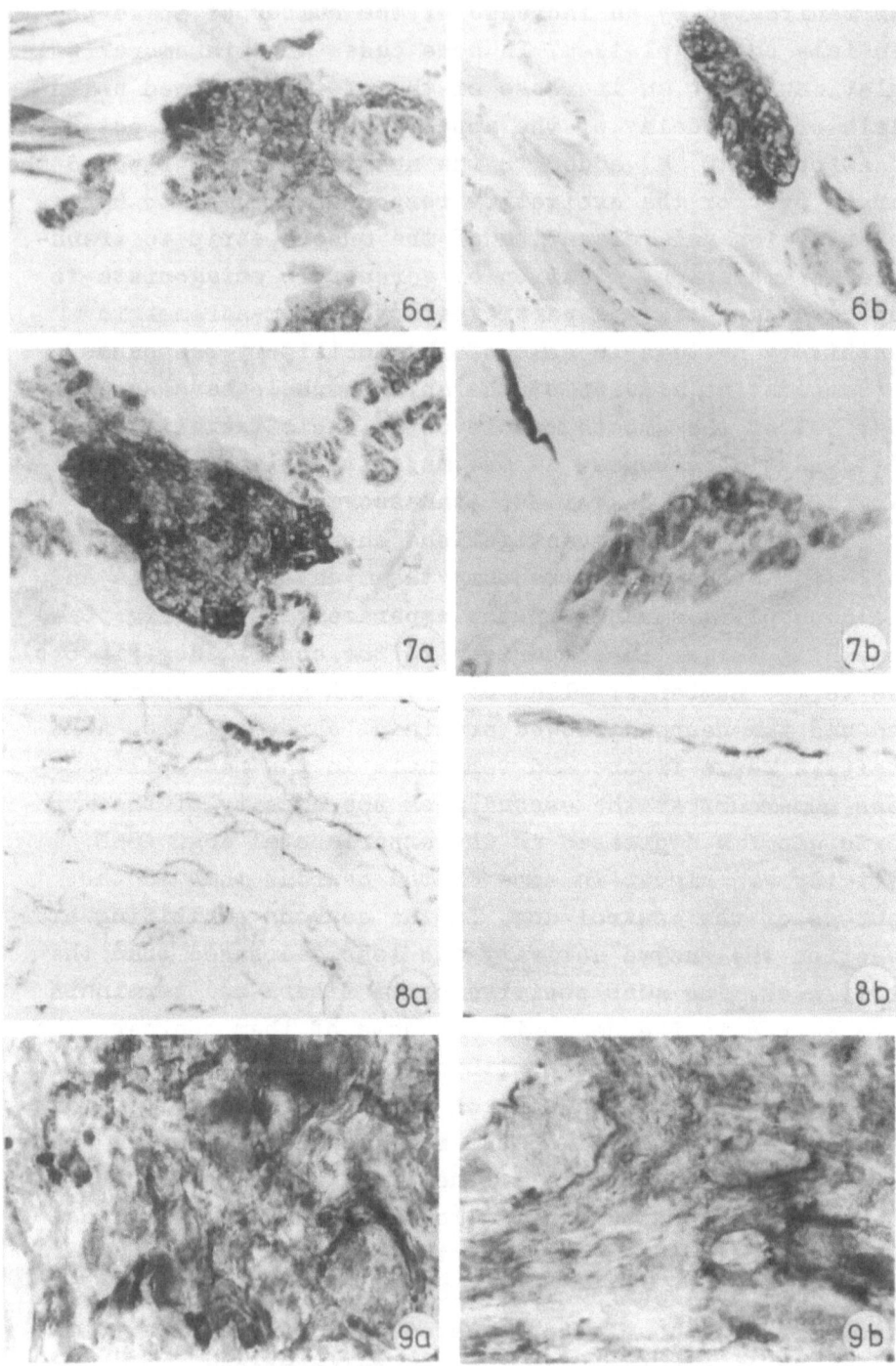

a hyperinnervation of the muscles in the distal regions of
both curvatures. In the second month the myenteric ganglia
were of higher density but of the same size in the distal
regions of the experimental dog as compared to the control
one. In the proximal part of the gastric remnant myenteric
ganglia were larger than those in the control dog though
their density was reduced. This period was characterized
by some rather large neurons exhibiting higher enzyme
activity and projecting large primary processes. The hyperinnervation of the muscles persisted in the distal regions.
The AChE positive fibers branched out forming richer net-
works in the experimental dog (Fig. 8 a) than in the
control one (Fig. 8 b). The proximal part of the gastric
remnant displayed a decreased number of fibers. In the
fifth and seventh month no differences were detected in
the density, size and form of the ganglia. In the fifth
month though there existed no noticeable differences in
AChE activity in the neurons and in the density of ACHE
positive fibers and terminals, some coarser and dark
fibers and large terminals were found in the ganglia of
the experimental dog (Fig. 9 a) as compared to the control
dog (Fig. 9 b). In the seventh month no differences was
noted AChE activity of the neuropil and in the number of
nerve fibers in the muscle coat

 DISCUSSION

   Our results suggest that the changes in the character
of the nerve transmission in the gastric remnant (2) are
realized in short terms after subtotal gastrectomy. The
excitatory responses increase significantly during the
first month after surgery, they still increase during the
second month and from the fifth month the nerve transmission resemble of this in the antrum of the stomach (3).
The increase of the biphasic responses shows the way of
changing the character of the transmission. The functional
changes occured in parallel to structural alterations com-
prizing all components of the myenteric plexus. The great
increase of the neurons and neuropil evidently is together

with the hyperplasia and hypertrophia of the smooth muscle
cells (1). The structural changes of the myenteric plexus,
partly described (5) in a previous paper, were followed in
the different stages after surgery. It is well known that
the AChE reaction is no a specific histochemical method
for localization of cholinergic neurons and fibers (4).
But the AChE reaction is a useful tool for vizualizing the
myenteric plexus and for studying the changes after gastric
resection. The functional as well the structural changes
occuring after subtotal gastrectomy suggest the great
regenerative and plastc possibilities of the enteric
nervous system.

References
1. Atanassova E., Jurukova Z. and Draganova E. (1978).
Transformation of the slow potential rhythm of the fundus
of the stomach after functional loading (Billroth I).
In:"Gastrointestinal Motility in Health and Disese" ed. by
H. Duthie, MTP, 495-505
2. Bayguinov O. and Atanassova E. (1981). Microelectrode
studies on single smooth muscle cells of the fundus before
and after functional loading. Adv.Physiol.Sci., 12,305-311
ed. by Gati, Szollar, Ungvary, Pergamon Press
3. Dobreva G., Bayguinov O. and Atanassova E. (1982).
Character of the nerve transmission in different stomach
regions. Acta Physiol.Pharmacol.Bulg., 8,3,45-51
4. Gershon M.D., Dreyfus D.F. and Rothman T.P. (1979).
The mammalian enteric nervous system: a third autonomic
division. In:"Trends in Autonomic Pharmacology" ed. by
S. Kalsner, Baltimore-Munich:Urban and Schwarzenberg,
1, 59-103
5. Lolova I. and Atanassova E. (1982). Histochemical
study of the myenteric plexus following gastric resection
on dogs. Z.mikrosk.-anat.Forsch., 96,2,269-288

19

Studies on the Process of Gastric Emptying

H. J. EHRLEIN, O. KEINKE and M. SCHEMANN

INTRODUCTION

The process of gastric emptying is incompletely understood.
It is not known which variables of the gastric and duodenal
motility play an important role in regulating gastric emptying, especially the function of the pylorus is unclear.
In recent studies on resistances controlling gastric emptying of liquid meals it was suggested that the resistance of
the small intestine might be the dominant factor in regulating gastric evacuation (1). However, the elimination of
gastric variables by the barostat method, by antrectomy or
pylorectomy might produce unphysiological results because
the function of the gastric, pyloric and duodenal motility
can be compensated by the others. In order to elucidate the
regulating mechanisms under physiological conditions we investigated the effect of nutrients and hormones on canine
gastric, pyloric and duodenal motility and on gastric emptying by transducer recordings and simultaneous radiography.

METHODS

In conscious dogs the antral and duodenal motility was recorded with chronically implanted strain gauge transducers
after the administration of a test meal. The transducers
were positioned on the antrum 2.5 cm (A1), 5cm (A2), and

7.5cm (A3) proximal and on the duodenum 2.5cm (B), 7.5cm
(D1), and 12.5cm (D2) distal to the pylorus. The external
diameter of the pylorus was measured with induction coils.
Radiography was used to measure gastric emptying, the
volume of the antrum and of the gastric fundus and body,the
internal pyloric diameter and the lumen of the proximal
duodenum. The test meals consisted of a mashed potato meal
or of an inert viscous cellulose meal (control) to which
barium sulfate as contrast medium and nutrients (glucose,
1 KJ/ml or oleic acid 0.5 KJ/ml) were added. The volume of
the meal was 200 ml, the viscosity was about 50 000 cps.
Hormones (pentagastrin 4 µg/kg · h; insulin 0.5 U/kg; 5-
hydroxytryptophane (5-HTP) 200 µg/kg·min) were given intravenously as infusion or bolus injection beginning ten minutes after the administration of the test meal. The motility
recordings were analysed with a computer.

RESULTS

Reservoir function of the gastric fundus and body

The gastric reservoir has three functions: 1. to receive
the swallowed food by an adequate receptive relaxation, 2.
to store the food over an adequate period of time so that
solids can be sufficiently ground and diluted by the antral
pump and nutrients can be absorbed by the small intestine,
and 3. to feed the antral pump with digesta.

In order to get information about the reservoir function
we measured the volumes of the antrum and gastric fundus
and body from radiographs taken at 10 min. intervals.During
gastric emptying of a viscous meal the volume of the antrum
remained constant, whereas the volume of the gastric reservoir decreased in close relationship to gastric emptying.
This result shows that the storage and evacuation of food
from the gastric reservoir is regulated in such a way that
the volume of the antrum is kept constant. The addition of
nutrients to the inert cellulose meal diminished significantly the rate of gastric emptying. The nutrient meals
were stored in the gastric reservoir over a prolonged

period of time in relationship to the delay of gastric evacuation. In contrast, the volume of the antrum was slightly decreased in comparison to the control (control 20.4 ± 10.0 ml, glucose 17.0 ± 8.6 ml ($p < 0.05$), oleic acid 18.4 ± 11.8 ml). These findings reflect the reservoir function of the proximal stomach; the prolonged relaxation adapts the emptying rate of the proximal stomach to that of the antral pump, thus being a pre-condition for the delay of gastric emptying. However, besides this effect the reservoir function did not seem to control gastric emptying because the diminution of the antral volume was very small and not significant with the oleic acid meal.

The role of the gastric reservoir in regulating gastric emptying can be demonstrated by the administration of pentagastrin, insulin and 5-HTP. With the viscous control meal there is a balance between the quantities of digesta swept from the gastric reservoir into the antrum and from the antrum into the duodenum (Fig. 1). Pentagastrin and vagal stimulation by insulin hypoglycaemia both increase the force of the antral waves, but produce simultaneously a profound relaxation of the fundus and body; the transfer of digesta from the reservoir into the antral pump is disturbed, the antral pump becomes empty and, thus, gastric evacuation

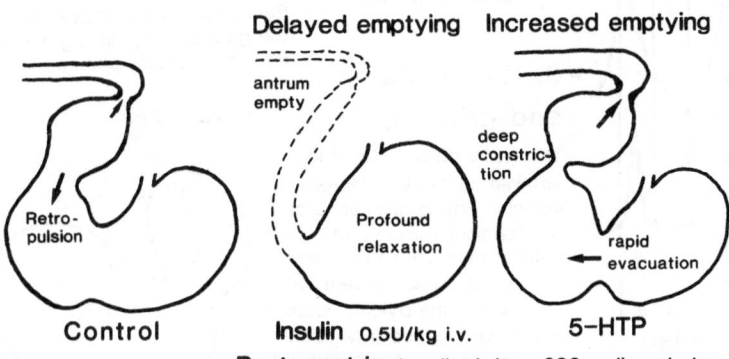

FIGURE 1 Effects of pentagastrin, insulin and 5-HTP on the gastric fundus and body.

is impaired inspite of the stimulated antral contractions.
In contrast, 5-HTP enhances both the evacuation of the
reservoir and of the antral pump so that gastric emptying
is increased (2).

Function of the antral pump

By simultaneous recording of motility and by radiography
the propagation of the antral wave can be differentiated
into three phases: 1. phase of propagation, 2. phase of

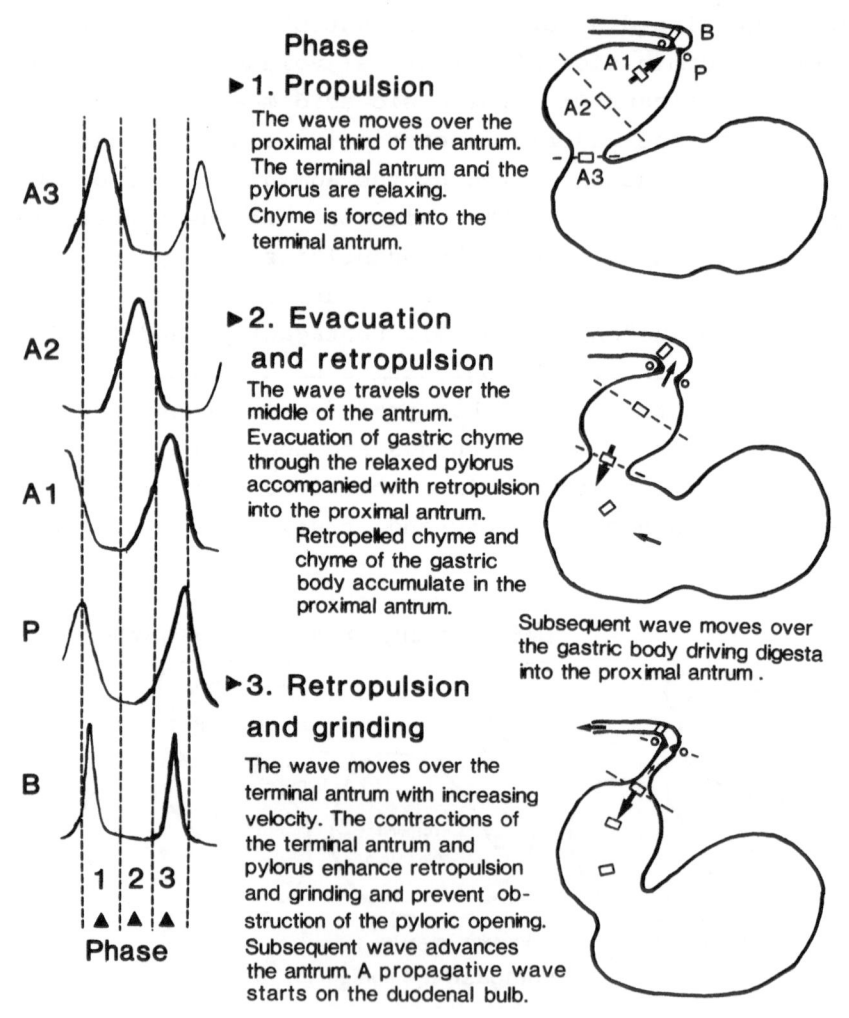

Phase

▶1. Propulsion

The wave moves over the
proximal third of the antrum.
The terminal antrum and the
pylorus are relaxing.
Chyme is forced into the
terminal antrum.

▶2. Evacuation and retropulsion

The wave travels over the
middle of the antrum.
Evacuation of gastric chyme
through the relaxed pylorus
accompanied with retropulsion
into the proximal antrum.
    Retropelled chyme and
    chyme of the gastric
    body accumulate in the
    proximal antrum.

Subsequent wave moves over
the gastric body driving digesta
into the proximal antrum.

▶3. Retropulsion and grinding

The wave moves over the
terminal antrum with increasing
velocity. The contractions of
the terminal antrum and
pylorus enhance retropulsion
and grinding and prevent obstruction of the pyloric opening.
Subsequent wave advances
the antrum. A propagative wave
starts on the duodenal bulb.

FIGURE 2 Relationship between gastric contractions and
         flow of digesta.

evacuation and retropulsion, and 3. phase of enhanced retropulsion and grinding. The three phases are illustrated
in Figure 2.

How do the antrum and pylorus control gastric emptying? The
flow of the gastric chyme into the duodenum occurs mainly
when the peristaltic wave spreads over the middle of the
antrum. In this phase the pylorus is relaxed (Fig. 2). Two
factors are important for the flow of digesta into the duodenum: 1. the depth of the antral constriction, and 2. the
degree of the pyloric relaxation. A deep constriction of
the antral wave produces a strong propagative force, whereas a shallow constriction reduces the forward flow of digesta and enhances the retropulsion through the central
orifice of the constricting ring. The depth of the antral
wave depends on the viscosity of the gastric contents (3).
With a saline meal the antral constriction occluds the
lumen so that the liquid in front of the wave is swept into
the duodenum. When the viscosity of the gastric content is
increased the constriction and the propulsive force of the
antral wave are reduced. Glucose and oleic acid entering
the small intestine also diminished the force of the antral
waves; the amplitude of the recording site A2 was 102.7%
in the control, 73.9% (p<0.01) with the glucose meal and

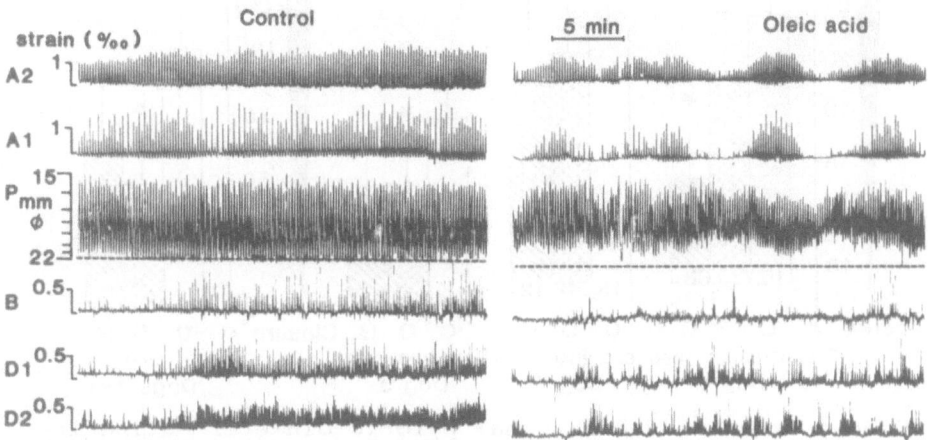

FIGURE 3 Gastroduodenal motility after administration of
an inert cellulose and oleic acid meal.

65.6% (p<0.01) with the oleic acid meal.

The measurement of the external pyloric diameter by induction coils and of the internal pyloric diameter by radiography revealed that the opening of the relaxed pylorus was
significantly diminished with the glucose and oleic acid
meal in comparison to the control (Fig. 3 and 4). The increase of the pyloric resistance also impaires gastric evacuation and enhances retropulsion of the gastric digesta.

We investigated four other factors which might effect
gastric emptying: 1. the rate and the propagative velocity
of the antral waves, 2. the sequence of the terminal antral
contractions, 3. the contractions of the pyloric sphincter,
and 4. the timing between antral and duodenal contractions.
A lower rate and a lower propagative velocity of the antral
waves could contribute to the delay of gastric emptying,
but neither the rate nor the velocity of the gastric waves
were altered significantly by the nutrients. In the literature a simultaneous contraction of the terminal antrum and
of the pylorus is described (4). The function of this contraction in controlling gastric emptying is not known. An
early contraction of the pyloric sphincter could increase

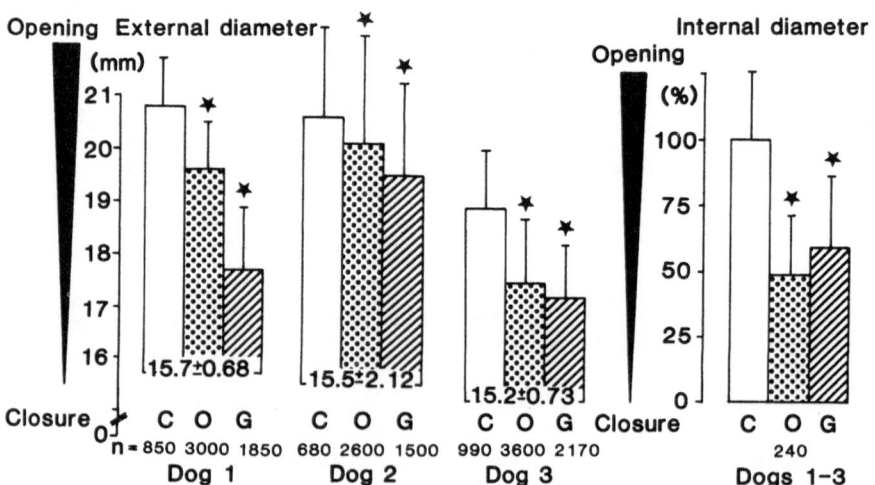

FIGURE 4 External and internal pyloric diameter during its
         phases of closure and opening. C = cellulose meal,
         O = oleic acid meal, G = glucose meal, n = number
         of data. ★p<0.05.

retropulsion, whereas a late contraction could prolong the
phase of gastric evacuation and enhance gastric emptying.
The analysis of the time difference between the contraction
maxima of the terminal antrum (site A1) and of the pylorus
showed no significant difference between the control and
the nutrient meals indicating that the sequence of the terminal antral contraction is of minor importance for the
control of gastric emptying. The degree of the pyloric
closure could also influence gastric emptying. The analysis
of the contraction maxima of the pyloric diameter revealed
a large variability but no significant difference between
the control and the nutrient meals (Fig. 4). The duodenal
bulb usually contracted simultaneously with the terminal
antrum (Fig. 2). An early contraction of the bulb could
impede gastric evacuation. The analysis of the time difference between the contraction maxima of the pylorus and
the bulb showed that the bulb contracted later with the
nutrient meals. Thus, these factors do not play an important role controlling gastric emptying.

Fluoroscopy revealed that two other factors of the duodenal motility were of great importance: 1. the relaxation
of the proximal duodenum, and 2. the pattern of the duodenal motility. In the control meal a profound receptive
relaxation of the proximal duodenum was present so that it
could receive large quantities of gastric chyme, whereas
the duodenal lumen was small in the nutrient meals due
to a tonic contraction (duodenal lumen: control meal =
100 $\pm$ 15.6%; glucose meal = 68.5 $\pm$ 18.9%, $p < 0.01$; oleic
acid meal = 54.3 $\pm$ 18.3%, $p < 0.01$). In the control meal the
duodenal contractions consisted predominantly of propagative waves driving the evacuated gastric chyme rapidly
into the jejunum. In the nutrient meals the rate and the
force of the propulsive duodenal contractions decreased
and local, segmental contractions became dominant.It is
likely that these contractions did not only retard the
transfer of the duodenal digesta but also impaired gastric
emptying.

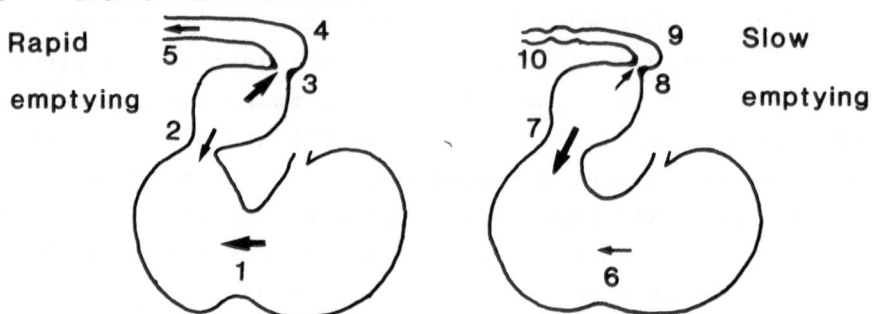

FIGURE 5 Factors producing rapid and slow emptying: 1. fast
evacuation of the reservoir, 2.deep constriction
of the antral wave, 3.wide opening of the pylorus,
4.receptive relaxation of the proximal duodenum,
5.propagative duodenal contractions, 6.prolonged
relaxation of the reservoir, 7.shallow constriction of the antral wave, 8.small opening of the
pylorus, 9.small lumen of the proximal duodenum,
and 10.segmental duodenal contractions.

SUMMARY

Several variables were found to be involved in regulating
gastric emptying. They are illustrated in Figure 5. The
pylorus plays a major role not by its contraction but by
its degree of relaxation and opening.

REFERENCES
1. Williams, N.S., Miller, J. and Meyer, J.H. (1982). Site
of chemoselective resistance to gastric emptying of
liquids. Gut, 23, A913-A914.
2. Pröve, J. and Ehrlein, H.J. (1983). Effects of 5-
hydroxytryptophane and insulin on gastric motility and
emptying in dogs. Q.J.Exp.Physiol., 68, 209-219.
3. Pröve, J. and Ehrlein, H.J. (1982). Motor function of
gastric antrum and pylorus for evacuation of low and high
viscosity meals in dogs. Gut, 23, 150-156.
4. Carlson, H.C., Code, C.F. and Nelson, R.A. (1966). Motor
action of the canine gastroduodenal junction: a cineradiographic, pressure, and electric study. Am.J.Dig.Dis., 11,
155-172.

The studies were supported by Deutsche Forschungsgemein-
schaft, grant Eh 64/2-2.

20

The Timing of Pyloric Closure in Man: Studies with Impedence Electrodes

I. A. EYRE-BROOK, G. E. LINHARDT, R. H. SMALLWOOD and A. G. JOHNSON

Although during gastric emptying the pylorus can close with terminal antral contractions (1, 2), the key question for the prevention of duodenogastric reflux is whether the pylorus can close in response to duodenal contractions when the antrum is relaxed.

We have studied the timing of pyloric closure using 4 silver wire electrodes 6 mm long mounted around the circumference of a Fogarty catheter (5FG 1.1 mm diameter) 5 mm proximal to the balloon. Impedence between opposite pairs of electrodes is measured at 100 KHz using a current of 100 µA. Pyloric closure is registered as a fall in impedence when all 4 electrodes are touched by the pyloric ring. The device is passed down the ACMI twin-channel gastroscope and positioned with the balloon just in the duodenum maintaining the electrodes in the pyloric ring ; a second Fogarty catheter records terminal antral contractions. The accuracy with which the impedence technique registers pyloric closure was confirmed during each study when the antrum was not contracting and the pylorus visible.

Twenty consenting, fasted patients without structural antro-duodenal disease were studied for a mean of 15 minutes each (under diazepam alone). During 300 minutes of good quality recording, active pyloric closure was observed on 193 occasions and was usually associated with antral or duodenal contractions. In 55.5 % of the 154 isolated duodenal contractions (no preceding antral contraction), the pylorus, which was closed before the contraction, remained closed ;

119

in 32 % the pylorus which was open, closed within 2 seconds of the contraction ; while in only 12.5 % was the pylorus open throughout.

These observations suggest that the pylorus is able to close in response to an isolated duodenal contraction.

1. CARLSON H.C., CODE C.F., NELSON R.A. (1966). Motor action of the canine gastroduodenal junction : a cineradiographic pressure and electrical study. Am. J. Dig. Dis., 11, 155-172.
2. WHITE C.M., POXON V., ALEXANDER-WILLIAMS J.   (1981). A study of motility in the normal gastroduodenal region. Dig. Dis. Sci., 26, 609-616.

21

Effect of Nervous Stimulation on Pyloric Resistance and Configuration

K. SCHULZE-DELRIEU, B. WRIGHT, C. LU and S. S. SHIRAZI

INTRODUCTION

The two loops formed by the circular muscle within the pyloric segment
(Figure 1) differ in their spontaneous and evoked mechanical activity: strips from the left canalis loop (or intermediate gastric sphincter) generate phasic contractions and stimulation of their nerves
evokes a contraction. Strips from the right canalis loop (the distal
sphincter) generate a high baseline tension and relax on nervous stimulation [1]. The mechanical end-result of nervous stimulation of the
entire pyloric segment is controversial: in manometric studies the
cat pylorus relaxes [2], whereas in studies of flow across the pylorus
stimulation produced a decrease of flow consistent with pyloric contraction [3].

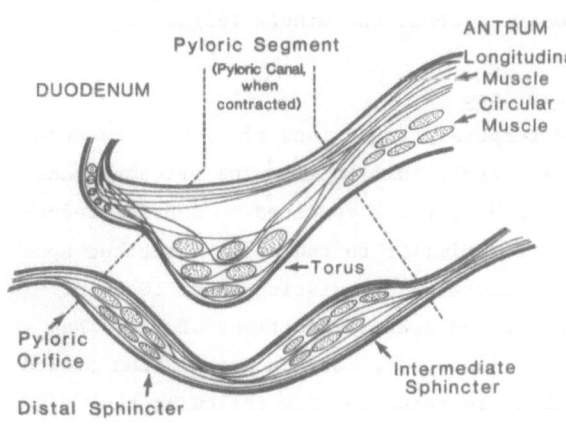

Figure 1: Longitudi-
nal section through
the gastroduodenal
junction giving a
scheme of its muscu-
lar anatomy.

Our radiographic and pyloric flow studies show that nervous stimulation leads to closure of the pylorus except when pyloric perfusion pressure is set very low. These changes resemble those that occur spontaneously at the end of gastric peristalsis [4-8].

METHODS

The gastroduodenal junction of 30 cats was removed and maintained in an organ bath as previously described [9]. A cannula was tied into the distal antrum to deliver Krebs' solution from a constant pressure reservoir directly to the pyloric segment. A second cannula in the proximal duodenum channeled pyloric output to a flow meter [3], to measure the resistance generated by the pyloric segment. The pressure head in the antral cannula was repeatedly adjusted so that a baseline flow rate of 30-60 ml/min was obtained [9]. For the radiographic studies, the Krebs' solution was replaced by barium suspension. Changes in pyloric configuration were recorded on videotape or on films every other second. Stimuli were delivered as 1 ms square wave pulses at 50V through electrodes across the pyloric segment.

RESULTS

Spontaneous changes in resistance and configuration

Rhythmic decreases of flow occurred at a rate of up to 5 cycles/ minute, but averaged 2 decreases/minute for the entire recording time (Figure 2). Most reduced flow briefly by about 10 ml min (Figure 2, Periods 1 and 5), but about one out of five reduced flow by half or more for several seconds (Figure 2, Period 6). These flow drops corresponded on radiographic observation to peristaltic waves terminating with pyloric closure. Less often, flow increased abruptly and returned to its original rate after about one minute (Figure 2, Period 2).

Evoked changes in pyloric resistance

Most nervous stimuli produced temporary reductions of flow. The duration of the flow reduction was proportional to stimulus frequency and train duration; stimulation at 2 Hz for 1 s resulted in a brief reduction of baseline flow by about 25% similar to the above described spontaneous decreases (Figure 2, Period 4). Stimulation above 10 Hz or for more than 4 s produced longer and deeper reductions of flow than occurred spontaneously. In some instances, nervous stimulation evoked a biphasic change in flow with an increase in flow following the

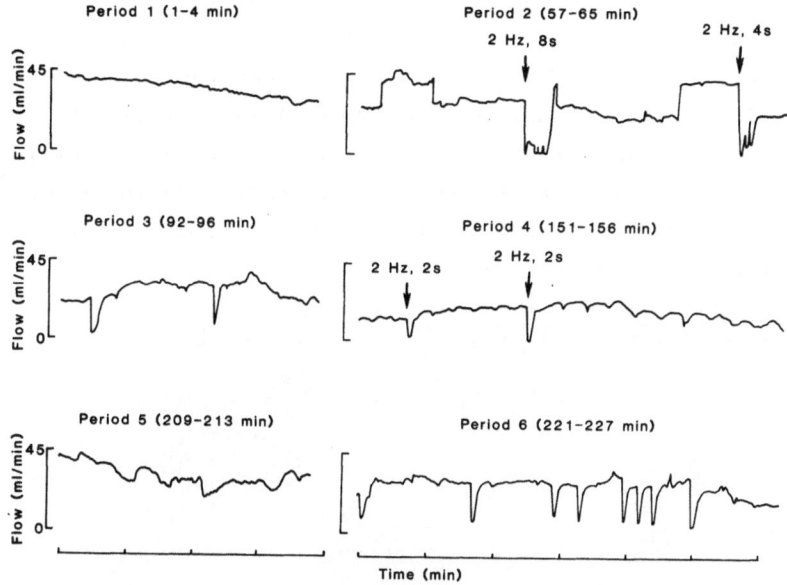

Figure 2: Flow record of one cat gastroduodenal junction in vitro. Electric stimulation is marked by arrows.

decrease (Figure 2, Period 2, First stimulus). Flow increases of similar magnitude as the flow decreases occurred only when baseline flow was below 20 ml/min. The decrease of flow was abrupt, but the nadir of flow occurred generally well after the end of the stimulus. Recovery of flow was gradual. Breakthrough flow occurred after about half a minute of continued stimulation (not shown).

Changes in pyloric configuration

When the perfusion pressure maintained a steady flow of barium, the pyloric segment was wide and no mucosal folds were recognized within its lumen (Figure 3, Frame 1). Nervous stimulation evoked pyloric closure similar to that occurring spontaneously; high threshold stimuli caused more pronounced changes for longer periods of time: the diameter of the gastroduodenal junction narrowed over a distance of at least 1.0 cm. This formation of the "pyloric canal" was accompanied by the appearance of longitudinal folds within its lumen (Figure 3, Frame 3). Following stimulation, the antral and duodenal cannulas also changed their position relative to each other. The duodenal bulb moved towards the center of the stomach, placing the duodenal cannula

closer and more orad to the antral cannula (not shown). Thus, the
gastroduodenal junction shortened and the "S" formed between the
antrum, pyloric segment and the duodenum was accentuated. Whereas
formation of the pyloric canal (pyloric closure) appeared almost
instantaneously, pyloric relaxation was a more gradual process with
straightening of the pyloric segment and disappearance of the longitudinal folds (Figure 3, Frames 5 and 6). Nervous stimulation never
widened the pyloric lumen.

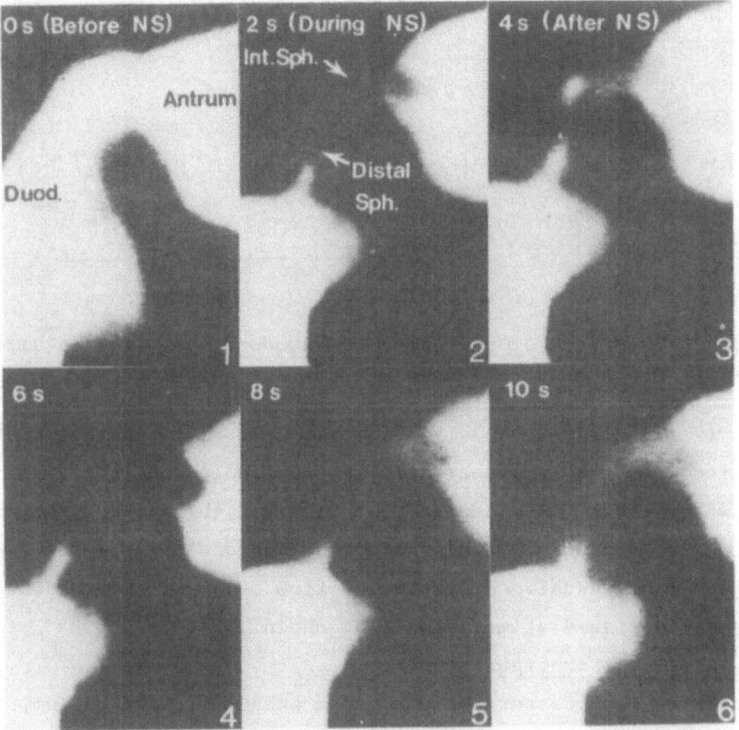

<u>Figure 3</u>: Radiographic appearance of the barium filled gastroduodenal
junction. Between frames 1 and 2, transmural electrical stimulation
was applied.

Fifteen intact cats were studied in addition. In these cats, flow
measurements showed similar reductions in pyloric flow on direct pyloric stimulation and on stimulation of the peripheral cut end of the
animal vagus nerve as described above for the isolated preparation.
Also, in five cats, changes in pyloric configuration <u>in</u> <u>vivo</u> were similar to those described above.

DISCUSSION

Our comparison between the effect of nervous stimulation on pyloric resistance and on pyloric configuration provide some explanation for the controversy that surrounds the pyloric response to nervous stimulation [1-4,11,12]. Using comparable stimulus parameters, some workers concluded that the pylorus relaxes [2] and others that it contracts [3]. Our radiographic studies showed that nervous stimulation led to formation of the pyloric canal: this closure of the entire pyloric segment accounts undoubtedly for the nerve-mediated increase in pyloric resistance described by Edin and coworkers [3] and confirmed here by us. Not reported by Edin [3] or others has been our finding that the pyloric perfusion pressure is critical to the direction in which pyloric resistance changes in response to nervous stimulation.

One conclusion to be drawn from our observations is that for the nervous control of pyloric resistance contraction of the proximal pyloric segment (or specifically the intermediate sphincter) is more relevant than relaxation of the distal pylorus (specifically the distal sphincter). Contraction of the proximal pylorus is clearly seen in the manometric recordings of Behar from the cat [2], and of Mir in dogs which had not received atropine [11]. In in vitro studies, strips from the pyloric segment contract except for strips from the most distal pylorus, (corresponding to the muscle fibers of the distal pyloric sphincter) which are inhibited [1,10]. The changes in pyloric configuration, in particular the formation of the lengthy pyloric canal, indicate that contraction of the intermediate sphincter had occurred. In the cat, most of the circular muscle of the pyloric segment is part of the broad intermediate sphincter loop. The distal sphincter loop occupies only a very narrow zone at the pyloric orifice [5,9]. The speed with which the pyloric canal forms and with which resistance to flow across the pyloric segment increases are also compatible with the time course of the contraction response of strips from the intermediate sphincter [1].

The similarity between spontaneous and evoked pyloric closure observed by us, both in the flow recordings and the radiographic studies, is also consistent with contraction of the intermediate pyloric sphincter. Intermediate sphincter muscle contracts intermittently and at the rates at which spontaneous flow drops or formation of the pylo-

ric canal occurred [1]. The importance of the intermediate sphincter
has been stressed in radiographic descriptions [5-7] of pyloric closure as it occurs at the end of gastric peristalsis (the so-called
terminal antral contraction). Contraction of the intermediate sphincter is seen to pull the entire pyloric segment shut. This is possible
because the intermediate sphincter loops obliquely across the pyloric
segment and fuses with the distal sphincter in the pyloric torus on
the lesser curvature [1,5,9]. Contraction of the intermediate sphincter leads to the formation of the pyloric canal and closure of the
gastric outlet by narrowing of the entire pyloric segment. Appearance
of longitudinal folds in the pyloric lumen is an integral part of spontaneous pyloric closure [5,7,8] and occurred also as we evoked formation of the pyloric canal by nervous stimulation. The longitudinal
folds present mucosa that bunches up within the pyloric lumen [8] as
the pyloric segment contracts.

According to our observations, the pyloric perfusion pressure is
critical for the direction in which pyloric resistance changes in
response to nervous stimulation. If a high baseline flow is maintained, stimulation decreases flow and if baseline flow is kept low,
nervous stimulation is more likely to decrease pyloric resistance.
This phenomenon probably relates to differences in the radial stretch
of the pyloric musculature: the stretch of muscle strips from the distal pyloric sphincter is critical to their mechanical response to nervous stimulation [1], with the largest relaxation response occurring
at intermediate degrees of stretch. When stretched further, these
strips cease to relax while strips from the intermediate sphincter
continue to contract. Differences in radial stretch of the pyloric
musculature could account for the discrepancy between manometric studies that reported pyloric relaxation [2] in response to vagal stimulation and flow studies which reported contraction [3]. In the flow
study the pyloric segment was probably wide open because of the large
cannulas and the high baseline flow rate used [3]. The catheter assembly used in the manometric study [2] was of comparatively small caliber and likely to produce only moderate pyloric stretch.

Another possible reason why the relaxation that occurs in pyloric
muscle strips [1,10] and in manometric studies of the pylorus [2,11]
only rarely increase flow across the pylorus is that the relaxation

does not really enlarge the pyloric diameter. All studies on nerve-mediated pyloric relaxation were performed under isometric conditions [1,2,9,10]. Even a large decrease in isometric tension of the pyloric muscle does not imply a large increase in its fiber length. No nerve-mediated increase in the diameter of the pyloric ring was observed by us radiographically. The abundant connective tissue within the pyloric wall and the high passive resistance that rings of the pylorus develop [12] makes it actually doubtful that the pylorus can enlarge much beyond its resting diameter. Decreased pyloric resistance on nervous stimulation might be equally well explained by contraction of the longitudinal pyloric muscle which shortens the pyloric resistance zone.

REFERENCES

1. Schulze-Delrieu, K. and Shirazi, S. S. (1983). Neuromuscular differentiation of the human pylorus. Gastroenterology, 84, 287-92

2. Behar J., Biancani P., and Zabinski, M. P. (1979). Characterization of feline gastroduodenal junction by neural and hormonal stimulation. Am. J. Physiol., 236(11), E45-51

3. Edin, R. (1980). The vagal control of the pyloric motor function. A physiological and immunohistochemical study in cat and man. Acta Physiol. Scand. Suppl., 485, 1-30

4. Carlson, H. C., Code, C. F., and Nelson, R. A. (1966). Motor action of the canine gastroduodenal junction: a cineradiographic, pressure and electric study. Am. J. Dig. Dis., 11, 155-72

5. Torgersen, J. (1945). The muscular build of the stomach and duodenal bulb. Acta Radiol. Suppl., 45, 1-187

6. Ehrlein, H. J. (1976). Gastric motility and emptying in rabbits. In: Vantrappen, G (ed). Proceedings of the Fifth International Symposium on Gastroduodenal Motility. pp. 284-89. (Herental, Belgium: Typoff Press)

7. Keet, A. D. (1957). The prepyloric contraction in the normal stomach. Acta Radiol., 48, 413-24

8. Williams, I. (1962). Closure of the pylorus. Br. J. Radiol., 35, 653-70

9. Schulze-Delrieu, K. and Wall, J. P. (1983). Determinants of flow across the isolated gastroduodenal junction of cats and rabbits. Am. J. Physiol., 245, 257-64

10. Anuras, S., Cooke, A. R., and Christensen, J. (1974). An inhibitory innervation at the gastroduodenal junction. J. Clin. Invest., 54, 529-34

11. Mir, S. S., Telford, G. L. Mason, R. G. (1979). Noncholinergic, nonadrenergic inhibitory innervation of the canine pylorus. Gastroenterology, 76, 1443-8

12. Biancani, P., Zabinski, M. P., and Behar, J. (1980). Mechanical characteristics of the cat pylorus. Gastroenterology, 78, 301-9

22

Small Intestinal Regulation of Gastric Emptying

B. CRANLEY and K. A. KELLY

The rate of gastric emptying varies as a function of the gradient in pressure between the stomach and the duodenum and the resistance to outflow across the pylorus (1). When the gradient increases, gastric emptying speeds, providing the pyloric resistance remains constant. In contrast, when the gradient decreases and pyloric resistance remains unchanged, gastric emptying slows.

After truncal vagotomy and distal, subtotal gastrectomy, regulation of intragastric pressure is impaired. Greater increases in intragastric pressure occur during gastric filling than are found in health. Hence, the gastrointestinal gradient increases. Moreover, the operation abolishes pyloric resistence. With the large gradient and the lack of pyloric resistence after the operation, gastric emptying is unusually rapid.

One way to slow the rapid gastric emptying after vagotomy and gastrectomy is to modify small intestinal contractile activity, increase enteric intraluminal pressure, and decrease the gradient. We found recently that retrograde pacing of the Roux loop in dogs with truncal vagotomy, distal gastrectomy and Roux-en-Y

gastrojejunostomy slowed gastric emptying of both isotonic and

hypertonic gastric instillates (2). The retrograde pacing resulted

apparently in orally moving jejunal contractions that increased

resistance to gastric outflow and so slowed emptying.

   The aim of this present study was to explore in more detail the

relationship between the frequency and direction of propagation of

small intestinal contractions and the rate of gastric emptying in

dogs after truncal vagotomy and Roux gastrectomy.

MATERIALS AND METHODS

Animal preparation

In 5 healthy female dogs weighing 15-18 kg, bilateral truncal

vagotomy and two-thirds distal gastrectomy with Roux-en-Y gastro-

jejunal reconstruction were performed. To construct the Roux loop,

the jejunum was divided 15 cm distal to the ligament of Treitz, the

distal cut end was closed, and an end-to-side gastrojejunal

anastomosis performed just distal to the site of closure. Jejunal

luminal continuity was restored by anastomosing the proximal cut end

of the jejunum to the side of the mid jejunum 40 cm from the

gastrojejunal anastomosis.

   Five monopolar silver-silver chloride recording electrodes were

implanted on the serosal surface of the Roux loop at 5 cm intervals

beginning 10 cm distal to the gastrojejunal anastomosis. Bipolar

pacing electrodes attached to an implantable pacing unit were sewn to

the Roux loop 5 cm proximal to the end-to-side jejunal anastomosis

and 35 cm distal to the gastrojejunostomy. Insulated wires from the

recording electrodes led to a radiotube socket mounted in a stainless

steel cannula. The cannula was positioned in the left abdominal wall

and sewn in place with wire sutures. The implantable pacing unit to
which the leads from the pacing electrodes were attached was placed
in a subcutaneous pocket on the right side of the abdomen.

Postoperatively, the dogs were maintained on a diet of 2 cans of
dog food per day. Tests were begun after a 2-week recovery period.

Conduct of tests

Sixteen gastric emptying tests were performed on each dog on
different days. In 8 tests, the emptying of a 100-ml gastric
instillate of 5% glucose was studied, while in the remaining 8 tests,
25% glucose was used. With each instillate, 4 tests with retrograde
pacing of the Roux loop alternated with 4 tests without pacing.

After a 24-hr fast, the conscious dog was placed in a Pavlov
sling. Leads from the monopolar recording electrodes were attached
to channels of an AC coupled chart recorder (Brush 360 Gould
Instruments; time constant, 1 sec). The abdominal cannula was used
as the indifferent electrode. Prior to giving the instillate, the
electrical activity of the Roux loop was recorded for at least 30
min.

An oro-gastric tube was inserted and 100 ml of the 5% or 25%
glucose solution marked with ^{14}C polyethylene glycol (PEG 450, New
England Nuclear, Boston, MA) was instilled. The tube was then withdrawn. Twenty minutes after the instillate was given, the orogastric
tube was reinserted and the gastric contents were aspirated. The
stomach was then washed with 100 ml water and the wash was recovered.

In experiments where retrograde pacing was employed, the frequency
of the pacesetter potentials in the Roux loop was first determined.
The frequency was usually 13-14 cycles/min, which, because of

transection of the jejunum, was a frequency slower than the 19-20

cycles/min characteristic of the intact canine proximal jejunum

(3,4). The direction of pacesetter potential propagation was usually

aborad (Fig. 1). The pacing unit was extrinsically activated 10-15

min before the instillate was given, and the pulse generator was

adjusted to provide stimuli of strength, duration and frequency great

enough to ensure capture of the jejunal pacesetter potentials. The

strength was usually about 8 ma, the duration 50 msec, and the

frequency 14-15 pulses/min. Propagation of pacesetter potentials

from the site of stimulation in an orad direction along the entire

loop was observed. Pacing was maintained for at least 10 min before

giving the instillate, was continued during the 20-min period in

which the instillate was in the stomach, and was terminated after the

gastric wash.

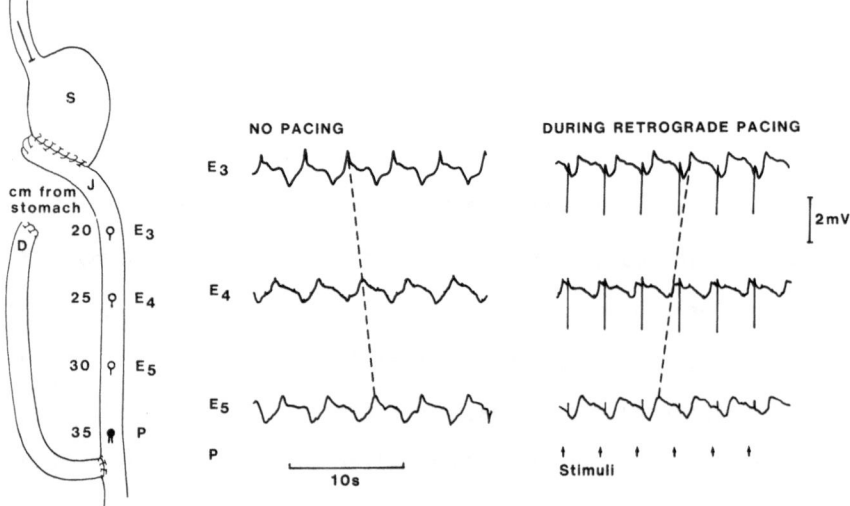

Figure 1.   Effect of pacing on electrical activity of canine jejunal
Roux limb. S=stomach, D=duodenum, J=jejunum, E=recording
electrode, P=pacing electrode. Dotted lines indicate
direction of pacesetter potential propagation.

Analysis of data

(a) Gastric emptying. The volume of gastric instillate emptied (VE) was determined in ml using the following formulae

$$VE = 100 - VR$$

$$VR = VA\frac{CA}{CI} + VW\frac{CW}{CI}$$

where VR is the volume (ml) of the original instillate remaining in the stomach after 20 min, VA is the volume (ml) of the gastric aspirate, VW is the volume (ml) of the gastric wash, and CI, CA, and CW are the concentrations of ^{14}C-PEG in the instillate, aspirate and wash, respectively. The concentration of ^{14}C-PEG was assessed by scintillation counting using a Beckman apparatus Model LS 3150 T.

(b) Jejunogastric reflux. To assess whether retrograde pacing of the Roux loop caused jejunogastric reflux, the concentration of ^{14}C-PEG in the gastric aspirate at the end of 20 min was measured and expressed as a percentage of the concentration of ^{14}C-PEG in the original instillate. If reflux occurred, a decrease in the percentage would be expected.

(c) Electrical recordings. The percentage of pacesetter potentials associated with action potentials (action potentials trigger contractions) was calculated for the 20-min period in which the instillate was in the stomach. A comparison was made between the percentage during periods of pacing and the percentage during periods without pacing. The occurrence of phase III of the interdigestive myoelectrical complex during the 20-min test period was also noted. The incidence of action potentials was correlated with the rate of gastric emptying.

(d) Statistical tests. The student's "t" test for paired data was used when comparing data from "pacing" and "no pacing" studies.

RESULTS

Gastric emptying

(a) No pacing. When 5% glucose was used, a mean±SEM of 70±10 ml of the instillate was emptied in 20 min (Table 1). When 25% glucose was instilled, a mean±SEM of 54±10 ml was emptied in 20 min, which was less than when 5% glucose was instilled ($P<0.05$).

Table 1. Effect of vagotomy, distal gastrectomy and Roux gastrojejunostomy alone or with pacing on caning gastric emptying

Type of 100-ml instillate	Mean±SEM ml emptied in 20 min**	
	No pacing	Pacing
5% glucose	70±10	53±10[+]
25% glucose	54±10[++]	35± 9[+]

**Of 5 dogs (n=5). Four tests were done on each dog.
[+]Differs from no pacing, $P<0.05$.
[++]Differs from value above, $P<0.01$.

(b) With pacing. With pacing the dogs emptied a mean of 53±10 ml of 5% glucose in 20 min, a volume less than the 70±10 ml emptied without pacing ($P<0.05$). The concentration of ^{14}C-PEG in the gastric aspirate with retrograde pacing was 71±4% of the original instillate and without pacing it was 66±7% ($P>0.05$). Thus, pacing slowed emptying without increasing dilution of the gastric marker.

With the 25% glucose solution, a mean of 35±9 ml was emptied in 20 min with pacing, which was less than the 54±10 ml emptied without pacing. The concentration of ^{14}C-PEG in the gastric aspirate was 56+4% of that in the original instillate with retrograde pacing and 53+6% in "no pacing" studies (P>0.05). Thus, pacing slowed emptying of 25% glucose instillates without increasing dilution of the gastric marker, just as was the case when 5% instillates were given.

Electrical activity

(a) Frequency of pacesetter potentials. Recordings from all the electrodes appeared similar. Therefore, only those from electrode 1, the electrode 10 cm distal to the gastrojejunal anastomosis, were analyzed in detail. In those tests without pacing of the Roux loop the frequency of the pacesetter potentials before giving the 5% instillate was 13.5+0.5 cycles/min and before the 25% instillate was 13.4+0.4 cycles/min. After giving either instillate, there was no consistent change in the frequency (P<0.05), nor did aspiration cause any change.

With retrograde pacing, the frequency of the pacesetter potentials increased from 13.3+0.4 cycle/min to 14.6+0.3 cycles/min when the 5% instillates were used (P<0.001) and from 13.3+0.3 cycles/min to 14.9+0.3 cycles/min when the 25% instillates were used (P<0.001). When pacing was discontinued, the frequency returned to pre-pacing rates with the 5% instillates, but remained slightly faster at 13.9+0.2 cycles/min with the 25% instillates (P<0.05).

(b) Action potentials. The relationship between the percentage of pacesetter potentials with action potentials during the 20-min period in which the instillates were in the stomach and the rate of gastric emptying was analyzed. We found, with or without retrograde pacing, that the greater the percentage of pacesetter potentials with

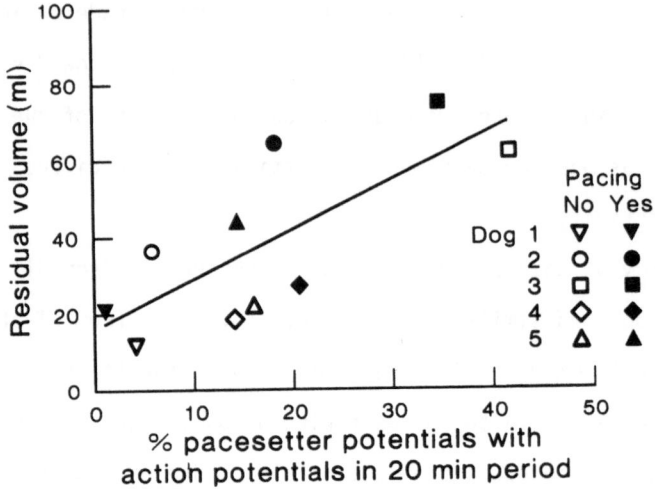

Figure 2.   Residual volume of 100-ml 5% glucose gastric instillate against percent of pacesetter potentials with action potentials.

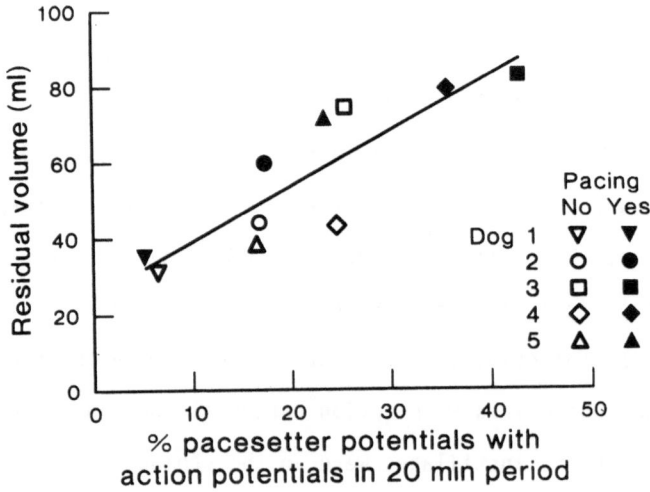

Figure 3.   Residual volume of 100-ml 25% glucose against percent of pacesetter potentials with action potentials.

action potentials, the slower the rate of gastric emptying. This was true for both 5% glucose instillates (Fig. 2, P<0.01) and 25% glucose instillates (Fig. 3, P<0.001). When the intense bursts of action potentials of phase III of the interdigestive myoelectric complex occurred in the Roux loop during the 20-min test period with pacing, gastric emptying was usually especially slow. Phase III occurred more often with the 5% instillate (5 times) than with the 25% instillate (2 times).

Retrograde pacing had no effect on the percentage of pacesetter potentials with action potentials during the 20-min period when the instillates were in the stomach. The percentages when the 5% glucose instillate and the 25% glucose instillate were in the stomach without pacing were $16\pm4\%$ and $19\pm3\%$, respectively, and these values did not differ from the corresponding percentages during pacing ($18\pm5\%$ and $26\pm5\%$, P>0.05).

DISCUSSION

We have shown in this study that retrograde pacing of a canine Roux loop after gastrectomy and Roux-en-Y gastrojejunostomy slowed the rate of gastric emptying of both 5% and 25% glucose instillates. Pacing likely exerted its effect on gastric emptying in part by increasing the frequency and reversing the direction of propagation of the pacesetter potentials in the Roux loop. The orally-moving jejunal contractions triggered by these orally-moving pacesetter potentials would have offered more resistance to gastric outflow, and so slowed emptying.

Pacing may have other, as yet undefined, effects on the bowel which could contribute to the slowing of gastric emptying, such as a pacing-induced alteration in the release of intestinal neural transmitters or hormonal regulators. However, pacing apparently did not exert its effect by altering the incidence of jejunal action potentials in the Roux loop; the incidence was similar during no pacing tests and pacing tests.

That is not to say that jejunal action potentials had no influence on the rate of gastric emptying in our preparation. On the contrary, the greater the incidence of action potentials in the Roux loop, the slower the emptying, an effect especially prominent when phase III of the interdigestive myoelectric complex was present in the loop.

These findings would seem, at first, to be at variance with those from previous studies carried out by us. We (5) showed that in dogs with an isolated, but myoelectrically continuous jejunal segment, transit of fluid through the segment was longest during phase I (no action potentials) and shortest during phase III (frequent action potentials) of the interdigestive cycles. One might have expected, therefore, that in the present study the increase in action potentials, especially as occurred during phase III, would have resulted in more rapid gastric emptying.

A clue to the explanation may be found in the experiments of Weisbrodt et al (6) and Bortolotti et al (7). Weisbrodt's group showed that when duodenal contractions were numerous and antral contractions infrequent, canine gastric emptying was slow, and vice versa. They explained this on the basis that duodenal contractions offered resistance to gastric outflow. Bortolotti et al (7) also demonstrated a relationship between duodenal contractions and gastric emptying. When they impaired duodenal contractions by a longitudinal duodenal myotomy, gastric emptying was speeded. They reasoned that the myotomy resulted in less resistance to gastric outflow. The same explanation may be applied to our findings where the rate of gastric emptying decreased as the incidence of action potentials, hence the amount of resistance offered by the Roux loop, increased.

It was also of interest to note that although pacing reversed the direction of propagation of the pacesetter potentials, phase III of the interdigestive cycles, which seemed to have a maximal slowing effect on gastric emptying, was always propagated in an aborad direction. This applied whether or not retrograde pacing of the Roux loop was employed. We also found in earlier tests (8) that phase III migrated distally through a segment of canine jejunum that was being paced in an oral direction.

We concluded that the rate of gastric emptying of glucose solutions after vagotomy, gastrectomy, and Roux gastrojejunostomy was regulated by the frequency and direction of propagation of the pacesetter potentials in the Roux loop and by the incidence of action potentials (contractions) in the loop.

ACKNOWEDGEMENTS

Statistical help from Alan R. Zinsmeister, Ph.D. and Anne C. Haddad, B.S. is gratefully acknowedged.

This research was supported by USPHS NIH Grant AM18278, the Wellcome Trust, the Ethicon Foundation, the Eastern Health and Social Services Board, Northern Ireland, and the Mayo Foundation.

REFERENCES

1. Kelly, K.A. (1981). Motility of the stomach and gastroduodenal junction. IN: Johnson, L.R., et al (eds). Physiology of the

Gastrointestinal Tract. pp. 393-410. (New York: Raven Press).

2. Cranley, B., Kelly, K.A., Go, V.L.W. and McNichols, L.A. (1983). Enhancing the anti-dumping effect of Roux gastrojejunostomy with intestinal pacing. Ann. Surg., in press.

3. Akwari, O.E., Kelly, K.A., Steinbach, J.H. and Code, C.F. (1975). Electric pacing of intact and transected canine small intestine and its computer model. Am. J. Physiol., 229, 1188-1197.

4. Bunker, C.E., Johnson, L.P. and Nelsen, T.S. (1967). Chronic in situ studies of the electrical activity of the small intestine. Arch. Surg., 93, 259-268.

5. Sarr, M.G., Kelly, K.A. and Phillips, S.F. (1980). Canine jejunal absorption and transit during interdigestive and digestive motor states. Am. J. Physiol., 239, G167-G172.

6. Weisbrodt, N.W., Wiley, J.N., Overbolt, B.F. and Bass, P. (1969). A relation between gastroduodenal muscle contractions and gastric emptying. Gut, 10, 543-548.

7. Bortolotti, M. Pandolfo, N. Nebiacolombo, C., Labo, G. and Mattioli, F. (1981). Modifications in gastroduodenal motility induced by the extramucosal section of circular duodenal musculature in dogs. Gastroenterology, 81, 910-914.

8. Sarr M.G., Kelly, K.A. and Gladen, H.E. (1981). Electrical control of canine jejunal propulsion. Am. J. Physiol., 240, G355-G360.

23

Vagal Osmosensitive Receptors Located in the Small Intestine. Role in Gastric Emptying

N. MEI, L. GARNIER and J. MELONE

Various kinds of receptors (mechanoreceptors, chemoreceptors, thermoreceptors) have been evidenced in the small intestine thanks to single recording techniques (1). We studied recently the intestinal osmosensitivity in anaesthetized cats using the microelectrode technique (2). We concluded that the vagal polymodal receptors were able to signal changes in intraluminal osmotic pressure. These endings are activated both by hypotonic (5 - 138mosmole) and hypertonic (550-1100mosmole) perfusions. Connected with unmyelinated fibres, they are located close to the epithelium as suggested by the short latency of their responses and by their sensitivity to mucosal stroking.

The aim of the present experimentation is to establish the possible involvement of the polymodal receptors in gastric emptying changes induced by intestinal osmotic pressure (see 3). For this purpose, electromyographic activities were recorded in cat stomach by means of Basmadjian electrodes. Perfusions of the first segment (duodenum) or the second segment (proximal jejunum) of small intestine were performed with the osmotic solutions which induce responses of the polymodal receptors (tap water and 3.2% NaCl solutions, in particular). In all cases, decrease in gastric EMG occurs quickly (within 3-10seconds) and persists several minutes. This effect is mediated by the vagus nerves since it disappears after cervical vagotomy.

Therefore it is concluded that : 1) the small intestine is endowed with nervous sensors capable of detecting changes in intraluminal osmolality, i.e. the polymodal mucosal receptors ; 2) these receptors are responsible for regulation of gastric emptying originating from intestinal area.

1. Mei, N. (1983). Sensory structures in the viscera. In: Ottoson, D. (ed). Progress in sensory physiology 4. pp. 1-42 (Springer-Verlag).
2. Garnier, L. and Mei, N. (1982). Do true osmoreceptors exist at intestinal level ? J.Physiol.(Lond.), 98, 327-397.
3.   Hunt, J.N. and Knox, M.T. (1968). Regulation of gastric emptying. In : Handbook of physiology, sect 6, vol 4. pp.1917-1935 (Washington DC)

24

Gastric Emptying in Asymptomatic Partial Gastrectomy (B-II) Patients

F. G. PASMA, L. M. A. AKKERMANS, H. Y. OEI,
A. J. P. M. SMOUT and P. WITTEBOL

INTRODUCTION

It is generally assumed that many of the postprandial symptoms occurring in patients after partial gastrectomy are caused by a disordered pattern of gastric emptying. Several studies reporting enhanced rates of emptying of liquids and solids after partial gastrectomy have been published ([1,2,3,4,5,6,8,9,10,11,12]) , but it should be noted, that differences in both measurement technique and patient selection render comparison of these studies impossible. In some studies patients with different types of resections were examined, in many studies the type of resection was insufficiently described, and in other studies vagotomized patients were included. Since the rate of emptying might be influenced by the size of the anastomosis ([13]) and will definitely be affected by vagotomy (highly selective or truncal) ([9,10]) the relevance of those studies is limited.

Radionuclide studies of gastric emptying in Billroth II patients (without vagotomy) are scarce. Heading et al. ([4]) found enhanced emptying rates of liquid and solid components of a mixed meal, while a difference between solid and liquid emptying rates could not be observed. MacGregor et al. ([9,10]) reported increased liquid emptying rates, but the patterns of emptying of solids in five patients with B-II resection were inconsistent. In these studies no attention was paid to the existence of a lag phase (i.e. the period between completion of the meal and the beginning of gastric emptying), as described

by Sheiner et al. ([14]) and ourselves ([7]). Although it is conceivable
that symptomatic and asymptomatic B-II patients have different emptying patterns, no studies are available in which asymptomatic B-II
patients were examined. Knowledge of the 'normal' emptying pattern of
the B-II gastric remnant must be considered a prerequisite for the
understanding of the postprandial symptoms in some B-II patients. The
aim of the present study was to determine pattern and rate of gastric
emptying of solids and semisolids in asymptomatic Billroth II
(Hoffmeister-Finsterer) patients.

METHODS

The patients were selected out of 93 patients who underwent
Billroth II resection in benign causes in the period 1971-1980.

All patients were operated by the same standard techniques. A two-
third partial gastrectomy was performed using the Schoemaker clamp,
to create a funnel shaped gastric remnant. The gastrojejunostomy was
made retrocolicly with a short afferent loop to the Hoffmeister-
Finsterer reconstruction.

These 93 patients were personally questioned by one of the authors
and a dietitian. According to Visick's criteria ([15]), 32 patients
were classified Visick I, having no gastrointestinal complaints and
using a normal diet. 15 patients out of this group, without systematic
disease or other major gastrointestinal surgery were selected for this
study. After an overnight fast the subjects received a 250 ml semi-
solid meal (porridge) and 2-3 days later a solid meal (pancake), both
labeled with Tc-99m tin colloid (9MBq).

The meals were energetically equivalent with similar concentrations
of protein, carbohydrate and fat ([7]). The patients were taking no
medication and were asked not to smoke 24 hours previously. The examination was performed in sitting position at an angle of 60° backwards.
With a gamma camera placed ventrally, time activity curves of the
gastric and small intestinal region were recorded continuously. In all
patients it was easily possible to localize the gastrojejunal junction
and no disturbing overprojection occurred. The recording started
during eating and was continued for about 60 minutes. After another
30 and 60 minutes recordings were made during 0.5 minutes in supine
position. Data analysis was performed with a digital computer system.

The duration of the lag time as well as the rate of subsequent gastric emptying were measured ([7]).

RESULTS

We reported earlier the gastric emptying pattern in 12 normal healthy volunteers ([7]). This emptying pattern shows two distinct phases: the lag phase and the emptying phase. For porridge the lag phase is 4.8 $\pm$ 1.4 min and for pancake 22.2 $\pm$ 4.4 min. The emptying rate is 47 $\pm$ 5 and 57 $\pm$ 6 %/hr, respectively. Fig. 1 shows the mean emptying patterns in the B-II patients for both meals. In all patients the lag phase for the porridge meal was reduced to zero. Sometimes, the emptying started already before the meal was finished. In 11 patients the emptying phase shows, at least for the first 45 min, an almost linear emptying pattern with a rate of 70.8 %/hr which is significantly ($p < 0.05$;

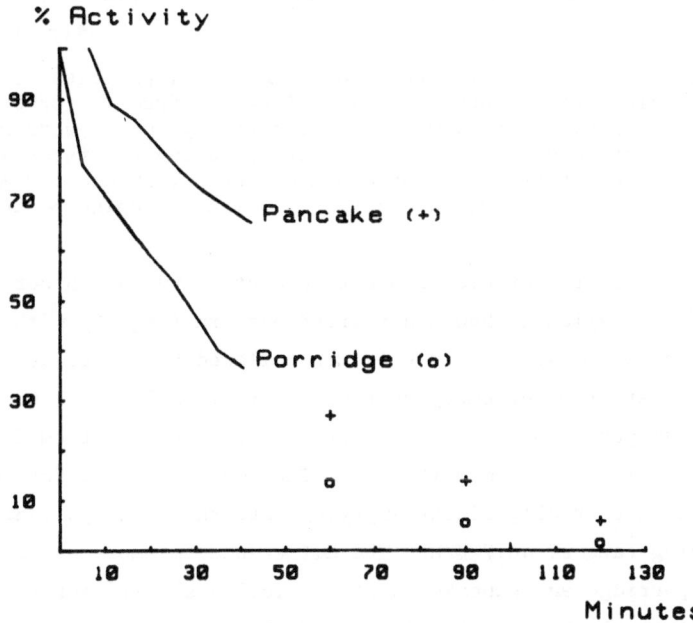

Figure 1. Mean emptying patterns of both meals in 15 B-II patients. Time activity curves were made continuously in sitting position during the first 45 min after start of the examination. At 60, 90 and 120 min recordings were made during 0.5 min in supine position.

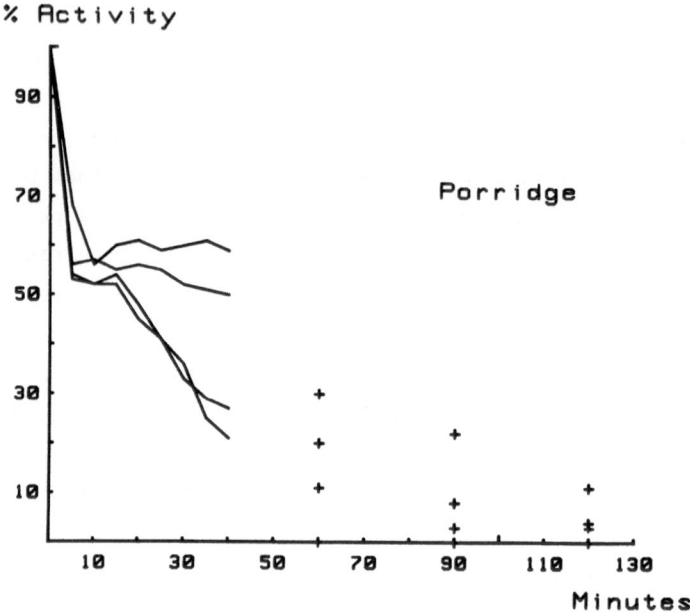

Figure 2. The emptying of a semi solid meal in 4 patients with a
distinct pattern which was different from the other 11
B-II patients examined. Time activity curves were made
continuously in sitting position during the first 45 min
after start of the examination. At 60, 90 and 120 min
recordings were made during 0.5 min in supine position.

Student-t-test) faster with respect to control values in our previous
study ([7]). 4 patients show a different pattern (Fig. 2) with a rapid
emptying of about 45-50 % in 6-10 min followed by a plateau phase of
10-35 min, after which emptying trails off. In all cases, there was
still a lag phase for solid food but this was reduced from 22.2 min
to a mean value of 6.5 min (Fig. 1). The emptying phase for solid
food shows a virtually linear emptying pattern in all patients with
an emptying rate of 46.7 %/hr. The difference in emptying rates
between porridge and pancake is statistically significant (p<0.05;
Student-t-test). Fig. 1 also indicates that 2 hours after ingestion
less than 5 % of both meals is still present in the stomach.

DISCUSSION
In this study the emptying rate of the semi solid meal is enhanced in

B-II patients. Two types of emptying pattern are seen: a) an almost linear rate in the first 45 min, and b) a rapid emptying of about 50 % (i.e., 125 ml) in the first 6-10 min, followed by a plateau phase, after which the emptying rate trails off. This last type of emptying is probably caused by the extra reduced capacity or disturbed adaptive relaxation of the gastric remnant in these patients who have, notwithstanding this rapid initial phase, no complaints.

Our experiments also show that there is a significant difference in emptying rates between semi-solid and solid food in B-II asymptomatic gastrectomy patients. In contrast to these results Heading et al. ([4]) reported that a B-II gastrectomy results in a loss of the ability to discriminate between solids and liquids as seen among normal individuals. MacGregor et al. ([10]) also reported that solid food empties precipitously with respect to normal controls. The difference in results may be caused by the type of gastroenterostomy. We used the Hoffmeister-Finsterer gastrojejunostomy, whereas in the studies of Heading and MacGregor the gastroenterostomy type is not mentioned, but the Pólya gastroenterostomy is most commonly used ([5]). We think that the technique of creating a funnel shaped gastric remnant with the Hoffmeister-Finsterer gastroenterostomy is greatly responsable for the almost normal emptying rate of solid food (pancake) in our asymptomatic B-II patients.

In 2 of these patients we performed manometric measurements in the gastric remnant and observed rather strong contractions with a frequency of about three per minute, which are typical of antral contractions. This might indicate that the distal part of the gastric remnant could function like 'antrum' in our patients. The fact that a lag phase still exists after the B-II gastrojejunostomy according to Hoffmeister-Finsterer in these patients is in favour of the view that an 'antrum'—like function exists in the gastric remnant.

CONCLUSION

Asymptomatic patients with a B-II partial gastrectomy and a Hoffmeister -Finsterer gastrojejunostomy show rapid emptying of semi solid food, but an almost normal emptying rate for solid food. This means, that the gastric remnant in these patients still differentiates between semi-solid and solid food. The existence of a lag phase in solid food emptying in these patients with an 'antrum'—like distal part of the gastric remnant, indicates that the lag phase is a major function of antral motility.

REFERENCES

1. Buckler, K.G., Gut, 1967, 8, 137-147.

2. Dozois, R.R., Kelly, K.A., Code, Ch.F., Gastroenterology, 1971, 61, 675-681.

3. Faxén, A., Berger, T., Kewenter, J., Kock, N.G., Scand.J.Gastroent., 1977, 12, 983-987.

4. Heading, R.C., Tothill, P., McLoughlin, G.P., Shearman, D.J.C., Gastroenterology, 1976, 71, 45-50.

5. Holt, S., Reid, J., Taylor, T.V., Tothill, P., Heading, R.C., Gut, 1982, 23, 292-296.

6. Horowitz, M., Cook, D.J., Collins, P.J., Harding, P.E., Shearman, D.J.C., Surg.Gynec.Obst., 1982 , 155, 737-744.

7. Jacobs, F., Akkermans, L.M.A., Oei, H.Y., Hoekstra, A., Wittebol, P., In: Wienbeck, M. (ed.), Motility of the Digestive Tract (Raven Press, New York), 1982, 233-240.

8. Kroop, H.S., Long, W.B., Alavi, A., Hansell, J.R., Gastroenterology, 1979, 77, 997-1000.

9. MacGregor, I.L., Parent, J., Meyer, J.H., Gastroenterology, 1977, 72, 195-205.

10. MacGregor, I.L., Martin, P., Meyer, J.H., Gastroenterology, 1977. 206-211.

11. Mayer, E.A., Thomson, J.B., Jehn, D., Reedy, T., Elashoff, J., Meyer, J.H., Gastroenterology, 1982, 83, 184-192.

12. Moberg, S., Carlberger, G., Bárány, F., Lundh, G., Rendic Gastroenterol., 1972, 4, 1-7.

13. Salessiotis, N.A., Am.J.Surg., 1975, 129, 656-660.

14. Sheiner, H.J., Quinlan, M.F., Thompson, I.J., Gut, 1980, 21, 753-759.

15. Visick, A.H., Ann.R.Coll.Surg., 1948, 3, 266-284.

25

Effects of Bombesin on Gastric Emptying of Solids in Normal and Antrectomized Subjects: Evidence for an Action at the Distal Stomach

C. SCARPIGNATO, B. MICALI, V. ALBANESE and G. BERTACCINI

INTRODUCTION

Intravenous infusion of bombesin produces a wide variety of actions in mammals. These concern gastrointestinal motility and secretions as well as numerous extra-gastrointestinal effects. Its activity
on gut motility is quite peculiar,including a predominantly stimulatory effect in the in vitro preparations and a predominantly inhibitory
effect in the in vivo experiments (for review see 1). An exception was
represented by the antrum and the pylorus which were always contracted by the peptide in all the species examined.

Gastric emptying of liquids or solids was shown to be delayed by
bombesin in rats (2),cats (Scarpignato & Vagne,unpublished results)
and humans (3,4). The inhibition of the contractility of the body and
the fundus (5) and the increase in frequency associated with the
decrease of amplitude of antral contractions (6,7) are likely to be
the major factors responsible for the slowed gastric emptying.

In order to further evaluate the relative importance of the
proximal and the distal stomach in the action of bombesin on gastric
emptying,we studied the effect of the peptide in seven antrectomized
patients and in seven age and sex matched controls. Results obtained
are reported here.

MATERIAL AND METHODS

Subjects

Seven healthy volunteers (5 males and 2 females,average age 36 years) without any gastrointestinal disease and seven patients (5 males and 2 females,average age 37 years) submitted to truncal vagotomy plus Billroth I gastrectomy because of duodenal ulcer were selected for the study. Written informed consent was obtained from all the subjects. All the patients have been operated at least six months before the study.

Experimental Design

After an overnight fast all the subjects underwent the test twice,having an intravenous infusion of bombesin on one day and a control saline infusion on the other,in a random order. Two indwelling intravenous cannulae were inserted in their forearms: one for the infusion of the peptide or saline and the other for blood sampling. Infusion of bombesin in saline (5 ng.kg^{-1}.min^{-1}) began 15 min before the meal and continued for 60 min. The synthetic peptide (mol. wt. 1619.92) was kindly supplied by Dr. Chiara De Paolis (Farmitalia-Carlo Erba Res. Labs., Milan, Italy). Blood samples for gastrin assay were withdrawn before and after (at 15,40,45,60 and 90 min) the test meal.

During the infusion of the peptide,in three healthy volunteers slight secondary reactions were observed. They consisted of nausea and abdominal discomfort which disappeared spontaneously after stopping the infusion. No side effects were reported by the patients.

Measurement of Gastric Emptying and of Plasma Gastrin Levels

Measurement of gastric emptying was made by a method previously described (4,8),using a standard mixed meal (containing 24 g of proteins) the solid component of which was labelled with 250 μCi of ^{99m}Tc sulphur colloid.In this investigation,however,two opposite scintillation detectors (Nuclear Accessories,Castiglione O.,VA,Italy) were used for recording radioactivity in the stomach.The geometric mean of anterior and posterior counts was used for calculations in order to minimize errors due to depth variations (9).

Plasma immunoreactive gastrin (IRG) was measured as previously detailed (4) using CIS reagents.

Evaluation of Data

There are many approaches to analysis and reporting of gastric emptying data. Plotting the emptying curves is the best way to examine and display the details of the emptying process. However, for comparison between different groups of subjects (namely healthy volunteers versus patients), the whole emptying curve rather than specific time points should be taken into account. Although a recent paper on the topic (10) concluded that residue area represents the most reliable parameter for testing differences between emptying curves, we feel that it masks manifest shape differences. Therefore we used the emptying index, firstly introduced by GRIMES and GODDARD (10) to describe each emptying curve. This was calculated according to the following formula:

$$E.I. = \left[\frac{100 - RR_{90}}{A_{90}} \right] \times 100$$

where RR_{90} represents the residual radioactivity (%) 90 min after the ingestion of the meal and A_{90} the area under the curve radioactivity-time. This index was adopted also because its use does not oblige us to perform a choice about the emptying pattern which may be different in healthy subjects and operated patients.

Quantitative evaluation of gastrin production was made by an integration of areas under the curve of immunoreactive gastrin in

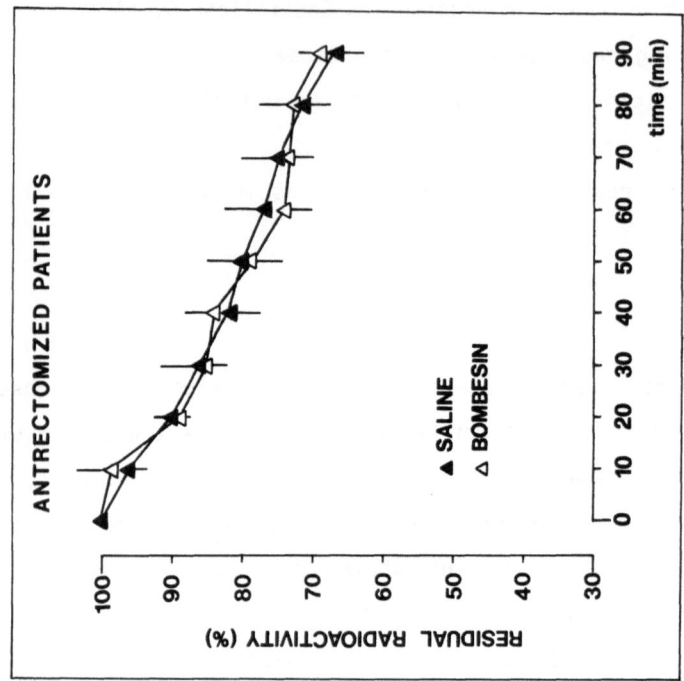

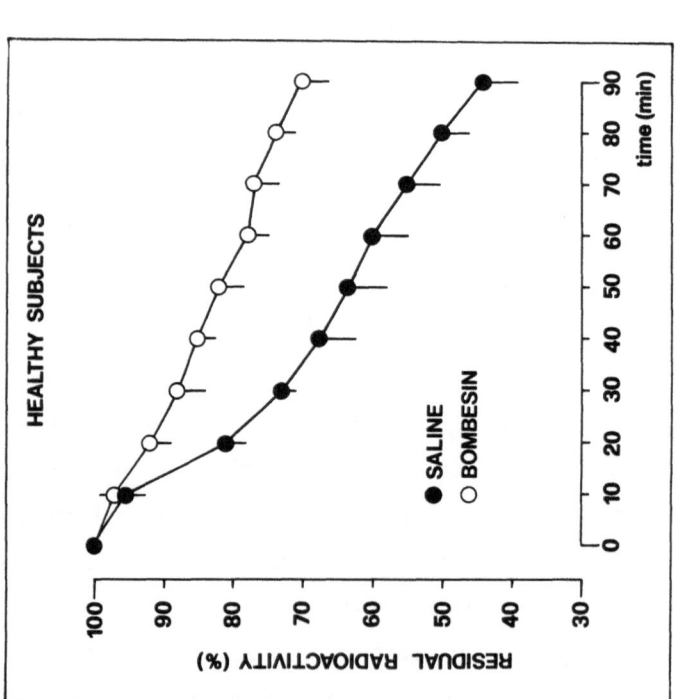

FIGURE 1   Time course of residual radioactivity in the stomach of healthy subjects and antrectomized patients during saline or bombesin infusion. Each point represents the mean of the values obtained from 7 subjects. Vertical bars are standard errors.

plasma, after subtraction of the basal values. From this an "IRG production rate" (in pg.ml^{-1}.min) was calculated by dividing the IRG area by 90 (time in min of the duration of the test).

All values are presented as a mean $\pm$ S.E.M.. The Student t test for paired or unpaired data was employed for determining statistical significance.

RESULTS

Bombesin, administered by intravenous infusion (5 ng.kg^{-1}.min^{-1}) to healthy volunteers caused a considerable delay in emptying of gastric contents (fig. 1). The emptying index changed from 0.93 $\pm$ 0.13 in saline-experiments to 0.42 $\pm$ 0.06 in bombesin-experiments (fig. 2), the difference being statistically significant.

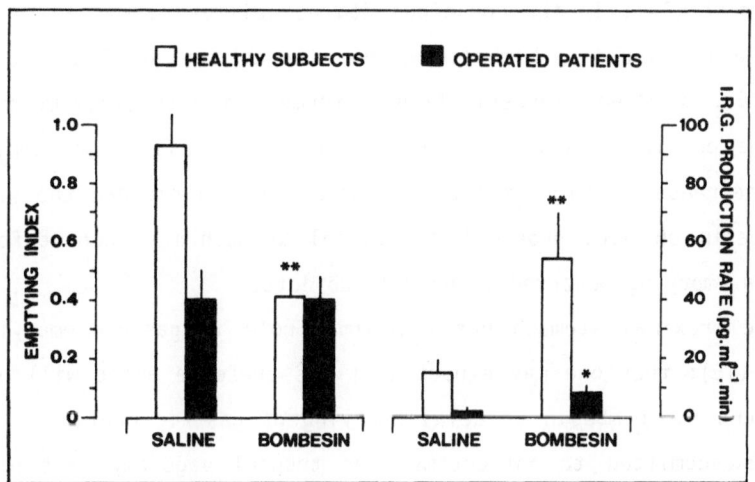

FIGURE 2   Emptying index and IRG production rate in normal subjects and antrectomized patients during saline or bombesin infusion. Each column represents the mean of the values obtained from 7 subjects. Vertical bars are standard errors. * = p < 0.02 , ** = p < 0.01

At variance with healthy subjects, in patients submitted to antrectomy and gastroduodenal anastomosis the infusion of the peptide
had no significant effect on gastric emptying (fig. 1), the emptying
index being 0.41 $\pm$ 0.10 and 0.40 $\pm$ 0.08 during saline and bombesin
infusion respectively (fig. 2).

As previously reported in dogs (12) and humans (4),bombesin
strongly increased gastrin response to food when administered to healthy subjects (fig. 2). This increase, although less pronounced, was
still evident also in antrectomized patients and probably reflects the
release of extragastric gastrin (13).

DISCUSSION

Inhibition of gastric emptying may be connected with a relaxant
effect on the proximal stomach and/or a contracting activity of the
distal part (14). In the conscious dog as well as in man the body and
fundus were relaxed by bombesin whereas the antrum was always contracted (5,6). A recent investigation,performed in cats (7),demonstrated
that the peptide produces in the antrum an increase of low-amplitude
and a decrease of high-amplitude contractions. Therefore the effects
of bombesin on both proximal and distal stomach may account for the
delay in emptying observed in normal subjects.

The proximal stomach has a minimal role in gastric emptying of
solids (15): thus one may expect that its presence alone will be not
sufficient for bombesin to delay emptying of gastric contents. In our
patients submitted to antrectomy plus truncal vagotomy gastric emptying of solids was delayed,in agreement with previous experimental
(15) and clinical (16) results. The emptying rate of these patients,
however,was not modified by the peptide. Thus,when antropyloric mechanism was removed by antrectomy,bombesin becomes unable to modify
gastric emptying. That vagotomy may affect the action of bombesin on
gastric motility is unlikely. Indeed the usual inhibitors (atropine,

hexamethonium or tetrodotoxin) did not significantly modify the effect of the peptide (5,17) and therefore it may be considered myogenic in nature (17).

In conclusion,results of the present investigation,strongly suggest that - in delaying gastric emptying - the pyloric antrum is the main site of action of bombesin.

ACNOWLEDGEMENTS

This work was supported by grants from M.P.I. and C.N.R. (Rome).

REFERENCES

1. Bertaccini, G. (1982). Bombesin. In: Bertaccini, G. (ed.). Handbook of Experimental Pharmacology, vol. 59/II, pp. 124-135. (Berlin: Springer-Verlag)

2. Scarpignato, C. and Bertaccini, G. (1981). Bombesin delays gastric emptying in the rat. Digestion, 21, 104-106

3. Walsh, J.H., Maxwell, V., Ferrari, J. and Varner, A. (1981). Bombesin stimulates human gastric function by gastrin-dependent and independent mechanism. Peptides, 2(Supll. 2), 193-198

4. Scarpignato, C., Micali, B., Vitulo, F., Zimbaro, G. and Bertaccini, G. (1981). The effect of bombesin on gastric emptying of solids in man. Peptides, 2(Supll. 2), 199-203

5. Bertaccini, G., Impicciatore, M., Molina, E. and Zappia, L. (1974). Action of bombesin on human gastrointestinal motility. Rend. Gastroenterol., 6, 45-51

6. Bertaccini, G., and Impicciatore, M. (1975). Action of bombesin on the motility of the stomach. Arch. Pharmacol.,289, 149-156

7. Vagne, M., Gelin, M.L., McDonald, T.J., Chayvialle, J.A. and Minaire, Y. (1982). Effect of bombesin on gastric secretion and motility in the cat. Digestion, 24, 5-13

8. Scarpignato, C. (1982). Radioisotopic measurement of gastric em-

ptying in man:a tool for assessing drug effect on gastric motility. In: Raynaud, C. (ed.). Nuclear Medicine and Biology, vol.I, pp. 265-269. (Paris:Pergamon Press)

9. Tothill, P., McLoughlin, G.P. and Heading, R. (1978). Techniques and errors in scintigraphic measurement of gastric emptying. J. Nucl. Med., 19, 256-261

10. Dugas, M.C., Schade, R.R., Lhotsky, D. and Vanthiel, D. (1982). Comparison of methods for analyzing gastric isotopic emptying. Am. J. Physiol., 243, G237-G242

11. Grimes, D.S. and Goddard, J. (1977). Gastric emptying of wholemeal and white bread. Gut, 18, 725-729

12. Modlin, I.M., Lamers, C. and Walsh, J.H. (1980). Mechanisms of gastrin release by bombesin and food. J. Surg. Res., 28, 539-546

13. Stern, D.H. and Walsh, J.H. (1973). Gastrin release in postoperative ulcer patients:evidence for release of duodenal gastrin. Gastro-enterology, 64, 363-369

14. Yamagishi, T. and Debas, H.T. (1978). Cholecystokinin inhibits gastric emptying by acting on both proximal stomach and pylorus. Am. J. Physiol., 234, E375-E378

15. Kelly, K. (1980). Gastric emptying of liquids and solids:roles of proximal and distal stomach. Am. J. Physiol., 239, G71-G76

16. Donovan, I.A., Owens, C., Clendinnen, B.G., Griffin, D.W., Harding, L.K. and Alexander-Williams, J. (1979). Interrelations between serum gastrin levels,gastric emptying and acid output before and after proximal gastric vagotomy and truncal vagotomy and antrectomy. Br. J. Surg., 66, 149-151

17. Mayer, E., Elashoff, J. and Walsh, J.H. (1982). Characterization of bombesin effects on canine gastric muscle. Am. J. Physiol., 243, G141-G147

26

Involvement of Endogenous Opiates in Radiation-Induced Suppression of Gastric Emptying

E. DANQUECHIN DORVAL, G. P. MUELLER, R. ENG,
A. DURAKOVIC, J. CONKLIN and A. DUBOIS

INTRODUCTION

The pathogenesis of radiation-induced suppression of gastric emptying is unknown. Therefore, we have determined the effects of ionizing radiations on gastric fractional emptying rate, on gastric basal electric rhythm and on plasma levels of β-endorphin.

MATERIAL AND METHODS

Twelve conscious, chair-adapted rhesus monkeys were studied on 3 separate days, once before and twice after a single 8 Gy cobalt-60 total body irradiation. Gastric fractional emptying rate (FER, %/min) was measured using a ^{99m}Tc-DTPA dilution technique.[1] Gastric basal electric rhythm (BER, waves/min) was recorded from 2 abdominal electrodes. The plasma concentration of β-endorphin (pg/ml) was determined using a standard radioimmunoassay.[2]

RESULTS

Irradiation significantly suppressed FER, decreased BER and increased plasma β-endorphin concentrations ($p < 0.01$; table 1; means

$\pm$ SE). These effects appeared within 30 min after exposure and had disappeared 2 days later. In addition, significant inverse correlations (p < 0.05) were found between β-endorphin and both FER (r = 0.63) and BER (r = 0.61).

Table 1. Effect of irradiation on β-Endorphin, BER and FER.

	β-Endorphin	BER	FER
Control Day	229+48.5	3.2+0.07	5.5+0.9
Irradiation Day	1447+228.2*	2.5+0.10*	0.2+0.2*
2 Days after Irradiation	159+43.3	3.1+0.08	4.7+0.7

*p < 0.01 compared to control day

CONCLUSIONS

Thus, total body irradiation transiently suppresses gastric emptying, decreases gastric BER, and increases plasma β-endorphin. These observations suggest that the radiation-induced suppression of gastric emptying may result from an alteration of the gastric basal electric rhythm induced by the release of β-endorphin.

REFERENCES

1. Dubois A, Van Eerdewegh P, Gardner JD: Gastric emptying and secretion in Zollinger-Ellison syndrome. J. Clin. Invest. 59: 255-263, 1977.

2. Mueller GP: Attenuated β-endorphin release in estrogen-treated rats. Proc. Soc. Exp. Biol. Med. 165: 75-81, 1980.

27

Gastrointestinal Contractile Activity Associated with Vomiting in the Dog

I. AIZAWA, K. NEGISHI, T. SUZUKI and Z. ITOH

INTRODUCTION

Vomiting, which seem's to be a protective function against ingested noxious materials, is one of the major pathophysiological phenomena in the gut. Gastrointestinal motility associated with vomiting had been studied with using contrast media in the stomach or duodenum (1), or electrodes on the intestine (2). However, mechanical movements during vomiting has not fully been elucidated, especially in the intestine, probably because of technical limitation. Contrast media in the intestine is not useful to follow its movement under fluoroscopy, and the electrical changes detected by electrodes on the intestine do not always reflect the strength of the intestinal contractions.

We have been studying gastrointestinal movements by means of chronically implanted force transducers which enable us to observe mechanical movements of various sites of the gastrointestinal tract at the same time and for a long period in the conscious state (3,4).

In the present study, we investigated the gastrointestinal mechanical movements during vomiting induced by three different stimuli, that is stimuli given through blood circulation and intraluminal space of the stomach and mechanical obstruction of the gut.

MATERIALS AND METHODS

   Five mongrel dogs were anesthetized and silicone tubing was implanted into the superior vena cava through the external jugular vein and was used for drug administration. Gastrostomy was constructed by implanting a silicone tubing into the stomach. In each dog eight force transducers were implanted on the serosal surface of the gastrointestinal tract. The sites of implantation were the gastric antrum and the intestine at 20 cm, 70 cm, 120 cm, 170 cm, 220 cm, 270 cm, and 300 cm distal to the ligament of Treitz. A C-shaped constricting device was implanted around the jejunum at 10 cm distal to the ligament of Treitz. This device has a balloon around the inner circle and when the balloon is inflated, the intestine is constricted from outside to constitute a reversible transient intestinal obstruction.

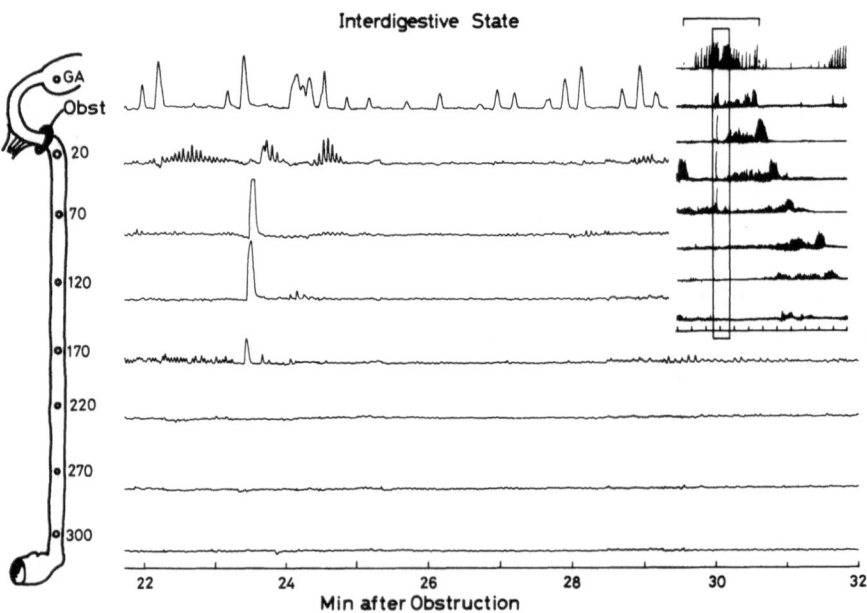

Fig. 1. Gastrointestinal motility after mechanical intestinal obstruction. A strong tonic contraction started from the mid-intestine 170 cm distal to the ligament of Treitz and migrated orally.

Experiments were performed in the conscious state after the dog recovered from the surgery and can eat normally and the motility tracing shows daily cyclic occurrence of the interdigestive migrating contractions after a certain period of feeding.

0.1 mg/kg of apomorphine dissolved in saline was injected subcutaneously.   20 mg/kg of copper sulfate dissolved in water was administered into the stomach through the implanted gastrostomy tubing.   A balloon of the constricting apparatus was inflated to make transient bowel obstruction.

The drug administration and the balloon inflation was carried out during the quiecent period of the interdigestive state in the stomach (4).

RESULTS

Mechanical obstruciton induced a strong tonic contraction which migrated orally to the gastric antrum 7.4 ± 2.9 min after

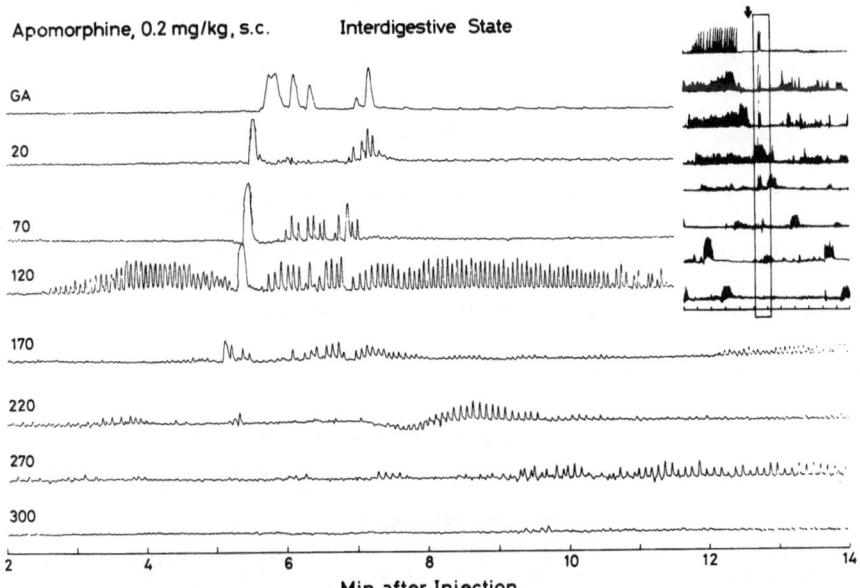

Fig. 2. Gastrointestinal motility after apomorphine injection.   Orally-migrating contraction started from the mid-intestine 170 cm distal to the ligament of Treitz, which is quite similar to changes after the mechanical obstruction.

creating the obstruction. (Fig. 1)   It usually originated at the mid-intestine, 170 cm distal to the ligament of Treitz, although the obstruction site was in the proximal jejunum.   Its velocity from the site of origination to the gastric antrum was 5.2 ± 0.6 cm/sec and the amplitude was 122 ± 42 % and 57 ± 15 % of the maximum amplitude of the interdigestive migrating contractions in the stomach and the small bowel, respectively.   After the strong retrograde migrating contraction reached the gastric antrum, vomiting was followed.

Injection of apomorphine induced the same motor pattern 5.8 ± 0.4 min after the injection as after the mechanical obstruction (Fig. 2).   Vomiting was always observed when the strong retrograde migrating contraction reached the stomach as in the case of the mechanical obstruction.

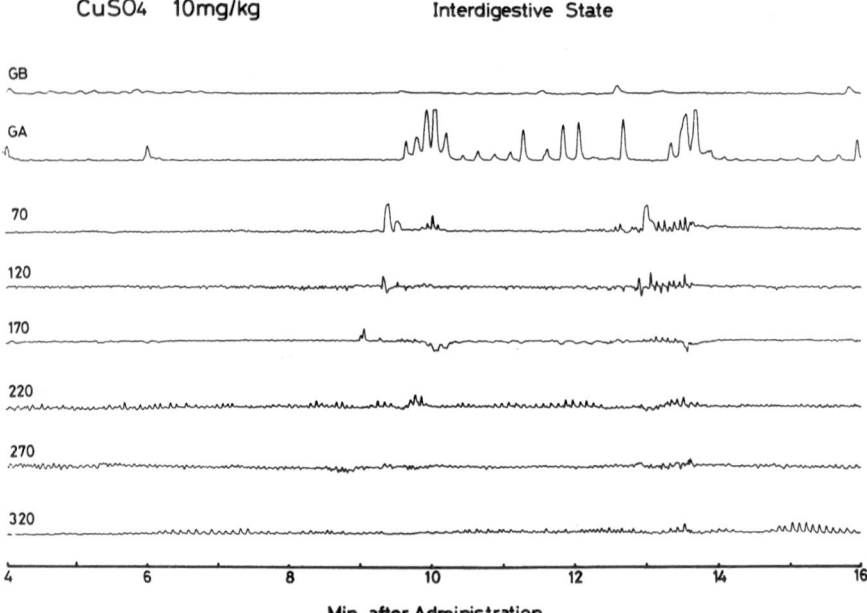

Fig. 3.   Gastrointestinal motility after copper sulfate instillation into the stomach. The amplitude of the orally migrating contraction was smaller than the mechanical obstruction or the apomorphine-induced contractions.   Ther initial contraction, however, initiated at 170 cm distal to the ligament of Treitz.

Instillation of copper sulfate into the stomach also induced an orally migrating contraction from the same site in the mid-intestine as in the case of mechanical obstruction (Fig. 3).

The migrating velocity and the amplitude of the contractions induced by apomorphine and copper sulfate were not significantly different from those observed after the mechanical obstruction.

Table. Comparison of velocity and contractile force.

	Velocity (cm/sec)	Contractile force (% of IMC)	
		Small intestine	Stomach
Obstruction	5.2 ± 0.6 (N=7)	122 ± 42 (N=15)	57 ± 15 (N=15)
Apomorphine	6.2 ± 2.9 (N=7)	150 ± 36 (N=12)	69 ± 21 (N= 9)
Copper sulfate	5.9 ± 0.4 (N=3)	77 ± 9 (N= 9)	52 ± 18 (N=3)

DISCUSSION

The present study is the first clear presentation of mechanical changes in the antiperistalsis associated with vomiting. With the aid of many force transducers on the intestine, we could observe motility changes at different sites of the intestine at the same time and compare the amplitude of retrograde migrating contraction to that of natural contractions in each corresponding sites of the gut. Stewart et al (2) has studied antiperistalsis in electromyograms of the intestine during vomiting and reported the similar electrical pattern with various emetic agents. We reconfirmed the presence of the intestinal antiperistalsis preceded somatic muscle reaction and added the fact that even the mechanical obstruction also evoked the similar mechanical intestinal antiperistalsis.

Orally migrating contractions of the intestine had less amplitude than the interdigestive migrating contractions, the strength itself being within a physiological range. The orally moving contractions consist of strong tonic contractions, however, we usually did not observe the decreased tone associated before the strong tonic contraction which Gregory found in the Thiry-Vella loop during apomorphine-induced vomiting (5). The fact the orally migrating contractions preceded the act of vomiting fits a physiological purpose of the vomiting --- that is to expel intestinal contents. Stewart et al (2) has reported that atropine abolished the intestinal reaction but not the emesis, however, it is necessary to solve the question whether the intestinal contraction is the earliest reaction in the various phases of vomiting, or the intestinal contraction itself is the initiator of vomiting.

Another point of interest is that the orally migrating contraction originated at the mid-intestine even when the vomiting was induced by mechanical obstruction at the upper intestine. After apomorphine injection the initial strong tonic contraction was observed at the mid-intestine. We have never observed that the contraction started from the upper intestine nor from the terminal ileum. It is suggested to exist a specific site in the small intestine where the orally migrating contraction initiates.

CONCLUSION

It is concluded that characteristics of the orally migrating strong contraction induced by peripheral stimuli were not different from those induced by apomorphine which is believed to act at the chemoreceptor trigger zone. This suggests that there exists a specific gastrointestinal motor pattern to vomiting regardless of the cause in the dog.

REFERENCES

1. Lumsden, K. and Holden, W. S. (1969). The act of vomiting in man. Gut. 10, 173-179.
2. Stewart, J. J., Burks, T. F., Weisbrodt, N. W. (1977). Intestinal myoelectric activity after activation of central emetic mechanism. Am. J. Physiol., 233, E131-E137

3. Itoh, Z., et al. (1976). Motilin-induced mechanical activity in the canine alimentary tract. Scand. J. Gastroent., 11. Suppl. 39, 93–110.

4. Itoh, Z., et al. (1978). Characteristic motor activity of the gastrointestinal tract in fasted conscious dogs measured by implanted force transducers. Am. J. Dig. Dis., 23, 229–238.

5. Gregory, R. A. (1947). Changes in intestinal tone and motility associated with nausea and vomiting. J. Pysiol. (London), 106, 95–103.

28

Vagal Control of Gastrointestinal Tract during Vomiting

J. P. MIOLAN, A. M. LAJARD, P. REGA and C. ROMAN

INTRODUCTION

Vomiting is characterized by a complex sequence of activities including salivation, spasmodic respiratory movements, forced inspiration and modifications of gastrointestinal motility. The neural coordinating mechanism for vomiting is located in the lateral reticular formation (1, 2). In addition, there is a separate chemosensitive area, responsible for the initiation of emesis by central emetic agents, and situated on the caudal margins of the fourth ventricle (Area postrema, Chemoreceptor Trigger Zone CTZ) (1, 2). The aim of the present work was to study the nervous efferent pathways involved in the control of the gastrointestinal tract during vomiting.

MATERIAL AND METHODS

This work was carried out on dogs in which electrodes for EMG recording were implanted in the stomach and along the entire small intestine during an aseptic surgical operation. The recording started one week after the surgical procedure and lasted two or three months. In some cases, the vagus nerves were severed in the thorax at the level of the diaphragm during a second surgical operation . Emesis was induced by flash intravenous injection of apomorphine chlorhydrate (10 - 50 µg.Kg^{-1}). The analysis of electrical tracing was done by

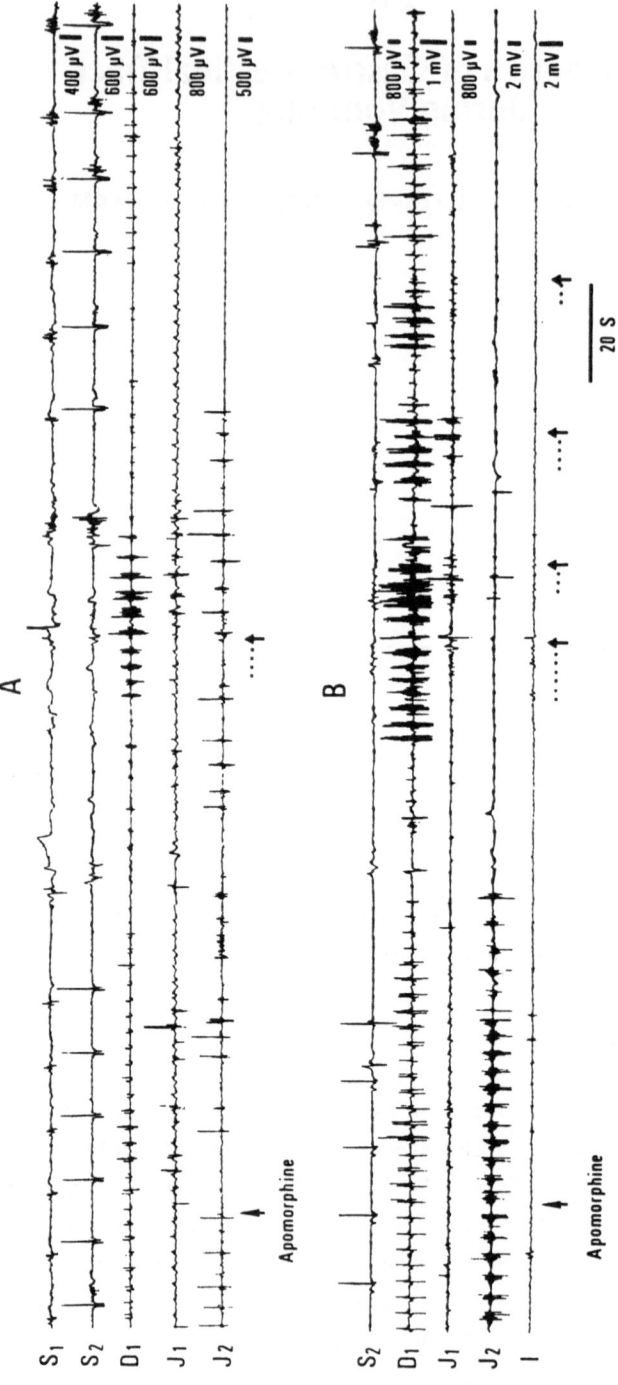

Fig. 1 : Modifications of gastrointestinal EMGs during vomiting induced in fed (A) or fasting (B) dog.
S_1, S_2, D, J_1, J_2, I : EMGs recorded by bipolar electrodes on the stomach (S_1, S_2), the duodenum (D), the jejunum (J_1, J_2) and the ileum (I).
Vomiting induced by IV injection of apomorphine chlorhydrate (25 μg.Kg^{-1} in A and 50 μg.Kg^{-1} in B), the dotted line indicates retching and the arrows expulsion of gastric content.

counting the number of fast activities (or spikes) per 30 sec., this
analysis started at least two minutes before and lasted 2-20 minutes
after the administration of the emetic substance.

RESULTS AND DISCUSSION

A. Modifications of gastrointestinal tract motility during vomiting.

The myoelectric activity of the gastrointestinal tract is characterized
by two types of potential changes : the slow waves (also refered to as
basic electric rythm, pacesetter potentials or electrical control
activity) and the spike potentials (also called action potentials, fast
activities, electrical response activities). The slow waves occur at an
uniform frequency for a given segment (from 4-5 cycles per min in the
stomach, 14-20 cycles per min at intestinal level), the spike potentials
are not always present. But when they occur they are superimposed on
the slow waves and associated with contraction of the muscle.

In the fasting dog, the stomach and the small bowel are affected
each 90-180 min. by a complex activity which migrates slowly in the
aboral direction and which constitues the so-called migrating myoelectric complex (MMC ; 3-4). After feeding, the electric activity of the
gastrointestinal tract is characterized by marked increase of fast
activities at both the gastric and intestinal level (post-prandial
pattern).

The intravenous injection of apomorphine chlorhydrate (10 to 50
μg.kg^{-1}) was always followed, after a delay of 30 to 90 seconds, by
the suppression of the fast activities when they were present on the
recordings (fig. 1). In the fasted dog, the hyperactivity of the phase
III of a MMC was stopped (fig. 1B), and this whatever the level of the
small intestine affected by the phase III. Later on, the gastric and
intestinal slow waves were dampened and even suppressed. The disappearance of the slow waves was well observed at the gastric level, but was
also noticed during a few seconds on the proximal part of the small
bowel (D fig. 1B). Thus, the injection of apomorphine induces, at first,
a suppression of all gastrointestinal motility. About 10 seconds after
the beginning of this inhibition, bursts of spikes appeared at intestinal level. When couples of electrodes were implanted a few centimeters
apart along the duodenum (fig. 2), it was observed that the first
contraction was propagated in an oral direction. This antiperistaltic

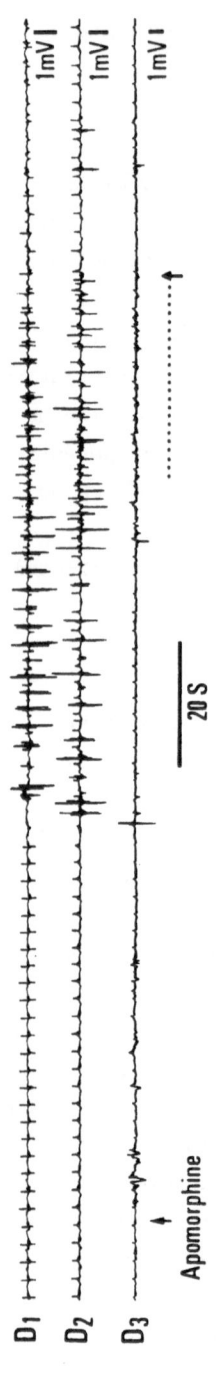

Fig. 2 : Duodenal EMGs during vomiting
D_1, D_2, D_3 : Duodenal EMGs recorded with bipolar electrodes 3 centimeters apart from each others.
Dotted line and arrow : same meaning as for fig. 1.
Note the bursts of spikes propagating orally from D_3 to D_2 and D_1.

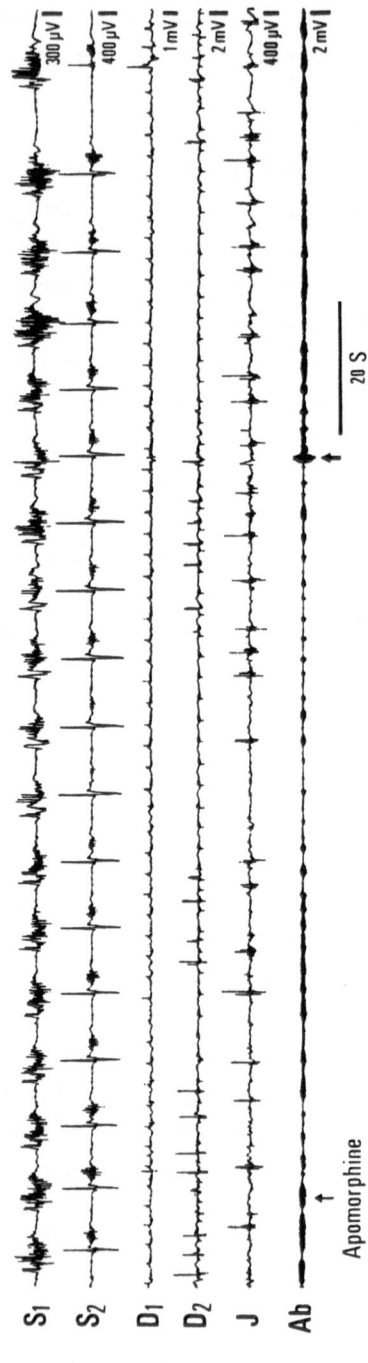

Fig. 3 : Gastrointestinal EMGs recorded during vomiting induced in bivagotomized dog.
S_1, S_2, D_1, D_2, J : same meaning as for fig. 1.
Ab : bipolar EMG of the abdominal wall (striated muscle).
Note that apomorphine injection, while being followed by respiratory changes and expulsion (arrow), does not induce on the gastrointestinal EMGs the changes characteristic of vomiting.

contraction was followed by a long lasting burst of action potentials (duration of 2-3 minutes). The duodenal antiperistalsis was contemporaneous with profuse salivation, swallowing and accelerated respiration. Then, it might be that antiperistalsis of the proximal intestine be associated with nausea. On a few occasions (n = 12 out of 140) the changes of gastrointestinal motility were not accompanied by retching and expulsion, but in most of the cases, retching and expulsion occured within 10 to 30 seconds after the duodenal antiperistalsis.

B. Nervous efferents pathways involved in vomiting

The modifications of GI motility occuring before and during vomiting were suppressed after injection of hexamethonium (10 mg.Kg^{-1}) or after section of the vagus nerves (fig. 3). From these results, it can be concluded that the vagus nerves are directly responsible for the excitatory and inhibitory events occuring during vomiting at the gastrointestinal level. Furthermore, all the digestive phenomena characteristic of vomiting were still present after intravenous injection of atropine (0.1 mg.Kg^{-1}) (fig. 4), and after administration of α and/or β adrenergic blockers (phentolamine 1 mg.Kg^{-1} ; propranolol .5 mg.Kg^{1}).

The inhibitory phenomena likely result from an activation of efferent vagal fibers, synapsing at intramural level, with inhibitory neurons producing inhibition of the muscle. Our results confirm the previous works of Abrahamsson et al. (5) showing that, in cat, the IV injection of apomorphine induced a receptive relaxation of the proximal part of the stomach. The intramural neurons involved in this inhibition are likely so-called non-adrenergic, non-cholinergic inhibitory neurons. Concerning the intestinal antiperistalsis, it cannot involve the classical cholinergic vagal pathway, since it is also present under atropine. This motor activity may result either from a post inhibitory rebound or from an excitatory non-adrenergic, non-cholinergic vagal pathway. The existence of such an excitatory non-adrenergic non-cholinergic (NANC) pathway has been demonstrated by electrical stimulations of the vagus (6) but its implication in a physiological process has never been established.

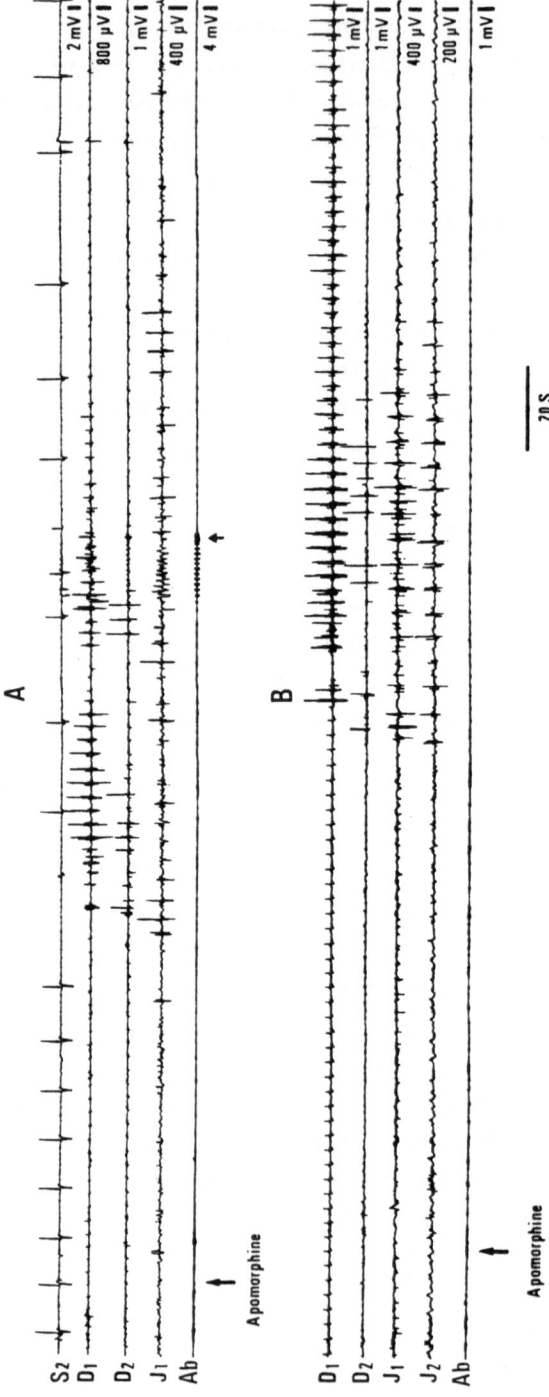

Fig. 4 : Gastrointestinal EMGs recorded in the atropinized dog.
  A. Vomiting is induced by IV injection of 20 μg.Kg⁻¹ of apomorphine.
  B. IV injection of apomorphine (30 μg.Kg⁻¹ IV) does not induce expulsion of the gastric content.
  Note that apomorphine is able to induce the same gastrointestinal modifications with or without
expulsion of the gastrointestinal content.

C. Pharmacological study of the nervous excitatory pathway involved in vomiting.

In order to evaluate the possible participation of a NANC excitatory pathway in the intestinal antiperistalsis preceding vomiting, various drugs interfering with enkephalinergic or monoaminergic mechanisms were tested.

1/ Is an enkephalinergic mechanism involved ?

Under atropine plus an opiate antagonist (Naloxone 4 mg.Kg^{-1}) the intestinal antiperistalsis is quite similar to that observed under atropine only. From this result it can be concluded that it is unlikely that an enkephalinergic mechanism be involved.

2/ Is a dopaminergic component involved ?

According to Anuras (7), dopamine is able to induce contractions in the duodenal smooth muscle of opossum. At low doses, Domperidone (.5 mg.Kg^{-1}), a dopaminergic blocking agent, depresses the CTZ and protects against vomiting induced by apomorphine, but has little effect on emesis produced by other stimuli. In order to appreciate the possible involvement of a dopaminergic mechanism in intestinal antiperistalsis, vomiting was induced by morphine under Domperidone plus atropine. In no instance was the duodenal antiperistalsis different from that observed under atropine only. In addition, Phenoxybenzamine (4 mg.Kg^{-1}) was unable to suppress the duodenal antiperistalsis. Thus it seems unlikely that dopamine acts as a peripheral transmitter during vomiting.

3/ Is a serotoninergic component involved ?

There is increasing evidence that serotoninergic neurons are components of the enteric nervous circuitry (8, 9), and that 5HT can act as an excitatory transmitter for the smooth muscle itself (10). Thus, it seemed worthwhile to investigate the possibility that 5HT may mediate the NANC intestinal contractions. In animals pretreated with an inhibitor of trypthophan hydroxylase (pCPA : 200 mg.Kg^{-1} and 300 mg. Kg^{-1} IP, 54 hours and 30 hours respectively before experiment), or in the presence of a serotoninergic blocking agent (Methysergide, 2 mg. Kg^{-1}), it was very difficult to induce emesis. But when vomiting occured, the duodenal antiperistalsis was reduced by about 50 % (fig. 5). From these results, it was difficult to appreciate whether the reduction of motility resulted from a decreased activity within the intra-

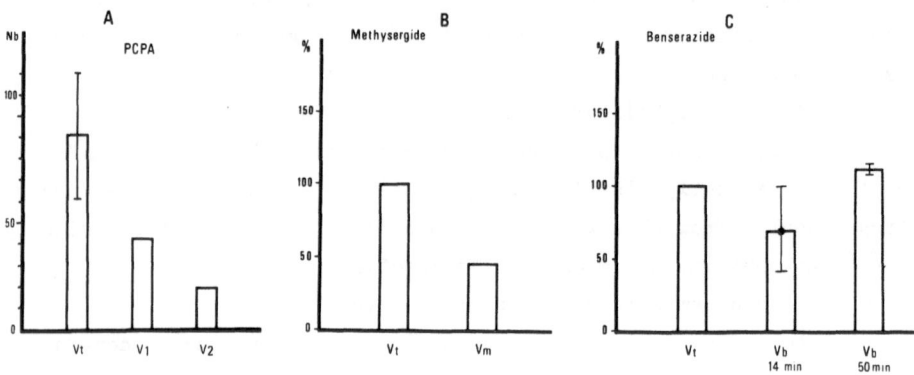

Fig. 5 : Modifications of duodenal spiking activity during vomiting
induced in presence of pCPA (A), Methysergide (B) and Benserazide (C).
 A.
  Nb : number of duodenal spikes.
  Vt : mean spiking and standard deviation during five
vomiting serving as reference.
  V_1, V_2 : first and second vomiting induced after pretreat-
ment with pCPA (25 µg.Kg^{-1} and 1 mg.Kg^{-1} apomorphine respectively).
 B.
  Vt : control recording (spiking activity = 100 %).
  Vm : vomiting induced in the presence of Methysergide
(2 mg.Kg^{-1}).
 C.
  Vt : control recording (spiking activity = 100 %).
  Vb + 14 min : vomiting induced 14 minutes after injection
of Benserazide (50 mg.Kg $^{-1}$, n = 5).
  Vb + 50 min : vomiting induced 50 minutes after injection
of Benserazide (50 mg.Kg^{-1}, n = 5).

mural circuitry, or from a reduction of the central outputs controlling the digestive changes of vomiting. To clarify this point, an inhibitor of the monoamine synthesis was used (Benserazide, 50 mg.Kg^{-1}).
This substance is less specific than pCPA, but has the advantage of
not crossing the blood-brain barrier. After pretreatment with
Benserazide a decrease of the atropine resistant antiperistalsis was
also observed (fig. 5). From all these results, it can be concluded
that a serotoninergic mechanism is, at least in part, involved in the
intramural circuitry organizing the antiperistaltic contraction preceding the expulsion of the gastrointestinal content.

SUMMARY

    - The modifications of gastrointestinal motility during vomiting
are composed of a complete inhibition of movements of the whole gastrointestinal tract, followed by an antiperistaltic contraction which
affects the proximal part of the small bowel just before a powerful
contraction of the abdominal wall, producing the expulsion of the gastric content.
    - The vagal nerves are responsible for all digestive phenomena
(inhibition and then, excitation) occuring during vomiting.
    - The inhibitory phenomena likely result from an activation of
the non-adrenergic non-cholinergic vagal pathway.
    - The antiperistaltic contraction of the small bowel occuring
just before the expulsion is likely controlled by a vagal excitatory
pathway including serotoninergic but not cholinergic nor adrenergic
intramural neurons.

This work was supported in part by a grant from the DRET 81/040.
The authors thank Mrs. E. Dussauze for typing the manuscript.

REFERENCES

1. Borison, H.L. and Wang, S.C. (1949). Functional localization of central coordinating mechanism for emesis in cat. J. Neurophysiol., 12, 305-313.

2. Borison, H.L. and Wang, S.C. (1953). Physiology and pharmacology of vomiting. Pharmacol. Rev., 5, 193-230.

3. Szurszewski, J.H. (1969). A migrating electric complex of the canine small intestine. Amer. J. Physiol., 217, 1757-1763.

4. Code, C.F. and Marlett, J.A. (1975). The interdigestive myoelectric complex of the stomach and the small bowel of the dog. J. Physiol., London, 246, 289-309.

5. Abrahamsson, H., Jansson, G. and Martinson, J. (1973). Vagal relaxation of the stomach induced by apomorphine in the cat. Acta Physiol. Scand., 88, 296-302.

6. Edin, R. (1980). The vagal control of the pyloric motor function : a physiological and immunohistochemical study in cat and man. Acta Physiol. Scand., Suppl. 485, 1-30.

7. Anuras, S. (1981). Effect of dopamine on opossum duodenal smooth muscle. Gastroenterology, 80, 51-54.

8. Dreyfus, C.F., Bornstein, M.B. and Gershon, M.D. (1977). Synthesis of serotonin by neurons of the myenteric plexus in situ and in organotypic tissue culture. Brain Res., 128, 125-139.

9. Gershon, M.D., Dreyfus, C.F., Piekel, V.M., Joh, T.H. and Reis, D.J. (1977). Serotoninergic neurons in the peripheral nervous system : identification in gut by immunohistochemical localization of tryptophan hydroxylase. Proc. Nat. Acad. Sci., 74, 3086-3089.

10. Furness, J.B. and Costa, M. (1973). The nervous release and the actions of substances which affect intestinal muscle through neither adrenoreceptors nor cholinoreceptors. Phil. Trans. Roy. Soc. London B, 265, 123-133.

Section 3
Biliary Tract

29

Enkephalins Mediate Cholecystokinin-Induced Gallbladder Contraction in the Guinea Pig

R. F. CROCHELT, E. SHAW and S. R. PEIKIN

Enkephalinergic nerves are present in the gallbladder but their role is not known. We examined the effect of the σ agonist met-enkephalin (ME), the μ agonist morphine (MS), and the κ agonist dynorphan (DYN) on circular muscle strips prepared from the guinea pig gallbladder.

RESULTS : ME(0.1-100 μM) caused a dose dependent increase in gallbladder tension with an ED50 of 1.7 μM. Although ME was less potent than cholecystokinin-octapeptide (CCK-OP) (ED = 1.9 nM), the peptides had similar efficacy. MS(1 μM-4mM) had no agonist activity. DYN caused a small but significant increase in tension, but was less potent than ME. Naloxone (NAL) caused a dose dependent inhibition of both CCK-OP and ME stimulated contraction. Half-maximal inhibition of contraction stimulated by 5 nM CCK-OP and 5 μM ME was achieved by 4 and 3 μM NAL, respectively. NAL did not alter contraction caused by acetylcholine. Atropine (0.1 mM), dibutyryl cyclic GMP (1.25 mM), methysergide (10 μM) and hexamethonium bromide (10 μM) did not inhibit ME (5 μM) induced contraction.

CONCLUSIONS : ME probably acts directly on gallbladder smooth muscle since muscarinic, CCK, serotoninergic, adrenergic and nicotinic antagonists did not alter ME induced contraction. In addition to a direct effect on gallbladder smooth muscle, CCK-OP may act indirectly by causing release of ME from intramural nerve fibers, since the opiate antagonist NAL inhibited CCK-OP stimulated contraction. ME or other endogenous opiates acting at the σ receptor may play an important role in mediating gallbladder contraction in the guinea pig.

29

Enkephalins Mediate Cholecystokinin-Induced Gallbladder Contraction in the Guinea Pig

R. T. JENSEN, E. SHAW and S. R. PEIKIN

30

Intramural Innervation of the Opossum Sphincter of Oddi

J. F. HELM, J. CHRISTENSEN, W. J. DODDS and S. SARNA

The predominate motor activity of the opossum SO, in vitro as in vivo, is spontaneous peristaltic contractions of myogenic origin that propagate antegrade toward the duodenum. We studied the response of the opossum SO in vitro to intramural nerve stimulation using SO segments from 15 animals. The SO segment, about 3 cm. long, was suspended in a muscle bath. Force transducers recorded circular muscle tension at four sites along the SO. To stimulate intramural nerves, 10–30 s trains of current pulses (16–40 ma, 0.5 ms duration, 5 hz) were delivered to one of three bipolar electrodes implanted along the SO. Antagonists were added to the bath to test their effects on SO responses to nerve stimulation. Results: Nerve stimulation in the proximal, mid or distal SO elicited repetitive peristaltic contractions that invariably originated in the proximal SO and propagated antegrade. These contractions were of similar wave form and duration (2-3 s) to spontaneous contractions. The repetitive contractions usually continued for the duration of the stimulus and occurred at a rate of 12-20/min. This rate was greater than the frequency of spontaneous contractions, 4-8/min. Atropine 10^{-6}M or tetrodotoxin 10^{-6}M completely blocked the excitatory response to nerve stimulation. After Atropine, nerve stimulation in the proximal SO inhibited spontaneous contraction throughout the SO for the duration of the stimulus. Nerve stimulation in the mid or distal SO did not inhibit spontaneous contractions at any site along the SO. The inhibitory response to nerve stimulation was completely blocked by tetrodotoxin, but unaffected by phenoxybenzamine, tolazoline, propranolol, hexamethonium, methysergide, pyrilamine, cimetidine, haloperidol or naloxone. We concluded: 1) Stimulation of intramural nerves at any site along the opossum SO elicits repetitive antegrade peristaltic contractions that resemble spontaneous contractions, but occur at a higher rate, 2) This excitatory response to nerve stimulation is mediated by cholinergic nerves, 3) Cholinergic blockade unmasks an inhibitory response elicited by nerve stimulation of the proximal SO, 4) This response is mediated by nonadrenergic inhibitory nerves.

31

The Relationship between Gastrointestinal Cyclic Motor Activity and Gallbladder Emptying in Humans

K. KRAGLUND, J. HJERMIND, F. T. JENSEN, E. ØSTER-JØRGENSEN,
H. STØDKILDE-JØRGENSEN and S. A. PEDERSEN

During the last decade, the fasting motor pattern of the proximal digestive tract in normal subjects has been shown to consist of periods of quiescence, alternating with contractile motor activity. Recently published studies have demonstrated a marked increase in biliary secretion during the 30 min. period preceding the phase III activity in the duodenum. The purpose of the present study was to investigate the relationshipbetween the interdigestive gastrointestinal motility and the emtying pattern of the human gallbladder and to answer two questions: 1) Does the human gallbladder empty in the fasting state, and 2) if so, is the emtying related to a specific phase of the activity in the gastrointestinal tract.

MATERIAL AND METHODS

The material consisted of 9 healthy volunteers and the motility recordings were done with a 4-lumen tube (COOK-Europe) and a perfused low compliance system. Gallbladder emtying was recorded by the use of scintigraphy with ^{99m}Tc-HIDA$^{(R)}$ (Solco).

RESULTS

The period of investigation ranged from 65 to 220 min. with a mean of 129 min. This rather large variation was in one case the result of a technical failure. ⌡ In the remaining

183

the differences were conditioned by the ability of each subject to keep still under the collimator. The total recording periodwas 19 hr and 25 min. During this period 11 activity fronts were observed and 7 periods of gallbladder
emtying were recorded. Reduction in counts over the gallbladder ranged from 8 to 32%. All emtyings took place in
connection with phase II activity in the intestine. Three
were in close proximity to the following phase III activity
and the remaining four occured early in a phase II. Four
activity fronts were not accompanied by output of bile. In
cases with gallbladder emtying early in Phase II, the duration of phase II was 105, 47, 66 and 54 min., respectively.
The remaining three emtyings corresponded to the entire duration of phase II which were 15, 15 and 36 min.

DISCUSSION

The present results confirm that bile output from the gallbladder varies cyclically according to the different phases
of the migrating motor complex. All emtyings took place in
connection with phase II activity of the intestine, but the
relationship to phase III activity was not constant. We recorded 7 periods of gallbladder emtyings and they all began
in the initial part of phase II activity period. If the phase II in question was short then the emtying continued during the whole period and in close connection with the following phase III. In cases with a longer duration of phase
II the emtying had finished well in advance of phase III
and a free interval of time with no gallbladder emtying
preceded phase III. Accordingly, it is not possible to give
an unequivocal answer to the question whether emtying from
the gallbladder contributes to the increase in bile output
to the duodenum in advance of phase three in the intestine.
In some situations the answer is confirmatory while in
others the emtying takes place to early to be included in
the late phase II duodenal bile output. Furthermore, in
some cases a total migrating motor complex was recorded
from the intestine without being accompanied by gallbladder
emtying. Other factors among which are cyclic secretion of

bile acids from the liver and changes in the resistance of the sphincter of Oddi are mainly responsible for the variations recorded in the bile output to the duodenum.

CONCLUSION

1) Bile output from the gallbladder occurs in fasting humans and 2) gallbladder emtying takes place in connection with phase II activity in the intestine but not always in close connection with the following phase III activity.

32

Defective Gallbladder Contractility Associated with Increased Bile Lithogenicity in Ground Squirrels and Prairie Dogs

J. S. DAVISON, T. M. FRIDHANDLER and E. A. SHAFFER

SUMMARY

Richardson ground squirrels were fed on either a trace cholesterol (control) diet or a 1% w/w cholesterol (test) diet. The lithogenic index of the gallbladder bile increased on the test diet from 0.52 ± 0.03 to 0.81 ± 0.04 ($p < 0.0001$). The isometric tensions generated *in vitro* by cholecystokinin octapeptide (CCK_8), acetylcholine (Ach) and depolarization by 70 mM K^+ solutions were significantly reduced by 50% though there was no shift in the normalized dose-response curve. In those animals which proceeded to the stage of cholesterol stone formation the defect in gallbladder contractility became even more severe. Ileal muscle from test animals showed no loss of contractility in response to any of the three stimuli. A similar defect occurred in prairie dogs associated with increased lithogenicity.

Thus, in these animal models, there is a clear and apparently specific defect in gallbladder contractility which onsets with early changes in bile lithogenicity and becomes progressively worse as cholesterol stones develop. This defect would contribute to gallbladder stasis which, in turn, might be a significant factor in the eventual formation of cholesterol gallstones.

INTRODUCTION

The production by the liver of bile supersaturated with cholesterol is recognized as being of primary importance in the aetiology of

cholesterol gallstone formation. However, this simple physico-
chemical explanation alone is inadequate. Cholelithiasis is accompanied by biliary stasis (1) which has long been considered to be a
potentially important factor since gallstones form almost exclusively
in the gallbladder even though other biliary compartments may contain
bile of equal or greater lithogenicity (2). This could be due as
much to the regulation of the enterohepatic circulation of bile salts
by the gallbladder as to the increased time available for the nuclea-
tion of cholesterol crystals.

One of the potential causes of biliary stasis is an increase in
cystic duct resistance which has been observed in the prairie dog
model of cholelithiasis (3). In that particular investigation,
malfunction of the gallbladder was largely discounted. The present
study demonstrates that a loss of gallbladder contractility is
associated with the early stages of cholesterol stone formation in at
least two animal models and may, therefore, be a highly significant
factor generally in this disease.

METHODS

Adult male ground squirrels (*Spermophilus richardsoni*) of mean weight
504g, trapped near Calgary, Alberta, were caged individually in
thermoregulated rooms at 23^0C on a 12/12 hr day/night light cycle.
After one month on a standard laboratory rat chow diet (cholesterol
content 0.027%), the animals were divided into two dietary groups for
an additional 14 days. The control group remained on the standard
diet, the test group had the same diet supplemented with cholesterol
(1%).

After 14 days the animals were fasted overnight for 16 hrs then
guilloteened. Each gallbladder was removed intact and set up in an
isolated organ bath for recording isometric tension changes along the
cystic duct-fundic pole axis. The bath contained modified Krebs-
Henseleit solution (4) at 37^0C, gassed with 95% O_2, 5% CO_2. The
initial resting tension was adjusted to 0.7g which in preliminary
experiments had been ascertained as being optimal for establishing
active tension changes in response to transmural electrical stimulation.

In the first series of experiments, responses to cholecystokinin octapeptide (CCK$_8$) in test and control animals were compared. In a second series of experiments, responses to CCK$_8$, Ach and high K$^+$ solutions were measured. In addition, in the second series, segments of terminal ileum were also removed and their responses to the same stimuli were observed.

Adult prairie dogs (*Cynomys ludovicianus*) were grouped into 6 control and 6 test animals and maintained on the same regimes as described for the ground squirrels. *In vitro* gallbladder responses to ED$_{100}$ CCK$_8$ were measured as described above.

Bile salts, cholesterol and phospholipids were measured in gall-bladder bile samples as described previously (2) and the lithogenic index calculated from the polynominal equations of Carey and Small at 37^{0}C with appropriate adjustment for total solid content (5). Results are given as mean±SE.

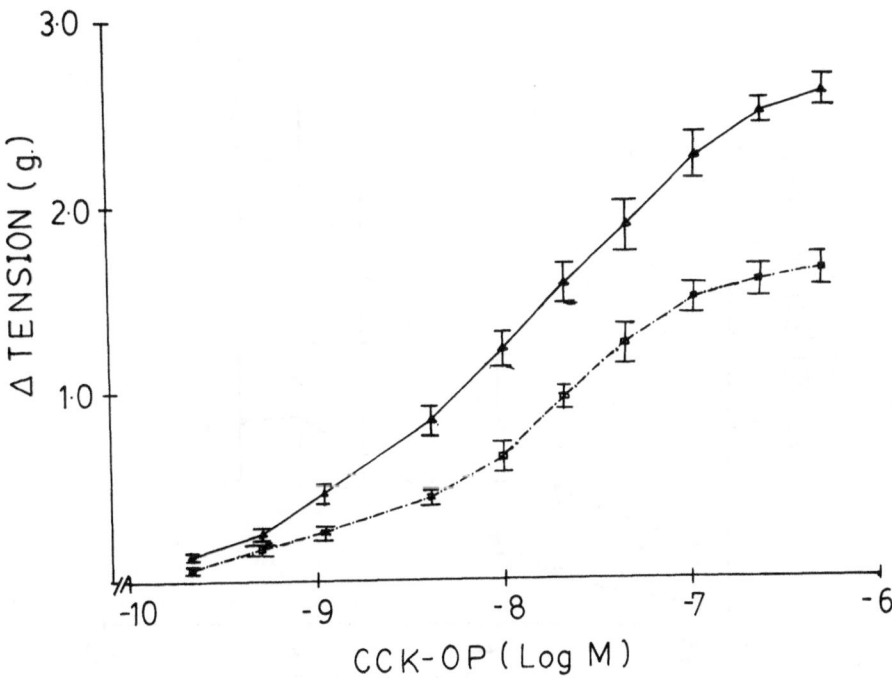

FIGURE 1   Response of isolated gallbladders to cholecystokinin
           octapeptide (CCK-OP).   Triangles - control animals;
           squares - test animals

RESULTS

Series 1   (12 test: 8 control animals)

The lithogenic index of gallbladder bile increased significantly
(p<0.0001) from a value of 0.52±0.03 in controls to 0.81±0.04 in
test animals (where a value of 1.0 represents saturation). None of
the animals developed microcrystals or stones. Serum cholesterol
increased from 293±26mg% in control animals to 491±61mg% in test
animals (p<0.005).

   Test animals showed a marked and significant reduction in tensions
generated *in vitro* in response to CCK_8 throughout the dose-response
curve (Fig 1). When the CCK_8 response curves were normalized to their
respective maximum (100%) activity, however, there was no significant
shift between the two groups. There was a linear correlation between
the lithogenic index or absolute cholesterol concentration and the
tension generated at ED_{50} CCK_8 : r = 0.6 (p<0.01) and r = 0.6 (p<0.05)
respectively.

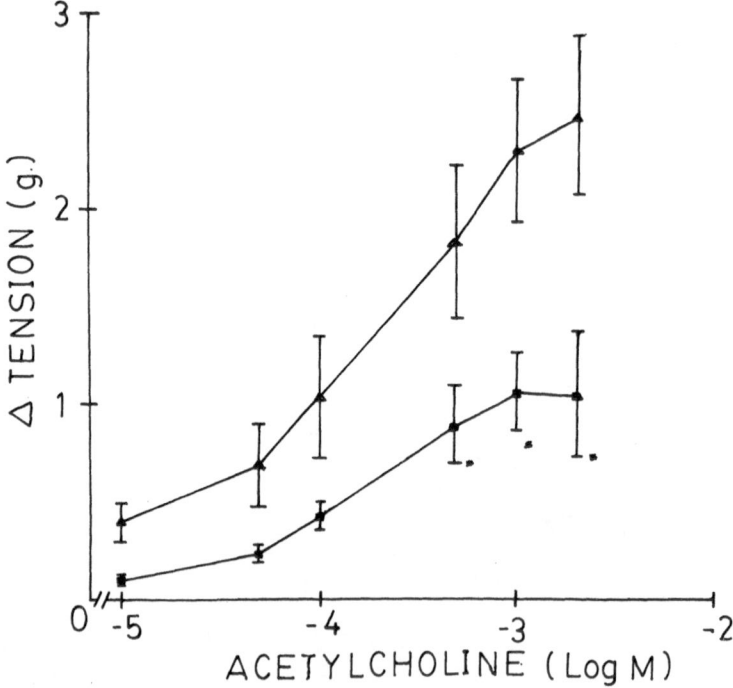

FIGURE 2   Response of isolated gallbladders to acetylcholine (Ach)
           Triangles - control animals; squares - test animals

Series 2   (6 control: 6 test animals)

A similar impairment of gallbladder contractility was seen in response
to Ach (Fig 2) and high K^+ solutions (Fig 3) in the test animals.
Again, however, normalized dose response curves were similar in
control and test animals. In this series, 3 animals on the test diet
developed cholesterol crystals and stones that were predominantly
cholesterol in composition (64%, 85%, 100%). Tensions generated in
response to ED_{100} CCK_8, Ach and high K^+ solutions showed a significantly greater deterioration at each stage of stone formation (Fig 4).

   Terminal ileum responses to all stimuli were similar in test and
control animals. Adult male prairie dogs fed a high cholesterol diet
also showed a significant increase in lithogenic index: control
0.72 ± 0.11; test 1.24 ± 0.16 ($p < 0.02$), and a significantly reduced
tension response to ED_{100} CCK_8 : control 4.2 ± 0.6g; test 2.8 ± 0.1g
($p < 0.02$).

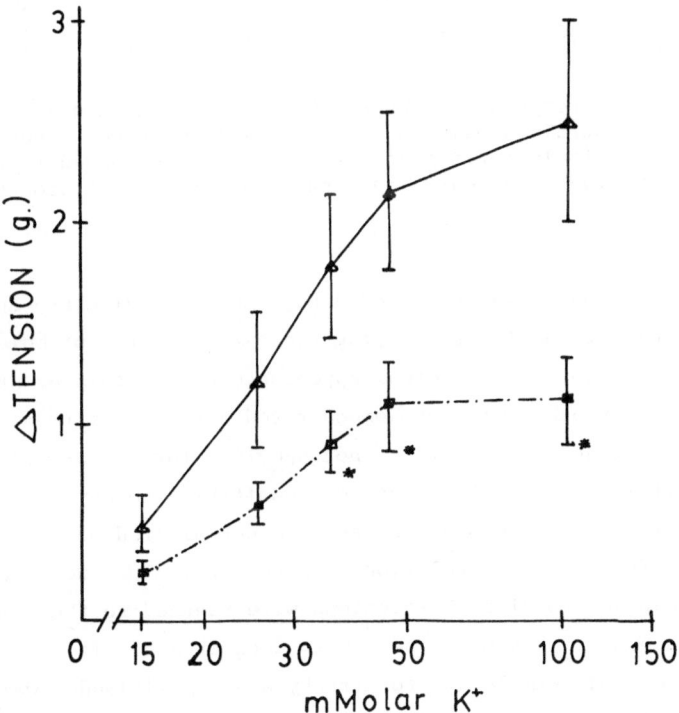

FIGURE 3 Responses of isolated gallbladders to high K^+ solution
       in presence of atropine (3.5×10^{-6}M)
       Triangles – control animals; squares – test animals

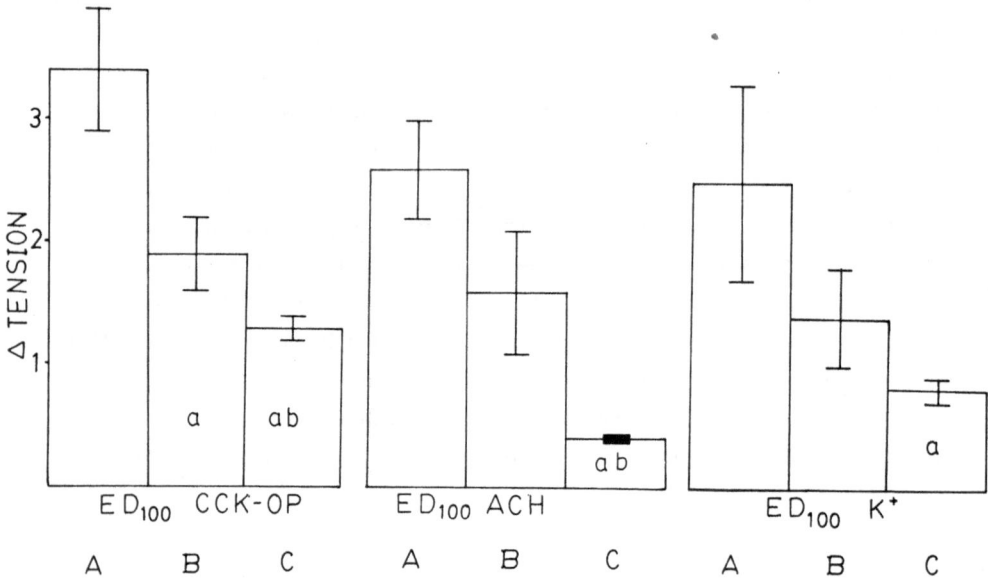

FIGURE 4   Tension responses to ED_{100} CCK-OP, Ach and high K^+ solutions.
A - control animals; B - test animals with no stones; C -
test animals forming stones.   a. $p<0.05$ compared to controls.
b. $p<0.05$ compared to test gallbladder without stones.

DISCUSSION

The Richardson ground squirrel, fed a high cholesterol diet, appears
to be an excellent model for studying the early events in cholesterol
cholelithiasis prior to the actual appearance of crystals or stones.
During this early phase we have demonstrated severe impairment of
gallbladder contractility that was not specific for any particular
stimulus. It was not due to a loss of sensitivity to any agonist
since normalized dose-response curves were not altered and could not
be accounted for by down regulation of receptors, since non-receptor-
mediated responses to high K^+ solutions were reduced to the same
extent as receptor mediated responses to CCK_8 or Ach. It is unlikely
that the defect was simply due to atrophy since gallbladder weights
were similar in both groups and light microscopy revealed no morphologic differences. The defect seems to be specific for gallbladder
muscle since responses of terminal ileum from animals on the test diet
showed no difference from controls in response to all three stimuli.

The less extensive study in the prairie dog, an established model for cholesterol cholelithiasis, produced the same picture of a generalized defect in gallbladder contractility occurring during the early stages of cholelithiasis.

In these animal models, therefore, it appears likely that a defective gallbladder would play a major role in the biliary stasis which accompanies cholesterol cholelithiasis. Moreover, because the defect occurs so early, and becomes progressively worse as stones develop, it is possible that stasis may be an even more significant factor in cholelithiasis than previously supposed.

The mechanism responsible for this defect can only be speculated upon at present, one potential candidate being prostaglandins. Cholesterol feeding in prairie dogs results in a striking increase in gallbladder mucin synthesis and secretion within five days, prior to the appearance of cholesterol gallstones (6). This accelerated release of mucin is markedly inhibited both *in vitro* and *in vivo* by aspirin (7) and by indomethacin (8), suggesting that prostaglandins might be involved. It would appear that in this animal model of cholesterol gallstone formation, mucin hypersecretion may be regulated in part by endogenous levels of prostacyclin, the major cyclo-oxygenase product in the prairie dog gallbladder epithelium. These events occur before stones develop. Curiously the only known physiological stimulus to mucin secretion in the gallbladder is CCK (9). The origin of the prostaglandin may be derived from hepatic bile which contains both arachidonic acid in phospholipids (10) as well as free prostaglandins (11). The possibility therefore exists that arachidonic acid in biliary phospholipids might be converted to prostaglandin and hence alter the mediation of gallbladder contraction.

REFERENCES

1. vonHelmsbach, M. (1856). In: Mikrugeologie. Berlin: Reimer
2. Shaffer, E. A. and Small, D. M. (1977). Biliary lipid secretion in cholesterol gallstone disease. The effect of cholecystectomy and obesity. J. Clin. Invest. 59, 828-40
3. Pitt, H. A., Doty, J. E., DenBesten, L. and Kuchenbecker, S. L. (1982). Stasis before gallstone formation: altered gallbladder compliance or cystic resistance? Am. J. Surg. 43, 144-9

4. Davison, J. S., Pearson, G. T. and Petersen, O. H. (1980). Mouse pancreatic acinar cells: effects of electrical field stimulation on membrane potential and resistance. J. Physiol. (Lond) 301, 295-305

5. Carey, M. C. and Small, D. M. (1978). The physical chemistry of cholesterol solubility in bile: relationship to gallstone formation and dissolution in man. J. Clin. Invest. 61, 998-1026

6. Lee, S. P., LaMont, J. T. and Carey, M. C. (1981). Role of gallbladder mucus hypersecretion in the evolution of cholesterol gallstones. Studies in the prairie dog. J. Clin. Invest. 67, 1712-23

7. Lee, S. P., Carey, M. C. and LaMont, J. T. (1981). Aspirin prevention of cholesterol gallstone formation in prairie dogs. Science 211, 1429-31

8. LaMont, J. T., Turner, B. S., DiBenetetto, D., Handin, R. and Schafer, N. A. I. (1983). Arachidonic acid stimulates mucin secretion in prairie dog gallbladder. Am. J. Physiol. 245, 992-8

9. Wahlin, T., Bloom, G. D. and Danielsson, A. (1976). Effect of cholecystokinin-pancreozymin (CCK-PZ) on glucoprotein secretion from mouse gallbladder epithelium. Cell Tissue Res. 171, 425-35

10. Ahlberg, J., Curstedt, T., Einarsson, K. and Sjovall, J. (1981). Molecular species of biliary phosphatidylcholines in gallstone patients: the influence of treatment with cholic acid and chenodeoxycholic acid. J. Lipid Res. 22, 404-9

11. Desphande, Y. G. and Kaminski, L. K. (1980). Identification and quantitation by radioimmunoassay of prostaglandin F_1 compounds in bile. Prostaglandins 20, 367-72

ACKNOWLEDGEMENTS

We are indebted to Dave Kirk, Shelley Wilson and Val Dickson for their expert technical support and to Jo Anna Swainger for typing the manuscript.

33

Prostaglandins Modulate Human Gallbladder Motility

C. KOTWALL, F. LENNON, A. S. CLANACHAN, H. P. BAER
and G. W. SCOTT

INTRODUCTION

The effects of prostaglandins (PGs) and related substances on gallbladder motility have been studied in several species. They produce concentration-dependent contractions of guinea-pig(1) and cat(2) gallbladder muscle. Responses of dog gallbladder are variable but concentration-dependent contractions occur after incubation of tissues in indomethacin(3), which inhibits the synthesis of PGs. Wood et al.(4) found that human gallbladder muscle, obtained from patients undergoing cholecystectomy, responded irregularly and only to high concentrations of PGs. This was also our initial experience, but we then found that a large part of the variability of responses could be related to the method of collecting the specimens from the operating room, the severity of the inflammatory and degenerative processes in the gallbladders and presumably to the level of endogenous production of PG-like substances. These factors were taken into account and controlled as far as possible in the present study.

MATERIALS AND METHODS

Portions of freshly removed gallbladders were obtained from 85 patients who had undergone cholecystectomy for cholesterol gallstone disease. The period of ischaemia was less than 20 min. The tissues were placed in ice-cold oxygenated Krebs solution and transported to the laboratory.   Each specimen was cut into 2 x 10 mm strips, mounted in 5 ml organ baths containing Krebs solution at 37°C and aerated with 95% O_2 and 5% CO_2.   The strips were adjusted to an initial tension of 0.5 g and allowed to equilibrate for 40 min under a slow Krebs wash.   Isometric contractions were recorded via Grass FTO3C force displacement transducers and Beckman multichannel recorders.   The contractile response to a maximally effective concentration of acetylcholine (1 mM) was recorded after the initial equilibration period and at the end of each experiment.   Following this initial stimulation, 30 min were allowed to elapse prior to studying the effects of PGs.   Half of the strips were incubated in Krebs solution containing indomethacin (10^{-5}M).   PGs were tested in a non-cumulative fashion and concentration-response curves were constructed; responses were expressed as a percentage of the maximal contraction of each strip.   Adjacent strips of each tissue were processed for histological examination and classified as having mild chronic cholecystitis, severe chronic cholecystitis or acute cholecystitis. This was based on the inflammatory and degenerative changes in the mucosa, muscle layer and subserosa.

Prostaglandins and sources were PGE_1, PGE_2, $PGF_2 \alpha$ (Sigma Chemical Co., St. Louis, Mo); endoperoxide analogue U-44069 (The Upjohn Co., Kalamazoo, Mich.); prostacyclin (Dr. J. Scholtholt, Hoechst AG, Frankfurt); leukotrienes B_4, C_4, D_4 (Dr. J. Rokach, Merck Frosst Canada Inc., Quebec).

RESULTS

Histologically, 50 of the gallbladders had mild chronic cholecystitis and 20 had severe chronic cholecystitis. Fifteen had acute cholecystitis, in which an acute inflammatory reaction, oedema and extravasation of red blood corpuscles were superimposed on chronic cholecystitis; there were marked degenerative changes in both the muscle and mucosal layers.

Approximately 90% of the muscle strips from each of these three grades of cholecystitis showed varying levels of spontaneous rhythmical contractions, occurring 2-3 times per min.   Indomethacin suppressed or abolished these spontaneous contractions in 90% of the muscle strips with chronic cholecystitis and in 60% of those with acute cholecystitis. Drug-induced contractile responses temporarily abolished spontaneous rhythmical contractions, thus allowing quantitation of responses.

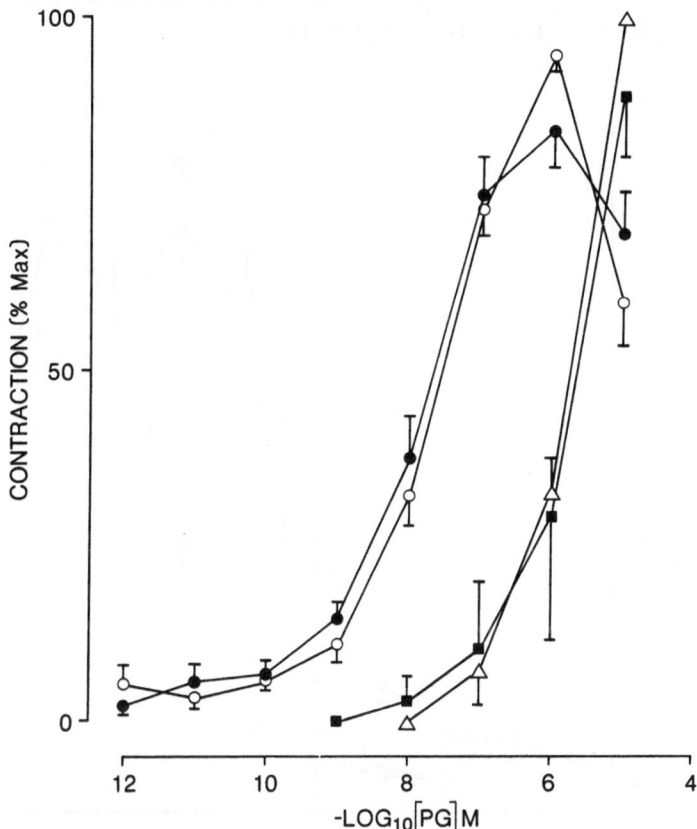

FIGURE 1   Contractile responses of strips of human gallbladders with chronic cholecystitis to PGs. The tissues were in Krebs solution containing indomethacin (10^{-5}M). Prostaglandins PGE_1 ($\bigcirc$), (n=17); PGE_2 ($\bullet$) (n=17); $PGF_2 \alpha$ ($\blacksquare$), (n=9); PGD_2 ($\triangle$), (n=6). The contractions are expressed as percentages of the maximal responses obtained. Note that maximal contractions were not obtained with $PGF_2 \alpha$ and PGD_2; these were plotted as percentages of the maximum obtainable contractions. Points are means ± SEM.

The responses of gallbladders with mild or severe chronic cholecystitis to PGs were similar, so they are grouped together. In 80% of these strips PGE_1 and PGE_2 produced concentration-dependent contractions. In the remainder spontaneous rhythmical contractions were marked and no responses were observed. However, after incubation with indomethacin, PGE_1 and PGE_2 produced concentration-dependent contractions in all strips (Figure 1). The mean maximal response to PGE_1, or PGE_2 was 0.5 g tension compared with a mean maximal response of 1.7 g to acetylcholine.

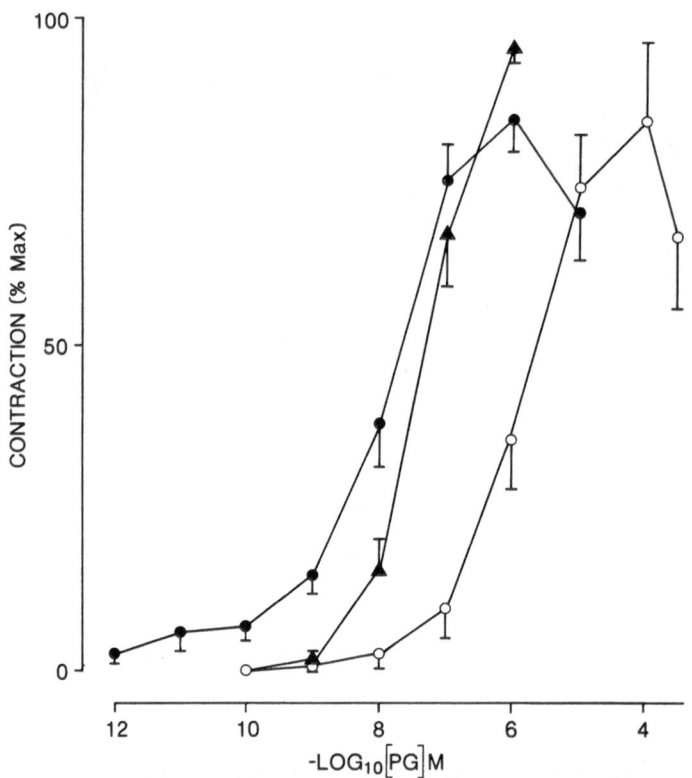

FIGURE 2   Contractile responses of strips of human gallbladders with chronic cholecystitis to PGs and related substances. The tissues were in Krebs solution containing indomethacin $(10^{-5}M)$. Prostaglandins PGE_2 (●), (n=17); PGB_2 (○), (n=7) and the synthetic analogue U-44069 (▲), (n=8). The contractions are expressed as percentages of the maximal contractions, but maximal responses were not obtained for U-44069. Points are means ± SEM.

$PGF_2\alpha$, PGD_2, PGB_2 and U-44069 produced concentration-dependent contractions in all strips regardless of their level of spontaneous activity and both in the presence and absence of indomethacin (Figures 1 and 2). Prostacyclin ($5.7x10^{-11}$ to 2.9×10^{-6}M) had no effect, but produced concentration-dependent contractions of guinea pig gallbladder strips in the presence or absence of indomethacin. Similarly, neither leukotriene (LT) C_4 nor LTD_4 showed any effects upon human gallbladders in the presence or absence of indomethacin

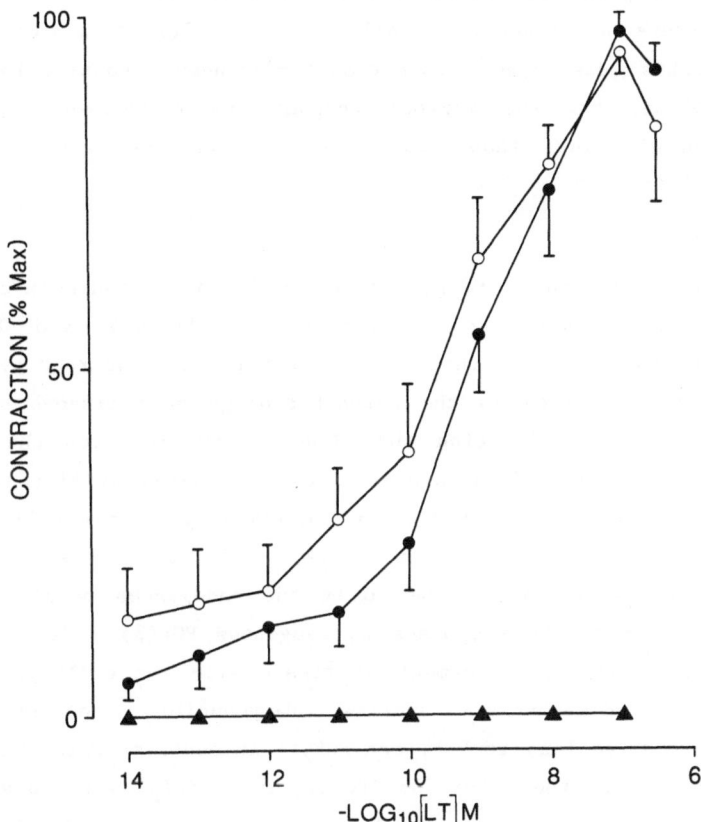

FIGURE 3   Contractile responses of strips of human gallbladders with chronic cholecystitis to leukotrienes C4 and D4 (▲), (n=6) and of strips of guinea-pig gallbladders to LTC_4 (●), (n=8) and LTD_4 (○), (n=8). The contractions are expressed as percentages of the maximal contractions. Points are means ± SEM. Note the lack of response of human gallbladder strips to these leukotrienes.

but produced contractions of guinea pig gallbladder (Figure 3). LTB_4 was inactive in both human and guinea-pig gallbladders, with or without indomethacin.

The 15 gallbladders with acute cholecystitis (superimposed on chronic cholecystitis) were remarkably poorly responsive. PGE_1 and PGE_2 produced either small relaxations or no responses; no contractile responses were seen. PGE_1 or PGE_2 in the presence of indomethacin produced concentration-dependent contractions in only two of these gallbladders. All of the gallbladders with acute cholecystitis displayed concentration-dependent contractions to acetylcholine, but the maximal response (mean tension=0.8g) was significantly less than that in the tissues with chronic cholecystitis.

DISCUSSION

The local production of PGs is increased in some chronic intestinal inflammatory diseases such as ulcerative colitis(5) and Crohn's disease(6) and may be increased in cholecystitis. Indirect evidence that PGs are involved in the pathophysiology of gallstone disease arises from the observation that indomethacin relieves the acute abdominal pain and tenderness associated with cholecystitis(7).

However, the effects of PGs on the motility of the gallbladder have been reported to be variable(4). A major cause of this experimental variability seems to be the endogenous production of PGs which obscure the responses to exogenous PGs(3). As shown in the present study, pretreatment of tissue with the cyclo-oxygenase inhibitor, indomethacin, unmasks reproducible concentration-dependent contractions to PGE_1 and PGE_2. In contrast with these two PGs, responses to the other PGs ($PGF_2 \alpha$, PGD_2, PGB_2) were consistent in the presence or absence of indomethacin. This might indicate that the endogenous production of PGs consists mostly of PGE_1 and PGE_2. Preliminary estimations (n=3) by high performance liquid chromatography of endogenous PG release indicate that PGE_2, LTB_4 and LTC_4 are released from tissues with chronic cholecystitis.

It is possible that endogenous production of PGs may contribute to spontaneous rhythmical contractions in gallbladders with chronic cholecystitis. However, as spontaneous contractions are abolished by indomethacin in only 60% of tissues with acute cholecystitis other, as yet unidentified mechanisms, may be involved. Furthermore, we do not believe that the lack of responsiveness of tissues with acute cholecystitis to PGs is due to diminished sensitivity. Rather, it appears to us that it is due to degenerative changes in the muscle and marked oedema of the tissues. There was a 53% reduction in the maximal responses to acetylcholine and this could have made it difficult to detect the much smaller responses to PGs.

Quantification of PG and LT release from diseased gallbladder tissues and the use of selective cyclo-oxygenase and lipoxygenase inhibitors may provide further evidence that these substances can modulate biliary motility in choleystitis.

ACKNOWLEDGEMENTS

Supported by MRC (Canada) and the Alberta Heritage Foundation for Medical Research. We thank Dawne Colwell for her expert technical assistance.

REFERENCES

1. Nakata, K., Osumi, Y. and Fujiwara, M. (1981). Prostaglandins and the contractility of the guinea-pig biliary system. Pharmacology, 22, 24-30

2. Thornell, E., Svanvik, J. and Wood, J.R. (1981). Effects of intra-arterial PGE_2 on gallbladder fluid transport, motility and hepatic bile flow in the cat. Scand.J.Gastroent. 16, 1083-88

3. Mroczka, J., Baer, H.P. and Scott, G.W. (1982). Effects of prostaglandins on isolated dog gallbladder and cystic duct. In: Weinbeck, M. (ed). Motility of the Digestive Tract. pp. 421-26. (New York:Raven Press).

4. Wood, J.R., Saverymuttu, S.H., Ashbrooke, A.B. and Stamford, I.F. (1980). Effects of various prostanoids on gallbladder muscle. In: Samuelsson, B., Ramwell, P.W. and Paoletti, R. (eds). Advances in Prostaglandin and Thromboxane Research. Vol. XIII: pp. 1569-71. (New York:Raven Press).

5. Sharon, P., Ligumsky, M., Rachmilewitz, D. and Zor, U. (1978). Role of prostaglandins in ulcerative colitis: enhanced production during active disease and inhibition by Sulfasalazine. Gastroenterology, 75, 638-40

6.   Rachmiliewitz D., Karmeli, F., Zifroni, A., Hawkey, C.J. and Sachar, D.B. (1982).   Enhanced intestinal prostanoid synthesis in Crohn's disease. Gastroenterology, 82, 1154.

7.   Thornell, E., Jansson, R. and Svanvik, J.   (1981). Indomethacin intravenously – a new way for effective relief of biliary pain: a double-blind study in man. Surgery 90, 468-72.

34

Fasting Canine Biliary Secretion and the Sphincter of Oddi

R. B. SCOTT, S. M. STRASBERG, T. Y. EL-SHARKAWY and N. E. DIAMANT

This study correlates the fasting delivery of bile acids into the duodenum with motility of the sphincter of Oddi (SO). Dogs were prepared with a functional cholecystectomy, a duodenal cannula for direct vision cannulation of the common bile duct, and 12 bipolar electrodes implanted from stomach to terminal ileum. In one set of experiments, a double lumen tube was positioned in the duodenum with one orifice at the level of the SO and a second 10 cm distally. The bile acid pool was depleted, and during a continuous IV infusion of Na taurocholate (20 uMole/min) bile acid delivery into the duodenum was assessed over 6 hours by a marker perfusion technique. In other experiments, a 2-lumen continuously perfused manometry catheter was placed to record motility in the bile duct, and SO for a period of 6 hours. Station pullthroughs of the SO were performed in each phase of the MMC.

RESULTS: Bile acid secretion rates fluctuated about the IV infusion rate during duodenal Phase I and II, peaked in late Phase II, and then fell to barely detectable levels during Phase III. Phasic contractions of the SO were intermittent during Phase I, increasingly frequent during Phase II, and continuous and maximal during duodenal Phase III of the MMC. Contractions were frequently peristaltic.

CONCLUSIONS: During fasting, the SO has a positive baseline pressure upon which phasic contractions are superimposed.   The occurrence and amplitude of phasic peristaltic contractions of the sphincter of Oddi are cyclically coordinated with the fasting intestinal motor pattern (MMC), and the cyclical variations in the delivery of bile acids into the duodenum.   This suggests that during fasting, the SO is a factor coordinating the cyclic delivery of bile acids into the duodenum with the MMC.   Both resting pressure and phasic contractions of the sphincter appear to play a role, with the net effect of intense phasic motor activity being that of impeding bile flow.

35

Stomach Motility Modulates Bile Flow in the Pig

V. RAYNER, G. WENHAM and P. C. GREGORY

INTRODUCTION

The secretory function of the upper digestive tract has been related
to the phases of the migrating myoelectric complex (MMC): in man the
pancreatic secretion of lipase and biliary secretion of bilirubin was
greatest during duodenal regular spiking activity (RSA)(1); in the dog
the amount of alkali secreted into the upper intestine progressively
increased during irregular spiking activity (ISA) to a maximum rate
just before the RSA in the duodenum (2) and the pH in the duodenum
reached its maximum value after the passage of the RSA through the
duodenum (3). However, it has been suggested that in the pig the pH
changes in the duodenum can be accounted for by the variations in
flow of acid digesta from the stomach with the phase of the MMC while
the rate of digestive secretion remains constant; there is no need –
at least as far as pH is concerned – to postulate a secretory
correlate of the MMC (4). In this paper we correlate the pattern of
bile flow as shown by X-ray screening with the pattern of myoelectric
activity and pH changes in the duodenum of the pig.

METHODS

Nichrome wire electrodes (120 μm diameter) were chronically implanted
in 4 pigs, weight 22-25 kg, in the stomach (10 and 20 cm before the
pylorus), the duodenal bulb and duodenum (2, 10 and 20 cm from the
pylorus), the common bile duct (CBD) and the body of the gall bladder.
A small PVC catheter (internal diameter 1.3 mm) was sewn into the

fundus of the gall bladder through which contrast medium was injected
(Biligram 35%, Schering). One of the four pigs was prepared with a
gastrojejunostomy and in another the mesenteric attachment of the CBD
to the stomach was severed. The other two pigs were fitted with
a catheter in the abdominal aorta to allow the infusion of
cholecystokinin octapeptide (CCK-OP).

Three pigs were prepared with electrodes as in the first series but
with half-bridge strain gauge transducers sewn to the gall bladder
and another 3 pigs had electrodes on the stomach and duodenum only but
with a large catheter (internal diameter 4mm) in the duodenal bulb.
Through this catheter a pH probe (Pye-Ingold type 140) was passed to
record variations of pH in the duodenal bulb at the choledochoduodenal
junction.

After recovery from surgery the pigs were placed in metabolism
cages and fed a barley-based meal twice daily. Myoelectric activity
was continuously recorded on a Grass model 7 polygraph using AC
preamplifiers with a time constant of 3 Hz; gall bladder movements
and pH measurements were recorded on the same polygraph using DC
preamplifiers. For the radiographic examination pigs were put in a
sling in front of an X-ray image intensifier and the polygraph was
reconnected. The gall bladder was emptied of bile and an equal
volume of contrast medium was injected. Screening was continued for
at least one MMC cycle.

RESULTS

Bile flow during periods of stomach motility

Contrast medium passed through the choledochoduodenal junction into the
duodenal bulb at all phases of the MMC in the duodenum. However flow
was modulated by stomach motility: before the stomach contraction
reached the middle one third of the pyloric antrum, the CBD remained
straight (Fig. 1a); as the wave of stomach contraction reached the
middle one third of the antrum, the contracted region of the lesser
curvature of the stomach pulled the mesenteric attachment of the CBD
causing the CBD to bend around the dilatation ahead of the contraction
(Fig. 1b) and bile was expelled entering the duodenal bulb just before
the bolus of stomach contents. The mixture of bile and digesta was
then propelled onwards by a contraction of the duodenal bulb
initiating a peristaltic rush through the duodenum.

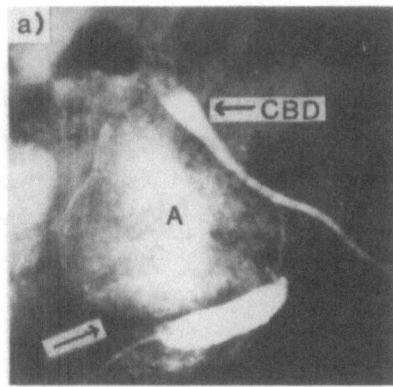 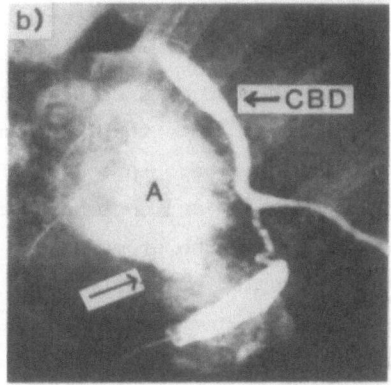

FIGURE 1   Relationship between antral contraction and bending
           movements of the common bile duct (CBD). a) CBD is
           straight when the stomach contraction (↗) is in the
           proximal one third of the pyloric antrum (A). b) The
           CBD is pulled ventrally to bend around the dilatation
           ahead of the contraction (↗) now in the middle third of
           the antrum (A).

In serial radiographs the bent CBD was observed to be 15% shorter than
the straight CBD. The frequency of bending of CBD is identical to the
frequency of stomach contraction. In the fasting pig the stomach
does not contract with every slow wave and contractions of the
stomach and bending movements of the CBD occurred in the same pattern
and at the same frequency (2.3 ± 0.1/min). When the pig was fed,
both stomach contractions and bending movements of the CBD occurred
with every slow wave (frequency 4.2 ± 0.1/min). A much greater
quantity of bile entered the duodenum and the gall bladder emptied of
contrast medium within 20 min of feeding.

   In the preparations in which the CBD was detached from the stomach
by gastrojejunostomy or severing the mesentery, no bending movements
were detected with stomach contractions. In one of the four
preparations peristalsis was seen along the length of the CBD at the
same frequency as gastric contractions. Histology showed some smooth
muscle fibres in the CBD. Low voltage slow waves and spikes (50-100µV)
were recorded in the CBD at the same frequency and in the same pattern
as stomach contractions (Fig. 2). It was still possible to record
these potentials in the preparation in which the mesentery had been
severed.

Bile flow during stomach quiescence

In the fasted pig, when an RSA occurred in the duodenum stomach motility ceased for 18.1 ± 0.8 min. At this time the bending movements of the CBD also ceased but bile flow did not. A slow flow of contrast medium into the duodenum continued throughout the period of stomach quiescence. After the RSA the duodenum and duodenal bulb were also quiescent and contrast medium entered the duodenal bulb and trickled back into the stomach. In fed pigs, although a duodenal RSA was seen within 100 min of feeding, the period of stomach quiescence was very short and no contrast medium trickled back through the pylorus.

The effect of cholecystokinin

The effects of intra-arterial injections of CCK-OP depended on the dose. Small amounts (0.5-2 µg) caused the CBD to clear of contrast medium, suggesting an increased rate of hepatic bile flow without any apparent gall bladder contraction. Higher doses (4-20 µg) caused progressively greater gall bladder contraction and expulsion of contrast medium. There was no change in the pattern of CBD movements when CCK-OP was injected.

Gall bladder motility

In both fasted and fed pigs phasic movements of the gall bladder were recorded from the transducer in the same pattern and at the same frequency (2.2 ± 0.1/min fasted, 4.2 ± 0.1/min fed) as stomach contractions (Fig. 2). The amplitude of these movements was greater in fed pigs (5-15 g versus 2-7 g in fasted pigs). In fasted pigs movements of the gall bladder ceased during periods of stomach quiescence after the RSA in the duodenum. Gall bladder tone slightly increased (3-7 g) during periods of stomach contraction in fasting pigs. In fed pigs gall bladder tone increased by 5-12 g within 20-30 min of feeding. Myoelectric activity of the gall bladder was difficult to record without artefact but myoelectric activity at stomach frequency was not usually seen.

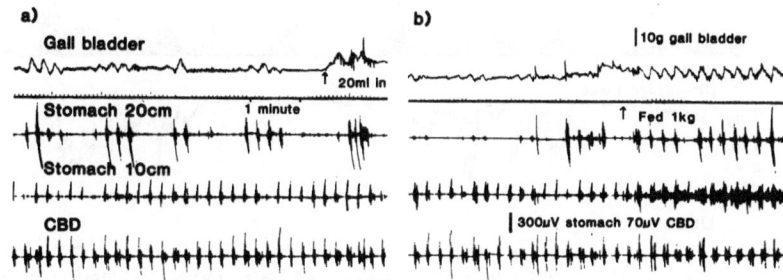

FIGURE 2   Relationship between gall bladder movements and myoelectric
           activity on stomach and CBD. Gall bladder movements are in
           the same pattern and frequency as stomach myoelectric activity
           20 cm from the pylorus. CBD and stomach myoelectric activity
           10 cm from the pylorus are similar. a) During ISA on
           duodenum b) at the end of duodenal and stomach quiescence
           and at the start of feeding.

pH changes with the duodenal MMC

The pattern of pH change was similar to that reported for the distal
duodenum beyond the pancreatic duct (4). In fasted pigs the duodenal
pH varied during ISA (minimum 2.3 $\pm$ 0.1, maximum 5.7 $\pm$ 0.1) rising to
6.9 $\pm$ 0.1 during the quiescent phase (Fig. 3). In fed pigs the pH
was higher (6.3 $\pm$ 0.2) throughout the MMC, the oscillations in pH
with the MMC progressively reappearing after feeding (average time
209 $\pm$ 25 min).

DISCUSSION

There has been some controversy whether peristalsis occurs in the CBD
and so makes a contribution to the transport of bile (5). The amount
and orientation of smooth muscle in the CBD varies with species and
some studies (6) have suggested that contraction of longitudinal
smooth muscle may be of greater importance than peristalsis involving
circular muscle fibres. Our experiments provided some evidence that
in pigs both weak peristaltic contractions of the CBD and lengthening
and shortening of the CBD occurred in phase with stomach contractions.
Myoelectric activity of the CBD occurred at the frequency of stomach
contractions as had been previously observed (7) and may be caused by
electrotonic transmission of stomach potentials. The influence of
such contractions on bile flow, however, may well have been less than
the effects of the conspicuous bending and straightening of the

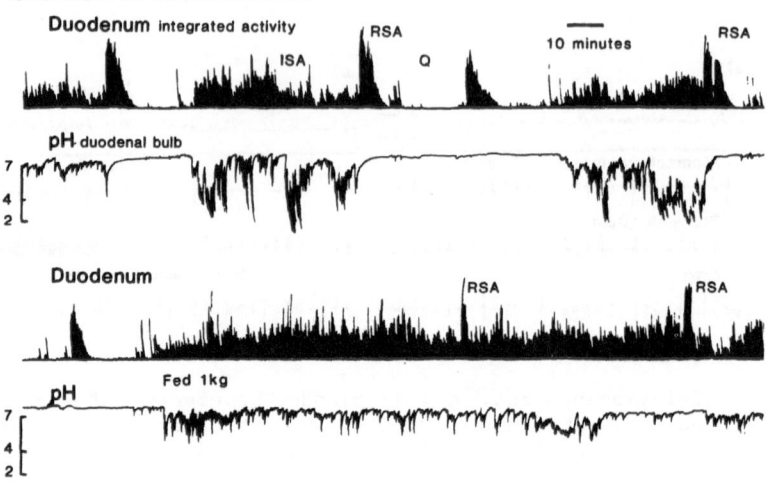

FIGURE 3 pH changes in the duodenal bulb with the phase of the MMC. The pH decreases when stomach contents enter the duodenum during ISA in the fasting pig and rises to 7.0-7.4 during quiescence after the RSA. In the fed pig the pH fluctuates from 5-7 with no change at the RSA.

CBD caused by the physical pulling of the lesser curvature of the stomach as each stomach contraction swept over the antrum. Gall bladder movements also occurred at the frequency of stomach contractions, as has been reported for the dog (8), and may also contribute to the pulsatile pattern of bile flow. Myoelectric activity of the gall bladder did not appear to be at the frequency of stomach contractions suggesting that the movements recorded reflect intra-abdominal pressure changes caused by the contraction of the stomach.

Although bile flow was modulated by stomach contraction, flow continued throughout the MMC cycle, albeit at a steady trickle during periods of stomach quiescence or after severing the mesentery between the lesser curvature of the stomach and the CBD. By radiology it was not possible to show quantitatively any differences on the rate of bile flow although our impression was that flow was less in periods of stomach quiescence. The pH values recorded at the site of bile entry 2 cm from the pylorus were similar to those reported previously in the pig's duodenum (4). The values support the view that variations in pH in the duodenum do not necessarily indicate a variation in the rate of entry of alkaline secretion with the MMC but may be brought about by a variable flow of acid digesta mixing with a relatively constant flow of alkaline secretion. If bile flow continues – even at a reduced rate – during the duodenal quiescent phase, this alkaline secretion will remain in the duodenum – and possibly reflux into the stomach – rather than being propelled onwards by duodenal motility. Our results may explain the finding in humans that duodenal pH rises after the RSA (3)'.

REFERENCES

1. DiMagno, E. P., Hendricks, J. C., Go, V. L. W. and Dozois, R. R. (1979). Relationships among canine fasting pancreatic and biliary secretions, pancreatic duct pressure, and duodenal phase III motor activity – Boldyreff revisited. Dig. Dis. and Sci., 24, 689-93

2. Lux, G., Femppel, J., Lederer, P., Rösch, W. and Domschke, W. (1979). Increased duodenal alkali load associated with the interdigestive myoelectric complex. Acta Hepato-Gastroenterol., 26, 166-9.

3. Vantrappen, G. R., Peeters, T. L. and Janssens, J. (1979). The secretory component of the interdigestive migrating motor complex in man. Scand. J. Gastroent., 14, 663-7

4. Bueno, L. and Fioramonti, J. (1982). Origin of the cyclical variations of the duodenal pH in pig. In: Weinbeck, M. (ed). Motility of the digestive tract pp 169-73. (New York: Raven Press)

5. Ryan, J. P. (1981). Motility of the gallbladder and biliary tree. In: Johnson, L. R. (ed). Physiology of the gastrointestinal tract. Vol. 1, pp 473-94. (New York: Raven Press)

6. Ludwick, J. R. (1966). Observations on the smooth muscle and contractile activity of the common bile duct. Ann. Surg., 164, 1041-50

7. Laplace, J. P. (1976). L'excretion biliare chez le proc 1) Electromyographie des voies biliaires extra-hepatiques. Rec. Med. Vet., 152, 33-43

8. Itoh, Z., Takahashi, I. and Suzuki, T. (1982). Contractile patterns of the gallbladder between meals in the dog. In: Weinbeck, M. (ed). Motility of the digestive tract. pp 405-13. (New York: Raven Press)

Section 4
Small Intestine and Migrating Myoelectric Complexes

36

Effects of Peptide YY and Porcine Pancreatic Polypeptide on Migrating Myoelectric Complexes in the Small Intestine of the Rat

A. AL-SAFFAR and K. TATEMOTO

INTRODUCTION

Peptide YY (PYY) is a novel peptide of 36 amino acid residue with an N--terminal tyrosine (Y) and a C-terminal tyrosine (Y) amide (1). PYY and pancreatic polypeptide (PP) possess distinct structural similarities and therefore it has been proposed that they belong to the same family of peptides (1). PYY is localized in endocrine cells of the open type in the intestinal mucosa of several mammalian species (2). PYY decreases secretin-stimulated pancreatic secretion (1) and inhibits jejunal and colonic motility (2). Recently, Suzuki et al (3) have shown that PYY inhibits the interdigestive migrating contractions in the stomach.

The present experiments were designed to investigate and compare the effects of PYY and porcine PP on the migrating myoelectrical complexes (MMC) in the small intestine of fasted conscious rats.

MATERIAL AND METHODS

Eleven male Sprague Dawley rats, 320-380 g, were anesthetized with pentobarbital sodium, 50 mg x kg^{-1} i.p. Three bipolar insulated nickel/chromium electrodes were implanted 2 mm apart into the wall of the small intestine, 5, 15 and 25 cm distal to the pylorus. Details of the implantation technique and recording of the myoelectrical activity have been published elsewhere (4). A jugular vein was provided with a silicon-rubber catheter.

The experiments were started after a recovery period of 7-10 days. Before an experimental run, the rats were housed in wire-bottomed cages and fasted for 24 h with free access to water.

PYY, prepared according to Tatemoto (1) and porcine PP (a gift from Dr. R.E. Chance, Eli Lilly Research Laboratoires, Indianapolis), were dissolved in a 0.9 % NaCl solution containing 0.2 % bovine serum albumin. The peptides were infused i.v. during 30-40 min. PYY was also administered as bolus injections 1-3 min after an activity front had passed the first electrode site.

The means of the interval, propagation velocity and the duration of at least three activity fronts immediately prior to the peptide administration were compared to those during and after peptide administration. The results were expressed as the mean $\pm$ standard deviation. Student's t-test for paired values was used for statistical analysis.

RESULTS

Intravenous infusion of PYY at a dose of 6 pmol x kg^{-1} x min^{-1} did not influence the MMC pattern (4 expts). At infusion rates of 12, 25 and 50 pmol x kg^{-1} x min^{-1}, PYY induced significant changes in the regular cycles of the MMC in the jejunum but not in the duodenum (Table 1). At a dose of 12 pmol x kg^{-1} x min^{-1}, PYY decreased the propagation velocity and increased the time interval between the activity fronts. At 25 and 50 pmol x kg^{-1} x min^{-1}, PYY inhibited the distal propagation of the duodenal activity fronts and the jejunal myoelectrical activity resembled the phase of slow waves of the MMC (Fig. 1).

Bolus injections of PYY (50, 100, 187 and 375 pmol x kg^{-1}) initiated a premature activity front within 10-300 sec (Fig. 2, Table 2). In comparison with spontaneously occurring activity fronts, the PYY-induced activity front was of longer duration in the duodenum and propagated at a slower velocity in the jejunum (Fig. 2, Table 2). In the jejunum, PYY increased the propagation velocity of the ongoing activity front as well as that following the PYY-induced activity front. The MMC pattern tended to return to that of the control within one hour period.

PYY (25, 50 and 100 pmol x kg^{-1} x min^{-1}) i.v. for 30 min or bolus injections (187 and 375 pmol x kg^{-1}) had no effect on the "fed" pattern of myoelectrical activity when administered 30-60 min after food intake (3 expts. each).

Table 1. Effect of i.v. infusion of PYY on the characteristics of the MMC in the small intestine.

PYY pmol × kg⁻¹ × min⁻¹	Intervals between the activity fronts (min)						Propagation velocity; duodenum to jejunum (cm × min⁻¹)		
	Duodenum			Jejunum					
	Control	During PYY	After[x] PYY	Control	During PYY	After[x] PYY	Control	During PYY	After PYY
12	12.6±3.4	13.5±2.3	15.0±4.9	14.3±2.3	17.3±3.3**	19.0±4.2**	2.37±0.44	1.2±0.32**	1.21±0.28**
25	11.9±3.6	13.5±3.2	13.0±3.0	15.4±1.7	NM	11.8±3.0	2.0 ±0.47	NM	1.36±0.47*
50	14.3±3.0	14.0±3.7	15.2±2.8	17.6±2.3	NM	17.0±4.6	2.46±0.56	NM	1.33±0.61*

Values shown are mean $\pm$ SD, 6 rats.
Duodenum (5 cm) and jejunum (25 cm) distal to the pylorus
x Time interval between first two activity fronts observed after cessation of PYY infusion
* denotes p<0.05; **denotes p<0.01.   NM = no migration.

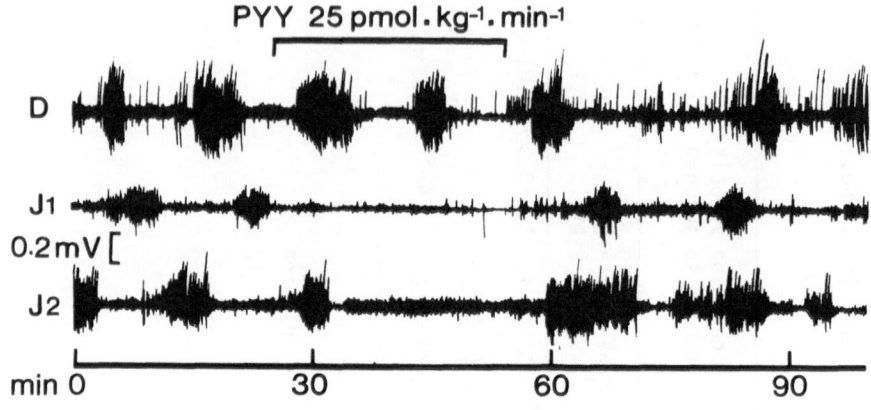

FIGURE 1.   MMC pattern before, during and after i.v. infusion of PYY.
Electrode positions are 5 (D), 15 (J1) and 25 (J2) cm distal to the pylorus. Note that the activity front fails to
migrate from the duodenum (D) to the jejunum (J1 and J2)
and only slow wave is recorded during PYY infusion.

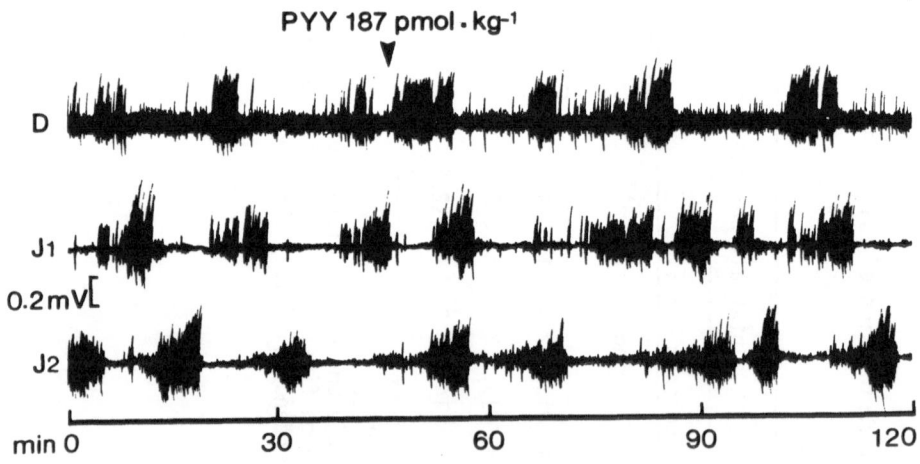

FIGURE 2.   Myoelectrogram showing that bolus injection of PYY initiates
a premature activity front within 15 sec. Note the increase
in migration time of the MMC following administration of
PYY. For further details see legend to Fig. 1.

Table 2.   Characteristics of the PYY-induced activity front (A.F.).

	Control	PYY pmol x kg^{-1}			
		50	100	187	375
Duration (min)^1	2.8±0.5	3.5±0.9*	3.6±0.55*	3.9±1.0	5.3±1.9*
Propagation velocity (cm/min)^2					
PYY-induced A.F.	2.6±0.65	1.7±0.5*	1.9±0.63	1.4±0.29**	1.1±0.15***
First A.F. after PYY		2.0±0.7	1.6±0.6**	1.7±0.48**	1.4±0.63**
Initiation of A.F. (sec)		192±44 (44-240)	146±85 (40-300)	77±64 (10-180)	19±7 (10-30)

Values shown are mean $\pm$ S.D.; 5 experiments in 4 rats. The figures in brackets indicate the range.
^{1}Measurements in the duodenum. ^{2}Measurements between first and third electrode sites.
* denotes p<0.05; **denotes p<0.01; ***denotes p<0.001.

Intravenous infusion of porcine PP did not influence the normal pattern of the MMC at a dose of 2.3 pmol x kg^{-1} x min^{-1} (4 expts.). At 12, 23 and 46 pmol x kg^{-1} x min^{-1}, porcine PP disrupted the MMC and

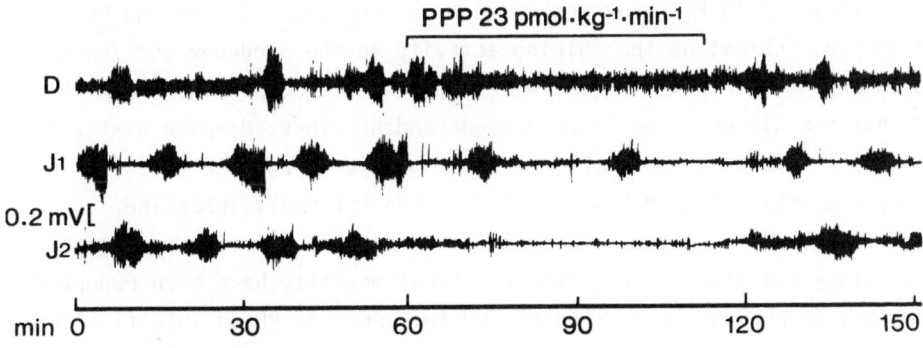

FIGURE 3.   Myoelectrogram showing that i.v. infusion of porcine PP (PPP) inhibits the activity front at the duodenum (D) and jejunum (J2) but not the recycling activity fronts at the middle electrode site (J1). For further details see legend to Fig. 1.

reduced the spiking activity in the duodenum and jejunum (5 expts. each)
The site of inhibition of the activity front occurred randomly in the
duodenum or jejunum (Fig. 3).

DISCUSSION
The present results show that bolus injections of PYY initiate premature
activity fronts in the duodenum that migrate onward to the jejunum. Previous studies have shown that motilin may initiate a premature activity
front with similar characteristics to the spontaneously occurring one
(5) and the stomach seems to be the target organ for motilin (6). In
contrast to motilin, PYY inhibits the interdigestive migrating contractions in the stomach of the dog (3), and in comparison with the spontaneously occurring activity front, the PYY-induced activity front was
of longer duration and propagated at a slower velocity. Thus, it seems
unlikely that the effect of PYY is mediated by the release of motilin.

In the jejunum, PYY inhibited the spiking activity and the propagation of the activity front and only slow wave activity was recorded.
The results suggest that in the jejunum PYY may contribute to the
occurrence of slow waves of MMC and inhibits the propagation of the
activity front in the small intestine. The inhibitory effect of PYY in
the jejunum confirms the finding of Lundberg et al. (2), who showed
that PYY causes a dose-dependent inhibition of jejunal and colonic motility in anesthetized cats.

In contrast to PYY, porcine PP induced irregularities in the MMC
pattern by inhibiting the spiking activity in the duodenum and jejunum
in an inconsistent way. Furthermore, the effects of porcine PP on the
MMC pattern did not seem to be dose-dependent. Thus, despite distinct
structural similarities between the two peptides, porcine PP exerts a
different action than PYY on the MMC in the rat small intestine.

Effects of PP has yielded conflicting results. Stimulatory (7) and
inhibitory (8) effects on gastrointestinal motility have been reported.
However, in none of these studies the influence of PP on intestinal motility have been studied in relation to the occurrence of the MMC.
Recently, Janssens et al. (9) have reported that in healthy subjects,
bovine PP administered at a low infusion rate (1 pmol $\times$ kg$^{-1}\times$ min^{-1})
does not influence the MMC. The effects obtained in the present study
and by others are not related to the occurrence of a defined pattern

of motility as the "fed" and "fasting" motility pattern. Thus, it is likely that the motility of the small intestine is not specifically influenced by PP.

In conclusion, PYY may be one of the factors which is of importance for the occurrence and propagation of the MMC. However, since information concerning release and circulating levels of PYY is not available, the physiological relevance of the present results has yet to be determined.

ACKNOWLEDGEMENTS

This study was supported by the Swedish Research Council (grant no. 3518).

REFERENCES
1. Tatemoto, K. (1982). Isolation and characterization of peptide YY (PYY), a candidate gut hormone that inhibits pancreatic exocrine secretion. Proc. Natl. Acad. Sci. USA, 79, 2514-2518
2. Lundberg, J.M., Tatemoto, K., Terenius, L., Hellström, P.M., Mutt, V., Hökfelt, T. and Hamberger, B. (1982). Localization of peptide YY (PYY) in gastrointestinal endocrine cells and effects on intestinal blood flow and motility. Proc. Natl. Acad. Sci. USA, 79, 4471-4475
3. Suzuki, T., Nakaya, M., Itoh, Z., Tatemoto, K. and Mutt, V. (1983). Inhibition of interdigestive contractile activity in the stomach by peptide YY in heidenhain pouch dogs. Gastroenterology, 85, 114-121
4. Al-Saffar, A. (1983). Analysis of the control of intestinal motility in fasted rats with special reference to neurotensin. Scand. J. Gastroent. (Accepted for publication).
5. Itoh, Z., Honda, R., Hiwatashi, K., Takeuchi, S., Aisaw, I., Talayanagi, R. and Couch, E.F. (1976). Motilin-induced mechanical activity in the canine alimentary tract. Scand. J. Gastroent., 11, suppl. 39, 93-110
6. Janssens, J., Vantrappen, G., Peeters, T. and Hellemans, J. (1982). The activity front of the migrating motor complex of the human stomach but not of the small intestine is motilin dependent. Gastroenterology, 82, 1093
7. Lin, T.-M. and Chance, R.E. (1978). Spectrum of gastrointestinal actions of bovine PP. In: Bloom, S.R. and Grossman, M.I. (eds). Gut

Hormones, pp 242-246 (Churchill Livingstone)

8. Lin, T.-M., Evans, D.C., Shaar, C.J. and Chance, R.E. (1979). Physiological versus pharmacological actions of bovine pancreatic polypeptide (BPP) on the pancreas, stomach, gallbladder, choledochal sphincter and intestine of dogs. In: Miyoshi, A. (ed.). Gut peptides, secretion, function and clinical aspects, pp. 175-181

9. Janssens, J., Hellemans, J., Adrian, T.E., Bloom, S.R., Peeters, T.L., Christofides, N.D. and Vantrappen, G.R. (1982). Pancreatic polypeptide is not involved in the regulation of the migrating motor complex in man. Reg. Pept., 3, 41-49

37

Motilin Release and the Migrating Myoelectric Complexes

S. SARNA, W. CHEY, R. CONDON, W. DODDS, T. MYERS
and T. CHANG

INTRODUCTION

The occurrence of phase III activity in the upper small intestine is generally associated with a peak in the plasma motilin level (1,2,3). Exogenous motilin, when injected during the relatively refractory state of an MMC cycle, initiates phase III activity prematurely (4,5). These two observations led some investigators to conclude that plasma motilin level cycles spontaneously and when plasma motilin level reaches a peak or a certain threshold, it initiates a phase III activity in the duodenum which then migrates distally.

There are, however, some flaws in this hypothesis, e.g., Rees (6) reported recently that on some occasions phase III activity that started in the upper small intestine was not accompanied by a corresponding increase in plasma motilin level. On the other hand, Lee (7) reported that when MMC cycling is disrupted by a meal or by synthetic human gastrin I or cholecystokinin-octapeptide infusion, fluctuations in plasma motilin levels continue. Thus, whereas a loose association clearly exists between the occurrence of phase III activity in the upper small intestine and the rise in plasma motilin level to a peak, the cause and effect relationship between these two events

has not yet been established, i.e. it is not established
whether motilin comes first or MMC comes first. The
objective of our study was to solve the mystery of the
chicken and egg issue, namely the relationship between
motilin release and MMC cycling (Fig. 1)

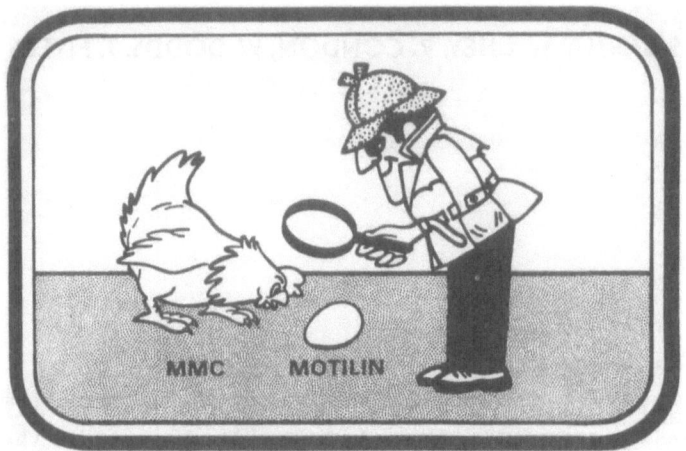

Fig. 1   *Which comes first? Motilin or MMC*

METHODS

The experiments were done on 5 healthy conscious dogs.
Each dog was surgically implanted under pentobarbital
sodium anesthesia with a set of 8 bipolar electrodes. The
first electrode E1 was 10 cm distal to the pylorus and the
last electrode E8 was 10 cm proximal to the ileocecal
junction. The remaining electrodes were spaced at equal
distances between E1 and E8. The dogs were fasted for 16-
18 hrs before each recording session. At least two
spontaneous phase III activities were recorded at electrode
E1 during the control period of each recording session.
The MMC period at the proximal duodenal electrode E1 was
determined and taken as 100%. Subsequent timings were then
referenced as a percentage of this cycle length (8).
Morphine bolus was used as a stimuls to initiate phase III
activity prematurely during the fasted and fed states (8).
    Peripheral blood samples of 4 ml were drawn at intervals
of 20 min during most of phase I activity, at intervals of
10 min during most of phase II activity, and at intervals

of 3 min from about 5 min before to 5 min after the
occurrence of phase III activity at E1. Similarly, blood
samples were drawn at intervals of 3 min from 5 min before
morphine injection at 40% of the MMC cycle to 5 min after
the end of premature phase III activity induced by morphine
at electrode E1. The plasma samples were assayed for
motilin in a blinded manner in Dr. Chey's laboratory.

RESULTS

The occurrence of spontaneous phase III activity in the
duodenum was always associated with a concommittent rise in
the plasma level of motilin. The motilin peak always
occurred after phase III activity had started at electrode
E1 in the duodenum as seen in Fig. 2. In this experiment,
phase III activity started at E1 96 min after the start of
the experiment, whereas the plasma motilin peak occurred 99
min after the start of the experiment. The mean time lag
between the onset of phase III activity at E1 in the
duodenum and the attainment of peak plasma motilin level in
5 dogs was 5.1 $\pm$ 2.3 SEM min.

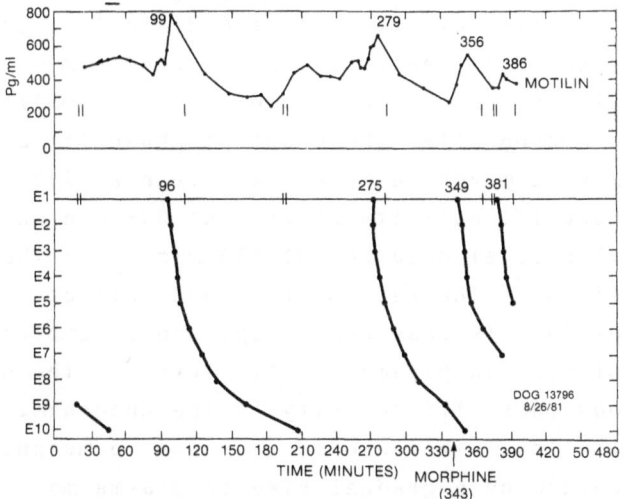

Fig. 2   Relation between plasma motilin and MMC cycles.
Numbers indicate the time in min from the start of the
experiment. Dots indicate the starting time of phase III
activities at the corresponding electrode sites.

In addition to this consistent temporal relationship
between the start of phase III activity in the duodenum and
the plasma motilin level peaks, two other relationships
between plasma motilin levels and MMC cycles were
consistently observed. These relationships are illustrated
in Fig. 2. Single and double vertical lines show the start
of phase I and phase II activities at E1. The plasma
motilin levels decreased more or less uniformly during
phase I activity in the proximal small intestine. The
plasma motilin levels started to increase only when phase
II activity started in the duodenum. The rise of plasma
motilin level during phase II activity was erratic. Thus
plasma motilin levels are related not only to phase III
contractions but also to phase I and phase II contractions.
The mean rate of decrease of plasma motilin concentrations
during phase I activity was 4.9 $\pm$ 1.4 SE pg/ml/min while
the mean rate of increase of plasma motilin concentration
during phase II activity was 4.1 $\pm$ 2.2 SE pg/ml/min.

A 200 μg/kg morphine bolus given at 40% of the MMC cycle
initiated premature phase III activity in all dogs and this
premature phase III activity migrated distally. The start
of premature phase III activity in the duodenum was
associated with a concomittent rise in plasma motilin level
which always peaked after the onset of phase III activity
at E1. In Fig. 2 morphine bolus was given at 343 min,
premature phase III activity started at 349 min while the
peak in motilin level occurred at 356 min after the start
of the experiment. The rate of rise and fall of plasma
motilin level in this case was abrupt and resembled the
sharp rate of rise in plasma motilin level at the beginning
of spontaneous phase III activity in the duodenum. The
plasma motilin level increase in response to morphine bolus
was not preceeded by a gradual rise in plasma motilin level
because there was no preceeding phase II activity before
the premature phase III activity.

In other experiments, the dogs were fed a meal (2 cans dog food ~ 1300 KCal at 20% of the MMC cycle) which disrupted further MMC cycling. During this disruption, morphine boluses were administered at 40% of the cycle and at 2 hrs after the meal (Fig. 3). In both cases morphine initiated phase III activity in the fed state at electrode E1 and this phase III activity migrated distally.

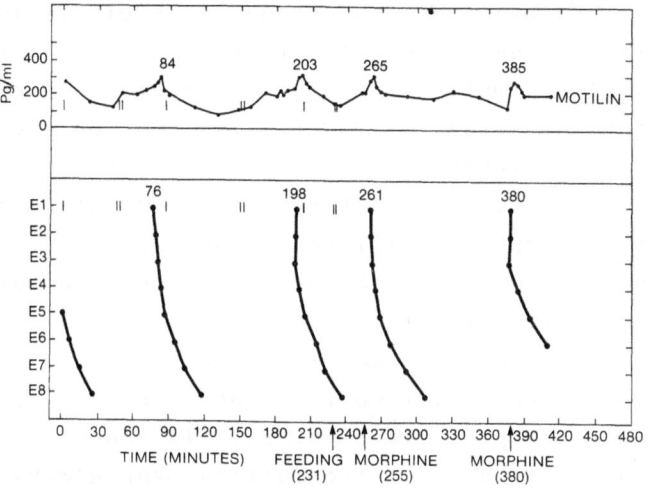

Fig. 3   Relation between plasma motilin level and mor-phine-induced phase III activity during the fed state.

The phase III activity in the fed state was also associated with a peak in motilin level which was significantly higher than the motilin level just prior to morphine adminis-tration.   The peak in plasma motilin level in the fed state always occurred after phase III activity had started in the duodenum.   On the contrary, even very large doses of moti-lin, e.g. 1.6 µg/kg, did not initiate a phase III activity in the fed state.   This finding implied that morphine did not release motilin to initiate phase III activity.

DISCUSSION

In the fasted state, the premature phase III activity initiated by morphine was associated with a significant increase in plasma motilin level.   This finding raised three possibilities:

1. Morphine released motilin which in turn initiated premature phase III activity.
2. Morphine initiated premature phase III activity which, in turn, released motilin.
3. Morphine released motilin and, concurrently, it initiated premature phase III activity.

The first possibility implies that motilin cycling is the cause of MMC cycling. The second possibility implies that motilin cycling is the effect of MMC cycling. The third possibility implies that motilin cycling is neither the cause nor the effect of MMC cycling, but both events may be controlled independently by another primary mechanism. The first possibility was ruled out because, in the fed state, morphine initiated phase III activity but motilin did not. Hence morphine did not release motilin to initiate phase III activity.

The second possibility that morphine initiated phase III contractions and phase III contractions, in turn, released motilin seems likely. This hypothesis is supported by the following observations: 1. The motilin peak always occurred a few minutes after the start of phase III activity in the duodenum when phase III contractions occurred over most of duodenum and proximal jejunum. 2. Motilin levels decreased uniformly during phase I activity in the duodenum and proximal jejunum where most of the endogenous motilin is stored in EC cells. 3. Motilin levels started to increase only with the start of phase II contractions in the duodenum and proximal jejunum.

The above hypothesis is further supported by our observations in some of the experiments that phase III activity that began in the distal jejunum was not accompanied by a significant peak in plasma motilin level because there were no phase III contractions in the duodenum and proximal jejunum (8).

Our hypothesis is supported by the observations of Achem-Karam (9) and his colleagues. These investigators reported that urecholine administration in man that initiates small intestinal contractions but not a phase III activity also significantly increases plasma motilin levels indicating that duodenal and proximal jejunal contractions release motilin.

The third possibility that morphine released motilin and concurrently initiated phase III activity or that MMC cycling and motilin cycling are both controlled by a third primary mechanism is also unlikely. In some experiments when the same dose of morphine was given during the absolutely refractory state so that no premature phase III activity was initiated, there was no concomittent release of motilin.

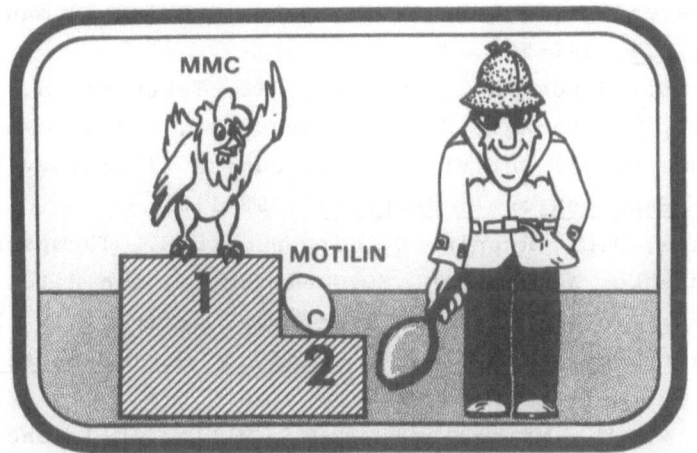

Fig. 4

CONCLUSIONS

We conclude that in the controversy between MMC and motilin, MMC wins, i.e. MMC comes first and then motilin (Fig. 4). In other words plasma motilin cycling is the effect of MMC cycling not the cause of MMC cycling. The mechanism of release of motilin by contractions remains to be determined but, it is possible that motilin may be released by MMC contractions simply by the squeeze of EC-cells. The physiological role of motilin thus released may be to coordinate the start of duodenal phase III activity with secretory and motor activity of other organs such as stomach, LES, and biliary tract.

REFERENCES

1.   Chey, W.Y., Lee,K.Y. and Tai, H.H. (1978). Endogenous plasma motilin concentration and interdigestive myoelectric activity of the canine duodenum. In: Bloom, S.R. (ed). Gut Hormones pp. 355-358. (Edinburgh: Churchill)

2.   Itoh, Z., Takeuchi, S., Aizawa, I., Mori, K., Taminato, T., Seino, Y., Imura, H. and Yanaihara, N. (1978). Changes in plasma motilin concentration and gastro-intestinal contractile activity in conscious dogs. Am. J. Dig. Dis., 23, 929-935.

3.   Vantrappen, G.R., Janssens, J., Peeters, T.L., Bloom, S.R., Christofides, N.D. and Hellemans, J. (1979). Motilin and the interdigestive migrating motor complex in man. Dig. Dis. Sci., 24, 497-500.

4.   Itoh, Z., Honda, R., Hiwatashi, K., Takeuchi, S., Aizawa, I., Takayanagi, R. and Couch, E.F. (1976). Motilin-induced mechanical activity in the canine alimentary tract. Scand. J. Gastroenterol. Suppl. 39, 93-110.

5.   Wingate, D.L., Ruppin, H., Green, W.E.R., Thompson, H.H., Domschke, W., Wunsch, E., Demling, L. and Ritchie, H.D. (1976). Motilin-induced electrical activity in the canine gastrointestinal tract. Scand. J. Gastroenterol., Suppl. 39, 111-118.

6.   Rees, W.D.W., Malagelada, J.-R., Miller, L.J. and Go, V.L.W. (1982). Human interdigestive and postprandial gastrointestinal motor and gastrointestinal hormone patterns. Dig. Dis. Sci., 27, 321-329.

7.   Lee, K.Y., Kim, M.S. and Chey, W.Y. (1980). Effects of a meal and gut hormones on plasma motilin and duodenal motility in dog. Am. J. Physiol., 238, G280-G283.

8.   Sarna, S., Chey, W.Y., Condon, R.E., Dodds, W.J., Myers, T. and Chang, T.M. (1983). Cause-and-effect relationship between motilin and migrating myoelectric complexes. Am. J. Physiol., 245, G277-G284.

9.   Achem-Karam, S.R., Funakoshi, A., Vinik, A.I. and Owyang, C. (1982). Dopaminergic regulation of the interdigestive migrating motor complex "independent" of motilin (Abstract). Gastroenterology, 82, 1005.

38

Motilin and Myoelectric Complexes in the Pig

J. C. CUBER, J. P. LAPLACE and J. A. CHAYVIALLE

INTRODUCTION

Amongst the humoral factors suspected to control myoelectric migrating complexes (M.M.C.), motilin has been postulated to be an important one. Exogenous motilin infusion was shown to induce M.M.C. like those naturally occurring in fasted dogs while it was without effect during the postprandial pattern (1). The hypothesis of a regulation of M.M.C. by circulating motilin was supported by low motilin levels during the postprandial pattern and synchronous variations of plasma motilin levels with M.M.C.: peak plasma motilin occurred with regular spiking activity (R.S.A.) phase and the lowest concentrations were found during quiescence in fasted dogs (2,3). Moreover, a dose of synthetic porcine motilin inducing a plasma motilin concentration similar to the peak values recorded in fasted dogs, could induce a R.S.A. like activity in the duodenum (2). As compared to that, controversial results were reported in the pig : motilin was found to be either released phasically with the M.M.C. in fasting pigs (4), or unrelated in any identifiable causal manner in association with M.M.C. according to others (5). In addition, infusions of natural or synthetic 13-Nle-motilin are unable to induce a premature M.M.C. (5). Such discrepancies, in the pig, might be related to inter-individual variations. It was indeed observed that motilin peaks may occur in dogs without M.M.C. being present, and as well M.M.C. may occur when motilin is undetectable (6). In the man too, though a statistical close

relationship was evidenced between M.M.C. and plasma motilin levels
(7), wide inter and intra individual fluctuations and also unrelated
M.M.C. and motilin peaks were recorded (8).

The present study, performed in the pig, was designed to reassess the
relationship between circulating motilin and M.M.C. in view of (i) the
contradictory data available in this species (ii) the wide inter-
individual variations evidenced by the results available in man and
dog.

MATERIALS AND METHODS

Animal preparation

Under halothane anesthesia, seven Large White hogs (mean live weight
69.4 ± 1.0 kg) were fitted with four groups of three chronic electrodes (nichromes wireş) on the duodenum every 10 cm distal to the pylorus, and a catheter in a carotid artery (medical grade silicone tubing;
I.D. 1.57 mm - O.D. 3.18 mm). After surgery, pigs were housed in individual cages for balance trials and allowed to a complete recovery
for ten days. They were fed twice a day at 9.00 a.m. and 4.00 p.m.,
1000 g of a well balanced diet diluted with 1000 g of water per meal.
The percentual composition of the diet was as follows : wheat flour
81.5, soyabean meal 12.0, cellulose 3.0, minerals and vitamins 3.5.

Experimental procedure

Pigs were fasted for 24 hrs before each recording session. The duodenal
electromyographic activity was recorded (bipolar derivation, time
constant 0.03 sec., Beckman[R] R611) from 9.00 a.m. After two full
M.M.C. cycles were recorded in the fasted state, the pigs were fed
(10 min. for intake of the meal) and recording continued over the
whole postprandial pattern (usually 2 to 3 hrs) and the first consecutive full M.M.C. cycle. During all this session arterial blood samples
were withdrawn every 5 or 10 min during quiescence and irregular spiking activity (I.S.A.), and every minute during R.S.A. Each pig was
tested twice on separate days.

Blood samples were collected in ice-chilled tubes containing 10 U
heparin and 500 U Trasylol[R] per ml of blood. Plasma was separated
from cells within 30 min and subsequently stored at -20°C until motilin
determination with a newly developed assay using : (i) a specific
rabbit antiserum (Quadralogic Tech., Vancouver) at a final dilution

of 1/54000; (ii) porcine motilin (Quadra Logic Tech.) as standard, and
for lactoperoxydase iodination followed by ion exchange chromatography
on a 1 X 10 cm SP-Sephadex C_{25} column (Pharmacia). Plasma samples were
tested as 200 µl duplicates in a final volume of 1.0 ml. The sensitivity limit was 2 to 4 pg per tube according to the plasma tested. The
within-and between-assays variations were 5.9 and 11.3 per cent respectively. All results were expressed as $pmol.1^{-1}$. The mean values of
plasma motilin concentration during each phase of M.M.C. (quiescence,
I.S.A., R.S.A.) were tested both in fasted and fed states and between
them as well by variance analysis.

RESULTS

On average (7 pigs X 2 experiments) fasted pigs displayed a significant cyclical variation of motilin (figure 1). Plasma motilin was
the lowest during quiescence (mean 7.7 $pmol.1^{-1}$), then rose significantly (P < 0.01) along the I.S.A. (mean over the duration of the
phase 16.0 $pmol.1^{-1}$). Motilin peaked at the onset of the R.S.A. (29.6
± 4.4 $pmol.1^{-1}$). The mean value over the whole R.S.A. was 22.5 $pmol.1^{-1}$,

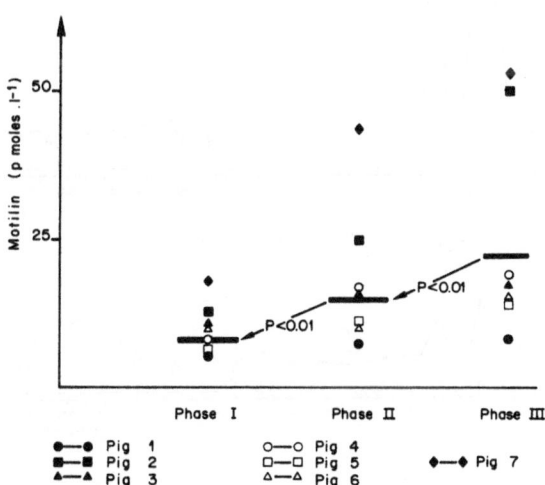

FIGURE 1 : Mean plasma motilin values for each phase of duodenal
electrical activity in seven 24 hrs-fasted pigs (2 experiments per pig). Horizontal bars indicate mean values.

i.e. significantly higher (P < 0.01) than the value for I.S.A. However, as shown in figure 1, there is a wide range of variation of mean values between pigs. This inter individual variation is illustrated by individual curves of motilin concentration (figure 2). In addition, there is also a large within animal variation from time to time (on consecutive M.M.C.) and from day to day (figure 3).

The meal intake induced a transient (10 min) increase (20.2 pmol.1^{-1}) of motilin. Then plasma motilin remained low (12 pmol.1^{-1}) during the whole duration of the postprandial pattern (2-3 hrs). The reappearance of M.M.C. was not associated with any typical cyclic variation of motilin. The mean values of motilin in fed pigs were indeed 6.5 , 6.4 , and 6.8 pmol.1^{-1} during quiescence I.S.A. and R.S.A.respectively.

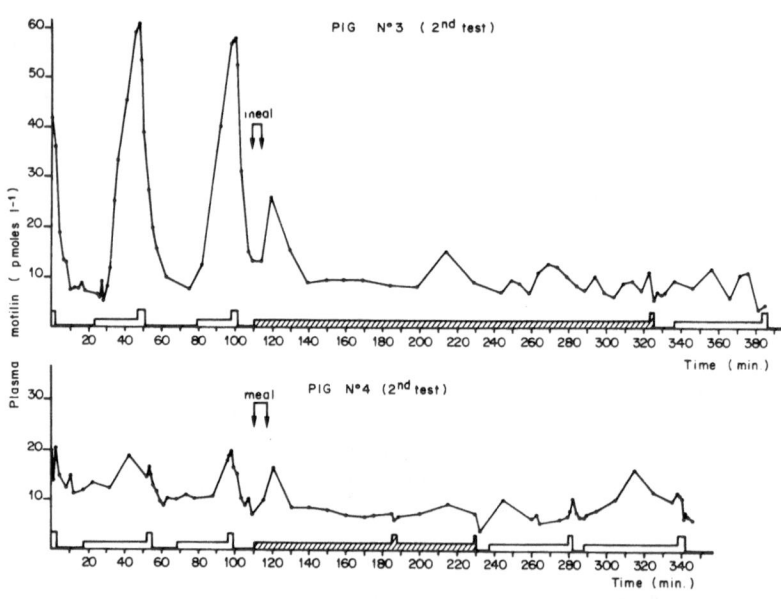

FIGURE 2 : Between pigs variation of motilin levels. Plasma motilin
concentration in 24 hrs-fasted and fed pigs (1000 g dry
matter, 1.5 l water), and duodenal electrical activity :
quiescence (——), I.S.A. (⊏⊐), R.S.A. (▯), postprandial pattern (▨).

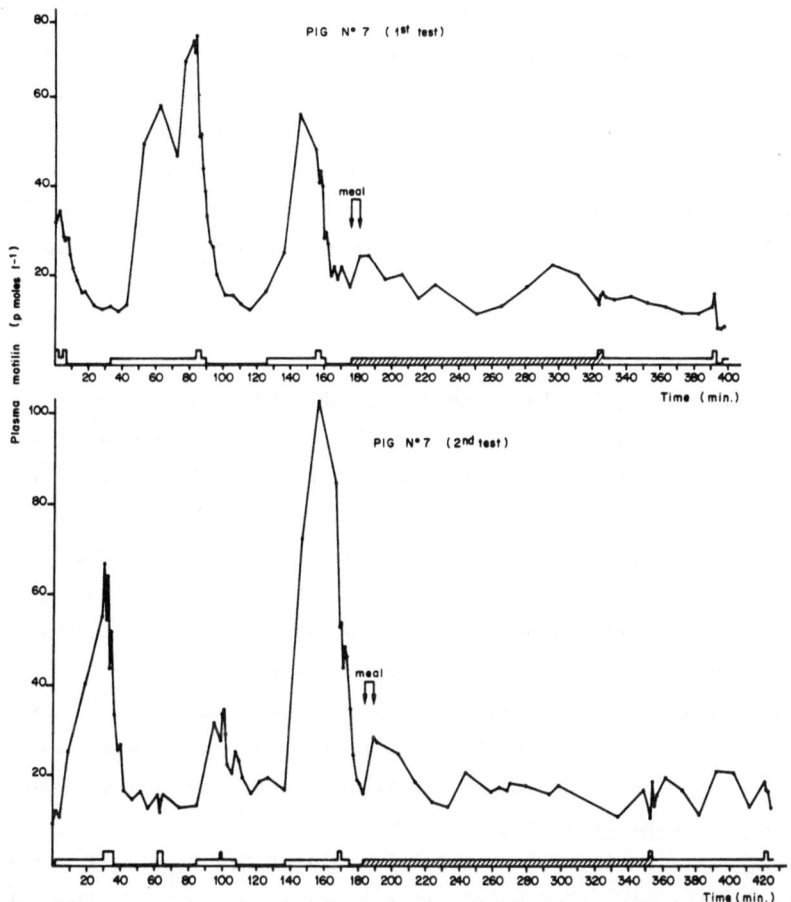

FIGURE 3 : Patterns of plasma motilin and duodenal electrical activity
(for explanation, see figure 2) in the pig n°7, on two
separate days, show a wide variation of motilin peaks from
M.M.C. to M.M.C. and from day to day.

DISCUSSION

The present work evidences wide between-animal as well as intra-
animal variations of plasma motilin levels. The occurrence of motilin
peaks related to the occurrence of R.S.A. is confirmed in the 24 hrs-
fasted pig, but in the fed state the early recurrence of M.M.C. occurs
without cyclic variations of motilin.

This is in good agreement with a previous work in the fasting young
pig (4) which indicates quite similar motilin levels at the end of

I.S.A. However, it is unlikely that motilin is the M.M.C.-inducing peptide in the fasted pig in view of (i) the unability of pure porcine motilin to induce M.M.C. in this species (ii) the wide within-animal and between-animal variations of plasma motilin peaks (iii) the absence of phasic release of motilin with M.M.C. in the fed animal. In the pig, cyclic variations of motilin concentration might be the consequence of a chain of events leading towards R.S.A. and involving presumably other regulatory peptides such as pancreatic polypeptide and/or somatostatin as suggested by a recent report (9).

REFERENCES

1. Itoh, Z., Honda, R., Hiwatashi, K., Takeuchi, S., Aizawa, I., Takayanagi, R., Couch, E.F. (1976). Motilin induced mechanical activity in the canine alimentary tract. Scand. J. Gastroent., 11, (suppl. 39), 93-110.

2. Lee, K.Y., Chey, W.Y., Tai, H.H., Yajima, H. (1978). Radio immunoassay of motilin. Validation and studies on the relationship between plasma motilin and interdigestive myoelectric activity of the duodenum of dog. Am. J. Dig. Dis., 23, 789-795.

3. Itoh, Z., Takeuchi, S., Aizawa, I., Mori, K., Taminato, T., Seino, Y., Imura, H., Yanaihara, N. (1978). Changes in plasma motilin concentration and gastrointestinal contractile activity in conscious dogs. Am. J. Dig. Dis., 23, 929-935.

4. Bloom, S.R., Christofides, N.D., Goodall, E.D., Rayner, V. (1982). Motilin and the migrating myoelectric complex in pigs. J. Physiol. (London), 322, 54 P.

5. Borody, T.J., Byrnes, D.J., Slowiaczek, J.G., Titchen, D.A. (1981). Motilin and migrating myoelectric complexes in pigs. J. Physiol. (London), 310, 37P-38P.

6. Fox, J.E.T., Track, N.S., Daniel, E.E. (1981). Relationship of plasma motilin concentration to fat ingestion, duodenal acidification and alkalinization and migrating motor complexes in dogs. Can. J. Physiol. Pharmacol., 59, 180-187.

7. Peeters, T.L., Vantrappen, G., Janssens, J. (1980). Fasting plasma motilin levels are related to the interdigestive motility complex. Gastroenterology, 79, 716-719.

8. Rees, W.D.W., Malagelada, J.R., Miller, L.J., Go, J.L.W. (1982). Human interdigestive and postprandial gastrointestinal motor activity and gastrointestinal hormone patterns. Dig. Dis. Sci., <u>27</u>, 321-329.

9. Bueno, L., Fioramonti, J., Rayner, V., Ruckebusch, Y. (1982). Effects of motilin, somatostatin, and pancreatic polypeptide on the migrating myoelectric complex in pig and dog. Gastroenterology, <u>82</u>, 1395-1402.

39

Somatostatin Induces Ectopic Activity Fronts of the Migrating Motor Complexes via a Local Intestinal Mechanism

J. HOSTEIN, E. SCHIPPERS, J. JANSSENS, G. VANTRAPPEN, M. VANDEWEERD, G. LEMAN and T. L. PEETERS

Somatostatin induces ectopic activity fronts of the migrating motor complex in man (1) and dog (2,3). It is not clear whether this is due to a central or to a peripheral effect of the hormone, because intraventricular administration of Somatostatin in the brain of rats (4) also increases the frequency of activity fronts in the small bowel. To study the peripheral effect of Somatostatin a tiny silastic catheter was implanted in 4 dogs in a ramification of an upper jejunal artery providing blood supply to a 5–10 cm jejunal segment 60 cm distally to the ligament of Treitz. In 3 dogs two catheters were implanted for segments 30 and 60 cm below Treitz. The catheter was kept open by a continuous perfusion (1,5 ml/24h) with a diluted heparinic solution (333 IU/ml) by means of an insulin infusion pump which was fixed to the animals protection jacket. After complete recovery of the dogs (at least two weeks after surgery) experiments were performed in conscious fasted animals. Small bowel motility was recorded by means of 10 implanted bipolar electrodes. After a control period with perfusion of saline (1 ml/min) 50, 100 and 200 ng/kg/h Somatostatin was added to the infusion. In the 3 dogs with two catheters 100 and 200 ng/kg/h Somatostatin was tested on each level separately. The Somatostatin perfusion lasted 5h and each dose was tested at least twice. I.v. infusions of Somatostatin followed the same protocol. Intra-arterial infusion of saline did not alter the characteristics of the MMC pattern in the perfused area. In all dogs Somatostatin induced 1-3 ectopic fronts. The induction was dose dependent: 50 ng/kg/h almost never and 200 ng/kg/h almost always induced ectopic activity fronts. The ectopic AF's always started during the initial period of the perfusion. They originated just distally to the perfusion site and progressed down at a normal propagation velocity 3.1 ± 0.3 cm/min vs. 3.4 ± 0.3 cm/min (mean + SEM). Later on and in spite of the continued Somatostatin perfusion normal AF's (starting in the gastroduodenal area) continued to occur.

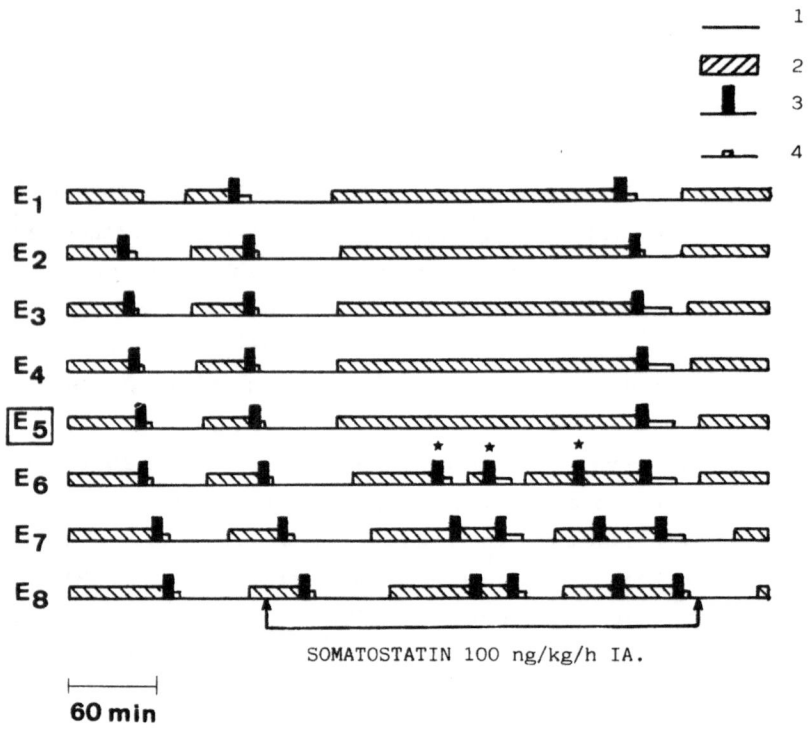

SOMATOSTATIN 100 ng/kg/h IA.

60 min

Figure 1 : Typical effect of intra-arterial infusion of Somatostatin (100 ng/kg/h) in a dog. E_5 is the electrode on the perfused segment. *Ectopic front.

The proximal part of the jejunum was more sensitive to the hormone than the distal one. 100 ng/kg/h Somatostatin almost always induced ectopic fronts (5 of 6 exp.) when infused into the prox. catheter but only rarely when infused into the distal one (2 of 6 exp.). During i.v. infusion of Somatostatin no ectopic fronts were induced.

In preliminary results with i.a. infusion of TTX at a local level of the small intestine ectopic fronts were also induced, starting below the perfused level.

Conclusion : Somatostatin may induce ectopic AF's via a local mechanism. The nature of this mechanism by which these "escape fronts" are produced remains to be determined. Because TTX has an almost similar effect the local effect of Somatostatin might be due to some interference with the innervation of the small intestine.

References

1. Peeters, T.L., Janssens, J., Vantrappen, G.(1983). Somatostatin and the interdigestive migrating motor complex in man. Regulatory Peptides, 5, 209-217.

2. Thor, P., Krol, R., Konturek, S.J., Coy, D.H., Schally, A.V. (1978). Effect of Somatostatin on myoelectrical activity of small bowel. Am. J. Physiol., 235, E249-E254.

3. Bueno, L., Fioramonti, J., Rayner, V., Ruckebush, Y. (1982). Effects of Motilin, Somatostatin, and Pancreatic Polypeptides on the migrating myoelectrical complex in pig and dog. Gastro-enterology, 82, 1395-1402.

4. Bueno, L., Ferre, J.P. (1982). Central regulation of intestinal motility by somatostatin and cholecystokinine octapeptide. Science, 216, 4127-1429.

40

Morphine Initiated Migrating Myoelectric Complexes in Post-Prandial State in Dog: Changes in Refractoriness of MMC Mechanism

S. K. SARNA and R. E. CONDON

ABSTRACT

The ingestion of a meal in nonruminants disrupts the cycling of MMC's for several hours. We investigated the initiation of phase III's during the post-prandial state by morphine to elucidate the mechanism of disruption of MMC's by a meal. Small intestinal recordings were made from 5 dogs by surgically implanted electrodes. Morphine boluses (5-400 µg/kg) were given during the fasted state and after a meal. Morphine initiated premature phase III's in the fasted state and it also initiated phase III's in the post-prandial state. Motilin did not initiate phase III's in the post-prandial state. The mean durations of morphine initiated phase III's in the fasted state and in the post-prandial state were not significantly different from that of spontaneous phase III's. However, morphine initiated phase III's in both the fasted and fed states propagated faster than spontaneous phase III's in the proximal half of small intestine but not in the distal half. The latent period for the initiation of phase III's was significantly greater 30-40 min after the meal than 2 hrs. after the meal. The minimum dose of morphine required to initiate a phase III 30-40 min after the meal was 3-4 fold higher than at a corresponding time in the fasted state. The minimum dose of morphine required to initiate a phase III decreased progressively after the initial increase till it reached fasted level 7-8 hrs after the meal. Spontaneous phase III's appeared after this period. We conclude that (1) morphine overcomes the disruption of MMC cycling after a meal; (2) morphine acts at different sites than motilin to initiate phase III's in the fed state; (3) the increased refractoriness of MMC mechanisms after a meal may play a role in the disruption of MMC cycling.

41

The Effect of Morphine on Motility, Flow and Transit in the Human Ileocolonic Junctional Region

E. M. M. QUIGLEY, S. F. PHILLIPS, M. WEINBECK and A. C. HADDAD

METHODS

We evaluated the effect of morphine on motility, flow and transit in the distal ileum and ICJ in 8 healthy volunteers who swallowed a multilumen tube (O.D. 8 mm) of 11 side holes. Six closely spaced side holes (intervals 1.5 cm) spanned the ICJ, one distal hole was located in cecum, 4 proximal ports recorded ileal activity. Tubes were located fluoroscopically; maintenance of position was monitored by frequency of rhythmic contractions. Ileal flows were assessed by marker dilution over a 20 cm segment, ileal to cecal transit by injecting lactulose and measuring breath H_2. Recordings lasted 5-6 hr fasting, 7-8 hr after drugs and 5-6 hr postprandially (plus drugs); mouth to ileal transit was marked by PEG in meals. A factorial design permitted assessment, double-blinded and randomized, of the actions of morphine sulfate (100 µg/kg i.v.), naloxone (40 µg/kg i.v. plus infusion of 10 µg/kg hrly) and atropine sulfate (7 µg/kg i.v. plus 4 µg/kg hrly).

RESULTS

Tube placement was maintained in all subjects. The 4 volunteers who received morphine demonstrated striking disturbances of motility. Frequent "MMC-like" activity was propagated in bursts during fasted and fed periods. Morphine retarded flow in the distal ileum during

245

fasting and markedly delayed (to 120-210 mins) the increase in postprandial flow (controls < 75 mins). A similar delay in mouth to ileal transit of PEG (> 225 mins vs controls 45-75 mins) was also observed postprandially. Morphine produced no consistent effect on breath H_2. Responses to morphine were attenuated but not abolished by naloxone. Atropine had no effect on the motility response to morphine but, itself, produced a profound diminution in distal ileal flow and PEG recovery.

CONCLUSION

Morphine induces MMC-like activity fronts in distal ileum while simultaneously retarding flow and transit.

42

Blockade of Migrating Myoelectric Complexes by Naloxone

G. L. TELFORD and J. H. SZURSZEWSKI

Prior experiments in our laboratory have shown that morphine initiates migrating myoelectric complexes (MMECs) in the small intestine in both fed and fasted dogs. Because it was therefore possible that endogenous opioids and opioid receptors could be involved in the control of endogenously initiated MMECs, we studied the effects of the opioid receptor antagonist naloxone. Naloxone (1-2 mg/kg, I.V., then 0.2-1.0 mg/kg/hr I.V. for 2.5-5.5 hrs) starting 30 to 60 minutes after the initiation of an MMEC in the duodenum, blocked the initiation of MMECs in the duodenum in 6 of 8 dogs. In 3 of the 6 dogs where the initiation of duodenal MMECs was blocked, jejuno-ileal MMECs were initiated prior to the return of an MMEC in the duodenum. Cycle times on the duodenum for the 8 dogs average 105 $\pm$ 9 min (mean $\pm$ SEM) prior to the infusion of naloxone and 235 $\pm$ 31 min (mean $\pm$ SEM) during the infusion of the antagonist. Naloxone (2 mg/kg I.V.) did not block the initiation of MMECs by exogenously administered motilin (400-500 mg/kg I.V.) when motilin was administered 5 minutes after naloxone (2 mg/kg I.V.) (n=4). To investigate the possibility that naloxone had an atropine like effect and was blocking cholinergic receptors rather than opioid

247

receptors, bethanechol (5 mg, subq.) (n=4) was administered during a standard naloxone infusion and during a saline infusion. There was a marked increase in spiking at all electrode sites with bethanechol with both the saline and naloxone infusions. In prior experiments we had demonstrated that this dose of naloxone completely blocked morphine's effect on the electrical activity of the gastrointestinal tract. We conclude: 1) endogenous opioids and their receptors may play a role in the control of initiation of duodenal MMECs, and 2) motilin does not act via opioid receptors. (Supported by NIH Grants AM 00741 and AM 17238.)

43

Effect of Intraduodenal Bile on Myoelectrical Activity of the Upper Gastrointestinal Tract and Sphincter of Oddi

I. TAKAHASHI, W. J. DODDS, H. AMMON and W. J. HOGAN

INTRODUCTION

Findings from a recent report suggest that infusion of biliary-pancreatic juice into the human duodenum initiates premature migratory motor complexes (MMC's) in fasted human volunteers.[1] The aim of this study was to determine whether intraduodenal injection of bile or bile diversion affected myoelectric activity of the upper gastrointestinal tract and sphincter of Oddi in unanesthetized, fasted opossums.

METHODS

We did a total of 95 studies in 6 animals, weighing 3.0 to 3.8 kg. At laparotomy, bipolar electrodes for chronic recording were implanted on the gastric antrum (GA), duodenum (sites D_1 and D_2), sphincter of Oddi (sites SO_1 and SO_2), proximal jejunum (J_1) and distal jejunum (J_2) by methods described previously.[2-4] After ligation of the distal common duct, a catheter was sutured into the gallbladder. We sutured a second catheter into the duodenum. When the gallbladder and duodenal catheters were brought to the skin and connected, bile flowed from the biliary tree into the duodenum. Disconnection of the two catheters allowed collection of bile or bile diversion from the intestine.

During 8-hr recording sessions that monitored myoelectrical activity in the upper gastrointestinal tract and sphincter of Oddi, hepatic bile was harvested continuously through the gallbladder catheter. The 10-20 ml of bile collected during a 6-8 hr period had an osmalality of 280 to 300 mOsm.

249

Several volumes of the animal's own bile, 2, 5 or 10 ml, or comparable volumes of saline, were injected into the duodenum 15 min after the onset of phase I of the duodenal MMC. For each volume of bile or saline, 3 or 4 observations were obtained in each animal. During some MMC cycles, bile was not diverted from the duodenum and neither bile nor saline was injected into the duodenum.

We also tested several potential pharmacological antagonists. In 4 animals the intraduodenal injections of bile or saline were injected 10 min after the administration of atropine (100 µg/kg i.v.) or hexamethonium (20 mg/kg i.v.).

The immediate effect of bile or saline on gastrointestinal spike burst activity ws determined by measuring the number of spike bursts per min for 4 min prior to and 4 min after duodenal injection. For each recording site the highest 1-min control value was compared against the highest 1-min post injection value. Cyclic length of the MMC was measured from site D_2. Analysis for statistically significant changes in spike burst rate or MMC cycle length was done using the Student's paired t-test.

RESULTS

Fasting Pattern of Myoelectrical Activity

The fasted opossums exhibited well-defined, migratory myoelectric complexes (MMC's) that generally originated in the stomach and propagated through the small bowel. Mean MMC cycle length recorded from the duodenum of 4 animals was 83 ± 5(SE) min. Consistent with previous findings,[2-4] variations in the rate of sphincter-of-Oddi spike bursts occurred synchronous with the duodenal MMC. The rate of sphincter-of-Oddi spike bursts became maximal at a rate of about 5 to 6/min, concurrent with passage of the phase III MMC activity front through the duodenal and decreased to a minimal rate of about 2/min during phase I of the duodenal MMC.

Bile Injection and Bile Diversion

Intraduodenal injection of bile during phase I of the duodenal MMC had an immediate effect on myoelectrical activity of the sphincter of Oddi and upper gastrointestinal tract whereas delayed effects on MMC cycle length were caused by bile injection as well as by bile diversion.

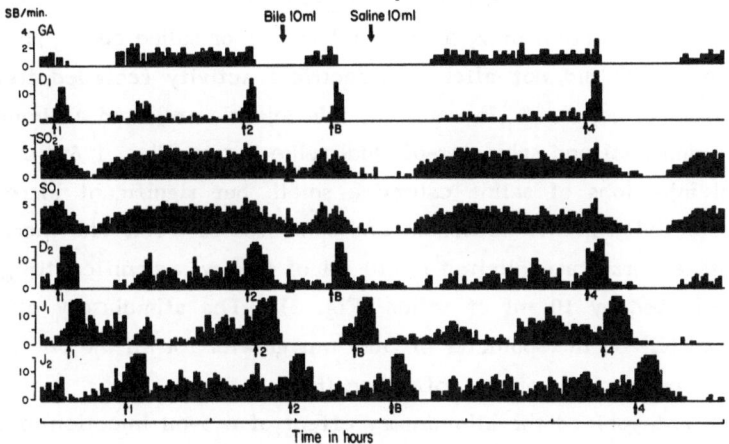

Figure 1. Histogram of gastrointestinal and sphincter-of-Oddi spike bursts obtained from an 8-hr recording. Spike-burst rate (No/min) shown for the gastric antrum (GA), duodenum (sites D_1 and D_2), sphincter of Oddi (sites SO_1 and SO_2), proximal jejunum (J_1) and distal jejunum (J_2). Intraduodenal injection of 10 ml bile elicited an immediate increase in spike bursts at sites D_2, SO_1 and SO_2. About 20 min later, a bile-induced premature MMC, notated B, began in the stomach and propagated through the small bowel. Saline injection elicited a weak immediate effect at site SO_2, but did not initiate a premature MMC. MMC's designated 1, 2 and 4 occurred spontaneously.

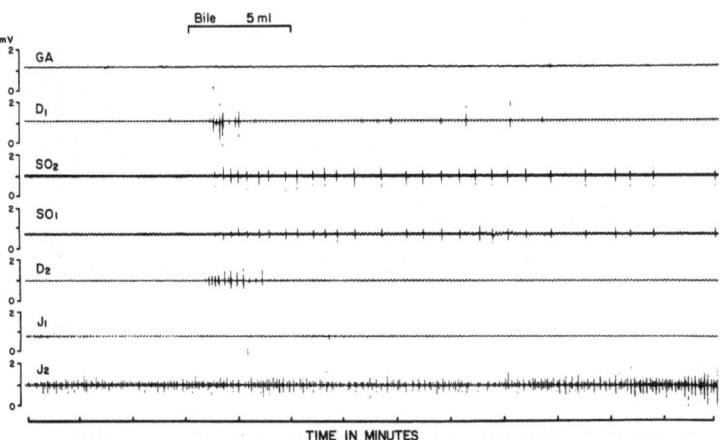

Figure 2. Myoelectrical recording. Intraduodenal injection of 5 ml bile elicited an immediate increase in the rate of duodenal and SO spike bursts while having no effect on the gastric antrum and jejunum.

IMMEDIATE EFFECTS

Intraduodenal injection of 2, 5 or 10 ml of bile or saline during phase I of the duodenal MMC did not alter myoelectrical activity recorded from the gastric antrum or jejunum. In contrast, bile injection elicited an immediate increase in duodenal and sphincter-of-Oddi spike bursts (Figs. 1 & 2). The 5 and 10 ml injections of saline caused a small, but significant increase of spike burst activity in the duodenum and sphincter of Oddi. The increase in duodenal spike burst rate elicited by 10 ml of bile was significantly greater than that elicited by 10 ml of saline (Fig. 3). The stimulatory effect of intraduodenal bile on the sphincter of Oddi was greater for all the bile volumes tested than comparable volumes of saline (Fig. 3).

A tropine antagonized the stimulatory effect of a 5-ml injection of bile or saline on spike burst activity of the duodenum whereas hexamethonium had no antagonistic effect.   In contrast, hexamethonium as well as atropine antagonized the stimulatory effect of intraduodenal injection of 5 ml bile or saline on the sphincter-of-Oddi spike bursts (Fig. 4).

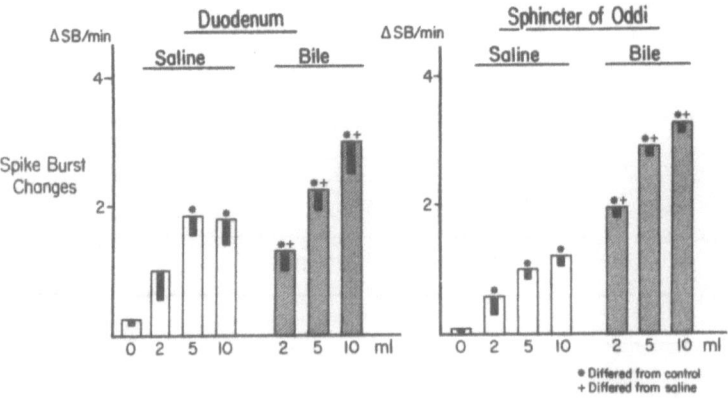

Figure 3. Increases in the rate of duodenal and sphincter-of-Oddi spike bursts elicited by intraduodenal injection of saline or bile.

A. Effect of Atropine

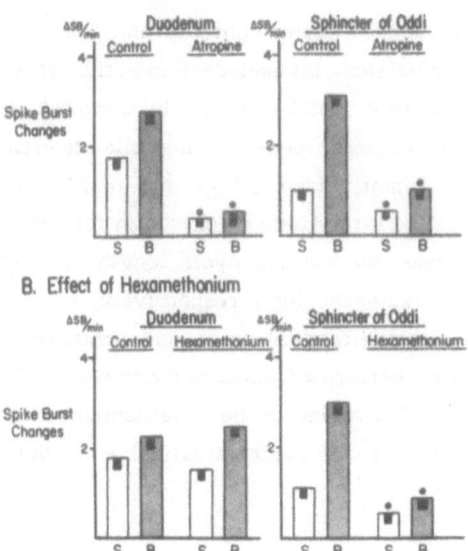

Figure 4. Effect of atropine and hexamethonium, respectively, on increases in the rate of duodenal and sphincter-of-Oddi spike bursts elicited by intra-duodenal injection of saline or bile.

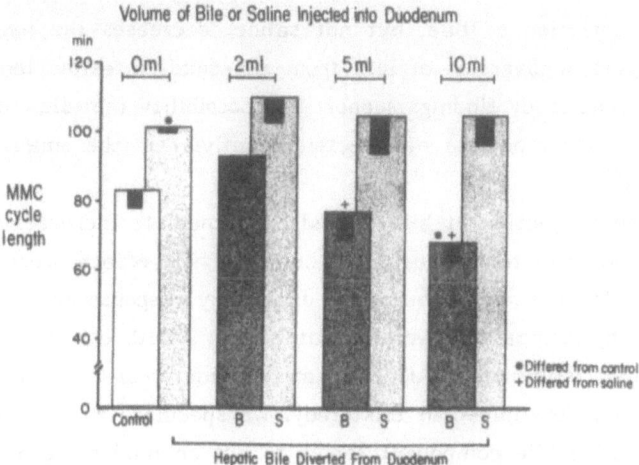

Figure 5. Effect of intraduodenal injection of bile (B) or saline (S) on the cycle length of the migratory myoelectric complex (MMC). During all conditions except the initial control, hepatic bile was diverted continuously from the duodenum.

DELAYED EFFECTS

As shown in Figure 5, diversion of bile from the gastrointestinal tract increased MMC cyclic length significantly from 83 ± 5 min to 101 ± 1 min (P<0.05). During bile diversion, intraduodenl injection of saline did not alter the length of the elongated MMC cycle. In contrast, the 5 and 10 ml intraduodenal injections of bile, given during bile diversion, decreased the MMC cycle length significantly from 101 ± 1 min to 77 ± 8 min and 68 ± 5 min, respectively, (P<0.05). The later value of 68 ± 5 min for the 10-ml bile injection was significantly less than the control cycle length of 83 ± 5 min (P<0.05).

Both atropine and hexamethonium, respectively, depressed myoelectrical activity in the upper gastrointestinal tract and sphincter of Oddi. In this circumstance, the fasting pattern of MMC activity was abolished and we could not evaluate the effect of atropine or hexamethonium on the delayed effect of bile on the fasting pattern of gastrointestinal and sphincter-of-Oddi myoelectrical activity.

DISCUSSION

The study findings indicate that in fasted, unanesthetized opossums: 1) iatrogenic installation of bile into the duodenum elicits an immediate increase in myoelectrical spike-burst activity in the duodenum and sphincter-of-Oddi that exceeds the excitation elicited by injection of comparable volumes of saline, 2) injection of bile, but not saline, decreases the length of the MMC cycle, and 3) diversion of bile from the small intestine lengthens the MMC cycle. The study findings support the possibility that flow of bile into the duodenum may modulate myoelectrical activity in the small bowel and sphincter of Oddi.

Intraduodenal injection of bile caused an immediate increase in duodenal spike bursts and sphincter-of-Oddi spike bursts. These effects were not caused by a volume effect alone because the excitatory response to bile exceeded that elicited by comparable volumes of saline. Although the active bile component that stimulates duodenal and sphincter-of-Oddi myoelectrical activity was not determined in this study, we speculate that it may be bile acids. The active bile component seems to act on mucosal chemoreceptors which are linked in series with motor nerves that act on intestinal smooth muscle. The excitatory effect of intraduodenal bile on duodenal and sphincter-of-Oddi spike bursts appears to be mediated by cholinergic nerves because the response was antagonized by atropine. Hexamethonium antagonized the excitatory effect on the sphincter of Oddi, but not on the duodenum. This later finding suggests that the cholinergic pathway to the sphincter of Oddi has one or more ganglionic connections that have nicotinic cholinergic transmission.

In addition to its immediate effect on the myoelectrical activity of the duodenum and sphincter of Oddi, intraduodenal injection of bile had a delayed effect of shortening the MMC cycle during intervals when endogenous bile was diverted from the duodenum. In association with the shortened MMC cycles, the periodic changes in the rate of sphincter-of-Oddi spike bursts remained synchronous with the duodenal MMC. We have observed similar finding for sphincter-of-Oddi spike bursts during premature MMC's elicited by motilin.[4] Injected volumes of saline, comparable to those of bile, did not alter the fasting pattern of MMC or sphincter-of-Oddi myoelectrical activity. The effect of atropine or hexamethonium on bile's delayed effect on the MMC and sphincter of Oddi could not be evaluated because both of these drugs abolished the fasting, cyclical pattern of the intestinal MMC and Sphincter-of-Oddi.

We estimate that in fasted opossums, bile enters the duodenum at a rate of about 0.05 to 0.2 ml per min, depending on the phase of the MMC and the degree of gallbladder contraction.[5-7] Thus, the rates of intraduodenal bile injection used in this study to elicit immediate increases in duodenal and sphincter-of-Oddi spike bursts, or decreases in the MMC cycle, were not physiological. The injection experiments, therefore, simply show that bile has the potential to enhance duodenal and sphincter-of-Oddi myoelectrical activity, but do not establish that this effect is physiological. However, a physiological role for bile as a modulator of intestinal myoelectrical activity is supported by the finding that diversion of bile from the intestine caused a significant increase in the length of the MMC cycle. The possibility exists, therefore, that bile acts as an excitatory modulator that decreases the relative refractory period of the gastrointestinal MMC cycle, thereby increasing the rate of MMC cycling.

REFERENCES

1. Owyang, C., Achem-Karam, S., Funakoshi, A. and Vinik, A.I. (1982). Pancreatico-biliary secretion stimulates motilin release and initiates the interdigestive migrating motor complex in man. Clin. Res., 30, 287.

2. Honda, R., Toouli, J., Dodds, W.J., Sarna, S., Hogan, W.J. and Itoh, Z. (1982). Relationship of sphincter of Oddi spike bursts to gastrointestinal myoelectric activity in conscious opossums. J. Clin. Invest., 69, 770-778.

3. Honda, R., Toouli, J., Dodds, W.J., Hogan, W.J., Geenen, J.E. and Itoh, Z. (1983). Effect of enteric hormones on sphincter of Oddi and gastrointestinal myoelectric activity in fasted conscious opossums. Gastroenterology, 84, 1-9.

4. Takahashi, I., Honda, R., Dodds, W.J., Sarna, S., Toouli, J., Itoh, Z., Chey, W.Y., Hogan, W.J., Greiff, D. and Matheny, K. (In press). Effect of motilin on the opossum upper gastrointestinal tract and sphincter of Oddi. Am. J. Physiol.

5. Hogan, W.J., Dodds, W.J., Toouli, J., Geenen, J.E., Helm, J. and Arndorfer, R.C. (1982). Motility of the choledochoduodenal junction. In: Wienbeck, M. (ed). Motility of the Digestive Tract. pp. 387-396. (New York: Raven Press).

6. Toouli, J., Dodds, W.J., Honda, R., Sarna, S., Hogan, W.J., Komorowski, R.A., Linehan, J.H. and Arndorfer, R.C. (1983). Motor function of the opossum sphincter of Oddi. J. Clin. Invest., 71, 208-220.

7. Hogan, W.J., Dodds, W.J. and Geenen, J.E. (In press). Motor function of the biliary-duct system. In: Christensen, J. and Wingate D.L. (eds). A Guide to Gastrointestinal Motility. (London: John Wright & Sons, Inc.)

44

Nocturnal Motor Activity of the Upper Gastrointestinal Tract, and Plasma Levels of Entero-Pancreatic Hormones and Primary Bile Acids in Man

F. BALDI, F. FERRARINI, M. SALERA, P. GIACOMONI, S. TOVOLI and L. BARBARA

INTRODUCTION

The data regarding the relationships between gastrointestinal motility and blood levels of many entero-pancreatic hormones in humans are still controversial. Motilin has been related with cyclic motor activity (1); however, this association has been mainly observed with duodenal motility (2) and has been recently put in doubt (3,4). Although less extensively studied, the similar association has been recently proposed between plasma pancreatic polypeptide (PP) and duodenal motor activity(5)

On the contrary, no data are available on the possible relationship between serum PBA and motor activity of the upper digestive tract.

The aims of our study were:

1) to characterize gastro-duodeno-jejunal motor activity during a prolonged period in resting conditions, following a standardized balanced liquid meal.

2) to investigate the relationships between this motor activity and plasma levels of motilin, PP, gastric inhibitory polypeptide (GIP), insulin and glucagon.

3) to monitor the enterohepatic kinetics of bile acids by evaluating serum PBA levels.

METHODS

The experiment was performed on 6 healthy men, 24-28 years of age. Informed consent was obtained from each volunteer. Motility was measured at 4 levels (corpus, antrum, descending duodenum and proximal jeju-

257

num) with a multilumen probe perfused at 3 ml/hr catheter by a low compliance system (pressure rise rate on sudden occlusion of the catheter: 300 mmHg/sec). The probe was connected to Statham P23 ID transducers and the pressures were recorded on a 6-channel polygraph (chart speed: 1.25 mm/sec).

Experimental design

The probe was positioned under fluoroscopic control. After a 12-hours fast, the subjects ate a standardized balanced liquid meal (300 ml, 570 Kcal, carbohydrates 55%, proteins 17%, fats28%), usually around 8 p.m.. The manometric recordings were started 5 min after the meal, with the subject lying supine, and continued for further 10 hours. During this period the subjects rested quietly in bed in a darkened room. Blood samples were drawn every 30 min during the first 1.5 hours and then every 10 min. Motilin and PP levels were measured in every blood sample, whereas GIP, insulin, glucagon and PBA were assessed every 30 min.

Motor activity

The fed pattern was considered to be present at each recording level until the appearance of an activity front (AF), identified according to the criteria proposed by Van Trappen et al (6). The following parameters were analyzed during the interdigestive period: 1) number of AFs/hr, 2) site of origin of the AFs, 3) percentage of the recording time occupied by phase 1 (motor quiescence), phase 2 (irregular but persistent contractions) and phase 3 (AF).

Hormones

Serum immunoreactive GIP, serum insulin and plasma glucagon concentrations were determined by specific radioimmunoassays, as previously described (7).

Plasma immunoreactive motilin was determined by the method described by Dryburgh and Brown (8) with minor modifications. Natural porcine motilin and motilin antiserum (GP 71) were kindly supplied by J.C. Brown, Vancouver, British Columbia, Canada. The antiserum was used at a final dilution of 1:30000. Scatchard analysis gave a binding affinity of 2.46 x 10^{-12} litres/mole in buffer solution and of 2.23 x 10^{-12} litres/mole in the presence of plasma. Motilin was labelled with ^{125}I by the chloramine T method and purified on a Sephadex G 25 column. The specific activity of the tracer was 342 µCi/µg. Incubation was performed at $4^{\circ}C$ for 72 hours in plastic tubes. The final 1 ml volume of incubation consisted of 100 μl of ^{125}I-motilin (3×10^3 cpm), 100 μl of standard porcine motilin or unknown samples, 100 μl of motilin antiserum and 700 μl of assay buffer (0.05 M phosphate buffer, pH 6.5; 1.5% bovine serum albumin; 0.625% aprotinin). Bound/free separation was obtained by dextran-coated charcoal. The lower detection limit was 16 pg/ml. Non-specific binding was estimated for each subject plasma and used in the calculation of the amount of motilin in the unknown samples. The interassay variability estimated from two pooled human plasma of approximately 50 and 250 pg/ml was 9.1% and 7.4% respectively; the intraassay variability was 4.8% and 3.9%.

Plasma immunoreactive PP was estimated by means of a specific RIA. Bovine PP (BPP) and antiserum anti BPP were obtained from Dr. R.E. Chance through the courtesy of Dr. E. Straus. The antiserum (lot n. 615-R110-146-10) was used at final dilution of 1:6.000.000. BPP was iodinated by the chloramine T method and purified by means of a Sephadex G-50 column. The specific activity of the tracer was 250 μCi/μg. BPP was used as standard. Incubation was carried out in 0.02 M Sodium Barbital (Veronal) pH 8.6, with 0.25% bovine serum albumin. Plasma was assayed at final dilution of 1:10. To obtain comparable incubation conditions, hormone-free plasma treated with charcoal was added to the standard curve. Separation was performed with charcoal. The experimental detection limit was 3 pg/tube. The intra and interassay coefficient of variation were 7.8% and 12.1% respectively. All samples were assayed simultaneously to eliminate possible interassay variability.

Bile acids

Serum levels of cholic (CCA) and chenodeoxycholic (CCDCA) acid conjugates were evaluated by a RIA technique, described in detail elsewhere (9). The assay was accurate and specific for each class of glycine-taurine-conjugated bile acids. Sensitivity was 1 pmol/tube, i.e. 0.05 μmol/litre for all assays,and was adequate to measure accurately minimal serum bile acid variation.

RESULTS

Motor activity

Gastric motility was evaluated considering only the antral recording site, since in some cases no motor activity was observed at the proximal recording level.

The interdigestive motor pattern began in the stomach, duodenum and
jejunum 302.7+61.5, 243.5+59.8 and 229.5+55.1 min (mv+SD) after the
meal, respectively. Overall, 23 migrating motor complexes (IMMCs) were
observed; 61% of them started in the stomach. The mean hourly number
of AFs decreased from the jejunum to the duodenum and to the stomach
(0.68+0.1, 0.59+0.2, 0.4+0.2, mv+SD; Figure 1). Phase 1 of the IMMC
was recorded in 63% and 50% of the recording time in the stomach and
duodenum-jejunum respectively; the corresponding figures of phase 2 are
29% and 41% (Figure 1). Phases 1 and 2 were simultaneously present in
the stomach and duodenum in 75.9% of the recording time.

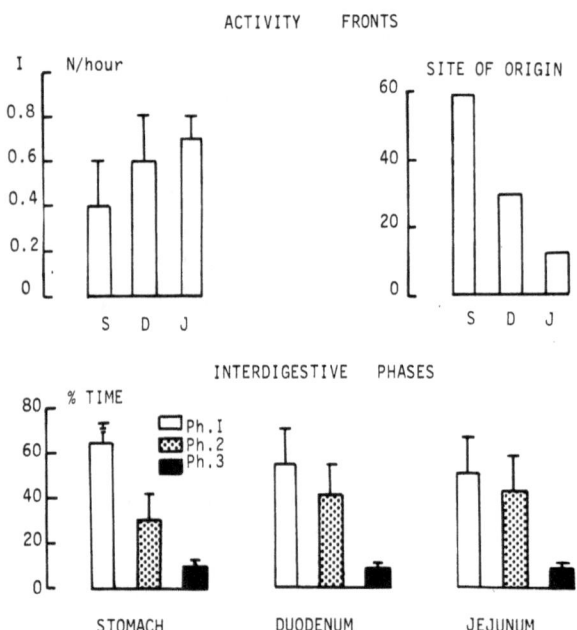

FIGURE 1 Analysis of the interdigestive motor pattern in 6 healthy
         men (mv+SD).

Hormones

In all the subjects the ingestion of the meal induced a sustained increase of GIP, insulin and PP (GIP from 221+31 to 774+1, insulin from
18+2.1 to 56+9.1 μU/ml and PP from 105+9.4 to 192+13 pg/ml; mv+SEM)
and a slight decrease of plasma levels of motilin and pancreatic glucagon (from 58+5.7 to 38+8.8 and from 106+9.5 to 88+8 pg/ml respectively; mv+SEM).

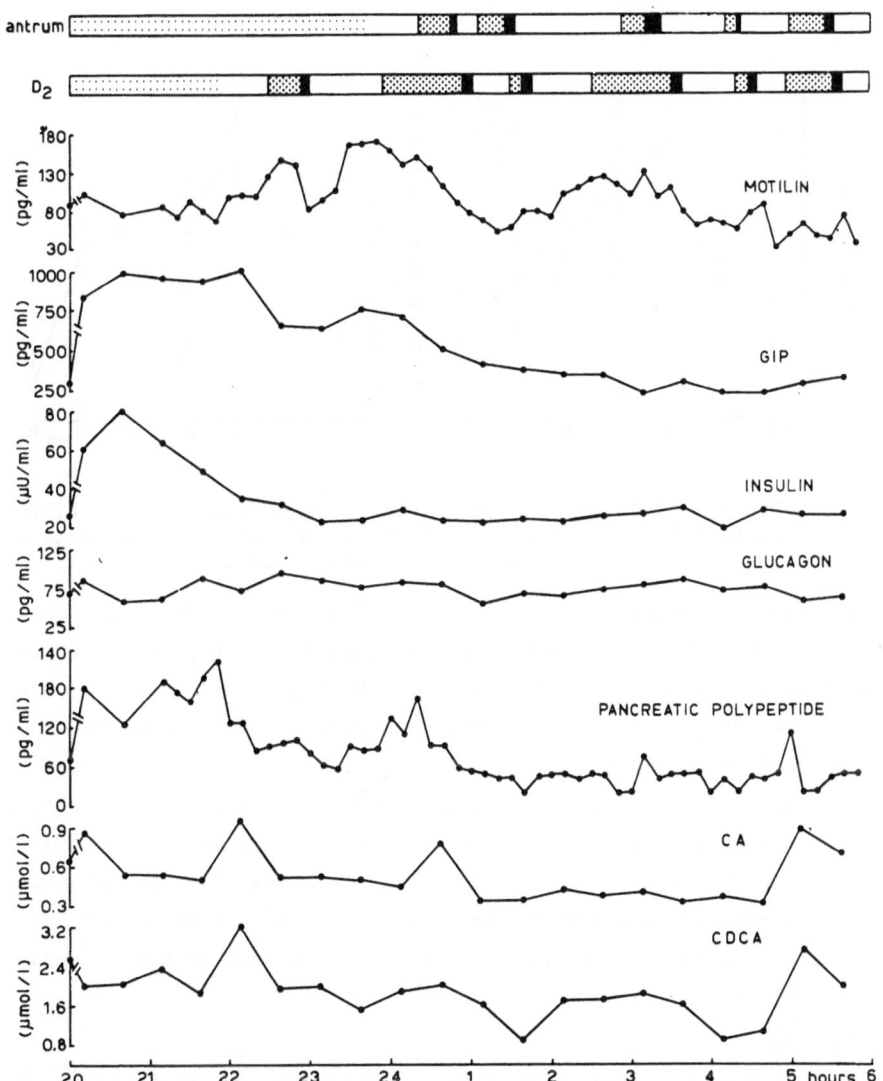

FIGURE 2 Schematic representation of gastroduodenal motility (::::::: fed pattern, ☐ Ph.1, ::::::: Ph.2, ▇▇ AF) and blood levels of the enteropancreatic hormones in a normal man.

During the interdigestive period GIP, insulin and glucagon showed minimal variations around the basal levels, whereas plasma PP and motilin showed relevant cyclic fluctuations (from 30 to 190 and from 16 to 170 pg/ml, respectively). Figure 2 represents the hormonal and motor pattern in one of the volunteers. In order to verify possible

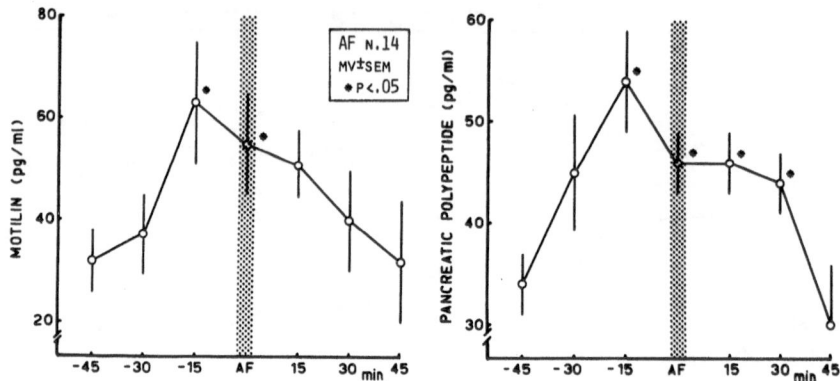

Figure 3 Plasma levels of motilin and PP (mv$\pm$SEM) evaluated.in 15 min
         periods before and after the AFs originating in the stomach
         (n. 14).   p <0.05   t test for paired data.

relationships between hormone levels and AFs, we considered the mean
plasma concentrations of motilin and PP during 15-min periods, starting from 45 min before to 45 min after the AFs. No relation was found
between PP and motilin plasma levels and AFs. We also investigated possible relationships between the site of origin of the cyclic motor activity and the hormone levels. We observed that the AFs originating in
the stomach were preceded by a significant increase of motilin and PP
plasma levels (Figure 3). However, of the 14 AFs arising in the stomach
only 11 (79%) were preceded by motilin peaks and 10 (71%) by PP peaks.
The corresponding figures for the AFs arising distal to the pylorus were 5 (56%) and 3 (33%).

Bile acids

Serum levels of PBA increased after the meal (CCDCA from 1.55$\pm$0.35 to
3.37$\pm$0.07 and CCA from 0.32$\pm$0.04 to 0.84$\pm$0.11 μmol/l; mv$\pm$SEM).

    During the interdigestive period PBA serum levels were lower but
showed cyclic fluctuations with the highest values corresponding to
phase 2 of the IMMC (CCDCA = 1.86+0.1 and CCA = 0.51+0.06 μmol/l;
mv+SEM) and the lowest values corresponding to phase 1 (CCDCA = 1.38+
0.07 and CCA = 0.32+0.03 μmol/l; mv+SEM). In Figure 2 the pattern of
serum PBA in one of the volunteers is shown.

DISCUSSION

In our experimental conditions (prolonged nocturnal recording after a standardized meal) the duration of digestive and interdigestive motor patterns differed when measured proximal or distal to the pylorus, as did also the rate of occurrence of the AFs (about 2/3 of them arising in the stomach and 1/3 in the duodenum). These differences should be taken into account in the analysis of upper GI motility.

As far as the relationship between entero-pancreatic hormones and upper GI motility is concerned, we observed that the plasma levels of motilin and PP were associated with the interdigestive motor activity. Both these hormones showed peak levels preceding the occurrence of the AFs; however this association was evident only for the cycles originating in the stomach and was not observed in 20-30% of them. This suggests that motilin and PP may play a role in the generation of IMMCs, especially of those arising in the stomach, but probably they are not the only factors involved.

Serum levels of PBA, and particularly of CCDCA, fluctuated ciclically during the interdigestive period, the highest values being associated with phase 2 of the IMMC. However, further studies, taking into account duodenal bile output and intestinal absorption, are needed to clarify the relationship between intestinal motility and the dynamics of the enterohepatic circulations of bile acids.

REFERENCES

1. Vantrappen, G., Janssens, J., Peeters, T.L., Bloom, S.R., Christofides, N.D. and Hellemans, J. (1979). Motilin and the interdigestive migrating motor complex in man. Dig. Dis. Sci., 24, 497-500

2. You, C.H., Chey, W.Y. and Lee, K.Y. (1980). Studies on plasma motilin concentration and interdigestive motility of the duodenum in humans. Gastroenterology, 79, 62-6

3. Daniel, E.E., Fox, J.E.T., Collins, S.M., Lewis, T.D., Meghji, M. and Track, N.S. (1981). Initiation of migrating myoelectric complexes in human subjects: role of duodenal acidification and plasma motilin. Can. J. Physiol. Pharmacol., 59, 173-9

4. Rees, W.D.W., Malagelada, J.R., Miller, L.J. and Go, V.L.W. (1982). Human interdigestive and postprandial gastrointestinal motor and gastrointestinal hormone patterns. Dig. Dis. Sci., 27, 321-9

5. Owyang, C., Achem-Karam, S.R. and Vinik, A.I. (1983). Pancreatic polypeptide and intestinal motor complex in humans. Gastroenterology, 84, 10-7

6. Vantrappen, G., Janssens, J., Hellemans, J. and Ghoos, Y. (1977). The interdigestive motor complex of normal subjects and patients with bacterial overgrowth of the small intestine. J. Clin. Invest., 59, 1158-66

7. Salera, M., Giacomoni, P., Pironi, L., Cornia, G.L., Capelli, M., Marini, A., Benfenati, F., Miglioli, M. and Barbara, L. (1982). Gastric Inhibitory Polypeptide release after oral glucose: relationship to glucose intolerance, diabetes mellitus, and obesity. J. Clin. Endocrinol. Metab., 55, 329-35

8. Dryburgh, J.R. and Brown, J.C. (1975). Radioimmunoassay for motilin. Gastroenterology, 68, 1169-76

9. Roda, A., Roda, E., Aldini, R., Festi, D., Mazzella, G., Sama, C. and Barbara, L. (1973). Development, validation and application of a single-tube radioimmunoassay for cholic and chenodeoxycholic conjugated bile acids in human serum. Clin. Chem., 23, 2107-13

45

The Development of Fasting Small Intestinal Motility in the Human Neonate

E. R. WOZNIAK, T. R. FENTON and P. J. MILLA

The ability of the human fetal and neonatal gut to move its luminal contents is well known, but knowledge regarding the development of intestinal motor activity is fragmentary, both in humans and in animals.

Using amniography, McLain (1) showed that there was no transit of contrast down the intestine of the human fetus until 30 weeks gestation and thereafter, there was increasing aboral transit and rate of propagation, as pregnancy progressed.

The development of a technique using chronically implanted electrodes in the fetal experimental animal (2) enabled small intestinal electromyographic recordings to be made in utero and after birth in the dog and sheep (3). Both species showed three gestation dependent stages of spiking activity - 1) disorganised activity, 2) groups of regular spike activity - 'the fetal pattern', 3) migrating motor complex pattern.

We have used perfused jejunal catheters in human premature and term neonates to determine whether similar developmental changes in the pattern of small intestinal motor activity occur in humans.

METHODS

Initial studies were performed on premature but otherwise healthy neonates, fed via 5 F.G. Silastic nasojejunal feeding tubes. Recordings were made after a six hour fast or after a feed, using a Gaeltec pressure transducer connected to the proximal end of the tube,

265

which was perfused at constant flow with normal saline or milk.

Six premature infants were studied in this way. They were born between 26 and 30 weeks gestation (mean 28.6 ± 0.7 SEM) and were studied longitudinally on three occasions on average, until a gestational age of 36 weeks.

Two further neonates born at 28 and 30 weeks gestation were studied at 30 and 33, and 36 weeks gestational age respectively. The first was studied using a vinyl 2mm O.D. 0.8mm I.D. triple lumen catheter inserted into the jejunum via a jejunostomy performed soon after birth for jejunal atresia. The second was studied with a Silastic nasojejunal feeding tube modified to provide two channels.

Three term infants were also studied using perfused triple lumen vinyl nasojejunal catheters in the fasting and fed state. Simultaneous recordings of the transmural potential difference across the intestine were made using silver/silver chloride electrodes connected to the jejunal saline column and a subcutaneous needle as a reference electrode.

RESULTS

Fasting Activity

The narrow lumen and compliant nature of the single lumen Silastic tube resulted in attenuation of recordings,and body movements such as arousals and startles resulted in considerable artefact even during sleep. However, differing patterns of motor activity at differing gestational ages were clear and three stages of development were seen (Table 1).

Table 1. Fasting small intestinal motility in the human neonate

Number studied	Gestation (weeks)	Pattern
6	26 to 30 (28.5±.7)	Disorganised random contractions
7	30 to 33 (31.2±.3)	Fetal complex
8	33 to 36 (34.1±.8)	Migrating motor complex pattern
3	Term (40.7±.5)	Migrating motor complex

Figures in parentheses denote mean ± standard error

In 6 neonates from 26 to 30 weeks (mean 28.5 ± 0.7 weeks)
gestational age contractions without regular periodicity or
rhythmicity were recorded. No multilumen recordings were made at this
stage of development and it is unknown to what degree this motor
activity is propagated.

From 30 to 33 weeks (mean 31.2 ± 3 weeks) repetitive groups of
regular contractions were seen in the seven neonates studied. These
consisted of 8 to 9 cycle per minute activity lasting 0.5 to 1.5
minutes and occuring every 3 to 5 minutes. In the neonate studied
at 30 weeks gestational age via the jejunostomy, this pattern of
activity was usually propagated aborally. 10% of these groups of
contractions were not propagated and there was no evidence of oral
propagation.

In the eight neonates studied from 33 to 36 weeks gestational age
(mean 34.1 ± 0.8 weeks) periods of 11 cpm activity which resembled
the migrating motor complex (MMC) pattern were seen. In the two
neonates studied at 33 and 36 weeks with multilumen tubes this
activity was always found to be aborally propagated. The duration
was very variable from 2.5 to 16.0 minutes with intervals between
complexes of 13 to 31 minutes.

In the three term infants studied, clearcut MMCs were recorded
with clearly defined phase II and phase III activity. The duration,
velocity of propagation and interval between phase III activity
fronts is shown in Table 2.

Table 2. Phase III migrating motor complex activity in three full
          term infants

Interval	44 ± 12 mins.
Velocity	3.1 ± 0.9 cm/min.
Duration	10.9 ± 3.0 mins.

During phase III MMC activity a rise in transmural potential
difference of 10.9 ± 1.1 mV was recorded in these three term infants.

Fed Activity

Prior to 33 weeks gestation there was no change in the pattern of
small intestinal activity in the fed state compared with the fasting
state. In the fed state, 2 out of 5 neonates of 33 to 36 weeks

gestational age and the three term neonates demonstrated irregular
motor activity typical of the post-prandial pattern, but phase III
MMC activity was not abolished.

Sucking

It was observed that the sucking reflex had not developed in the
premature infants with disorganised random contractions and the fetal
complex pattern of small intesinal motor activity. Development of the
migrating motor complex pattern of activity was associated with
gaining the ability to suck in all infants.

DISCUSSION

With improving ability to provide the respiratory support for
premature infants, problems with nutritional support have aroused
increasing interest in the ontogeny of human gastrointestinal function.
Our studies have shown a clearcut developmental progression of small
intestinal motor activity in the human neonate. The three stages of
disorganised, fetal and MMC patterns resemble the three stages of
spiking activity described in animals by Bueno and Ruckebush (3).

The disorganised pattern in animals is characterised by random
spikes with only occasional   aboral propagation and occurred from
0.6 to 0.8 of term in sheep and from 0.8 to 0.9 of term in dogs. In
the human neonate studied from 26 to 30 weeks gestational age (0.65 to
0.75 of term) random contractions were seen which were unaffected by
feeding. It is not clear whether this activity in the human is
propagated or capable of propulsion of intestinal contents, but
McLain's data (1) would suggest it is not. In clinical practice, it
is this very premature group in which difficulty in establishing
enteral feeds is commonly encountered.

Stage 2, the fetal pattern in sheep and dogs, consisted of regular
aborally propagated spike bursts lasting approximately 4 minutes and
recurring at 12 to 15 minute intervals. This pattern was seen from
0.8 to 0.95 of term in sheep and from 0.9 of term to 15 days after
birth in dogs. This pattern is similar to the short repetitive groups
of regular, usually aborally propagated contractions demonstrated
in fasted and fed human neonates from 30 to 33 weeks gestational age
(0.75 to 0.83 of term) although in human neonates the duration and
interval between these 'fetal complexes' is about one third of that
in sheep and dogs. Certainly this pattern appears to be an

intermediate stage between disorganised activity and development of
MMCs.

From 0.95 of term in sheep and from 15 days after birth in the dog
MMCs occurred similar to those seen in adult animals but propagated
more slowly. MMC like activity was seen in human neonates from 33
weeks gestational age (0.83 of term) and at term, clearly defined
phase II and III MCC activity is present. The propagation of phase III
activity is also slower than in adults.

MMC activity in humans appears at an earlier gestational stage
than in animals and may reflect a species difference in neurological
maturation since the coincident development of the sucking reflex
was striking. As the animals were studied in utero and the humans
after birth, postnatal adaptation to extrauterine life may also be
an important factor.

The earlier development of these three phases of intestinal motor
activity in human neonates compared with fetal and postnatal sheep
and dogs, is illustrated in Table 3.

Table 3.   Development of small intestinal motility in humans
           compared with dogs and sheep (Bueno & Ruckesbusch (5))

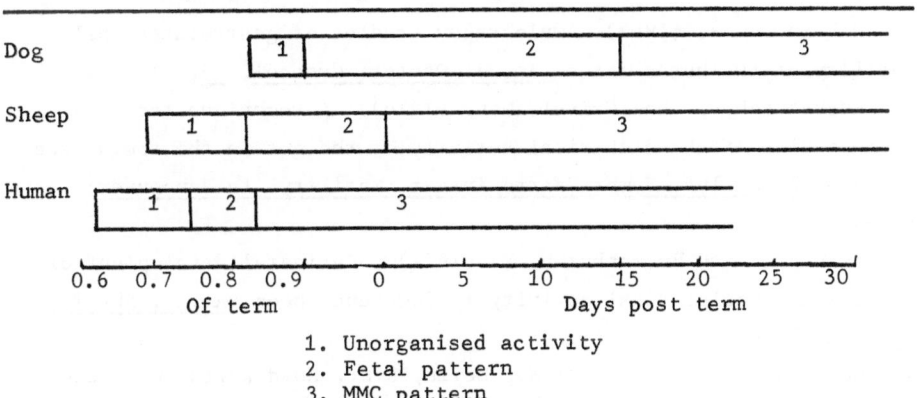

1. Unorganised activity
2. Fetal pattern
3. MMC pattern

The onset of development of postprandial activity in response to
food occurred after 33 weeks gestation in human neonates and coincided
with the development of MMC activity and of the sucking reflex.
Unlike normal adults and children, however, this activity was not
abolished by feeding. The abolition of MMCs by food may be a

developmental phenomenon which occurs at a later stage of maturity.

Ruckebusch and Bueno (5) have shown that pigs fed one or two feeds a day had periods of postprandial activity with abolition of MMC activity whereas pigs fed 'ad lib' and having several feeds a day had little postprandial activity and the number of periods of phase III MMC activity per day was the same as in the fasted animal.

Human neonates are fed by continual milk infusion or by bolus feeds every 1 to 3 hours and it is possible that the persistence of MMC's during the postprandial period is related to this frequent feeding pattern, which does not change until weaning occurs.

CONCLUSION

Postnatal development of small intestinal motor activity in premature human neonates occurs in three stages similar to that demonstrated in animals in utero.

1) From 26 to 30 weeks gestation,disorganised activity occurs.

2) From 30 to 33 weeks gestation,repetitive short groups of propagated contractions termed the fetal complex occurs.

3) From 33 weeks gestation, migrating motor complex activity and the sucking reflex start to develop.

REFERENCES

1. McLain , C.R. (1963). Amniography studies of gastrointestinal motility of the human fetus. Am. J. Obstet. Gynecol, 86, 1079-1087.

2. Ruckebusch, Y. and Grivel, M.L. (1974). A technique for long term studies of the electrical activity of the gut in the foetus and neonate. Proc. Int. Symp. Gastro intest. Motility 4th Vancouver, 428-434.

3. Bueno, L. and Ruckesbusch, Y. (1979). Perinatal development of intestinal myoelectrical activity in dogs and sheep. Am. J. Physiol, 237, (i) E61-67.

4. Read, N.W., Smallwood, R.H., Levin, R.J., Holdsworth, C.D. and Brown, B.H. (1977). Relationship between changes in intraluminal pressure and transmural potential difference in the human and canine jejunum in vivo. Gut, 18, 141-151.

5. Ruckesbusch, Y. and Bueno, L. (1976). The effect of feeding on the motility of the stomach and small intestine in the pig. Br. J. Nutr., 35, 397-405.

ACKNOWLEDGEMENT

E.R.W., and T.R.F., gratefully acknowledge Duphar - B.V. for their financial support.

46

Feeding Behaviour and the Migrating Myoelectric Complex

F. CRENNER, G. FELDER, A. LAMBERT and J. F. GRENIER

INTRODUCTION

Many food intake studies have been performed, concerning feeding behaviour (1,2,3), the role of the nervous system (4) or the role of some peptides (5,6,7), especially cholecystokinin (8,9,10). A wide litterature is also existing about factors of all kinds acting on the intestinal motility and the occurence of the MMC ; few works however concern psychic mechanisms (11).

But the relationships between appetite and intestinal motility is very poorly known. The purpose of our study was to investigate if there was a correlation between the occurence of the MMC and feeding in dogs which had permanent access to food.

MATERIAL AND METHODS

Four male mongrel dogs (12-18 kg) were surgically preparated for intestinal electromyography with totally implantable multichannel telemetry systems. Six Ag-AgCl monopolar electrodes were serosally sewn on the duodenum, jejunum and ileum. Wires from the electrodes led to a 6 channel miniature radiotransmitter implanted in the abdominal cavity. The telemetry range was 5 meters, the battery life was 1000 hours and the device could be switched on and off by external telecontrol. The electromyographic signals were provided by a receiver and a decoder to a graphic recorder (Beckman Dynograph R411) ; the bandwidth for the whole recording line was 0,16 - 80 Hz (-3dB points) - equivalent time

constant : 1 second. The timing and the weight, i.e. the amount of calories, of each food intake of the dog was transduced and registered
on the graphic recorder.

A 20 days recovery period was allowed after the operation.
Then, a 4 weeks non-stop recording was performed in each dog while it
was free to move in a 4 m^2 cage. The animals had permanent access to
water and to food (standard dog can food : 57 % protein, 38 % fat, 4 %
carbohydrate). A 12 hours/12 hours rythm was observed for the light-
dark alternance.

A permanent activity period on the electromyographic tracing
was considered as the phase III of an MMC only if it propagated from
the duodenum to the terminal ileum. The time of occurence of an MMC was
registered when the phase III was present on the duodenum. A food intake was counted if it represented more than 30 kcal.

RESULTS

The experiments provided 3000 hours of tracing, and 1000
meals were recorded. The dogs were in good health at the time of the
study and their weight was constant all over the experiment. The dayly
caloric intake was 700 to 3000 kcal/day and the number of meals was 3
to 15 per 24 hours : there were large variations between animals, and
even in the same dog, the amount of food eaten varied, in a smaller
proportion, from one day to an other. Figure 1 shows two extreme examples of the dayly number of MMC's : the dog n° 1 almost always interrupted the MMC, when the dog n° 2 was in fasting state (on an electromyographic point of view) more than half of the time. Dogs n° 3 and
n° 4 presented intermediate behaviours.

80 % of the total number of meals occured when the MMC was
absent : it was already interrupted by a previous food intake. 20 % of
the meals where taken as the MMC existed ; in this situation, food intakes occured for 22 % during phase I, 70 % during phase II and 8 %
during phase III. No correlation could be observed between the occurence of the meals or their importance and the MMC.

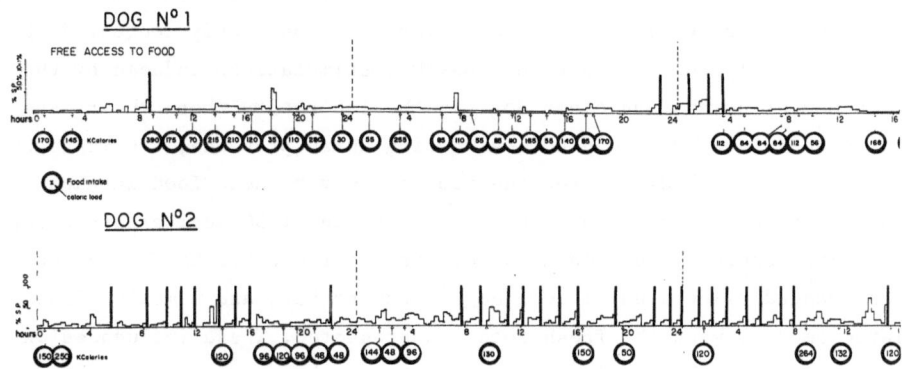

FIGURE 1   Electromyographic recordings obtained on the duodenum (percentage of slow waves superimposed by spike bursts versus
time). The black strips correspond to a phase III of the MMC
propagated from the duodenum to the terminal ileum. Pastilles
under the tracing indicate the time of occurence of meals and
their caloric load.

DISCUSSION

        The method used for our experiments was very simple, but
the results could not be expressed in a synoptical way : we were unable to discern general rules correlating the MMC and the meals. For
instance, when many MMC's occured consecutively, i.e. after a rather
long fasting period, the first meal can consist in a large as well as
in a small amount of food. Or during a fed period, a large food intake
can be followed by a long period without meal, and maybe by MMC's, as
well as by a renewed consistent meal.

        Most of the meals occured when the MMC was already inter-
rupted : the dogs did not wait after a food intake to be fasted to eat
again. When the animals eat as the MMC was present, the distribution
of the meals over the different phases of the MMC was comparable with
the temporal distribution of these phases on an electrode : the time
of occurence of the food intake seems to be random and uncorrelated
with the MMC's phases. This random distribution was observed on every
electrode placed along the bowel.

The animals under experiment did not suffer any material or technical inconvenience, owing to the implanted telemetric device used for the recordings : the dogs were alert and apparently contented. But they certainly received external psychic stimulations induced by the presence of humans and other dogs in the laboratory where their cage was placed. Some dogs did not eat during human presence, others begun to eat when somebody entered the room ; however these food intakes were very poor in calories, and the threshold of 30 kcal observed for counting generally removed these errors. On the other hand, the food was changed twice a day : some dogs begun to eat, and sometimes for a large amount, when the fresh food was presented. These influences on the animals can be considered as important ; but the experiment was performed on animals in "normal" psychic conditions, i.e. in temporary human presence for dogs accustomed to man.

The problem that concerns that kind of behavioural study on dogs is to know exactly the level of the observation : are physiological regulatory mechanisms delegated a minor role compared to the psychological factors which determine when and how much the animal eat ? And on another hand, is the MMC with the associated phenomenons able to initiate a hunger-satiety signal ?

CONCLUSION

The procedure of this study was very simple : we performed intestinal electromyographic recordings in dogs that had access to food ad libitum. Technical problems brought by long lasting experiments were overcome by an implantable telemetry system and an automatic recording of the food intakes. Our particular experiment did not show any correlation between the occurence of food ingestion and the intestinal electromyographic recording. We conclude that the MMC takes no obvious part in the control of feeding behaviour in dogs.

REFERENCES

1. Bernstein, I.L. (1975). Relationship between activity, rest and free feeding in rats. J. Comp. Physiol. Psychol., 89, 253-257.
2. Bernstein, I.L., J. Zimmerman, C. Gzeisler and E. Weitzman (1981). Meal patterns in "free-running" humans. Physiol. Behav., 27, 621-623.

3. Armstrong, S. (1978). A chronometric approach to the study of feeding bahavior. Neurosci. Behav. Reviews, 4, 27-53.

4. Grijalva, C. (1982). The role of the autonomic nervous system in hypothalamic feeding syndromes. Appetite, Journal for Intake Research, 3, 111-124.

5. McLaughlin, C. (1982). Role of peptides from gastrointestinal cells in food intake regulation. J. Anim. Sci., 55, 1515-1527.

6. Sanger, D. (1981). Endorphinergic mechanisms in the control of food and water intake. Appetite, Journal for Intake Research, 2, 193-208.

7. Morley, J., A. Levine, G. Yim and M. Lowy (1983). Opioid modulation of appetite. Neurosci. Behav. Reviews, 7, 281-305.

8. Baldwin, B., T. Cooper and R. Parrot (1982). Effect of cholecystokinin octopeptide on food intake in pigs. Proc. Nutr. Soc., 41, 119-121.

9. Rehfeld, J. (1980). Cholecystokinin as a satiety signal. Int. J. Obesity, 5, 465-469.

10. Hsiao, S. and C. Wang (1983). Continuous infusion of cholecystokinin and meal pattern in the rat. Peptides, 4, 15-17.

11. Steinbach J. and C. Code (1980). Increase in the period of the interdigestive myoelectric complex with anticipation of feeding. Gastrointestinal Motility, J. Christensen (ed.) pp. 247-252 (Raven Press).

47

Does Exercise Affect the Migrating Motor Complex in Man?

D. F. EVANS, G. E. FOSTER and J. D. HARDCASTLE

INTRODUCTION

The existence of the fasting migrating motor complex (MMC) of the small
intestine in man has now been well established. Recently there has been
considerable interest in the internal controlling mechanisms that
regulate the onset and timing of the MMC. The periodicity of the
MMC has been shown to be influenced by sleep (1,2) and also psychological stress (3) but nothing is known of any effects of physical
activity, this partly due to the difficulty of monitoring small
intestinal pressures during prolonged physical exertion.

We have used a tethered pressure sensitive radiotelemetry capsule
(RTC) (4) and a portable receiving system (5) to monitor fasting
small intestinal motility in a group of subjects undergoing a period
of prolonged physical activity. Pressures in the proximal jejunum and
intervals of the MMC have been compared with a similar group of rested
fasting control subjects.

SUBJECTS AND METHODS

Twenty healthy volunteer subjects (mean age 25.5 years $\mp$ 6.5sd) without any history of gastrointestinal problems were recruited into the
study. The subjects were fasted overnight for at least twelve hours
prior to the start of the study.

On the study day each subject swallowed a pressure sensitive radiotelemetry capsule (RTC) attached to 100cm of fine silk thread. This
became positioned after a variable time (Table 1) in the proximal

jejunum. The position of the RTC was confirmed by the length of
thread, identification of small intestinal pressure waves and a
negative cold water swallow (6). Pressures were detected by a
three aerial abdominal belt and a portable receiver (5) recording
onto a standard 4 channel miniature body borne tape recorder (Oxford
Medical Systems, Oxon) (Fig. 1)

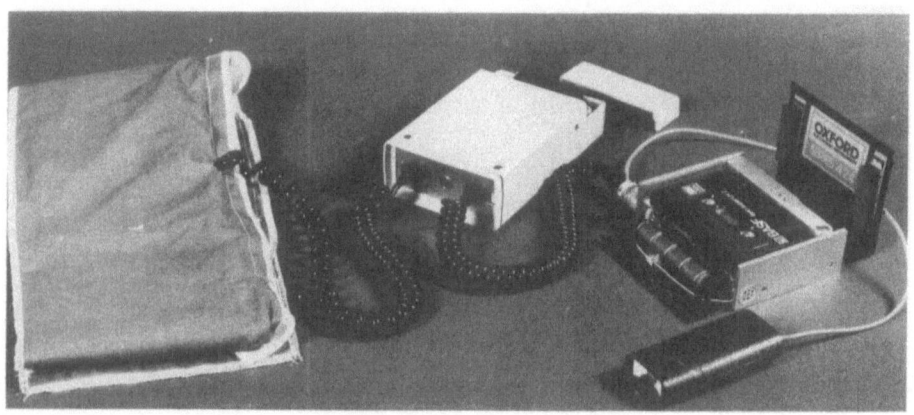

Fig. 1.   Aerial belt, portable receiver and cassette tape recorder
           for ambulatory monitoring of small bowel motility.

After the passage of a phase III activity front in the jejunum,
subjects were randomly divided into two groups. One group (n=10)
continued to sit quietly in the laboratory for the duration of the
test (Fig. 2(a)) the other group (n=10) commenced a 12 mile walk
along a route predetermined by the investigators. (Fig. 2(b)).
Jejunal pressures were continuously monitored using the portable
system throughout the test period.

The route was designed with suitable inclines such that the subject
would be tired by completing it in the four hours allowed. At the end
of the four hour period the test was ended in both groups by releasing
the tethering thread, the capsules being subsequently recovered per
rectum.

Recordings were analysed for the incidence of fasting jejunal activity
fronts in both groups and the results compared.

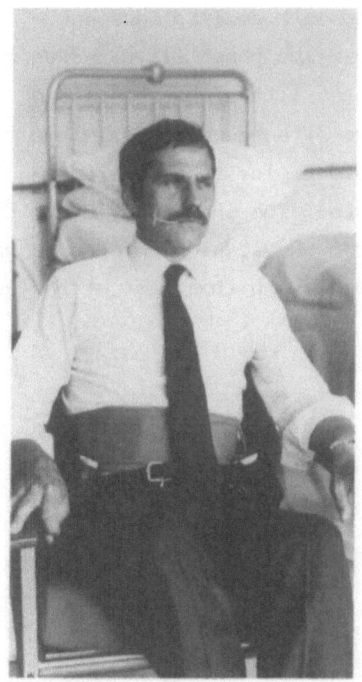 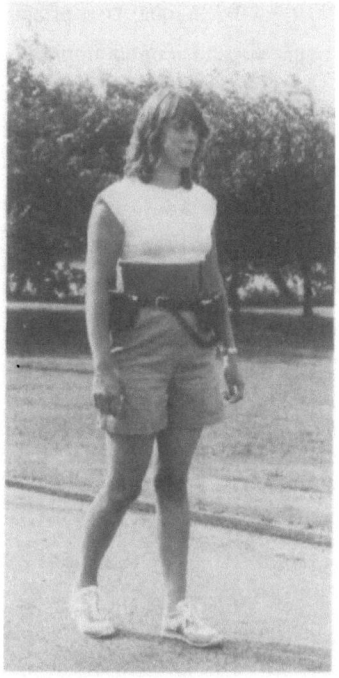

Fig. 2   (a)   (b)
(a) Subjects in the resting control and exercise groups (b).
Tethered RTC and recording equipment allow for unrestricted activity.

RESULTS

All subjects recorded a jejunal activity front prior to the walk.
The median time between swallowing the RTC and the appearance of
the activity front was 115 minutes, (range 20-200) for the exercise
group and 102 minutes, (range 15-170) for the controls, there being no
significant difference between the groups. The wide range demonstrates
the variability of the time taken for the RTC to leave the stomach.
This usually happened as a result of the migration of an antral
activity front, this appearing at an indeterminant time after the
capsule had been swallowed.

Activity fronts were easily recognised in the jejunum during the
exercise period. They were clearly distinguishable from any artefact
caused by movement during the exercise and it was also possible to
identify phase I and II periods. Fig. 3 is an example of an ambulatory
recording after high speed replay. A jejunal phase III activity front
can be clearly seen. This follows a period of phase II activity and

is followed by a quieter phase I period with smaller movement artefacts superimposed upon the record. The phase III was seen as a period of high frequency pressure waves with a characteristic elevation above the baseline. This was often seen in real time recordings but was enhanced by the rapid replay technique and assisted in the identification of fronts. The inset portion of Fig. 3 illustrates the 11 cycle per minute frequency typical of the jejunal activity front, this was obtained by replaying this part of the record at a faster paper speed.

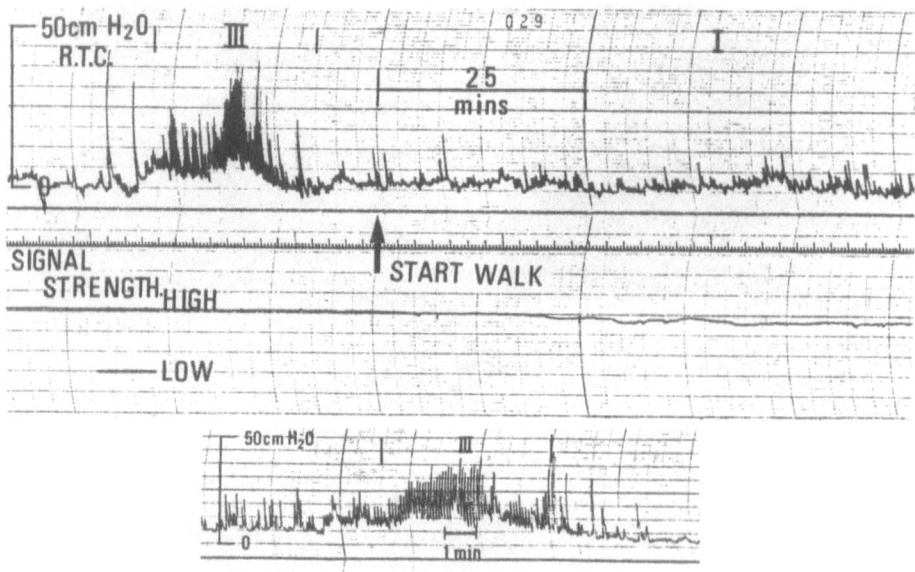

Fig. 3.   Ambulatory recording of jejunal pressures during exercise.
Signal strength channel allows for identification of
artefact during periods of low transmission of capsule.
Inset portion shows an activity front in the jejunum.

A comparison of the results of the exercise group and the rested controls can be seen in table I. All the subjects in the control group had at least one jejunal activity front during the 240 minute test period with a median number of two. In the exercised group six out of the ten subjects experienced jejunal activity fronts during the four hour exercise period. The median number of fronts seen during this period was one. This difference was significant using the Mann Whitney U test (u=21, p=0.02). Of those subjects who had activity fronts, the median interval during the exercise period was 150 minutes (range 75-240) compared with 100 minutes (range 66-144) for the equivalent time period in the control group. This difference was again significant (u=42, p=0.01). If, however the results for all the exercise group was included (those who did not experience activity would therefore record a time of greater than 240 minutes, this being the total exercise period) the median jejunal phase III interval was 177 minutes (range 75-240) (Fig. 4).

Signal loss in the ambulatory studies is important and might account for missed activity fronts. The signal loss was found to be acceptable with a median value of 7.5 minutes (range 0-40), this was equivalent to only 3.5% of the total exercise period. Typical losses were less than five minutes for the whole test.

COMPARISON OF JEJUNAL ACTIVITY FRONT INTERVALS. EXERCISE v. RESTED CONTROLS

	Fasted Resting Controls (n = 10) Median (range)	Exercise Group (n = 10) Median (range)
Time to first jejunal activity front	* 102 mins (15 - 170)	* 115 mins (20 - 200)
Number of activity fronts during test period	20	10
Median number per subject	** 2 (1 - 3)	** 1 (0 - 2)
No. of subjects who had activity fronts during tests	10	6
Interval between activity fronts during test period	*** 100 mins (66 - 144)	*** 150 mins (75 - 240)
Signal loss on ambulatory recording		7.5 mins (3.5%) (0 - 40)

$$* \; u = 130 \quad p = NS$$
$$** \; u = 21 \quad p = 0.02$$
$$*** \; u = 42 \quad p = 0.01$$

Table I. A comparison of intervals of the MMC between the control and exercised groups.

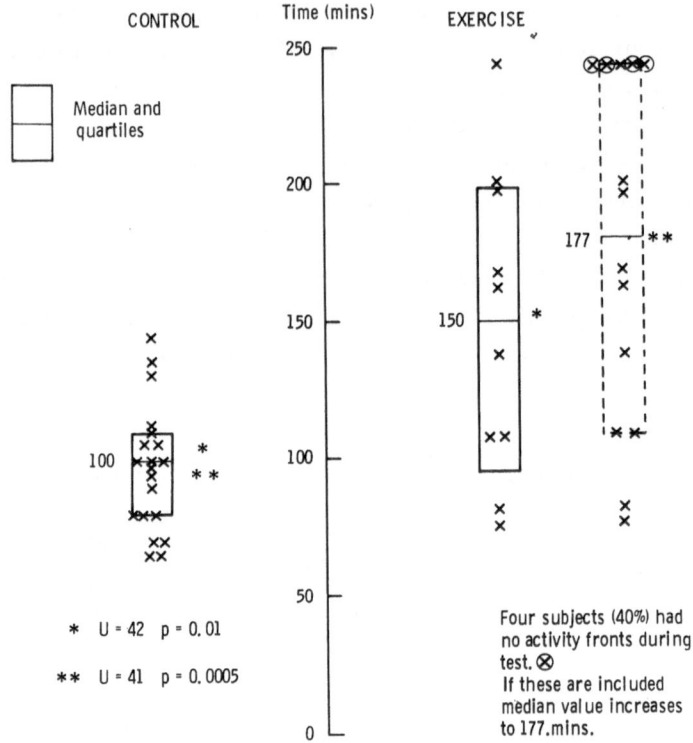

COMPARISON OF JEJUNAL ACTIVITY FRONT INTERVALS

Intervals between jejunal activity fronts were analysed for both groups. There was a significantly longer interval during the exercise period than seen in the resting controls. This was increased if those subjects with no activity fronts during exercise were also recorded.

Fig. 5.   A comparison of jejunal activity fronts between control and exercised subjects. Inclusion of times from those subjects with no fronts during exercise elevates the median interval to 177 minutes.

DISCUSSION

Radiotelemetry capsules and a portable receiver have been used to measure gastrointestinal motility in a group of subjects undergoing continuous exercise. The system has proved reliable and comfortable with little signal loss and can be adapted to many different situations where ambulation is necessary.

Phase III activity fronts of the MMC were easily recognised, there being a significant increase in the interval between fronts in the exercised group when compared to resting controls.

40% of the exercised group failed to show any phase III activity during the test period, in the control group however, all the subjects had at least one active phase during the test.

Modification of the timing of the migrating motor complex in this study may be controlled by a number of factors. The MMC rate may be modulated by a central control mechanism which inhibits gastro-intestinal activity during periods of physical exertion. An alternative explanation could be that of a hormonal modulation caused by a reduction of local gastrointestinal polypeptides such as motilin, a hormone known to be important in regulation of the MMC cycle (7). A third, but more simple explanation might be an overall reduction in gastrointestinal motility caused by reduction in blood flow to the gastrointestinal tract during sustained physical activity.

More work is needed to elucidate these mechanisms and to investigate further modifying influences of migrating motor activity in the small intestine.

REFERENCES:

1. Finch, P.M., Ingram, D.M., Henstridge, J.D. and Catchpole, B. (1982) The relationship of sleep stage to the migrating gastrointestinal complex in man. Gastroenterology, 83, 601-612

2. Evans, D.F., Foster, G.E. and Hardcastle, J.D. (1981). Motility patterns of the human antrum and jejunum and their association with sleep studies using a radiotelemetry system. Gut, 22, A424.

3. Valori, R.M., Patrick, M.P.H., Raiman, A., Parnham A. and Wingate, D.L. (1982). Prolonged and Intermittent stress inhibits human fasting motor complexes (M.C.'s). Gut, 23, A214.

4. Watson, B.W., Ross, B. and Kay, A.W. (1962). Telemetering from within the body using a pressure sensitive radio pill. Gut, 3, 181-186

5. Slater, E.J., Evans, D.F., Foster, G.E. and Hardcastle, J.D. (1982) A portable radiotelemetry receiver for ambulatory monitoring. J. Biomed. Eng., 4, 247-251.

6. Evans, D.F., Foster, G.E. and Hardcastle, J.D. (1982). The motility of the human antrum during the day and during sleep. An

investigation using a radiotelemetry system. ln: Wienbeck (ed).
Motility of the digestive tract. pp. 185-193. (New York: Raven Press)
7. Vantrappen, G., Janssens, J., Peeters, T.L., Bloom, S.R.,
Christofides, N.D. and Hellemans, J. (1979). Motilin and the interdigestive migrating motor complex in man. Diseases and Science.
24, 497-500.

48

Sham Feeding Amplifies the Secretory Component of Interdigestive Activity

T. L. PEETERS, G. VANTRAPPEN and J. JANSSENS

Sham feeding stimulates gastric secretion and the release of gut hormones, but the effect on motility is less documented. We studied the effect of sham feeding on motility, gastric acid, motilin and PP. In two groups of six volunteers' motility was assessed manometrically. In group I, gastric juice was aspirated, in group II no gastric collection was performed. Blood samples were taken every 10 minutes and analysed for PP and motilin. After one cycle of the migrating motor complex had been recorded a sham feeding (a steak of 150 g) was given by the chew and spit method, and the experiment was further continued for at least 3 hours. In both groups fluctuations of motilin and PP correlated to the motility cycle during the control period. Sham feeding did not interrupt the motor cycle nor the motilin fluctuations, but PP rose significantly. In group I acid output in the 30 min period preceding an activity front (AF) was higher than in the following 30 min period (0.64 vs. 0.28 mEq/30 min, $p < 0.05$). This secretory component was amplified after sham feeding (1.89 vs. 0.62 mEq/30 min, $p < 0.05$) and persisted although to a smaller extent during the second cycle after sham feeding (1.42 vs. 0.68 mEq/30 min). In group I the period of the MMC was 70 + 10 min. Interestingly, the period was larger in the second group during the control period (114 + 15 min) and still larger after sham feeding (142 + 24, $p < 0.05$). These data confirm the existence of a link between secretory and motor phenomena. Sham feeding mainly amplifies the secretory component. They also suggest that an increased basal acid secretion, lengthens the interdigestive cycle.

48

Sham Feeding Amplifies the Excitatory Component of Interdigestive Activity

J.F. ERPELL, G. VANTRAPPEN and JANSSEN

49

Jejunal Motility in Dystrophia Myotonica: a Manometric Study of Migrating Motor Complex

D. COUTURIER, S. GRANDJOUAN, L. ELOUAER-BLANC, A. VERDURON, B. TRAVERS, J. C. TURPIN, P. BOUCHE and J. GUERRE

Dystrophia Myotonica (DM) is a hereditary disease characterized mainly by progressive muscular atrophy and myotonia involving skeletal muscles with progressive muscle wasting and weakness. The electrophysiological feature of the disease is repetitive discharges of striated muscle cell membrane observed after voluntary or induced contractions. Cataract, testiculus atrophy, mental deficiency and fronto-parietal baldness are the more commun extramuscular symptoms of the disease (1, 2, 3). Cardiac muscle is commonly involved and conduction defects are observed. Gastrointestinal smooth muscle may also be involved : oesophagus (4, 5), stomach (6, 7), colon (8) and anal sphincter (9).

Small bowel involvement has been suggested by clinical (pseudoobstruction syndrome) (10) and radiological (dilatation of loops, delayed transit) (6) observations. Since the description of the interdigestive myoelectrical motor complex in man, possible abnormalities in pathological conditions where the gastrointestinal tract may be involved, should be seeked. Manometric investigation of gastric and duodenal motility in a patient with Dystrophia Myotonica has showed contractions of reduced amplitude in the fasted state and the occurence of migrating motor complex in the basal state (11). In a manometric study of jejunum in patients with DM, motility index of fed pattern was reduced and phase 2 of MMC was prolonged (12).

METHODS

The study was performed on 7 healthy volunteers (3 males, 4 females)

287

aged 24-33 years (mean 26 years) and 6 DM patients (2 males, 4 females) aged 14-46 years (mean 32 years). All 6 patients had a history of progressive muscular atrophy and myotonia with electromyographic features of the disease. Clinical symptoms of digestive involvement were systematically looked for : out of 6 patients, dysphagia was observed in one, abdominal pain in two and delayed digestive transit in one. Informed written consent was obtained from control subjects and patients.

PROCEDURE

Intraluminal pressure in the proximal jejunum was measured by means of three perfused tubes (maximal outer diameter of the catheter bundle 4 mm) bonded together with tetrahydrofuran. Side holes were 5 and 10 cm above the most distal side hole. A sealed mercury unit of 30 g weight was attached to the tip of the polyvinyl tube in order to facilitate its position_ing in the proximal jejunum. The tubes were continuously perfused with 0,9 % saline at a flow rate of 0.6 ml/min by an Arndorfer constant infusion pump ; pressures were recorded by statham P23 series transducers ; the write-out was on a Beckman R 511 A dynograph.

In another session oesophageal motility was evaluated manometrically using a three-tubes-probe and a recording system as described above. To evaluate the functional capacity of jejunal absorption a D-Xylose test was performed : blood level was measured one hour after a 25 g ingestion.

Experimental design

After overnight fasting, the probe was passed by nosetrip at 8 a.m then a controled low residue food intake of 200 cal was given. After about three hours, the probe was positioned fluoroscopically until the mercury unit was 15 cm distal to the ligament of Treitz and was fixed externally in order to prevent more progression. The onset of the recording was four hours after the 200 cal meal intake. Motor activity in the proximal jejunum was then continuously recorded for 4-5 h from noon to 4-5 p.m. During the recording time, the subjects adopted a semi reclining posture.

Motility recording analysis

Each jejunal recording was scanned to determine wether or not a cyclic pattern of motor activity was present. Phase 3 motor activity (P3) was defined as the period of intense and recurring motor activity lasting more than 2 min and distally propagated. The following data were measured.

- Total number of P3 (which were reported to the total duration of recordings to determine the mean duration of interdigestive cycles).

- The duration of phase 3 (min) from the onset of regular contractions to quiescence was calculated for each study. A mean value was obtained in each group.

- The velocity of migration (cm. min-1) of the MMC was assessed by dividing the distance transversed by the migrating phase 3 by the time taken to cross the three recording sites.

- Pressure wave maximal frequency was measured during phase 3 (No/min).

Peristaltic wave amplitudes were measured on the manometric oesophageal recordings, the mean amplitude of contraction was then calculated for the upper part (striated muscle area) and the lower part (smooth muscle area) of the oesophagus. The resting pressures within the uppser and lower oesophageal sphincters were measured and relaxation phases were evaluated. Significance of quantitative data was evaluated by the Mann and Whitney test.

RESULTS

Table 1 : Fasting jejunal motor activity in DM patients compared to that of a healthy control group by evaluation of Phase 3 migrating motor complexe characteristics (Values are mean ± sm).

	Healthy subjects	Dystrophica Myotonica	Statistical significance (Mann and Whitney)
Mean number of Phase 3 per hour of recording	0.75 n = 7	0.18 n = 6	$P < 0.05$
Duration of the Phase 3 (min)	5.99 ± 0.49 n = 5	3.41 ± 0.251 n = 4	$P < 0.01$
Velocity of Phase 3 propagation (cm.min-1)	8.73 ± 0.909 n = 5	4.96 ± 1.073 n = 4	$P < 0.02$
Maximum jejunal contraction rate (No./min)	11.65 ± 0.047 n = 5	11.67 ± 0.103 n = 4	NS

Oesophageal and/or intestinal functionnal disturbances : In one patient (GUI) a moderate dysphagia associated with dysphonia appeared 3
years after the firt signs of Dystrophia Myotonica ; in two patients
(AUD, CAB) erratic abdominal pain associated in one case with intestinal transit disorders suggested gut involvement.

Table 1 indicates that a cyclic pattern of jejunal motor activity
was present in 6/7 healthy controls and in 4/6 DM patients. To compare
the mean duration of interdigestive cycle in both groups, the total
number of phase 3 was reported to the total duration of recordings and
the mean number of P3 per hour of recording was calculated.

The phase 3 occurrence is significantly reduced in the DM patients
group (0.18) in comparison with the healthy control group (0.75) (P <
0.05). Considering the characteristics of phase 3, the mean duration
is shorter in DM patients group (3.41 ± 0.251 min) than in controls
group 5.99 ± 0.491 min) (P < 0.01) ; the time taken for phase 3 to
travel through the studied jejunal loop was 4.96 ± 1.073 in DM group
(control 8.73 ± 0.909 - P < 0.05). Amplitude and frequency of jejunal
contractions during P3 in DM patients were not different from normal.

In 4 out of 6 DM patients recordings, when P3 was identified, we
tried to distinguish the other phases of the cyclic activity : in 2
cases Phase 1 which is characterized by an absence of contractions, is
short or absent ; and in the other 2 cases phases 1 were observed, but
such a "silent" period was observed recurrently and not consecutively
to a P3 period.

In two out of 6 DM patients recordings where P3 were not observed,
the motor activity was sustained and consisted in series of bursts of
contractions, the frequency was near the maximum rate but bursts of
contractions do not travel distally along the jejunal loop.

The results of manometric evaluation of oesophageal motility are
presented in Table 2.

As already mentioned, the most consistent abnormalities in DM patients are a decrease in UOS resting pressure and in amplitude of peristaltic contractions of the proximal oesophagus. Two DM patients
(FOU, GUI) presented an important decrease of peristaltic contraction
of the distal oesophagus while a slight decrease was observed in the
remainder. In one case (FOU) a reduced LOS resting pressure was associated suggesting a major involvement of the smooth muscle portion of

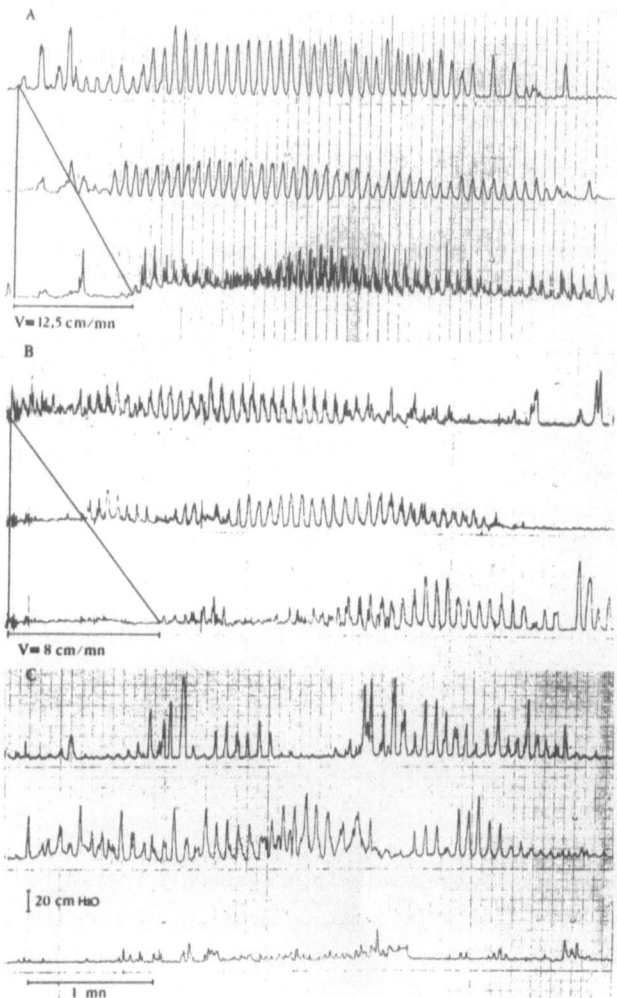

FIGURE 1 Manometric recordings of fasting jejunal motility. The
first three figures show from top to bottom : the proximal,
the mean distance catheter recording and the distal catheter recording.
A - Phase 3 in a healthy control subject.
B - Phase 3 in a DM patient (CAB).
C - Sustained motor activity comprising series of bursts of
contractions, not clearly propagated, in a DM patient
(TAU).

the oesophagus (13). Two others patients (AUD, TAU) presented a prolonged relaxation phase of the UOS while each of them had a normal relaxation phase of the LOS. In one case (FOU) the cyclic fasting jejunal motility was absent during recording suggesting an .important
small bowel involvement. In this case, the xylose test was at the lower limit of the normal range. In 5/6 DM patients, D xylose test value
was within normal range excluding an important jejunal malabsorption.

Table 2 : Manometric evaluation of oesophageal motility (UOS : upper
oesophageal sphincter ; LOS : lower oesophageal sphincter ;
N : normal ; ↗ : increase induration).

	UOS resting pressure (cm H_2O)	UOS relaxation	LOS resting pressure (cm H_2O)	LOS relaxation	Amplitude of peristaltic contractions (cm H_2O) Proximal: 10 cm	Distal 10 cm
GUI	32	N	30	N	5	10
AUD	30	↗	20	N	20	30
TAU	25	↗	36	N	15	20
DEV		N	32	N	8	25
CAV	10	N	31	N	8	20
FOU			10		5	15

DISCUSSION

Involvement of smooth muscle is a less well recognized aspect of
DM. There is very little information available about the pattern of
small bowel motor activity in these patients in contrast to the oesophagus.

The present study revealed that fasting motor activity in proximal
jejunum is abnormal in DM patients. In two of these patients, a cyclic
pattern of motor activity was not identified. Whereas, bursts of marked contractions alternated with short quiescent phases occuring during
5-6 hour recordings. Kerlin, in a recent study in healthy subjects
(14), reported that the mean period between two successive phases 3
migrating motor complexes was variable with a wide range from 15 min
to > 3 h.

As suggested by others, phase 3 activity was the most readily defi-

ned facet of fasting motility. The evaluation of P3 characteristics -
when occurred- demonstrated the marked reduction in cyclic fasting
jejunal activity in our patients compared to control subjects as previously reported (12). The mean duration of P3 activity was shorter
and then jejunal propagation velocity was slower. In contrast, the maximal rate of rythmic contractions and their mean amplitude measured
during P3 occurrence was normal. In a study of duodenal myoelectrical
activity in a DM patient, Daniel and Lewis (11) showed that a migrating motor complex occurred in the basal state. It was no different
than seen in normal subjects apart from the maximal frequency of contractions which was as high as 18.5/min and as low as 11.0/min. The
difference observed between this previous work and ours should be explained by the differences in calculating methods. In the present
work, the maximal rate was evaluated only during P3 activity while the
short periods of fast contractions were taken into account in the
previous study. However, this value in normal subjects decreased from
duodenum to ileum (14).

As previously notified in the upper gastrointestinal tract, there
is no parallelism between clinical and manometric disturbances. All DM
patients presented abnormalities of their fasting cyclic pattern while
only 2 developed clinical signs. The absence of phase 3 activity was
noted in 2 patients without symptoms of small bowel involvement while
2 other patients with abdominal signs demonstrated manometric features
of cyclic activity. In this studied group, there is no correlation between manometric results and the severity of striated muscle alterations
or the length of disease history.

The recording of UOS showed similar findings to those previously
reported (5). A decrease of peristaltic contraction amplitude in the
distal part of the oesophagus was noted in every DM patient more markedly in two and with a decrease of LOS resting pressure in one of the
latter. An absence of peristalsis or a reduced amplitude has been mentioned in half of the DM patients in a previous study (5) while the
LOS resting pressures were normal. It is of interest to note that the
patient who developed an abnormal LOS resting pressure in our study had
the longest disease history. Garret et al (15) documented similar abnormalities and also found a reduced resting pressure at the gastro-
oesophageal junction. Two of our DM patients presented a prolonged re-

laxation phase of their UOS while it was normal in the LOS. This feature already pointed out by Siegel (13) suggested that myotonia of the
oesophageal muscle was involved as well as simple failure of its action.

As in sclerodermia, it has been notified long ago that manometric
disturbances of the oesophagus usually precede dysphagia. This fact
appeared very clearly in this study since only one of our DM patients
presented with dysphagia while all of them demonstrated abnormalities
of oesophageal peristalsis.

Our aim was to relate oesophageal and small bowel manometric disturbances. One of the two patients with a major decreased amplitude
of peristaltic contractions in distal oesophagus showed absence of cyclic activity in proximal jejunum. Such an association suggested an
important smooth muscle involvement of the disease. For the remainder
in DM group, it appeared that the smooth muscle manometric alterations
were not homogeneous in all parts of the digestive tract. We observed
that none of our DM patients presented jejunal malabsorption tested by
D-xylose.

The maximum rate of contractions in proximal jejunum being normal
for our patients,the electrical control activity seemed unchanged in
DM. It is likely that the other changes of P3 characteristics are related to muscle cell histological alterations (e.g., dystrophy and
fatty infiltration) (8).

It is known that while fasting, flow of intestinal contents is intermittent and variable with the presence of absence of P3. The phase
3 activity periods contributed to 50 % of total fasting flow (16). Our
results could explain that when shorter and more slowly propagated,
the phase 3 may contribute to delayed transit of barium (8).

In conclusion, gastrointestinal motility was throuroghly investigated
in 6 patients with Dystrophia Myotonica. The abnormal fasting motor
activity of jejunum demonstrated here   indicates a possible mechanism by which intestinal stasis and clinical disturbances of intestinal transit might arise.

BIBLIOGRAPHIE

1 - Nowak T.V., Ionacescu V., Anuras S. (1982). Gastrointestinal mani-
     festations of the muscular dystrophies. Gastroenterology, 82, 800-
     810.

2 - Turpin J.-C., Morice J. (1980). La gravité de la dystrophie myo-
pathique myotonique de Steinert. Sem. Hôp. Paris, 56, 335-340.

3 - Tome F.M.S., Fardeau M. (1976). Dystrophie myotonique de Steinert. Encycl. Med. Chir., Paris, Neurologie, 17178 B-10.

4 - Siegel C.I., Hendrix T.R., Harvey J.C. (1966). The swallowing
disorder in myotonia dystrophica. Gastroenterology, 50, 541-550.

5 - Swick H.M., Werlin S.L., Dodds W.J., Hogan W.J. (1981). Pharyn-
goeosophageal motor function in patients with myotonic dystrophy.
Ann. Neurol., 10, 454-457.

6 - Simpson A.F., Khilnani M.T. (1975). Gastrointestinal manifestations of the muscular dystrophies. Am. J. Roentgenol. Radium Ther.
Nucl. Med., 125, 948-955.

7 - Kuiper D.H. (1971). Gastric bezoar in a patient with myotonic
dystrophy. Dig. Dis., 16, 529-534.

8 - Bertrand L. (1949). Le megacolon dans la maladie de Steinert.
Rev. Neurol. Paris, 81, 480-486.

9 - Shuster M.M., Tow D.E., Sherbourne D.H. (1965). Anal sphincter
abnormalities characteristic of myotonic dystrophy. Gastroenterology, 49, 641-648.

10 - Faulk D.L., Anuras S., Christensen J. (1978). Chronic intestinal
pseudo obstruction. Gastroenterology, 74, 922-931.

11 - Lewis T.D., Daniedl E.E. (1981). Gastroduodenal motility in a
case of dystrophia myotonica. Gastroenterology, 81, 145-149.

12 - Nowak T.V., Brown B.P., Green J.B., Ionasescu V.V., Anuras S.
(1982). Jejunal manometry in patients with myotonic dystrophy.
Gastroenterology. (abst.), 82, 1139

13 - Siegel C.I., Henrix T.R., Harvey J.C. (1966). The swallowing disorder in myotonia dystrophica. Gastroenterology, 50, 541-551.

14 - Kerlin P., Phillips S. (1982). Variability of motility of the
ileum and jejunum in healthy humans. Gastroenterology, 82, 694-
700.

15 - Garret J.M., Dubose T.D.,Jackson J.E., Norman J.R. (1969). Oesophageal and pulmonary disturbances in myotonica dystrophica.
Arch. Intern. Med., 123, 26-32.

16 - Kerlin P., Zinsmeister A., Phillips S. (1982). Relationship of
motility to flow of contents in the human small intestine.
Gastroenterology, 82, 701-706.

50

Modification of the Interdigestive Migrating Motor Complex (IMMC) in Patients with Partial Gastrectomy and Gastrojejunostomy

M. BORTOLOTTI, G. BERSANI, A. LONGANESI, T. CALLETTI,
S. FOSCHI and G. LABÒ

The interdigestive motor activity of the stomach and proximal jejunum was recorded with a manometric probe in 8 patients who underwent partial gastrectomy and gastrojejunostomy (Billroth II) for duodenal ulcer (PG group), in 9 normals (N group) and in 5 patients with duodenal ulcer (DU group). The latter two groups were considered as controls. In the PG group the motor activity was recorded from the gastric remnant and from the efferent loop, and the results were compared with recordings at similar levels in the other two groups. The probe catheters were perfused with bubble free water by using a low-compliance pneumo-hydraulic pump and were connected to transducers P 23 Db and a polygraph. The recording was carried out after 14 hours of fasting and lasted at least 180 minutes each.

Results. In control groups the IMMC phase III activity fronts began from the stomach sweeping through the small intestine with a mean time interval of 107 min (range 69-120 min) in the N group and 121 min (range 95-138 min) in the DU group. In the PG group the gastric remnant did not show any cyclic pressure variation that could be ascribed to IMMC phase III activity fronts. Conversely, the efferent loop showed phase III activity fronts at a mean time interval of 41 min (range 20-64 min). The mean propagation velocity of these activity fronts was 3.1 cm/min (range 2.5-4.8 cm/min) whereas that of the control groups was 5 cm/min (range 4.5-6.8 cm/min). The duration of the activity front in the PG group was 4.8 min (range 3.5-5.6 min), whereas in the control groups it was 6.5 min (range 4.4-7.2 min). In addition, in the PG groups there was a clear prevalence of phase II, lasting approximately 5/6 of the entire cycle, whereas in the control groups phase II activity lasted about 3/4 of the entire cycle.

Conclusion. The removal of the gastric antrum following the Billroth II procedure is associated with clear modifications of the characteristics of the intestinal IMMC, and in particular with a striking increase in the frequency of the phase III activity fronts as observed either after truncal vagotomy with splancnicectomy (1) and after complete denervation of an autotransplanted intestinal loop (2). So we may conclude that the nervous inhibitory mechanism, that in normal conditions continuously slows down the idio-intestinal IMMC frequency at the level of the gastric IMMC, requires the presence of the gastric antrum, where the inhibition likely originates.

References
1) Ruckebusch Y.,Bueno L. Gastroenterology 73:1309-1314,1977.
2) Sarr M.G.,Kelly K.A. Gastroenterology 78:1251   1980.

51

Disorganisation of the Interdigestive Small Bowel Motility by *E. coli* Endotoxin in the Rat

S. GUSTAVSSON, B. RÖNNBERG, E. STÅHLE and T. WADSTRÖM

INTRODUCTION

There is a growing awareness that enteropathogenic bacteria can mediate intestinal dysfunction not only via effects on secretion but also by affecting intestinal motility. Thus, in the rabbit ileal loop model, a number of bacteria and bacterial toxins - Vibrio cholerae, cholera toxin, enteroinvasive E.coli, heat-stable (ST) E.coli enterotoxin etc - are known to produce alterations in the myoelectric pattern (1-3).

ST is a common etiological factor in E.coli diarrhoea and in the present investigation we are studying whether this enterotoxin interferes with the interdigestive small bowel motility, i.e. one proposed mechanism for clearance of the intestinal lumen from noxious elements.

MATERIAL AND METHODS

Motility experiments

Male Sprague-Dawley rats (150-200 g b.w.) were provided by a central venous catheter the day before the experiment. The small bowel motility pattern was studied in fasting animals by intravenous infusion of a bile-excreted radiopharmaceutic (^{99}Tc^{m}-HIDA, Solco Nuclear, Basle). Immediately after the end of the infusion period (1 hour) the gastrointestinal tract was excised in continuity, stretched out on a Perspex plate and scanned for radioactivity (4). In fasting control animals the radioactivity along the small bowel is distributed in distinct

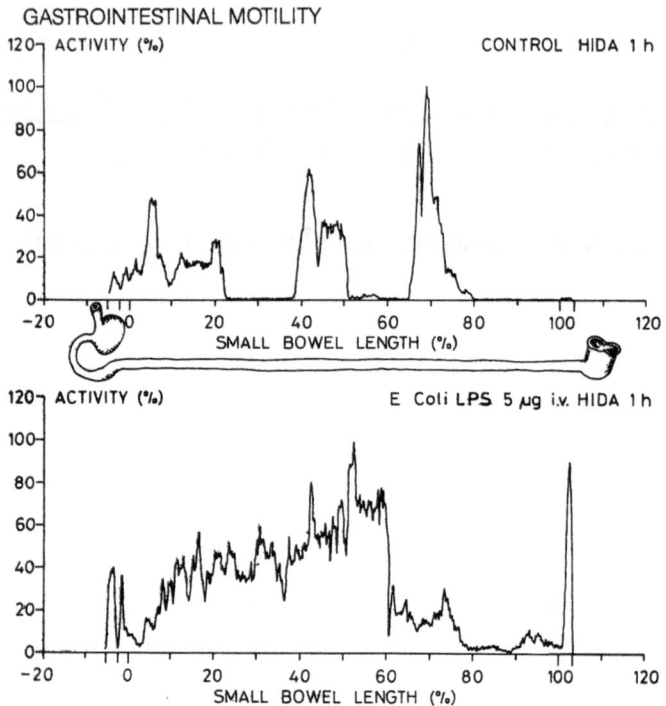

Fig. 1. Distribution of radioactivity along the excised gastrointestinal specimen. The bile-excreted radiopharmaceutic ^{99}Tc^m-HIDA has been
infused for 1 hour. The curves have been normalized to 100 % at their
maximum point. In fasting control animals (upper panel) the radioactivity is distributed in a few separate portions. After i.v. injection of crude ST or endotoxin (lower panel) no distinct portions are
recognized (disorganised interdigestive motility **pattern**).

portions separated by fairly long completely empty segments (Fig. 1,
upper panel). The number of portions (3-4 in 1 hour) corresponds well
with the reported frequency of the migrating myoelectric complex (MMC)
in this species (5). Further, by combining the HIDA-method with electro-
myographical recordings we have proven that the development of the portions of intestinal contents is a result of muscular contractions induced by phase III of the MMC (6).

Bacterial products

Crude ST was produced by cultivating an E.coli strain (C57/26C$_2$) in
a 10 litre broth fermentor culture. The supernatant was filtrated
through a Millipore filter and heat-treated (80° for 20 min).

Semi-purified ST was produced by ultrafiltration of crude ST on an
Amicon filter (cut off mol weight 10 000). The filtrate was further
purified by hydrophobic interaction chromatography on Octylsepharose
CL-48 (Pharmacia Fine Chemicals, Uppsala, Sweden) (7). The amount of
semi-purified ST giving a positive gut-body ratio (> 0.09) in the suck-
ling mouse assay was 5 ng (one effective dose).

Toxin preparations. Endotoxin E.Coli 0.55:B5, smooth strain lipo-
polysacharide (LPS) was purchased from List Biological Laboratories,
California. The LD_{50} in 20 gram mice for this preparation is 250 ug.
Highly purified cholera toxin was purchased from Schwartz/ Mann Inc.,
Spring Valley, New York.

RESULTS

Enteral administration

Neither of the bacterial products were capable of changing the
interdigestive small bowel motility pattern from normal when admin-
istrered perorally (by orogastric intubation in light ether anesthesia)
or intraduodenally (via an indwelling catheter). Maximum doses used:
Crude ST = 1 200 mouse doses, endotoxin = 1 000 µg, cholera toxin =
150 µg.

Parenteral administration

Intravenous and intraperitoneal administration of crude ST resulted
in a complete change in the normal fasting motility pattern. As exempli-
fied in Fig. 1 lower panel there are neither distinct portions nor empty regions between the portions. After successive purification of the
crude ST preparation the effect on motility diminished. We found that
the effect was related to the endotoxin content, as measured by KDO
determination (Ståhle, Gustavsson, Rönnberg, Wadström, to be published).

Semi-purified ST had no effect on the normal interdigestive motility
when administered in doses as high as 900 mouse doses intravenously or
intraperitoneally.

E-Coli LPS iv Dose (μg/animal)	Interdigestive motility pattern Normal(n)	Disorganized(n)
0.5	1	0
1.0	1	0
2.0	0	3
2.5	1	1
5.0	2	5
10.0	0	10
50.0	2	8
Pretreatment with Indomethacin 20mg/kg 50.0	7	1

Endotoxin. According to the Table endotoxin administered intravenously changed the normal small bowel motility pattern from normal when
administered in doses of 5 μg and above. After pretreatment with indomethacin (20 mg/kg) the effect of endotoxin on motility was abolished.

Cholera toxin (200 μg/kg b.w.) had no effect on the interdigestive
small bowel motility pattern when administered 12-24 hours before the
motility recording.

DISCUSSION

Our preliminary findings suggested that crude ST inhibited the normal interdigestive small bowel motility in our rat model (8). However,
ST seemed to be effective only after intravenous or intraperitoneal
administration but not after intraluminal inocculation, a route of
administration used by Mathias et al. (3). Further, after each successive purification step of our crude preparations the effect on motility
diminished indicating that also other factors beside ST in the preparations may affect the development of interdigestive motility complexes.
In fact the present study indicates that the effect of ST on motility,
if any, is weak in comparison with other bacterial products in the crude
preparations.

The reason for the discrepancy between our findings and those obtained in the ileal loop model concerning ST and cholera toxin may well
be explained in differences in methodological approach. The sensitivi-

ty for bacterial toxins is known to vary between different species.   In
the rabbit ileal loop model the animal is in general anaesthesia and
the motility is recorded immediately after a laparotomy.   Further, the
electric phenomenona described in the ileal loop model have no similarity with classical MMC-complexes as they orginally were described by
Szurziewski (9).

Clearly the findings that minimal amounts of endotoxin given systematically induce a complete disorganisation of the normal interdigestive pattern, warrant further studies.   It is known that endotoxin
Can affect gastric emptying (10) but the effect of endotoxin on small
bowel motility has not been studied as known to us.   We think that the
effect of endotoxin on interdigestive motility may be of clinical
importance since it occurs already at doses where circulatory and hema-
tological parameters of the animals are unchanged.

At present we cannot state whether the effect of endotoxin on
motility is a direct one or whether it is mediated by activation of
cascade phenomena.   The capability of indomethacin, a prostaglandin
synthesis inhibitor, to inhibit the effect of endotoxin may indicate
one possible mediator for the effect (8).

We speculate that the effect of endotoxin on gut motility may be
of clinical importance in some conditions where there is a defect in
the mucosal barrier giving rise to resorption of endotoxin from the
gut lumen.   Endotoxin effects on motility may also contribute to intestinal paralysis in intestinal ischema, postoperative inhibition and
mechanical ileus.

REFERENCES

1. Mathias, J.R., Carlson, G.M., DiMarino, A.J., Bertiger, G.,
Morton, H.E. and Cohen, S. (1976) Intestinal Myoelectric Activity in
Response to Live Vibrio Cholerae and Cholera Enterotoxin. J. Clin.
Invest., 58, 91-96
2. Burns, T.H., Mathias, J.R., Martin, J.L., Carson, G.M. and
Shields, R.P. (1980). Alteration of myoelectric activity of small
intestine by invasive Escherichia coli. Am. J. Physiol., 238, G57-G62
3. Mathias, J.R., Nogueira, J., Martin, J.L., Carlson,G.M. and
Giannella, R.A. (1982). Am. J. Physiol., 242, G360-G363

4. Wilén, T., Gustavsson, S. and Jung, B. (1980). Study of Small Bowel Transport Pattern in Fasted, Conscious Rats with an Intact Gastrointestinal Tract. A Methodological Study with Bile-Excreted $^{99}Tc^m$-Solco-HIDA. Eur. surg. Res., 12, 283-293

5. Ruckebusch, M. And Fioramonti, J. (1975). Electrical spiking activity and propulsion in small intestine in fed and fasted rats. Gastroenterology, 68, 1500-1508

6. Wilén, T., Gustavsson, S. and Jung, B. (1983). Evidence for a Propulsive Function of the Migrating Myoelectric Complex (MMC) in Rats. Eur. surg. Res., in press

7. Rönnberg, B. and Wadström, T. (1983) Improved Method for Purification of Human Escherichia coli Heat-Stable Enterotoxin by Hydrophobic Interaction, Molecular-Sieve and High Performance Liquid Chromatography. Prep. Biochem., in press

8. Gustavsson, S., Rönnberg, B., Ståhle, E., Wilén, T. and Wadström, T. (1983). Disorganisation of the Small Bowel Transport Pattern by E.Coli Heat-Stable (ST) Enterotoxin in a Rat Model. Experimental Bacterial and Parasitic Infections, eds. Keusch and Wadström, pp 219-223

9. Szurszewski, J.H. (1969) A migrating electric complex of the canine small intestine. Am. J. Physiol., 217, 1757-1763

10. van Miert, A.S.J.P.A.M and van Duin, C.Th.M. (1980). Endotoxin-Induced Inhibition of Gastric Emptying Rate in the Rat. The Effect of Repeated Administration and the Influence of some Antipyretic Agents. Arch. int. Pharmacodyn., 246, 19-27.

ACKNOWLEDGEMENT

Financial support was obtained from the Swedish Medical Research Council (project no 17X- 3498 and 16X- 4723).

52

Abnormal Gastrointestinal Motility in Diabetics and after Vagotomy

G. E. FOSTER, D. F. EVANS, J. R. ARDEN-JONES, A. BEATTIE and J. D. HARDCASTLE

INTRODUCTION

The most widely performed operation for peptic ulcer disease is a truncal vagotomy and drainage procedure. Intermittent diarrhoea is seen in 20% of cases following this operation and this can be prolonged and incapacitating in 5% of individuals (1) overshadowing any direct benefit due to the surgery. A number of subjects with well controlled diabetes mellitus suffer from the gastrointestinal side effects of bloating after food and intractable diarrhoea, often of a very urgent nature (2). Two clinical conditions can thus coexist with severe abnormalities of gastrointestinal motility. We have previously described abnormal fasting jejunal rhythms in such subjects (3) but studies that have endeavoured to identify a specific site or sites of abnormal activity have been few (4) (5).

We have studied fasting and fed gastrointestinal motility patterns in a group of patients suffering from postvagotomy diarrhoea and in a group of diabetics with functional gastrointestinal motor abnormalities. In addition gastric emptying studies of both solids and liquids have been performed and results obtained have been compared to those recorded from a group of normal volunteer subjects.

SUBJECTS & METHODS

Subjects:

Studies have been performed on eight diabetics (mean age 36.6 yrs $\mp$ 6.5 s.e.m.) all with proven neuropathy and gastrointestinal symptoms of pain, diarrhoea, alternating bowel habit, gustatory sweating and

305

nausea and vomiting. Autonomic denervation had been confirmed in
this group by standard physiological testing (6).

Nine patients with postvagotomy diarrhoea were studied (mean age
48.1 yrs $\mp$ 10.5 s.e.m) all of whom had symptoms for at least twelve
months. Studies in the patient groups were compared with results from
nine normal subjects (mean age 24 yrs $\mp$ 4.7 s.e.m). Informed consent
was obtained from all patients and volunteers in the study and all
methods were approved by the Nottingham Hospitals Ethical Committee.

Methods:

Gastrointestinal motility and gastric emptying:

Long term studies of fasting gastric and jejunal motility were
performed as previously described by us (3) using a linked pressure
sensitive radiotelemetry capsule (RTC). After a period of fasting
activity of at least two MMC cycles had been recorded subjects were
fed a standard meal. Whilst motility patterns continued to be
recorded, dual phase solid and liquid gastric emptying was monitored
as described below and the time taken for fasting MMC activity to
return was noted.

Gastric emptying:

The test meal given to the patients consisted of a pre-cooked roast
chicken dinner. The meal also contained 30gm of chicken liver labelled
with 5mCi 99m technetium sulphur colloid, this constituted the solid
phase of the meal. The liquid phase of the meal was 2C0ml of fresh
orange juice labelled with 119 indium. The two phases of the meal
were differentially imaged using a computer controlled gamma camera.
Times for 50% (T_{50}) and 90% (T_{90}) of each phase to leave the stomach
were calculated. In some cases, especially in those patients with
delayed emptying the T_{90} time was obtained by extrapolation. Results
from the patient group were compared to those from the nine normal
subjects.

STATISTICAL ANALYSIS

Results were compared using the standard t test or the Mann Whitney U
test as appropriate according to data distribution.

RESULTS

Small intestinal motility

The intervals between jejunal phase III activity fronts were compared
in each of the three groups and are summarised in Table I

Table I. Jejunal phase III interval.

Group & number of fronts analysed	Mean interval (mins)	s.e.m.	Median	Range
Normal n=117	105.5 ***	4.1	101	12-240
Vagotomy n=57	88.6 *	6.4	76	13-286
Diabetic n=41	83.00**	6.9	80	23-247

Student t test

*   p< 0.05

**   p< 0.01

In both the vagotomy (p< 0.05) and diabetic group (p< 0.01) the intervals between phase III fronts were significantly shorter than those of the control subjects.

Also recorded was the time to appearance of the first phase III activity front following feeding (Table II), this too was significantly shorter in both the vagotomy (=0.03) and diabetic group (p=0.003) than that of the asymptomatic normal controls.

In one of the diabetic subjects and two with post vagotomy diarrhoea sporadic bursts of high frequency, high amplitude activity were seen in the jejunum which we have termed 'Q' complexes (3) and in each case these were associated with an absence of any phase III activity fronts

Table II. Return of fasting jejunal activity after food.

Group & number of subjects	Median return of fasting activity front (mins)	Range
Normal n=9	348 ***	108-564
Diabetic n=8	168 *	66-281
Vagotomy n=9	239 **	138-436

Mann Whitney U Test

*   u=17 p=0.003

**   u=32 p=0.03

Gastric Emptying

The results of the gastric emptying studies are summarised in Table III and shown graphically in Figure 1. In the diabetics, emptying rates for both liquid (p< 0.02) and solid (p< 0.002) components at the T_{90} (90% emptying) level were significantly slower than those seen in normal

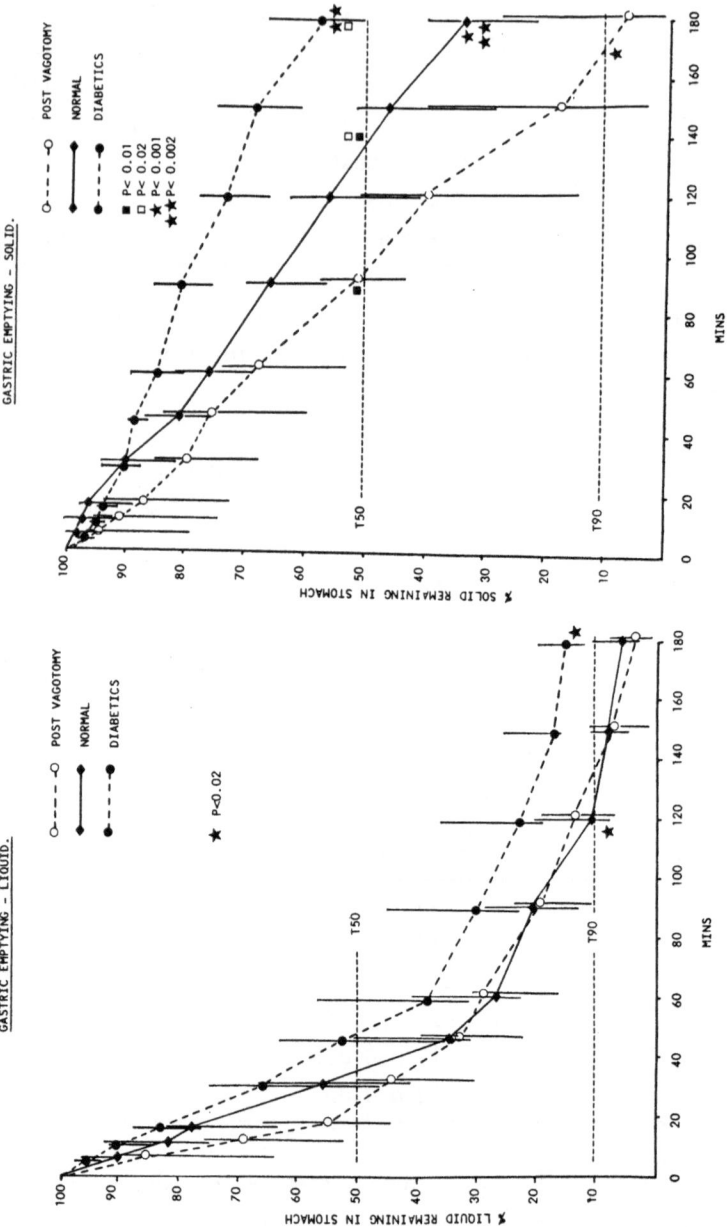

Fig. 1. Gastric emptying of the test meal in post vagotomy, diabetics and normal controls

subjects and significant amounts of solid (25%) remained in the
diabetic stomach when 'fasting' MMC activity resumed. In contrast
to the diabetics,in the vagotomy subjects solids emptied
significantly faster both to 50% T_{50} (p$<$0.01) and 90% T_{90} (p$<$0.001)
than from the stomachs of the normal group.

Table III. Gastric emptying of solids and liquid components of meal.

	Normal n=9	Diabetic n=8	Vagotomy n=9
Liquid 50% median (range) mins	34 (22-57)	40 (20-90)	20 (10-60)
Liquid 90% median (range) mins	*120 (100-170)	*220 (180-240)	130 (90-180)
Solid 50% median (range) mins	+140 (85-200)	*200 (180-225)	+ 94 (45-140)
Solid 90% median (range) mins	++220 (165-260)	++320 (250-450)	**170 (110-234)

$$* \quad p<0.02 \qquad + \quad p<0.01$$
$$** \; p<0.001 \quad ++ \; p<0.002$$

DISCUSSION

In this study similar jejunal motility patterns were seen in post
vagotomy patients with diarrhoea and diabetics with functional
motility disorders. In both groups the fasting MMC cycled more
frequently than in normal subjects, a conflict with that of previous
workers (7) who found no difference between the fasting activity of
four vagotomy patients with diarrhoea and a number of normal subjects.
A faster return from a fed jejunal pattern with a fasting MMC was also
seen in the vagotomy patients, this possibly due to the more rapid
gastric emptying of solids and liquids seen in this group. By
contrast the diabetic patients also had a shorter fed pattern of
activity, in them however, the fasting MMC resumed when significant
amounts of food still remained in the stomach. Differences between
the two groups may be due to an added sympathetic denervation
demonstrable in the latter.

Objective gastrointestinal motility patterns have been demonstrated
in groups of patients with functional motility disorders. Jejunal
recordings were made using a convenient and patient acceptable radiotelemetry method, none of our subjects failing to or refusing to

swallow the RTCs, side effects were minimal. Methods such as these
should begin to play a part in the investigation of functional
motility disorders in man.

REFERENCES

1. Barnes, A.D. and Cox, A.G. (1969). Diarrhoea. In: Williams and
Cox (eds). After Vagotomy. pp 211-219. (London: Butterworth)

2. Atkinson, M. and Hosking, D.J. (1983). Gastrointestinal
complications of diabetics mellitus. Clinics in Gastroenterology, 12,
633-650.

3. Foster, G.E., Arden-Jones, J.R., Evans, D.F., Beattie, A.B., and
Hardcastle, J.D. (1982) Abnormal jejunal motility in gastrointestinal
disease. In: Wienbeck (ed). Motility of the digestive tract. pp 427-432
(New York: Raven Press)

4. McNally, E.K., Reinhard, A.E. and Schwartz P.E. (1969). Small
bowel motility in diabetics. Am. J. Dig., 14, 163-169.

5. Whalen, G.E., Soergel, K.H. and Geenen, J.E.   (1969). Diabetic
Diarrhoea. A Clinical & Pathophysiological study. Gastroenterology, 56,
1021-1032.

6. Hosking, D.J., Bennett, T.B. and Hampton, J.R.   (1978) Diabetic
autonomic neuropathy. Diabetes, 27, 1043-1055.

7. Thompson, D.G., Ritchie, H.D. and Wingate, D.L. (1982). Patterns
of small intestinal motility in duodenal ulcer patients before and
after vagotomy. Gut, 23, 517-523.

53

Stimulation of Action Potential Complexes by Fluid Distension of Rabbit Small Intestine – Evidence that Migrating Action Potential Complexes are a Non-specific Myoelectric Response

R. W. SJOGREN, M. WARDLOW and L. G. CHARLES

Migrating action potential complexes (MAPC's) are an abnormal motility pattern that have primarily been associated with certain bacterial enterotoxins.[1-5] It has been reported that sudden luminal distension in vivo does not result in MAPC's.[1] However, the peristaltic reflex due to sudden in vitro luminal distension has been reported to result in aborally propagating action potentials and contraction rings.[6-8] Neither approach has studied the effects of gradual luminal distension which would be more likely to occur in clinical diarrheal illness. An association of action potential bursts with fluid production has been reported in rabbits infected with Salmonella in vivo, but the contribution of luminal distension per se was not assessed.[9] The purpose of this study was to describe the effect of gradual in vivo luminal distension on myoelectric activity.

MATERIALS AND METHODS

Male New Zealand white rabbits were studied. Anesthesia was induced with ketamine and xylazine and maintained with intermittent intravenous pentobarbital. In 12 healthy animals a 15 cm loop was constructed in the terminal ileum 10 cm orad to the mesenteric attachment of the appendiceal tip (Figure 1). Drainage catheters were placed into the distal portion of the loop and into the ileum immediately proximal to the loop. An injection catheter was placed into the proximal portion of the loop. Three $Ag-AgCl_2$ bipolar electrodes were sutured to

311

the serosa of the loop at 2 to 3.5 cm intervals at least 2.5 cm from
catheter tips.   39°C intraperitoneal temperature was maintained with a
hydrothermal blanket.   Fluid output was measured volumetrically.

FIGURE 1:   SCHEMATIC DIAGRAM OF IN VIVO RABBIT ILEAL LOOP

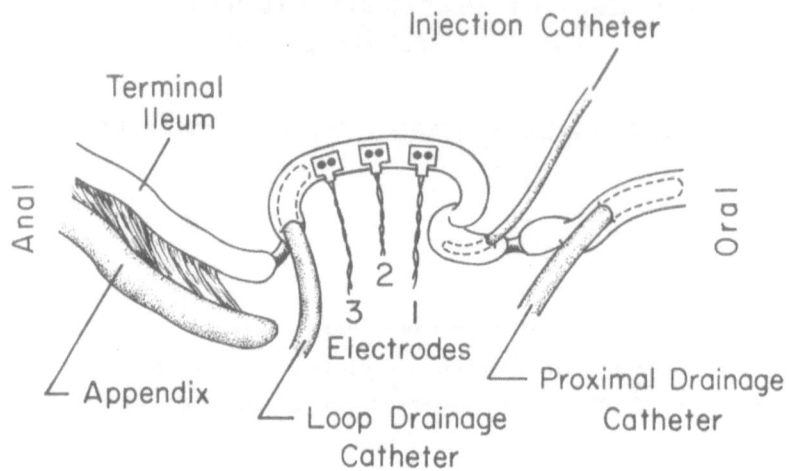

Following surgery and a 30 minute postoperative stabilization period, continuous recordings began.   After the 30 minute pre-test period,
continuous 2.4 ml/hr perfusion of phosphate buffered saline at pH 7.4
was begun.   The perfusion rate of 2.4 ml/hr was selected to correspond
with fluid output obtained in response to 100 µg of cholera toxin
(Calbiochem, La Jolla, CA) in preliminary studies.   The outflow cannula in six of the animals was obstructed resulting in gradual loop
distension, while in the remaining six it remained patent.   All animals were recorded for the 6 hour test period following which obstruc-
tions were relieved and recording continued in both groups of animals
for the 1 hour post-test period.   After the study, the ileum was removed and electrode positions measured with the loop under a constant
10 gm stretch.   Transmural biopsies were obtained between electrodes
and from ileum immediately proximal to the loop for light microscopy.

Taped data was computer analyzed.   Analog data was amplified and
band pass filtered at 0.16-30 Hz for slow waves and at 5.3-30 Hz for
spikes.   For slow wave analysis, 1 Hz analog to digital conversion was
performed for the first 256 consecutive seconds of each 10 minute

period and a fast fourier transform run on these non-overlapping points.[10] The slow wave frequency chosen for each 10 minute period was the frequency with the greatest power in the 12-25 cpm frequency bracket and compared to manual counts obtained at 15 minute intervals. This frequency bracket was chosen from a 3 dimensional representation of successive power spectra and found free of aliasing.[11]

For spike analysis, analog to digital conversion was continuously performed at 100 Hz. A spike was defined as any voltage above a threshold that subsequently returned below that threshold. A time offset was included to prevent double counting of biphasic spikes.[12] Spikes were grouped as a single burst until a gap of 2.5 seconds without spike activity occurred. The spike burst was then closed out and a summary of the electrode, burst onset time, number of spikes in the burst and burst duration was stored. The threshold spike voltage for each electrode was determined by periodic observation of the analog signal. Movement artifacts were deleted from digital records by hand editing.

Spike bursts were divided according to duration and numbers of spikes into action potential complexes (those spike bursts lasting $\geq$ 2.5 seconds and having > 9 spikes) and unpatterned spike activity (the remaining unanalyzed spike activity or USA). As shown in Figures 2

FIGURE 2: ANALOG RECORD OF MIGRATING ACTION POTENTIAL COMPLEX

A migrating action potential complex is a spike burst lasting $\geq$ 2.5 seconds that apparently migrates between leads. Lead 1 is proximal and lead 3 is distal. Each lead is separated by a distance of about 2.5 cm.

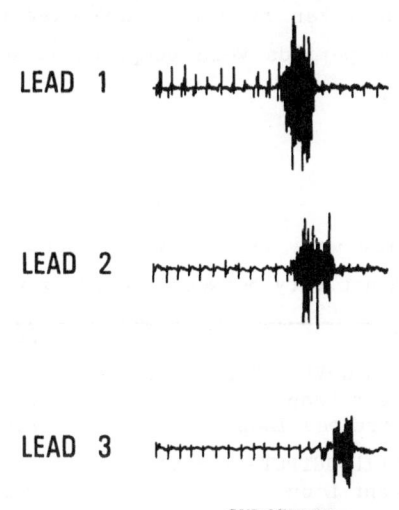

LEAD 1

LEAD 2

LEAD 3

ONE MINUTE

FIGURE 3: ANALOG RECORD OF STATIONARY ACTION POTENTIAL COMPLEX

LEAD 1

A stationary action poten-
ial complex is a spike
burst lasting ≥ 2.5 seconds
that does not migrate.
Lead 1 is proximal and lead
3 is distal. Each lead is
separated by a distance of
approximately 2.5 cm.

LEAD 2

LEAD 3

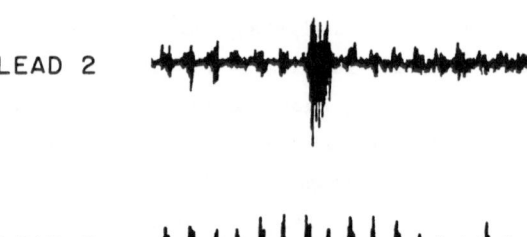

├────── I MINUTE ──────┤

and 3, action potential complexes were subdivided into those that
propagated in a velocity range of 0.2-10.0 cm/sec (migrating action
potential complexes or MAPC's) and those that did not (stationary
action potential complexes or SAPC's). For analysis of propagation
the two electrodes with the best signal-to-noise ratio on the analog
record were chosen. For each experiment, all reported myoelectric
data was taken from the same electrode. Mean values between groups
and time periods were compared using appropriate paired and unpaired
t-tests.

RESULTS

Mean slow wave frequency for both groups was 17.2 cycles per minute
and did not vary between groups or with study period (Table 1).

TABLE 1:	Pre-Test	Test	Post-Test
MEAN SLOW WAVE FREQUENCY (#/min)			
Patent Loop	17.6 ± 0.6	17.2 ± 0.2	16.9 ± 0.5
Obstructed Loop	16.9 ± 0.4	17.3 ± 0.2	18.5 ± 0.5
MEAN FLUID OUTPUT (ml/hr)			
Patent Loop	0.5 ± 0.3	2.7 ± 0.3*	
Obstructed Loop	0.0 ± 0.0	2.6 ± 0.4*	

* $p < 0.05$ compared to pre-test period

For fluid output (Table 1), the test and post test periods are combined because fluid output during the test period into an obstructed loop could only be measured when the obstruction was relieved, i.e. in the post-test period. The increase in fluid output due to perfusion was not statistically different from the sum of the 2.4 ml/hr perfusion rate and the pre-test output. Transient intestinal obstruction did not alter this crude measurement of net fluid output.

Compared to the unperfused pre-test period, loop perfusion had no effect on spike activity in the patent loops (Table 2). Although unpatterned spike activity tended to decrease during perfusion, the response was variable and not statistically significant. There were statistically significant increases in MAPC and SAPC frequency during the test period in obstructed loops. Although the MAPC frequency response to obstruction was statistically greater than the SAPC frequency response (p <0.05) both responses to luminal distension were dramatic (MAPC 1000 fold, SAPC 15 fold).

TABLE 2:	Pre-Test	Test	Post-Test
MEAN MAPC FREQUENCY (#/hr)			
Patent Loop	0	0.0 ± 0.0	0
Obstructed Loop	0	34.3 ± 7.0 *	1.0 ± 0.5 †
MEAN SAPC FREQUENCY (#/hr)			
Patent Loop	0	1.4 ± 0.9	1.8 ± 1.0
Obstructed Loop	0.2 ± 0.2	21.7 ± 7.6 *	4.3 ± 3.0 †
MEAN USA FREQUENCY (#/sec)			
Patent Loop	0.07 ± 0.05	0.05 ± 0.03	0.03 ± 0.01
Obstructed Loop	0.23 ± 0.15	0.11 ± 0.03	0.04 ± 0.01

* $p < 0.05$ compared to patent loop,   † $p < 0.05$ compared to test period

The time from the beginning of the pre-test period to the first MAPC averaged 102 ± 23 minutes and to the first SAPC averaged 118 ± 30 minutes. During loop obstruction there was a gradual increase in action potential complex frequency reaching a maximum during the third and fourth test period hours (Table 3).

TABLE 3:	CHANGE OF ACTION POTENTIAL COMPLEX FREQUENCY WITH DURATION OF TEST PERIOD IN OBSTRUCTED ILEAL LOOPS					
	HR 1	HR 2	HR 3	HR 4	HR 5	HR 6
MAPC FREQUENCY (#/hr)	7.7	23.8	36.7	54.8	50.2	32.5
SAPC FREQUENCY (#/hr)	6.7	19.2	29.3	26.7	28.8	19.5

Following relief of obstruction at the end of the test period, frequency of action potential complexes quickly returned to levels seen in patent loops (Figure 4).

FIGURE 4:   CESSATION OF ACTION POTENTIAL COMPLEXES AFTER RELIEF OF
OBSTRUCTION IN A PERFUSED ILEAL LOOP

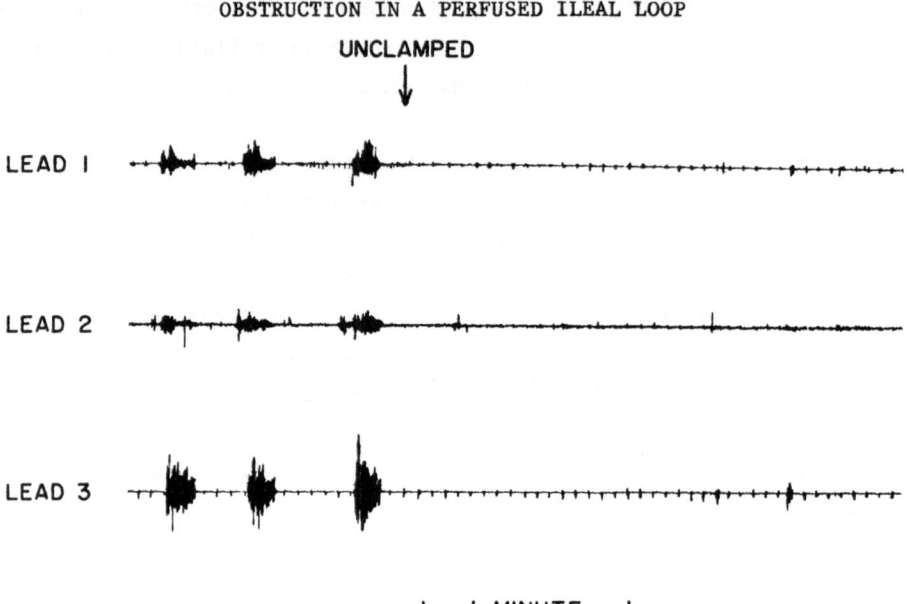

Table 4 reports action potential complex parameters for the test period in the obstructed loops.   The duration and spike density of MAPC's and SAPC's were remarkably consistent and did not statistically differ.   MAPC propagation velocity was also consistent and did not vary with direction of propagation.   Approximately two-thirds of MAPC's propagated aborally.

TABLE 4: MEAN ACTION POTENTIAL COMPLEX PARAMETERS
(test period, obstructed loop)

	MAPC	SAPC
Duration (sec)	6.5 ± 0.9	7.2 ± 1.6
Density (spike/sec)	9.0 ± 2.0	7.6 ± 1.0
Velocity (cm/sec)	2.0 ± 0.0	---
% Aboral	64 ± 11	---

Hematoxylin and eosin stained sections of each loop and of ileum immediately proximal to each loop were normal.

DISCUSSION

This study employed a comprehensive computer analysis of myoelectric activity from an <u>in vivo</u> ileal loop preparation.   The analysis identified a group of action potentials with prolonged duration (action potential complexes) that were associated with luminal distension. Action potential complexes were subdivided based on propagation into migrating action potential complexes (MAPC's) which have been extensively described[1-4,13-15] and stationary action potential complexes (SAPC's) which have not been previously described. Although MAPC frequency was statistically greater than SAPC frequency following luminal distension, both types of action potential complexes responded vigorously to the stimulus. MAPC's and SAPC's could only be separated based on propagation, their other characteristics being indistinguishable. The observation that luminal distension is a strong stimulus for action potential complexes would be the same if either subgroup were considered alone.

Perfusion of patent ileal loops with fluid volumes similar to those produced by cholera toxin failed to induce spike activity. However, perfusion coupled with luminal distension by obstructing outflow resulted in striking stimulation of action potential complexes. The effects of luminal distension were rapidly reversed by decompression. We conclude that MAPC's may be induced by luminal distension resulting from fluid accumulation comparable in volume to that produced by cholera toxin stimulation. Although the models are different, we suggest that MAPC's resulting from gradual luminal distension in vivo may represent a response similar to the peristaltic reflex resulting from acute luminal distension in vitro.[6-8]

The list of factors capable of inducing MAPC's is growing: bacterial enterotoxins[1-3], enteroinvasive bacterial infections[4,9,16], prostaglandins[13] ricinoleic acid[14] and mucosal injury[5,15]. Many of the factors in this list may coexist in the setting of diarrhea. We conclude that luminal distension should be added to this list and that MAPC's should be considered a non-specific myoelectric response to a variety of stimuli. Studies reporting the occurrence of MAPC's should consider the role played by luminal distension.

REFERENCES

1. Mathias JR, Carlson GM, DiMarino AJ, Bertiger G, Morton HE, Cohen S. Intestinal myoelectric activity in response to live Vibrio cholerae and cholera enterotoxin. J Clin Invest 1976;58:91-6.
2. Burns TW, Mathias JR, Carlson GM, Martin JL, Shields RP. Effect of toxigenic Escherichia coli on myoelectric activity of small

intestine. Am J Physiol 1978;235:E311-15.
3. Sinar DR, Charles LG, Burns TW. Migrating action-potential complex activity in absence of fluid production is produced by B subunit of cholera enterotoxin. Am J Physiol 1982;242:G47-51.
4. Mathias JR, Carlson GM, Martin JL, Shields RP, Formal S. Shigella dysenteriae I enterotoxin: proposed role in pathogenesis of shigellosis. Am J Physiol 1980;239:G382-6.
5. Justus PG, Mathias JR, Martin JL, Carlson GM, Shields RP, Formal S. Myoelectric activity in the small intestine in response to Clostridium perfringens A enterotoxin: correlation with histologic findings in a in vivo rabbit model. Gastroenterology 1981;80:902-6.
6. Yokoyama S, North RA. Electrical activity of longitudinal and circular muscle during peristalsis. Am J Physiol 1983;244:G83-8.
7. Yokoyama S, Ozaki T. Effects of gut distension on Auerbach's plexus and intestinal muscle. Jap J Physiol 1980;30:143-60.
8. Kottegoda SR. An analysis of possible nervous mechanisms involved in the peristaltic reflex. J Physiol (London) 1969;200:687-712.
9. Weisberg PB, Carlson GM, Cohen S. Effect of Salmonella typhimurium on myoelectrical activity in the rabbit ileum. Gastroenterology 1978;74:47-51.
10. Brigham EO. The Fast Fourier Transform. New Jersey: Prentice-Hall, 1974.
11. van der Schee EJ, Smout AJPM, Grashius JL. Application of running spectrum analysis to electrogastrographic signals recorded from dog and man. In: Wienbeck M, ed. Motility of the Digestive Tract. New York: Raven Press,1982:241-50.
12. Sinar DR, Charles LG. Glucose is the major component controlling irregular spike activity after feeding in primates. Gastroenterology 1983;85:in press.
13. Mathias JR, Carlson GM, Bertiger G, Martin JL, Cohen S. Migrating action potential complex of cholera: a possible prostaglandin-induced response. Am J Physiol 1977;232:E529-34.
14. Mathias JR, Martin JL, Carlson GM, Burns TW. Ricinoleic acid effect on motility of the small intestine in rabbits. J Clin Invest 1978;61:640-4.
15. Sjogren RW, Curry RG, Sinar DR. Patterned myoelectric response to graded mucosal damage in ricin-treated rabbit small intestine. Gastroenterology 1983;84:1313.
16. Burns TW, Mathias JR, Martin JL, Carlson GM, Shields RP. Alteration of myoelectric activity in small intestine by invasive Escherichia coli. Am J Physiol 1980;238:G57-62.

ACKNOWLEDGEMENTS

The authors with to thank Dr. D. R. Sinar, East Carolina University School of Medicine, Greenville, N.C. for his encouragement and constructive thoughts on the conduct and analysis of this study and Dr. E. C. Boedeker, Walter Reed Army Institute of Research, Washington, D.C. for his review of the manuscript.

The views expressed herein are those of the authors and do not necessarily represent those of the United States Army or the Department of Defense.

54

Electrical Activity of an Intrinsically Denervated Jejunum of the Unanesthetized Rat

D. A. FOX, M. L. EPSTEIN and P. BASS

INTRODUCTION

The enteric nerves and their respective mediators have been
postulated to be involved in the intestinal intrinsic reflex (1),
motility, modulation of intestinal blood flow, water and electro-
lyte transport, absorption of nutrients, and secretion from endocrine and paracrine cells (review see 2). Selective ablation of
different portions of the enteric nervous sytem would facilitate
characterization of the function and site of action of both
endogenous substances and drugs.

Experimental attempts have been made to destroy the enteric
neurons. Hukuhara has shown that arterial perfusion of a loop of
bowel in the dog for four hours (i.e., making the bowel anoxic)
elicits degenerative changes in the intamural ganglion cells and
abolition of the enteric reflexes without markedly altering smooth
muscle function (1). Szurszewski et al. utilizing the Hukuhara
preparation have demonstrated alterations in electrical and mechanical properties of the gut after enteric neuronal ablation (3,4).
Experiments using both arterial perfusion and intraluminal administration of mercuric chloride have also caused enteric nerve damage
(5,6). Sato et al., employing a much simpler technique, produced
aganglionosis in the colon and anorectum of the rat by serosal application of the cationic surfactant benzalkonium chloride (BAC)
(7,8). Recently, we have shown that serosal application of BAC, as

well as other surfactants to the rat jejunum, selectively ablates
the ganglion cells in the myenteric plexus sparing those of the
submucoal plexus (9). In addition, this treatment reduces the
substance P, somatostatin, met-enkephalin, and vasoactive intestinal peptide-like immunoreactivity only in the myenteric plexus,
further demonstrating selectivity.

In this presentation, we elucidate the alterations in intestinal
electrical activity associated with selective myenteric neuronal
ablation.

METHODS

Methods for BAC-induced myenteric neuronal ablation have been previously described (9). Briefly, various concentrations of BAC were
applied to the serosal surface of a 2-3 cm segment of rat jejunum
every 5 minutes for one-half hour (6 applications). The serosa was
then thoroughly rinsed with saline, and the animals were allowed to
recover. Thirty days after treatment, the treated and an untreated
segment of jejunum were removed and examined histologically.

To examine changes in smooth muscle electrical activity associated with BAC treatment, 3 silver monopolar electrodes, one orad
to, at, and caudad to the BAC-treated jejunal area, were chronically implanted. In these studies, 0.062% BAC was utilized. This
concentration of BAC was shown to destroy greater than 90% of the
myenteric neurons in the rat jejunum. In addition, 3 electrodes
were implanted in control rats in the same position as those in the
treated animals. Myoelectric activity was recorded while the rats
were unanesthetized, unrestrained, and fasted for at least 20
hours.

RESULTS

The effect of BAC was concentration dependent. Thirty days after
treatment with 0.062% BAC, there was a loss of neurons in the area
of the myenteric plexus as depicted in Figure 1B, in contrast to
the normal tissue, Figure 1A. However, the ganglion cells in the
submucosal plexus were still present. This effect was noted over
the concentration range of 0.015 to .25% BAC. At higher concentra-

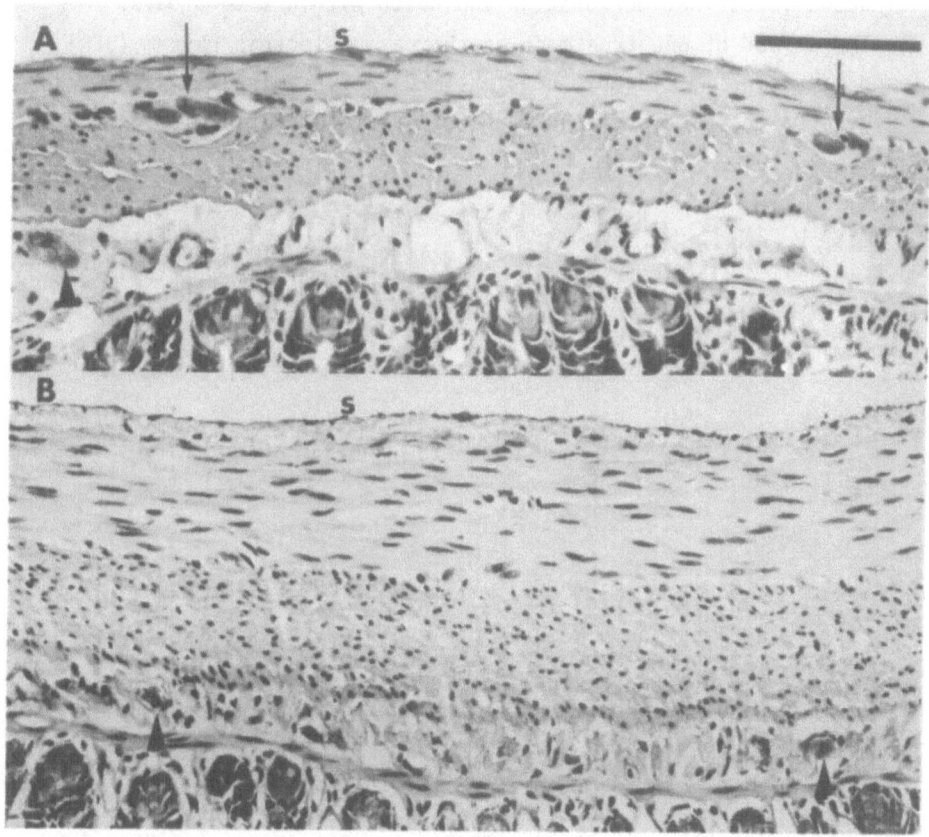

FIGURE 1   Effect of serosal application of benzalkonium chloride
(BAC) on the rat jejunum. Sections were cut in the
longitudinal axis and stained with hematoxylin. A) Untreated sections of jejunum showing the normal distribution of ganglion cells in the myenteric (arrow) and
submucosal plexuses (arrowhead). B) Section treated with
0.062% BAC. Note the absence of ganglion cells in the
area of the myenteric plexus and the presence in the submucosal plexus (arrowhead). S, serosa of the intestine.
Calibration bar, 100 µm. (Adapted from Fox et al., J.
Pharmacol. Exp. Ther., in press.)

tions, selectivity was lost, and a generalized tissue damage was
observed. 0.5% BAC produced a disruption of the muscle layers and
a lymphocytic infiltration. Concentrations of 1% BAC or higher

induced intestinal perforation and death within 2 to 3 days.

The effect of BAC treatment on the basic electric rhythm (BER) and migrating myoelectric complex (MMC) was examined. As shown in Figure 2, the BER in the BAC-treated area was eratic with an un-

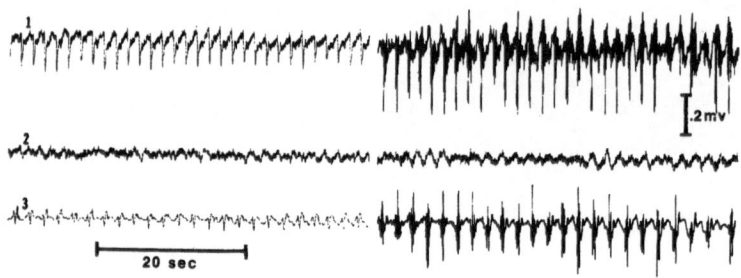

FIGURE 2   The electric response of the jejunum of an unanesthetized rat, above (1), at (2), and below (3) the site of BAC application. Record obtained 7 days after treatment. Left panel represents electrograms made during a period of quiescence, when only BER is observed. The right panel depicts electrograms during a period of gut contractility as indicated by the spike activity. Electrograms 1 and 3 are associated with the area orad and caudad, respectively, to the treated area 2. Note the lack of a regular cyclic BER pattern and absence of spike activity in the BAC-treated jejunal area. (Adapted from Fox et al., J. Pharmacol. Exp. Ther., in press.)

defined pattern. The region orad to the BAC-treated area had a normal BER frequency of 38 cycles/min, while the BER in the caudad areas was significantly reduced to 30 cycles/min.

Spiking activity in the areas orad and caudad to the BAC-treated area appeared in bursts beginning 3-4 days postsurgery. In contrast, spike potentials were absent in the BAC-treated area for approximately 2 weeks after treatment. On days 13-17, spikes appeared but were of greater duration and shorter frequency than the areas orad and caudad to it and were not always associated with remnants of BER seen in this area.

Propagation of bursts of spike potentials at the orad electrode began between days 6-9. From this time until approximately day 13, the MMC began on the orad electrode and skipped to the caudad electrode without any spiking on the aganglionic region. On days 13-17, when irregular spiking on the aganglionic segment appeared, its incidence coincided with the orad burst and was followed by a caudad burst. There appeared to be an apparent propagation through the aganglionic region. Once this pattern was initiated in an animal, its regularity persisted until the animal was sacrificed (as long as 2 months). In addition, when compared to control animals with 3 electrodes positioned as those of the treated animals', there was not a significant difference among the controls and the orad and caudad area of the treated animals with respect to burst duration, interval between bursts, period, or propagation velocity of the MMC.

DISCUSSION

We have demonstrated a chemical ablation selective for the myenteric nerve plexus. It is a simple, useful technique for studying the function of the myenteric neurons. Our data indicate that ablation of the myeneteric neurons disrupts the BER but not the MMC propagation in the rat. Regarding the BER, it has been shown that 4 hours of hypoxia in a loop of bowel in the dog destroys or causes vacuolization of the ganglion cells in the myenteric plexus (1,10). Meissner's (submucosal) plexus was less sensitive to the hypoxia. Szurszewski et al. utilizing this technique have demonstrated a decrease in BER and contractile frequency associated with myenteric neuronal disruption at and below the site of treatment (3,4). Our results are in agreement with Szurszewski, in which BAC-induced myenteric denervation disrupted the BER in the aganglionic area and reduced its frequency caudad to the denervation.

Intrinsic nervous control of the MMC has been postulated. Sarna et al. have shown that close intra-arterial mesenteric injections of atropine, hexamethonium, and tetrodotoxin block the propagation of the MMC in the dog (11). Also, it has been demonstrated that after a series of intestinal transections and rearastomoses the onset of the burst (phase 3) of the MMC in the resulting intestinal segments are independent of one another (12). Sarna's studies, as well as those of Heppell et al. (13), which also utilize intestinal transection, support the notion that enteric nerves are instrumental in the initiation and propagation of the MMC.

In contrast to the above three studies (11,12,13), the present investigation suggests that the myenteric plexus is not involved in the control of the MMC in the rat. After chemical ablation of the myenteric neurons, there is a normal propagation of the MMC. In addition, the burst duration, interval between bursts and burst propagation velocity in intestinal areas both orad and caudad to the aganglionic areas, are not different from control animals. The discrepancy between our results and those of others may suggest that both the myenteric and submucosal plexuses must be altered to affect the MMC or that the submucosal plexus is more important in its control. Our method selectively ablates the myenteric neurons, whereas the methods employed in the above studies would alter both intrinsic nerve plexuses.

In conclusion, the present investigation has demonstrated that the myenteric neurons play a modulatory role in the generation and propagation of the BER. In contrast, humoral factors or the submucosal neurons may be more important than the myenteric neurons in the control of the MMC.

REFERENCES

1. Hukuhara, T., Sumi, T., and Kotani, S. (1961). The role of the ganglion cells in the small intestine taken in the intestinal intrinsic reflex. Jap. J. Physiol., 11, 281-88
2. Costa, M. and Furness, J. B. (1982). Nervous control of intestinal motility. In: Bertaccini, G. (ed). Mediators and Drugs in Gastrointestinal Motility I. pp. 279-382. (Berlin Heidelberg New York: Springer-Verlag)
3. Szurszewski, J. and Steggerda, F. R. (1968). The effect of hypoxia on the electrical slow wave of the canine small intestine. Am. J. Dig. Dis., 13, 168-177
4. Szurszewski, J. and Steggerda, F. R. (1968). The effect of hypoxia on the mechanical activity of the canine small intestine. Am. J. Dig. Dis. 13, 178-185
5. Okamoto, E., Iwasaki, T., Kakutani, T., and Ueda, T. (1967).

Selective destruction of the myenteric plexus: Its relationshp to Hirschsprung's disease, achalasia of the esophagus and hypertrophic pyloric stenosis. J. Ped. Surg., 2, 444-454

6. Imamura, K., Yamamoto, M., Sato, A., Kashiki, Y., and Kunieda, T. (1975). Pathophysiology of aganglionic colon segment: An experimental study on aganglionsis produced by a new method in the rat. J. Ped. Surg., 10, 865-873

7. Sato, A., Yamamoto, M., Imamura, K., Kashiki, Y., Kunieda, T., and Sakata, K. (1978). Pathophysiology of aganglionic colon and anorectum: An experimental study on aganglionsis produced by a new method in the rat. J. Ped. Surg., 13, 399-405

8. Sakata, K., Kunieda, T., Furuta, T., and Sato, A. (1979). Selective destruction of intestinal nervous elements by local application of benzalkonium solution in the rat. Experientia, 35, 1611-1612

9. Fox, D. A.,, Epstein, M. L., and Bass, P. Surfactants selectively ablate enteric neurons of the rat jejunum. J. Pharmacol. Exp. Ther. In press

10. Nagata, T. and Steggerda, F. R. (1963). Histological study on the deganglionated small intestine of the dog. Physiologist, 6, 242

11. Sarna, S., Stoddard, C., Belbeck, L., and McWade, D. (1981). Intrinsic nervous control of migrating myoelectric complexes. Am. J. Physiol., 241, G16-22

12. Sarna, S., Condon, R. E., and Cowles, V. (1983). Enteric mechanism of initiation of migrating myoelectric complexes in dogs. Gastroenterology, 84, 814-22

13. Heppell, J., Kelly, K., and Sarr, M. (1983). Neural control of canine small intestinal interdigestive myoelectric complexes. Am. J. Physiol., 244, G95-G100

55

Evidence for a Muscarinic Inhibitory Brake Activated by Peptides in the Canine Small Intestine

J. E. T. FOX, E. E. DANIEL, T. J. MacDONALD, J. JURY and K. H. ROBOTHAM

INTRODUCTION

Acetylcholine (ACH) injected intraarterially (ia) contracts the canine gut by a tetrodotoxin-(TTX) and hexamethonium-insensitive, atropine-sensitive mechanism. Field stimulation (40V, 0.5ms, 1-5Hz) produces phasic and tonic contractions which are slightly reduced by hexamethonium, almost eliminated by atropine (1) and blocked by TTX. Thus the major endogenous stimulant released by field stimulation is ACH which stimulates activity via a muscarinic receptor on the smooth muscle. Phasic and tonic contractions can be elicited after atropine by ia motilin and appear to represent release of a non-muscarinic transmitter to the smooth muscle (2).

Two inhibitory neural pathways in the canine gastrointestinal tract are known, the non-adrenergic non-cholinergic pathway and the adrenergic pathway releasing norepinephrine to α_2 receptors (3). In the guinea pig ileum, excitation of muscarinic receptors inhibits synaptic transmission in the myenteric plexus as demonstrated by measuring release of ACH (4,5). Furthermore, this inhibition occurs with nerve stimulus parameters expected to release very small amounts of ACH as demonstrated by intracellular recordings and probably constitutes an important negative feedback loop (6).

Our initial studies showed that ACH when injected ia into the electrical field stimulated, or ia motilin stimulated small intestine produced a short tonic contraction followed by a prolonged inhibition

of phasic contractions. McNeil A343 (Mn) the putative muscarinic
(M_1) ganglionic agonist (7) produced inhibition only. We thus propose
that a third inhibitory pathway, a muscarinic inhibitory pathway, also
exists in the canine small intestine and some peptides which stimulate
ACH release may release it in the vicinity of this receptor and thus
produce inhibition. The peptides tested were substance P (SP) and
bombesin.

METHODS

The terminal arteries to the small intestine in anaesthetized dogs were
cannulated in 2 to 4 sites (jejunum and ileum) and strain gauges and
electrodes applied as described previously (3). To test for inhibition,
increasing concentrations of agonists were injected ia to the actively
contracting segment until complete inhibition was obtained. The
concentration of drugs producing 50% inhibition was calculated by
plotting the % inhibition against the $\log_{10}$ of the concentration
injected. Drugs used in this study were acetylcholine bromide,
substance P, atropine sulphate (30 µg/kg iv and 100 µg ia at each site),
hexamethonium bromide (10 mg/kg iv) (Sigma); McNeil A343 (gift of
McNeil); bombesin (gift of Bachem); reserpine (0.5 mg/kg iv, 24 and 4
hrs prior to experimentation, a regime which blocked the inhibition of
phasic activity of proximal intestine by distention or activation of
distal intestine) (CIBA); tetrodotoxin (10-30 µg ia to the site)
(Calbiochem); and pirenzipine (64 µg/kg iv) (gift of Boehringer
Ingelheim). Paired and unpaired t-tests were used as appropriate.

RESULTS

Increasing concentrations of ACH, Mn, SP and bombesin inhibited field
stimulated activity (Fig. 1). This was not blocked by hexamethonium
but was eliminated by TTX (data not shown) suggesting a neural
mechanism. Prior treatment with reserpine did not alter the response
to ACH and bombesin but increased the ED_{50} for SP and Mn (Fig. 2).
Pirenzipine the putative M_1 antagonist (7) did not block field
stimulated responses but shifted the inhibitory ED_{50} for all agonists
and slightly reduced the inhibitory response to ACH (Fig. 3). The
excitatory response to ACH was blocked by atropine (30 µg/kg iv)
subsequently. Following excitation of the non-muscarinic excitatory
pathway by ia motilin after atropine, the ED_{50} for each agonist
increased (Fig. 4).

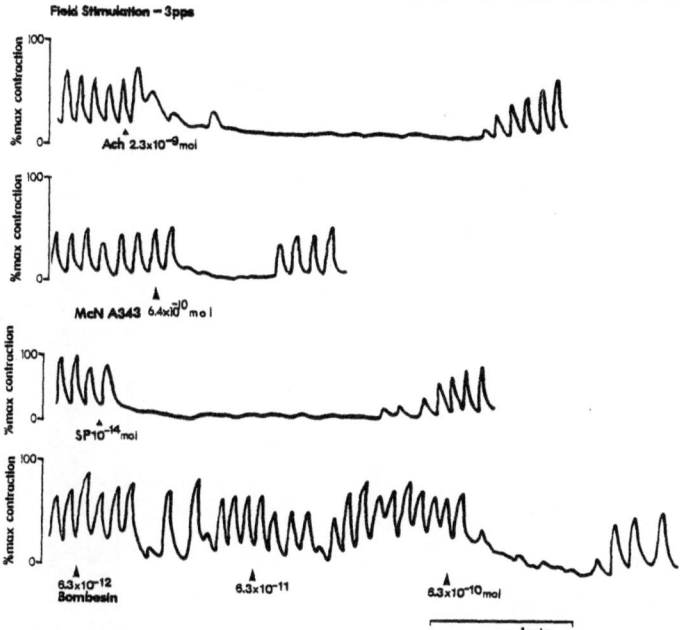

FIGURE 1   Dynograph tracing showing the inhibitory effects of
intraarterial (ia) injections (at arrows) of acetylcholine
(ACH), McNeil A343 (McN), substance P (SP), and bombesin in
mols on field stimulated contractions of the canine ileum.
Bars show percent of maximum acetylcholine contractions and
time in minutes.

DISCUSSION

The present study demonstrates the presence of a potent inhibitory
pathway in the canine small intestine which is stimulated by ACH.   That
this is via muscarinic receptors is suggested by its insensitivity to
hexamethonium, its stimulation by McNeil A343 the putative M_1 agonist
(8) and its sensitivity to pirenzipine the putative M_1 antagonist (7).
The presence of a muscarinic inhibitory receptor in the myenteric
plexus is well established for the guinea pig ileum (4,5,6).   Our
findings suggest that this receptor would be M_1 (on nerves) rather than
M_2 on smooth muscle, since McNeil A343 does not produce excitation and
pirenzipine does not block field stimulated contractions or smooth
muscle excitation by ACH.   Furthermore, the extreme sensitivity of the
response and the prolonged duration of its action i.e., a single
stimulus can reduce the response to a second stimulus, suggests that
ACH released in the plexus would serve as negative feedback to its own
transmission.

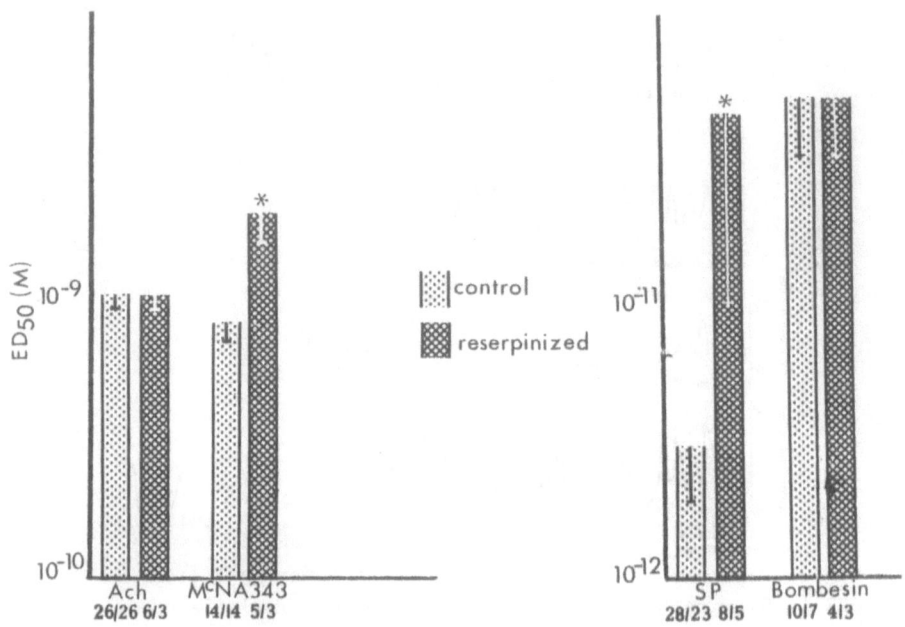

FIGURE 2   The effect of prior reserpine treatment on the ED_{50} of
inhibitory responses of the agonists on field stimulated
contractions of the ileum.   Bars = mean ± SEM.   Numbers at
the bottom of the columns = the number of sites tested/
number of animals tested.   * = significantly different,
p < 0.05 by unpaired t-test.

Our findings also suggest that the peptides, SP and bombesin also

can release ACH to this receptor and that when each of these peptides

is given ia this is the most sensitive response (Fig. 1).   Both SP

and bombesin-like nerves have been identified in the canine myenteric

plexus (9 and Daniel, Costa and Furness, unpublished data), and thus

the ACH released may act directly at that site and not diffuse to the

smooth muscle.   In the case of SP the neural excitatory response,

release of ACH to smooth muscle (3) could be mediated via spill-over of

ACH from the plexus or stimulation of the cholinergic terminals in the

smooth muscle itself.

Besides the muscarinic inhibitory pathway which is capable of

inhibiting field stimulated activity there is also the adrenergic

pathway releasing norepinephrine to an α_2 receptor (10).   Our results

from the reserpinized animals suggest that ACH and bombesin do not

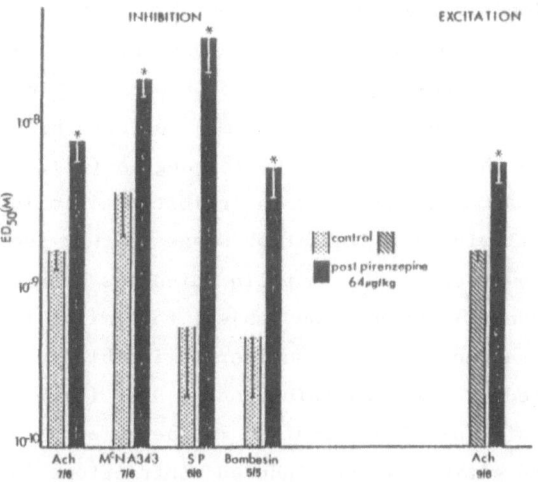

FIGURE 3   The effect of pirenzipine treatment on the ED_{50} of
inhibitory responses on field stimulated contractions of the
ileum for the agonists. * = significant differences,
$p < 0.05$ by paired t-test.

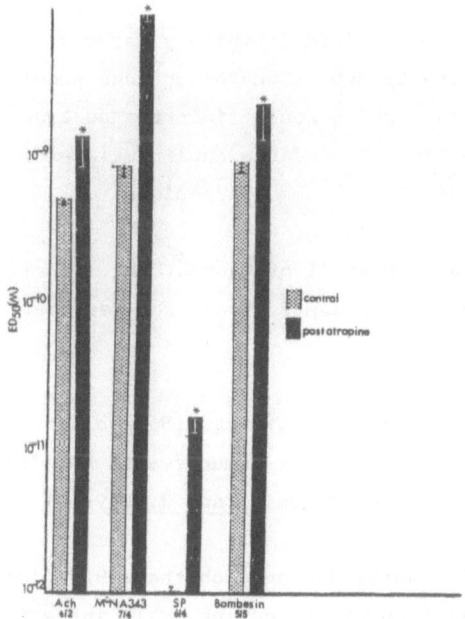

FIGURE 4   The effect of sufficient atropine treatment to block ACH
excitatory responses on the ED_{50} for inhibitory responses of
the agonists on ia motilin induced contractions
* = significant differences, $p < 0.05$ by paired t-test.

effect inhibition via this route but that SP and Mn can stimulate this pathway as well. Stimulation of adrenergic nerves by SP has also been suggested for the guinea pig colon (11), also Mn may not stimulate cholinergic receptors exclusively and may reflect the high affinity binding found in the canine sympathetic ganglia (12).

The capacity of these agonists to inhibit motilin induced contractions following atropinization suggests that the non-muscarinic cholinergic pathway excited by motilin which has been shown to have a nicotinic synapse (2) may also be subject to similar inhibition in this case by the non-adrenergic non-cholinergic inhibitory transmitter which can be stimulated by the nicotinic agonist DMPP (8). In fact in very preliminary studies all four agonists may be able to induce inhibition of atropine-insensitive motilin induced contractions in the absence of adrenergic input, i.e., after reserpinization. However, further quanification is required. Since we do not know the nature of this we can only infer by elimination that all agents are able to release this unknown inhibitor.

The presence of a sensitive muscarinic inhibitory pathway in the canine intestine stimulated both by ACH or neuro-peptides provides a natural feedback inhibitory brake which would limit the contractile responses to activation of cholinergic and non-cholinergic excitatory nerves and would prevent or reduce maximum contractions.

ACKNOWLEDGEMENTS

Supported by the Medical Research Council of Canada. Dr. J.E.T. Fox is a MRC Scholar. The authors wish to thank R. Vonau for secretarial assistance.

REFERENCES

1. Fox, J.E.T., Daniel, E.E., Jury, J., Track, N.S. and Chiu, S. (1983). Cholinergic control mechanisms for immunoreactive motilin release and motility in the canine duodenum. Can. J. Physiol. (in press)

2. Fox, J.E.T., Daniel, E.E., Jury, J., and Robotham, H. (1983). The mechanism of motilin excitation of the canine small intestine. Life Sci. (submitted)

3. Daniel, E.E., Gonda, T., Domoto, T., Oki, M. and Yanaihara, N. (1982). The effects of substance P and met-enkephalin in dog ileum. Can. J. Physiol. Pharmacol., 60, 830-840

4. Sawynok, J. and Jhamandas, K. (1977). Muscarinic feedback inhibition of acetylcholine release from the myenteric plexus in the guinea pig ileum and its status after chronic exposure to morphine. Can. J. Physiol. Pharmacol., 55, 909-916

5. Szerb, J.C. (1980). Effects of low calcium and of oxytremosine on the kinetics of the evoked release of ^{3}H acetylcholine from the guinea pig myenteric plexus: comparison with morphine. Naunyn Schmiedebergs Arch Pharmac., 311, 119-127

6. Morita, K., North, R.A. and Tokimasa, T. (1982). Muscarinic presynaptic inhibition of synaptic transmission in myenteric plexus of guinea pig ileum. J. Physiol., 333, 141-149

7. Hammer, R., Berrie, C.P., Bridsall, N.J.M., Burgen, A.S.V. and Hulme, E.C. (1980). Pirenzipine distinguishes between different subclasses of muscarinic receptors. Nature, 283, 90-92

8. Goyal, R.K. and Rattan, S. (1975). Nature of the vagal inhibitory innervation to the lower esophageal sphincter. J. Clin. Invest., 55, 1119-1126

9. Oki, M., and Daniel, E.E. (1980). Distribution of substance P like immunoreactivity in both intrinsic and extrinsic nerves of the gastrointestinal tract. Nippon Heikatonkin Gakkai Zasshi, 16, 75-77

10. Daniel, E.E., Sakai, Y., Jury, J. and Fox, J.E.T. (1982). Mode of action of neurotensin on gastrointestinal motility. In: Wienbeck, M. (ed). Motility of the Digestive Tract. pp. 87-93. (N.Y.: Raven Press)

11. Krier, J., and Szurszewski, J.H. (1983). Effect of substance P on colonic mechanoreceptors motility and sympathetic neurones. Am. J. Physiol., G259-G267

12. Hammer, R. (1980). Muscarinic receptors in the stomach. Scand. J. Gastroenterol., 15: Suppl. 66, 5-11

56

The Ileal Brake: a Potent Mechanism for Feedback Control of Gastric Emptying and Small Bowel Transit

N. W. READ, A. McFARLANE, R. I. KINSMAN and S. R. BLOOM

INTRODUCTION

The absorption of nutrients in the small intestine depends on both the efficiency of the epithelial transport mechanisms and the length of time that nutrients remain in contact with the absorptive epithelium [1, 2]. The existence of neurohumoral mechanisms controlling either of these functions has never been established. The aim of the present study was to investigate the possible existence of a feedback mechanism, whereby the presence of nutrients in the distal small intestine might control small intestinal transit, allowing optimal time for absorption to occur.

MATERIAL AND METHODS

Subjects

Experiments were carried out on 43 healthy subjects (9 female, 34 male, aged 19 to 31).

Effects of infusion of nutrients on transit time of lactulose

Small bowel transit time of lactulose was measured during infusion of 0.9% saline or isosmotic solutions of either fat emulsion or protein hydrolysate or glucose into either the jejunum, ileum or colon, using a polyvinyl double lumen tube positioned fluoroscopically with its proximal orifice at the ligament of Treitz, and its distal port either at the ligament of Treitz, the ileum or the colon.

335

In the ileal and colonic experiments, 100 ml of either isotonic saline (pH = 6.5) or an isosmotic solution of either fat emulsion {Intralipid; Kabivitrum, Ealing, London}, protein hydrolysate {Bacto Peptone, Oxoid Ltd} or glucose was infused through the distal port at a rate of 1.2 ml per minute for 85 minutes.   Each subject underwent an infusion of saline and at least one other nutrient solution. The infusions were carried out on separate test days in the same subjects and the order was randomised.   Twenty minutes after the commencement of the nutrient infusions, lactulose syrup {Duphulac, Duphar BV. Weesp, Holland} was injected into the jejunum via the proximal port at a rate of 2 ml every thirty seconds.

Small bowel transit time (SBTT) was estimated by measuring the increase in breath hydrogen concentration that occurred when the unabsorbable carbohydrate marker, lactulose, reached the colon and was fermented by colonic bacteria [3,4].

Venous blood samples (10ml) were taken throughout each experiment for assay of neurotensin and enteroglucagon.

In a separate series of experiments carried out on 7 healthy male volunteers, the effect of intralipid on the small bowel transit of lactulose was investigated during continuous intravenous infusion of naloxone (20ug/Kg/h) or isotonic saline.

Effects of infusion of nutrients of transit time of a meal

Further experiments carried out in five healthy volunteers investigated the effects of infusing intralipid or saline into the ileum on the passage of a solid test meal [4] (mashed potato, three frankfurter sausages, baked beans and a dessert consisting of homogenised pineapple in custard) labelled with 25 microcuries of ^{99m}Tc-sulphur colloid through the stomach and small intestine. The infusion was commenced 20 minutes before eating the meal and continued for 185 minutes. Gastric emptying was measured by counting the radioactivity over the surface of the stomach with a single crystal scintillation detector [4], and small bowel transit time was measured by breath hydrogen analysis [5].

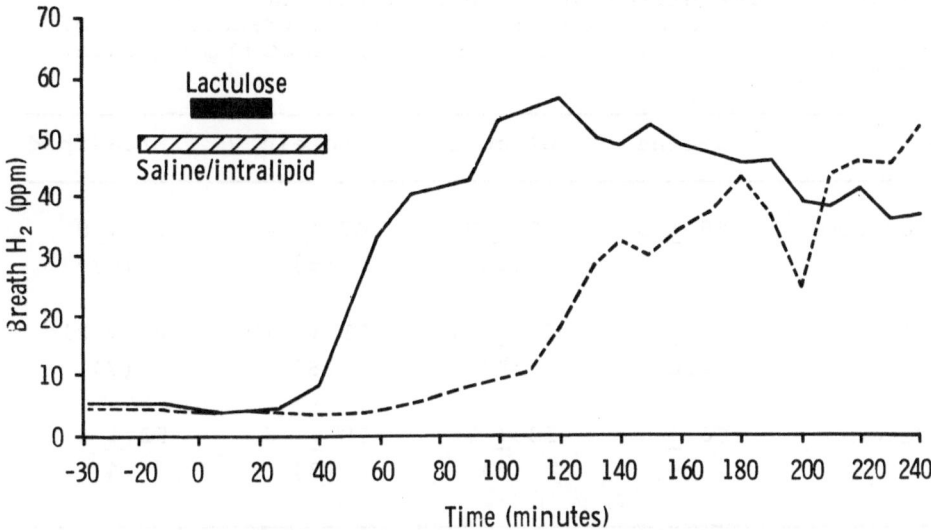

FIGURE 1   The effect of infusion of intralipid (dashed line) and
saline (solid line) on the average breath hydrogen profiles
from 7 normal subjects after infusion of 100ml 10%
lactulose at the ligament of Treitz.

RESULTS

Small bowel transit time of lactulose

Figure 1 shows that the profile of breath hydrogen excretion appeared
to be shifted to the right during ileal infusion of intralipid compared with isosmotic saline.   This was associated with significant
delays in small bowel transit time (p<0.02 {Table 1}).   There were no
significant differences in SBTT, or breath hydrogen profile during
infusion of intralipid into the jejunum or colon compared with
infusion of saline into the same regions.

Infusion of protein into the ileum also caused a significant delay
in SBTT compared with saline although this delay was not as pronounced
as that seen with ileal fat infusion (Table 1).   Infusion of glucose
into the ileum and infusion of glucose and protein into the colon or
jejunum had no effect on small bowel transit time of lactulose.

Plasma levels of neurotensin and enteroglucagon

Although ileal infusion of intralipid and protein slowed the transit
of lactulose through the small bowel, this was not accompanied by any

Table 1.   The effect of jejunal, ileal and colonic
infusion of nutrients on the small bowel transit time of
the head of a bolus of lactulose infused at the ligament
of Treitz

	Saline	Glucose	Protein	Intralipid
Jejunum	55 + 3 (12)	42 + 8 (5)	47 + 4 (5)	51 + 8 (6)
Ileum	50 + 3 (20)	56 + 11 (5)	71 + 11[a] (5)	125 + 21[b] (7)
Colon	66 + 8 (9)	53 + 3 (5)	78 + 16 (3)	52 + 4 (4)

Results are expressed as mean + SEM with the number of experiments in
brackets. Degree of significance compared with infusion of saline
into a corresponding intestinal site is   indicated by superscripts
(a = p <0.05;   b = p <0.02)

significant elevation in plasma levels of enteroglucagon or neurotensin, compared with infusion of saline (Fig. 2).   Conversely,
significant increases in plasma enteroglucagon and neurotensin were
observed approximately 80 minutes after the start of the infusion of
intralipid in the jejunum (Fig. 2) although this was not associated
with any alteration in the small bowel transit time of lactulose.
Jejunal infusion of glucose or protein and ileal or colonic infusion
of glucose, protein or intralipid had no significant influence on
plasma levels of enteroglucagon and neurotensin (Fig. 2).

Effect of Naloxone

Infusion of naloxone abolished the delay in SBTT induced by ileal
intralipid infusion in 5/7 subjects, though it had no influence on the
small bowel transit time during infusion of saline (Fig. 3).

Gastric emptying and SBTT of a solid meal

Ileal infusion of intralipid significantly prolonged the half-time for
gastric emptying (intralipid vs saline;   184 + 33 vs 79 + 10 min;
Mean + SEM; p <0.02) and the small bowel transit time (intralipid vs
saline;   456 + 29 vs 245 + 32 min;   p <0.02) of the solid meal.

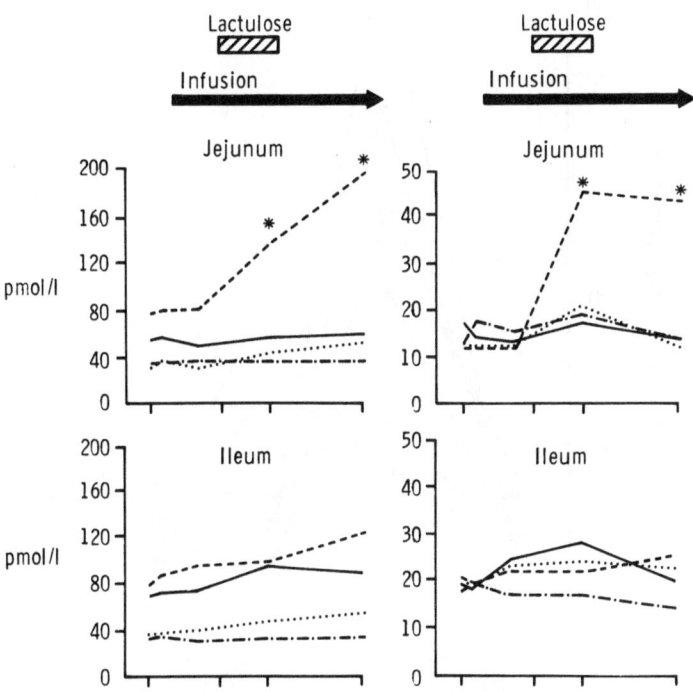

FIGURE 2 The effect of infusion of saline (solid line), intralipid (dashed line), protein (dotted line) and glucose (dashed and dotted line) into the jejunum (top) and ileum (bottom) on plasma levels of enteroglucagon (left) and neurotensin (right). Asterisks indicate results that are significantly different from saline control.

In 2 out of 5 subjects, gastric emptying did not appear to commence until the fat infusion was complete.

DISCUSSION

This study supports the existence of a feedback mechanism whereby the presence of unabsorbed fat or protein in the ileum delays the passage of material through the small intestine. This phenomenon has been confirmed by Spiller and his colleagues [6] who found that infusion of semi-digested intralipid at a point 170 cm from the teeth delayed transit of bromosulphthalein through a simultaneously perfused 30 cm length of human jejunum.

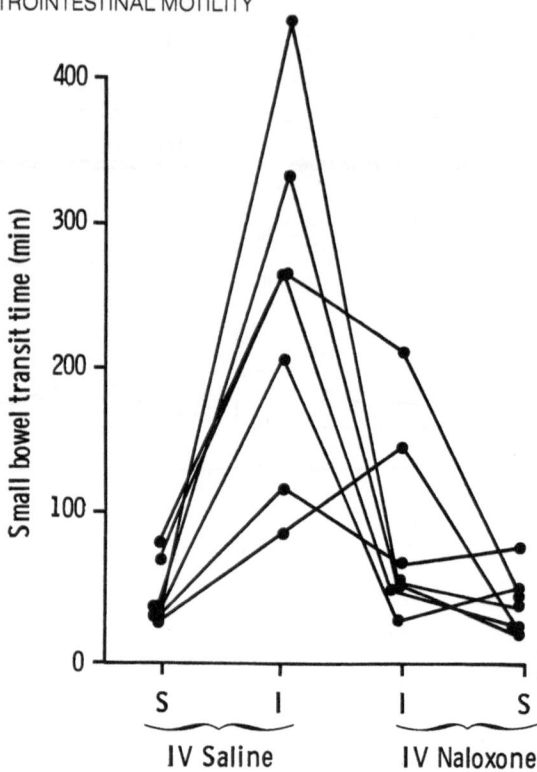

FIGURE 3. The effect of ileal infusion of saline and intralipid on
small bowel transit time of lactulose in 7 subjects during
intravenous infusion of saline (right) and naloxone (left)

The mechanism whereby ileal fat delays small bowel transit time is
unknown.   Although circumstantial evidence implies mediation by the
candidate hormones, neurotensin and enteroglucagon [7,8,9,10], our
results strongly indicate that these peptides do not mediate the
'ileal brake', since ileal infusion of fat and protein hydrolysates
slowed small bowel transit of lactulose without causing any significant rise in these peptides while jejunal infusion of nutrients
released neurotensin and enteroglucagon without slowing transit. The
lack of any increase in enteroglucagon and neurotensin after ileal
infusion of intralipid may at first sight appear surprising since fat
is thought to be a potent releaser of the both of these ileal peptides. This discrepancy may be explained if enteroglucagon and neurotensin are released by the fatty acid rather than the triglyceride

[11,12] since intralipid is largely in the form of triglyceride. The observation that naloxone abolishes the effect of intralipid on small bowel transit in 5/7 subjects suggests that endogenous opioid peptides are involved in the mechanism in at least some subjects.

The profound delay in gastric emptying induced by the presence of fat in the ileum has not, to our knowledge, been previously described, as most studies have concentrated on the influence of interaction of nutrients with duodenal and jejunal receptors on gastric emptying. Its possible importance is as a mechanism to signal the fact that the small intestine is becoming overloaded with nutrients and reduce the input of further food material from the stomach.

REFERENCES

1. Holgate, A.M. and Read, N.W. (1982). Can a rapid small bowel transit limit absorption? Gut, 23, A912.

2. Johansson, C. (1975). Studies of gastrointestinal interactions. V. Characteristics of the absorption pattern of sugar, fat and protein from composite meals in man. A quantitative study. Scand. J. Gastroent. , 10, 33–42.

3. Bond, J.H. and Levitt, M.D. (1974). Investigation of small bowel transit time in man utilising pulmonary H_2 measurements. J. Lab. Clin. Med., 85, 546–559.

4. Read, N.W., Miles, C.A., Fisher, D., Holgate, A.M., Kime, N.D., Mitchell, M.A., Reeve, A.M., Roche, T.B., and Walker, M. (1980). Transit of a meal through the stomach, small intestine and colon in normal subjects and its role in the pathogenesis of diarrhoea. Gastroenterology, 79, 1276–1282.

5. Corbett, C.L., Thomas, Read, N.W., Hobson, N., Bergman, I. and Holdsworth, C.D. (1981). Electrochemical detector for breath hydrogen determination: measurement of small bowel transit time in normal subjects and patients with the irritable bowel syndrome. Gut, 22, 836–840.

6. Spiller, R.G., Bloom, S.R., Silk, D.B.A., Frost, P.G., Brown, B.E., Lee, Y.C. and Ghatei, M.A. (1983). The ileal brake – a compensatory slowing of jejunal transit following ileal fat infusion in man. Clin. Sci. Mol. Med., 63, 53P.

7. Holst, J.J. (1978). Extrapancreatic glucagons. Digestion, 17, 168-190.

8. Rosell, S. and Rokaeus, A. (1979). The effect of ingestion of amino acids, glucose and fat on circulating neurotensin-like immuno-reactivity (NTLI) in man. Acta. Physiol. Scand., 107, 263-267.

9. Besterman, S., Sarson, D.L., Blackburn, A.M., Cleary, J., Pilkington, T.R.E. and Bloom, S.R. (1978). The gut hormone profile in morbid obesity and following jejuno-ileal by pass. Scand. J. Gastroenterol., Suppl. 49, 15.

10. Holst, J.J., Sorensen, T.I.A., Andersen, A.N., Stadil, F., Andersen, B., Lauritsen, K.B. and Klein, H.C. (1979). Plasma entero-glucagon after jejuno-ileal by-pass with a 3:1 or 1:3 jejuno-ileal ratio. Scand. J. Gastroenterol., 14, 205-207.

11. Go, V.L.W. and Demol, P. (1981). Role of nutrients in gastro-intestinal release of immunoreactive neurotensin. Peptides, 2 (Suppl. 2), 267-269.

12. Ferris, C.F., Hammer, R.A. and Leeman, S.E. (1981). Elevation of plasma neurotensin during lipid perfusion of rat small intestine. Peptides, 2 (Suppl. 2), 263-266.

57

Comparison of Neurotensin and Fat on Myoelectric Activity Pattern of the Small Bowel

P. J. THOR, J. W. KONTUREK, R. SENDUR and S. J. KONTUREK

INTRODUCTION

Neurotensin (NT) is a tridecapeptide localized in the N cells of the jejunal and ileal mucosa (1). The physiological role of NT has not yet been identified but it has been shown to have a wide range of biological actions on gastrointestinal motility, secretion and circulation (2). Several nutrients, particularly fat, were reported to increase plasma levels of NT, suggesting that their gastrointestinal effects were mediated by endogenous release of NT (3).

The aim of this study was to compare the actions of NT and fat on myoelectric activity of the small bowel and plasma level of immunoreactive NT in dogs.

METHODS

Experiments were performed on four mongrel dogs weighing about 15 kg. Animals were anesthetized with thiobarbital sodium (15 mg/kg) and at laparatomy under aseptic conditions eight monopolar silver electrodes were sutured to the serosal surface of the small bowel and spaced proximately 30 cm apart from duodenum to ileum. A silver needle placed subcutaneously at the back of the animal served as a reference electrode. Recordings were made with a Beckman R-611 recorder through the resistance capacitance input of 9853 A couplers at a time constant of 1 s and high frequency cutoff at 100 Hz. All experiments were performed in conscious dogs that were fasted for at least 18 h. All dogs were provided surgically with duodenal and gastric fistulas.

A polyethylene catheter (PE-50) inserted into the leg vein was connected to a peristaltic pump (Unipan Poland) and i.v. infusion of saline alone (rate of 40 ml/h) in control experiments or NT (UCB-Bioproducts, Bruxelles, Belgium) dissolved in saline was administered. NT was either infused i.v. or injected i.v. in single bolus doses (range 0.15 - 2.5 µg/kg). In tests with fat, sodium oleate (100 mM) or 20% intralipid (lipofundin, Braun, Melsungen, Germany) was administered intraduodenally (i.d.) at rates 2 - 8 mmol/h and 20 - 80 ml/h, respectively. Recordings were manually analyzed to determine the time of occurrence of the four phases of the migrating myoelectric complexes (MMCs). On each test day, at least two cycles of duodenal MMCs were recorded and then i.v. NT or i.d. fat was administered.

In tests with atropine, NT was given by a constant i.v. infusion or fat was administered i.d. at a constant rate for 2-3 h and then atropine was added to i.v. infusion in a bolus dose of 20 µg/kg followed by a constant dose of 10 µg/kg-h for the rest of the experiment.

Blood samples were withdrawn before and during i.v. NT or i.d. fat administration for radioimmunoassay of NT-like activity as described previously (4).

RESULTS

A typical pattern of myoelectric activity in the fasting state were observed in all dogs. Intravenous infusion of NT at dose of 2.5 µg/kg -h completely abolished the MMCs at all levels of the small bowel (Fig. 1). These effects were established 2 - 4 min after commencement of the NT infusion and continued throughout the entire period of its infusion. NT-induced pattern of myoelectric activity was characterized by increased spiking similar to that seen in fed animals.

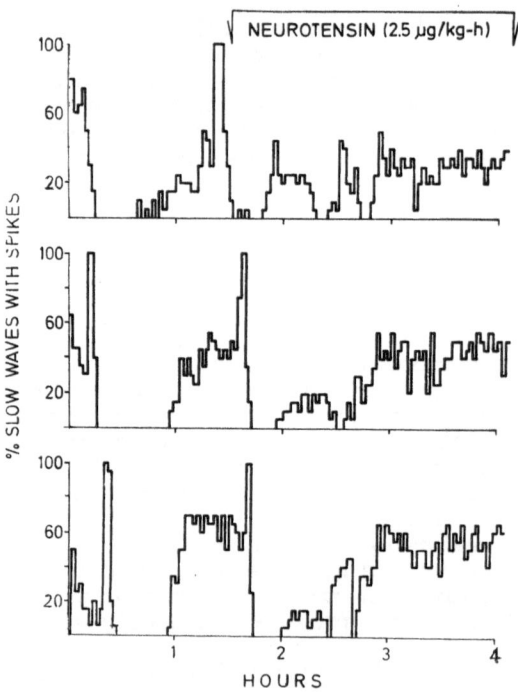

FIGURE 1. Temporal distribution of slow waves with spike potentials at three sites of the small bowel (duodenum, jejunum and ileum) during fasting period and after i.v. infusion of neurotensin at a dose of 2.5 µg/kg-h. Similar responses were obtained in each animal.

However, during infusion of NT at lower doses of 0.15 - 0.6 µg/kg-h, not all phases of MMCs were abolished; phase III of MMC could be easily distinguished on the recordings shown on Fig. 2.

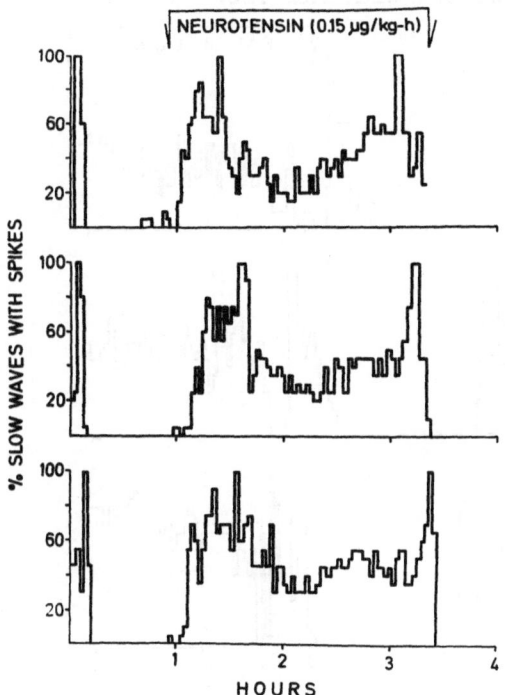

FIGURE 2. Temporal distribution of slow waves with spike potentials at three sites of the small bowel (duodenum, jejunum and ileum) during fasting period and after i.v. infusion of neurotensin at a dose of 0.15 µg/kg-h.

Intravenous bolus injection of NT in doses ranging from 0.15 to 0.6 µg/kg caused an increase in spike activity on each bowel level. This increase in spike activity was not dose-dependent and subsided after 10 min, however, the next phase III of MMC was delayed by about 20%. In one of the four dogs bolus injection of NT as well as commencement of NT infusion at a constant dose caused induction of phase III of MMC which started in the duodenum or middle portion of the small bowel.

Atropine tended to decrease the spike activity induced by NT but failed to abolish it completely (Table 1).

In tests with i.d. sodium oleate given at doses of 2 - 8 mmol/h or 20% intralipid at a rate of 10 - 80 ml/h, the occurrence of MMCs was completely abolished and typical fed-pattern was induced (Fig. 3).

Atropine given i.v. partly decreased the spike activity of the small bowel induced by i.d. fat (Table 1).

Plasma levels of NT increased dose-dependently with both i.v. NT and i.d. fat. In tests with i.d. oleate or intralipid, plasma NT reached the values comparable to those seen at the lowest dose (0.15 µg/kg-h) of exogenous NT. Higher doses of NT (2.5 µg/kg-h) inducing similar motility pattern as i.d. fat raised plasma NT about 10 times about the value obtained with i.d. fat.

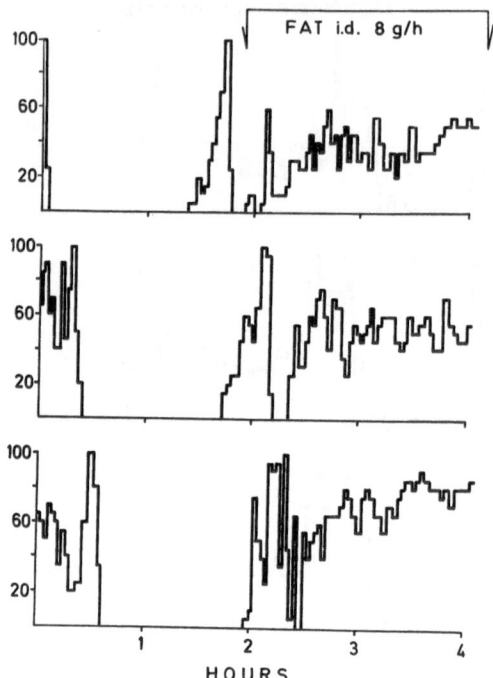

FIGURE 3. Temporal distribution of slow waves with spike potentials at three sites of the small bowel (duodenum, jejunum and ileum) during fasting period and after i.d. infusion of fat (8 g/h).

Table 1. Plasma NT levels and spike activity recorded at midjejunum after i.v. infusion of NT or i.d. instillation of fat with and without i.v. administration of atropine

Treatment	Plasma levels of NT (pM)	Slow waves with spikes (%)
Fasted	7.2 ± 1.3	14.8 ± 2.1
NT 0.6 µg/kg-h	53.4 ± 6.7	28.2 ± 5.4
2.5 µg/kg-h	449.0 ± 58.3	43.2 ± 7.3
Oleate 8 mmol/h	42.6 ± 7.5	38.5 ± 6.2
NT 2.5 µg/kg-h Atropine	517.4 ± 74.8	$21.3 \pm 3.8^*$
Oleate 8 mmol/h Atropine	$16.3 \pm 4.7^*$	$18.4 \pm 3.9^*$

* Significant decrease below the control value

DISCUSSION

The results of this study demonstrate that NT given i.v. increased intestinal spike activity at all doses tested but abolished the occurrence of MMCs only at higher doses. Intraduodenal fat abolished intestinal cyclic activity and increased spike activity while raising plasma NT to the level observed after lower doses of exogenous NT.

The mechanism responsible for the initiation of MMCs and their disrupture after feeding with a replacement by a fed-type motility pattern is not clear. Both nervous and hormonal factors seem to be involved. Several exogenous gut hormones such as gastrin (5), CCK (6) and insulin have been shown to induce the fed-like motility pattern but these effects appear to represent pharmacological rather than physiological actions because of the high doses of the peptide used. Wingate (7), who compared intestinal motility pattern after feeding and after infusion of exogenous gut peptides including gastrin, CCK and secretin found that they failed to reproduce the digestive motility pattern and concluded that none of them is hardly likely to be responsible for the change from a fasting to fed motility pattern.

Recently, NT was reported to abolish the MMCs in rats (8) and in humans (9) and to induce a motility pattern resembling that seen after ingestion of fat but no study compared the effects of NT and fat on intestinal motility and plasma NT levels in the same species and under similar experimental conditions.

The results of this study confirm that NT in conscious dogs increases the spike activity of the small bowel but complete inhibition of MMCs, similar to that observed after a fatty meal, can be achieved only at higher doses (2.5 µg/kg-h) of NT that raised plasma NT far above the physiological levels. Lower doses of NT (0.15 - 0.6 µg/kg-h) which increased plasma NT to the levels comparable to those observed after a fatty meal increased the spike activity of the small bowel but failed to affect MMCs. In fact, in some experiments, NT injection was followed by the appearance of the premature MMCs starting from the duodenum or jejunum.

It is of interest that atropine failed to suppress completely the increased spike activity induced by both NT and fat, suggesting that the muscarinic receptors are not involved in the action of NT and fat on intestinal smooth muscles.

These results indicate that NT may contribute to but cannot be fully responsible for the alteration of interdigestive to a digestive motility pattern observed after a fatty meal.

REFERENCES

1. Helmstaedter, V., Taugner, C.H., Feurle, G.E., and Forsmann, W.G. (1977). Localization of neurotensin-immunoreactive cells in the small intestine of man and various mammals. Histochemistry, 53, 35-41.
2. Rosell, S., Rokaeus, A., and Theodorsson-Norheim, E. (1983). The role of neurotensin in disease. Scan. J. Gastroent. 18 (Suppl. 82), 59-67.
3. Rosell, S., and Rokaeus, A. (1979). The effects of ingestion of amino acids, glucose and fat on circulating neurotensin-like immunoreactivity (NTLI) in man. Acta Physiol. Scand. 107, 263-267.
4. Konturek, S.J., Jaworek, J., Cieszkowski, M., Pawlik, W., Kania, J., and Bloom, S.R. (1983). Comparison of effects of neurotensin and fat on pancreatic secretion in dogs. Am. J. Physiol., 244, G590-G598.

5. Weisbrodt, N.W., Copeland, E.M., Kearley, R.W., Moore, E.P., and Johnson, L.R. (1974). Effect of pentagastrin on the electric activity of the small intestine of the dog. Am. J. Physiol., 227, 425-429.

6. Mukhopadhyay, A.K., Thor, P., Johnson, L.R., Copeland, E.M., and Weisbrodt, N.W. (1977). Effect of cholecystokinin on myoelectric activity of small bowel of the dog. Am. J. Physiol. 232, E44-E47.

7. Wingate, D.L., Pearse, E.A., Hutton, M., Dand, A., Thompson, H.H., and Wunsch, E. (1978). Quantitative comparison of the effects of cholecystokinin, secretin and pentagastrin on gastrointestinal myoelectric activity in the conscious dogs. Gut, 19, 593-601.

8. Al-Saffar, A., and Rosell, S. (1981). Effects of neurotensin and neurotensin analogues on the migrating myoelctric complexes in the small intestine of rats. Acta Physiol. Scand., 112, 203-208.

9. Thor, K., Rosell, S., Rokaeus, A., and Kager, L. (1982). (Gln^4)-Neurotensin changes the motility pattern of the duodenum and proximal jejunum from a fasting-type to a fed-type. Gastroenterology 83, 569-574.

58

Modulation of Rat Small Bowel Motor Activity by Food and Peptides

M. R. E. HUTTON and D. L. WINGATE

INTRODUCTION

Contractile activity and propulsion in the small intestine can both be studied but changes in one cannot always be correlated easily with changes in the other.

METHOD

The conscious rat is convenient for the study of intestinal motility using intestinal electromyography and studying the distribution of marker (^{51} Cr) 30 minutes after intraduodenal bolus injection (1,2,3).

In this study, rats were implanted with either 2 monopolar serosal electrodes, on the jejunum and mid-ileum, or an intraduodenal catheter, under Hypnorm (fentanyl) anaesthesia. All animals were allowed 5-7 days to recover from surgery.

RESULTS

Bursts of regular spiking activity (RSA) preceded by irregular spiking activity (ISA) recur at frequent intervals 14.1 $\pm$ 0.6 min (Fig 1) and the timing of these bursts is not altered by iv infusion of motilin.

SMALL BOWEL EMG IN THE CONSCIOUS RAT

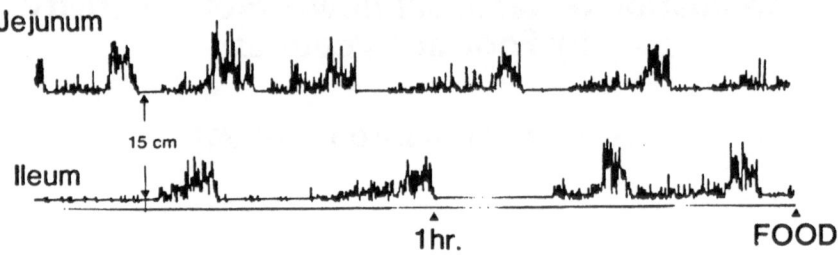

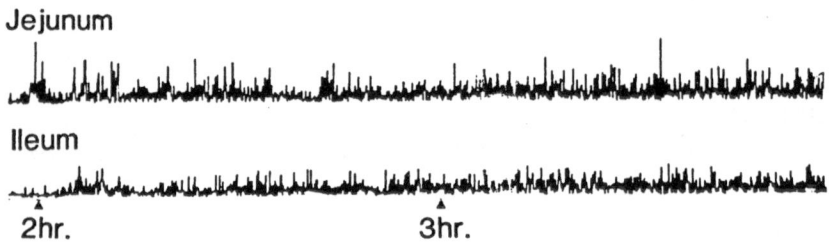

Fig. 1

2 ug/Kg/hr or by subcutaneous morphine (4 mg/Kg); both morphine and
D-Ala D-Leu enkephalin (DADLE), however, abolish fasting ISA.

Periodic activity is replaced by continuous ISA for 2-3 hours after
food (rat chow ad-lib) (Fig 1) during iv infusion of pentagastrin

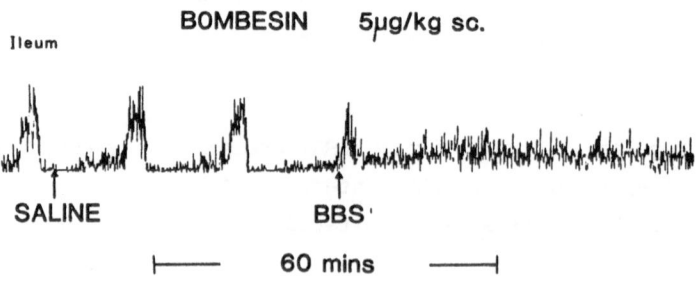

Fig. 2. Effect of bombesin on the fasting EMG

5 ug/Kg/min. Bombesin (50 ug/kg/hr iv for 1 hour) induced an initial abolition of all spikes followed by continuous ISA for 2-3 hours. As in other species, morphine and DADLE abolish postprandial ISA replacing it with regular bursts of RSA.

Patterns of spike activity are not well correlated with the distribution of marker along the small bowel; both in fasting and after food, the marker is aggregated into peaks (Fig 3), although fewer peaks occur after food (p<0.001).

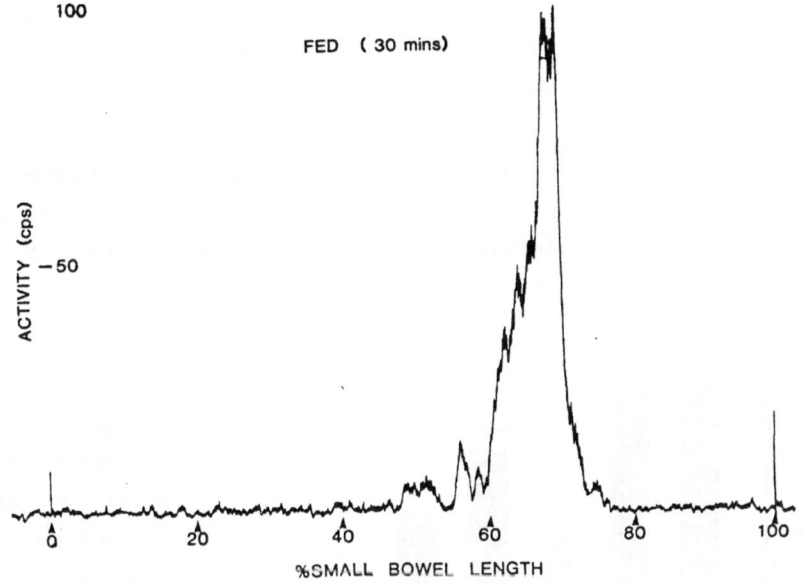

Fig 3a. Distribution of marker injected into the duodenum 15 minutes after food

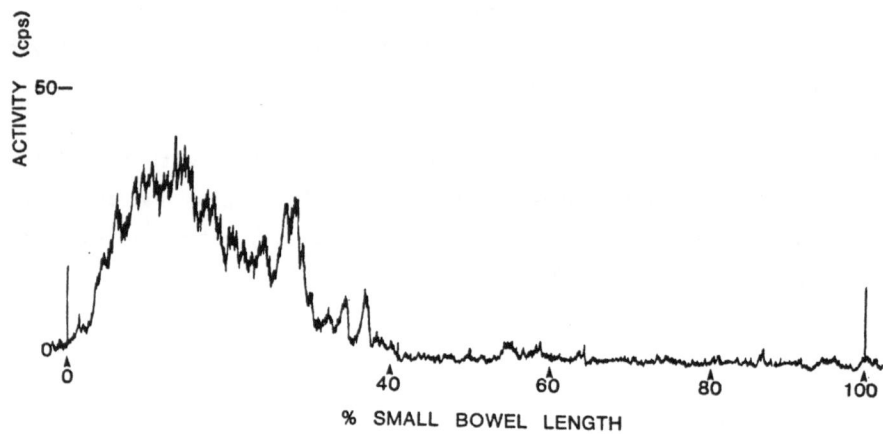

<u>Fig 3b.</u> Distribution of marker injected during pentagastrin infusion.

However, morphine and DADLE retard marker transit and reduce ISA in both fasted and fed animals; it seems that in rats ISA has a significant role in propulsion. Fig 4 summarises the effects of peptides and opioids on intestinal transit (4).

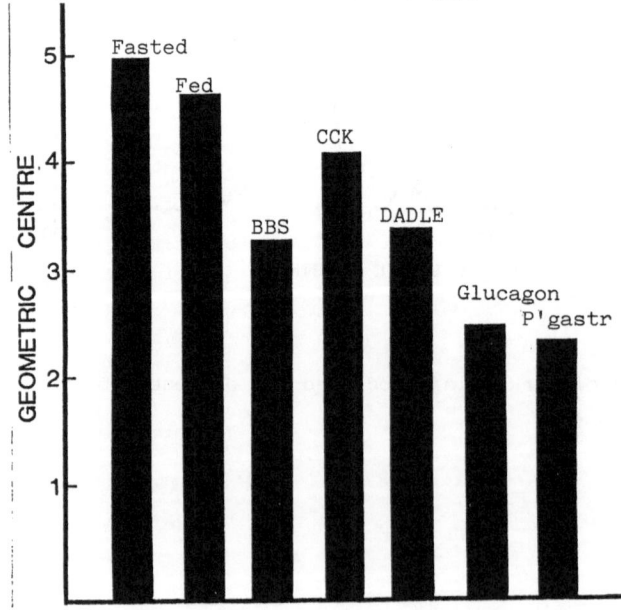

Fig. 4
Quantitative effect of peptides on marker transit as shown by mean values for geometric centre.

CONCLUSION

In terms of intestinal motility, the rat resembles dog and man in the effects of food, of peptides which mimic the response to food and also of opioids.   Qualitative and quantitative differences in periodic activity suggest differences in control mechanisms from those of dog and man.

REFERENCES

1   Ruckebusch M and Fioramonti J. (1975) Electrical spiking activity and propulsion in small intestine in fed and fasted rats. Gastro-enterology 68 1500–1508

2   Gustavsson S. (1978) Studies on the transport of small bowel contents. Upsala J Med Sci 83 167–173

3   Bueno L, Ferre JP, Ruckebusch M, Genton M, Pascaud X. (1981) Continuous electrical and mechanical activity recording in the gut of the conscious rat. J Pharmacol Methods 6 129–136

4   Miller M, Galligan JJ, Burks TF. (1980) An evaluation of methods for measurement of intestinal transit. Digest Dis Sci 26 722

59

Dose-Dependent Effects of Ceruletide on Jejunal Motor Activity and on Experimentally Induced Pain in Healthy Humans

G. STACHER, H. STEINRINGER, G. SCHMIERER, C. SCHNEIDER, S. WINKLEHNER, G. MITTELBACH, C. De PAOLIS and C. PRAGA

Ceruletide stimulates the contractile activity of the distal duodenum and the jejunum and accelerates small intestinal transit. Recently it was found that the peptide also exerts analgesic effects. This study investigated whether i.m. doses of 5, 10, and 20 µg ceruletide (Farmitalia Carlo Erba, Milan, Italy) would, in comparison with placebo, both stimulate jejunal motility and alleviate experimentally induced pain. Sixteen healthy men (age 20 - 32 yr) participated each in four experiments one week apart and received, in random double-blind fashion, all of the treatments. Jejunal pressures were recorded continuously by three perfused catheters with orifices spaced 3 cm apart and positioned 10 to 20 cm beyond the ligament of Treitz. The pressure recordings were analysed by computer. Chains of square wave constant current impulses of increasing intensity administered to the subjects' earlobe and constant intensity, variable time radiant heat stimuli applied sequentially to six spots on the forearm were used to induce pain. Each experiment lasted 150 min, 30 before and 120 min after drug administration. Ceruletide dose-dependently increased phase II ($P < 0.001$) and decreased phase I type activity ($P < 0.001$) and the occurrence of activity fronts (Fig. 1). The number and amplitude of contractions as well as the area under the pressure curve (Fig. 2) increased significantly and dose-dependently ($P < 0.001$). Ceruletide also increased dose-dependently threshold ($P < 0.001$) and tolerance ($P < 0.001$; Fig. 3) to electrically induced pain and threshold to thermally induced pain ($\underline{P} < 0.05$; Fig. 4). All effects lasted dose-dependently for 60 to more than 120 min. Only mild sedative and other side effects occurred; respiration, heart-rate, and blood pressure remained unaffected.

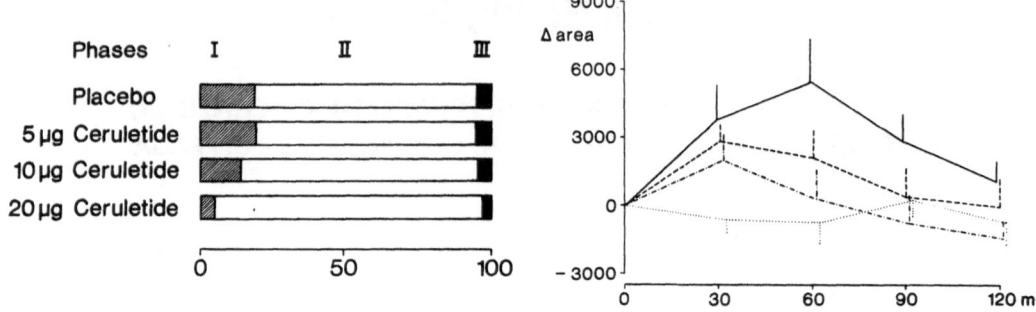

FIGURE 1   Percent distribution of MMC-phases in the 120 min after drug administration.

FIGURE 2   Area under the pressure curve. Change $\pm$ SEM from basal values after administration of 20 µg ceruletide (——), 10 µg ceruletide (----), 5 µg ceruletide (— · —), and placebo (····).

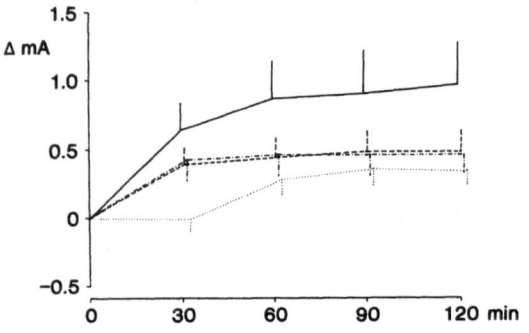

FIGURE 3   Tolerance to electrically induced pain. Change $\pm$ SEM from basal values after administration of 20 µg ceruletide (——), 10 µg ceruletide (----), 5 µg ceruletide (— · —), and placebo (····).

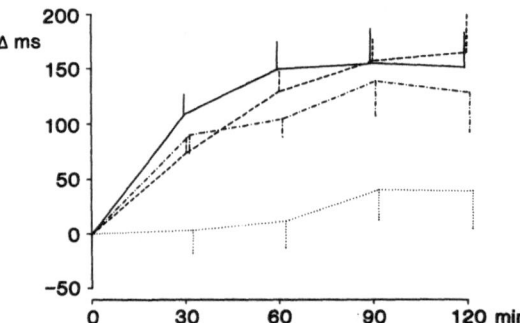

FIGURE 4   Threshold to thermally induced pain. Change $\pm$ SEM from basal values after administration of 20 µg ceruletide (——), 10 µg ceruletide (----), 5 µg ceruletide (— · —), and placebo (····).

Conclusion: Ceruletide, in the doses tested, both stimulates jejunal motility and alleviates pain. A further investigation of these effects in post-operative patients suffering from intestinal atonia and pain seems indicated.

60

Indomethacin-Induced Spiking Activity in Rabbit Ileum: *in Vivo* Interactions of Prostaglandins and Cholinergic Neurotransmission

K. L. KOCH and A. DWYER

INTRODUCTION

Prostaglandins may modulate intestinal tone and motility. Prostaglandin E_2 causes contraction of longitudinal muscle and relaxes circular muscle, whereas prostaglandin $F_2\alpha$ elicits contraction of both layers in in vitro studies.[1] Indomethacin, a potent inhibitor of prostaglandin synthesis,[2] would be expected to affect intestinal motility. In vitro studies show indomethacin relaxes the longitudinal muscle layer in response to a variety of stimuli,[3] and causes contraction of circular muscle.[4] Few studies have assessed the effects of indomethacin on in vivo gut motility. Mathias[5] reported indomethacin induced spiking activity and disrupted migrating action potential complexes stimulated by cholera toxin in anesthetized rabbits; Sanders[6] showed indomethacin increased luminal pressure in the ileum of anesthetized cats; Konturek[7] found that indomethacin caused diffuse spiking activity throughout the small intestine in conscious dogs. These in vivo studies suggest that indomethacin induces excitatory and contractile motility events and are consistent with in vitro effects of indomethacin on circular muscle reported above.

We have further characterized the electromechanical effects of indomethacin in in vivo rabbit ileum and have attempted to delineate the mechanism of spiking activity induced by indomethacin.

357

METHODS

Male New Zealand White rabbits weighing 2.0-3.0 kg were used in all
studies. Pentobarbitol sodium, 30 mg/kg, was given via an ear vein.
A tracheostomy was performed on each animal. A jugular vein catheter
and carotid artery catheter were inserted to administer additional
anesthetic or drugs and to monitor systolic pressure, respectively.
Body temperature was maintained at $38^{\circ}C$ throughout each experiment
by a heating blanket. The ileum was identified through a midline
abdominal incision and 3 Ag-AgCl monopolar electrodes were sewn to
the ileal serosa 2 cm apart. The electrodes were connected to a
rectilinear recorder (Beckman R612) through 8353A couplers. Recorder
sensitivity was 0.05 mV/mm, high frequency cut-off was 30 Hz and low
frequency filter setting was 0.16 Hz.

A basal or equilibration period of 90 min elapsed before any drug
was administered. Indomethacin, 5 mg/kg I.V., or saline were then
given, and myoelectric activity was recorded for 4-6 hours.

In other experiments, when spiking activity was maximum 30-60
minutes after injection of indomethacin, one of the following drugs
was administered intravenously: scopolamine hydrobromide, 0.08 mg/kg,
phentolamine mesylate, 3 mg/kg; propranolol hydrochloride, 2 mg/kg;
hexamethonium bromide, 10 mg/kg, and prostaglandin E_2, 18 ug/kg.
In additional experiments, bilateral cervical vagotomy was performed
during the period of maximal indomethacin-induced spiking activity
by transecting previously isolated vagal nerves.

Slow-wave frequency and spiking activity were determined during
10-minute periods 30 and 60 minutes after indomethacin or were determined during 5-minute periods immediately before (time 0) and 3 and
20 minutes after each autonomic nervous system blocking agent,
prostaglandin E_2, or vagotomy. Where appropriate, results were
compared using unpaired or paired Student's t-test.

RESULTS

Figure 1 shows a control recording obtained from three electrodes in
rabbit ileum. Slow-wave frequency averaged 18.0 ± 0.6 and few spikes
or action potentials are seen. This pattern was observed for 6 hours.

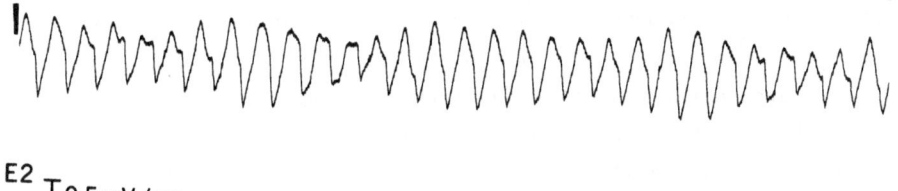

E2 $\underline{\mathrm{I}}$ 0.5mV/cm

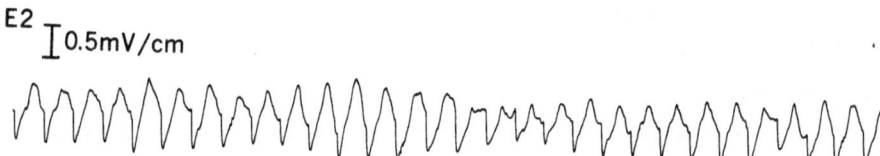

E3

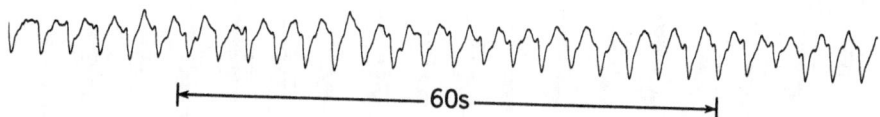

|←————— 60s —————→|

FIGURE 1   Myoelectric recording from control rabbit.   E1 denotes
           the proximal and E3 the distal electrode sites.

        Thirty minutes after administration of indomethacin, spiking
   activity occurred on all three electrodes as shown in Figure 2.

E1

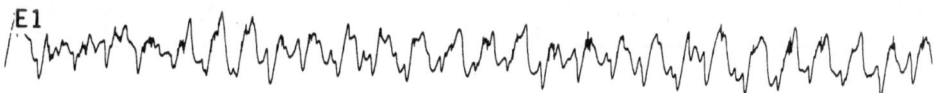

E2 $\underline{\mathrm{I}}$ 0.5mV

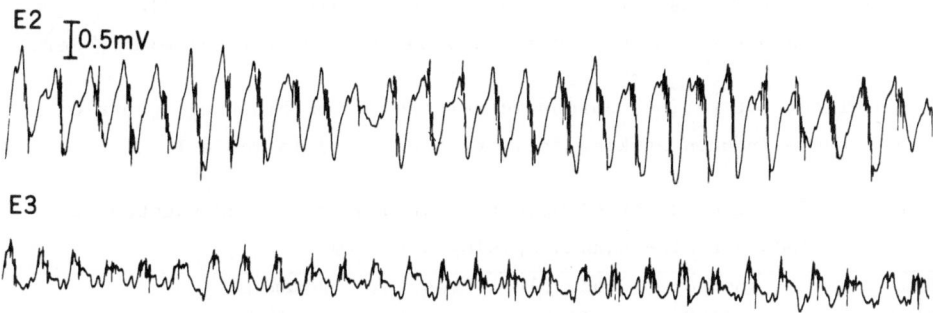

E3

|←————— 60s —————→|

FIGURE 2   Spiking activity on slow waves induced by indomethacin,
           5 mg/kg, I.V.   E1 denotes the proximal and E3 the distal
           electrode sites.

Spiking activity commenced on discrete portions of each slow wave.
The percentage of slow waves with spikes increased significantly 30
and 60 minutes after injecting indomethacin compared with controls
(57% and 69% versus 0.1% and 0%, p <0.01, respectively). Onset time
to spiking was 19 ± 4 minutes, duration of spiking was 190 ± 22 minutes,
and spiking activity was associated with phasic increases in intraluminal pressure.

Figure 3 illustrates the close correlation of indomethacin-induced
spiking activity and phasic contractions of the ileum.

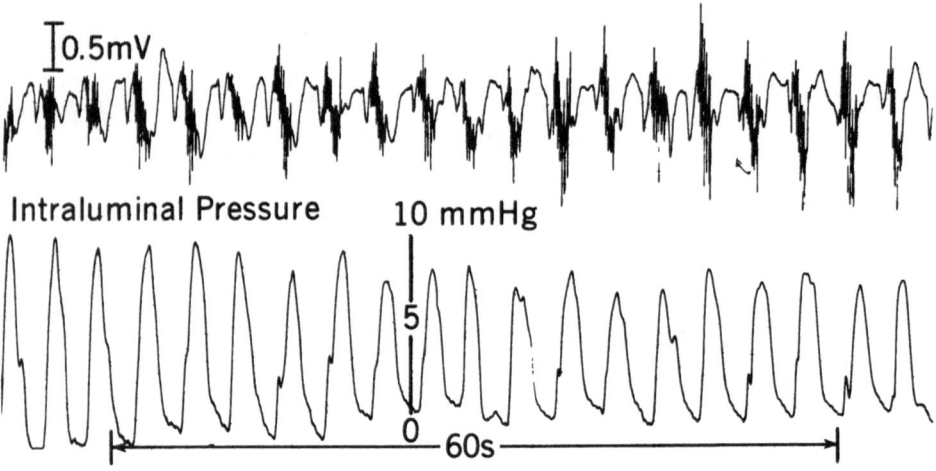

FIGURE 3   Electromechanical effects of indomethacin in rabbit ileum.
Intraluminal pressure was measured with saline-filled
catheter (PE 200) positioned beneath the serosal electrode.

The effects of various autonomic nervous system blocking agents on
indomethacin-induced spiking activity are listed in Table 1.

Table 1.   Effect of prostaglandin E_2, various drugs, and vagotomy on
indomethacin-induced spiking activity

Time (min)	PGE_2	Scopol- amine	Phentol- amine	Propran- olol	Hexameth- onium	Vagotomy
0	84 ± 6	63 ± 3	75 ± 6	82 ± 6	82 ± 5	75 ± 9
3	14 ± 6*	41 ± 9	79 ± 9	77 ± 8	82 ± 12	62 ± 10
20	78 ± 8	25 ± 6*	85 ± 6	72 ± 8	79 ± 9	68 ± 16

* p <0.01

Scopolamine reduced spiking activity on slow waves from 63% to 25%
20 minutes after injection (p <0.01); whereas phentolamine, propranolol and hexamethonium had no effect on spiking activity, although
phentolamine and hexamethonium reduced systolic blood pressure by 50%.
Prostaglandin E_2 (18 ug/kg) reduced spiking activity from 84 to 14 at
3 minutes after injection (p <0.01). This effect lasted approximately
10 minutes and spiking returned to baseline activity (78%) 20 minutes
later. As shown, bilateral cervical vagotomy had no effect on spiking
activity induced by indomethacin.

Slow-wave frequencies were reduced to 15.9 ± 0.3 60 minutes after
indomethacin. With exception of PGE_2 or propranolol, these frequencies
were unchanged after autonomic blocking agents. Three minutes after
propranolol slow wave frequency decreased from 15.3 ± 0.4 to
15.0 ± 0.4 (p <0.05). In contrast, PGE_2 increased slow-wave frequency
from 17.0 ± 0.3 to 19.7 ± 0.5 three minutes after injection (p <0.01).
By 20 minutes after PGE_2, slow-wave frequency approached baseline
(18.1 ± 0.5 cycles/min).

DISCUSSION

Intestinal tone and motility may be modulated by the endogenous
production of prostaglandins. PGE_2 decreases circular muscle contractility,[1] whereas indomethacin increases contraction of the circular
layer in vitro.[4] Because PGE_2 or prostacyclin inhibits indomethacin-
induced "motility" or spiking activity in vivo, it has been hypothesized that these endogenously synthesized prostaglandins inhibit
circular muscle contraction.[6,7] Our studies support this hypothesis:
after a lag period of approximately 19 minutes, indomethacin induced
intense spiking activity on slow waves; and, the spiking was abolished
by infusion of PGE_2. Similar spiking activity has been observed in
rabbit ileum after administration of acetylsalicylic acid.[8] That
two dissimilar cyclo-oxygenase inhibitors produce rhythmic spiking
activity suggests the spiking results from a deficiency of endogenous
prostaglandins (i.e., inhibition of cyclo-oxygenase) and not from
nonspecific drug effects. The deficiency of prostaglandins presumably
allows expression of an excitatory pathway.

A major finding of this study is that the indomethacin-induced
spiking activity is suppressed by scopolamine mesylate. This observation suggests a cholinergic neuromuscular pathway mediates the

excitatory circuit represented by spiking activity. Standard doses of adrenergic and ganglionic blocking agents had no effect on the indomethacin-induced myoelectric activity. Furthermore, bilateral cervical vagotomy did not alter spiking activity; thus, parasympathetic central nervous system control of the scopolamine-sensitive pathway was excluded. Taken together, these findings suggest indomethacin "unmasks" a postganglionic or enteric cholinergic neural circuit which mediates rhythmic spiking activity in the ileum.

Prostaglandins appear to modulate autonomic nervous system function in other tissues.[9] By depressing release of norepinephrine, prostaglandin D_2 and D_3 affect sympathetic neurotransmission in nictitating membrane.[10] By linking calcium, a receptor site(s) and acetylcholine-containing vesicles, prostaglandins may modulate acetylcholine release from guinea pig myenteric plexus.[11] Thus, prostaglandins may facilitate or depress autonomic neurotransmission, either cholinergic or adrenergic, depending upon the particular organ, and the quantity and proportion of various prostaglandins that are present at the receptor site. Our in vivo observations imply that ongoing synthesis of prostaglandins affect enteric nervous system function in rabbit ileum in that indomethacin "unmasks" a scopalamine-sensitive, vagotomy-resistant, excitatory neuromuscular pathway. Conversely, our observations also suggest that endogenous prostaglandin production suppresses this excitatory circuit.

The precise site(s) of prostaglandin modulation of enteric nervous system function and intestinal smooth muscle activity remains to be determined. The physiologic significance of indomethacin-induced spiking activity is unknown at present, but the interactions of endogenous prostaglandins and cholinergic neurotransmission may be relevant to local control of in vivo intestinal motility.

REFERENCES

1. Bennett, A. and Fleshler, B. (1970). Prostaglandins and the gastrointestinal tract. Gastroenterology, 59, 790-800
2. Vane, J. R. (1971). Inhibition of prostaglandin synthesis as a mechanism of action for aspirin-like drugs. Nature, 231, 232-5

3. Bennett, A., Eley, K. G., Stockley, H. L. (1975). Modulation by prostaglandins of contractions in guinea-pig ileum. Prostaglandins, 9, 377-84

4. Sanders, K. M. and Szurszewski, J. H. (1981). Does endogenous prostaglandin affect antral motility? Am. J. Physiol, 241, G191-5

5. Mathias, J. R., Carlson, G. M., Bertiger, G., Martin, J. L. and Cohen, S. (1977). Migrating action potential complex of colera: A possible prostaglandin-induced response. Am. J. Physiol, 232, E529-34

6. Sanders, K. M. and Ross, G. (1978). Effects of endogenous prostaglandin E on intestinal motility. Am. J. Physiol., 234, E204-8

7. Konturek, S. J., Thor, P., Pacolik, W., Gustaw, P. and Dembinski, A. (1982). The role of prostaglandins in the myoelectric, motor, and metabolic activity of the small intestine in the dog. In: Wienbeck, M. (ed). Motility of the Digestive Tract. pp. 437-44. (New York: Raven Press)

8. Koch, K. L., Dwyer, A. and Jeffries, G. H. (1983). Electro-mechanical effects of acetylsalicylic acid and sodium salicylate on in vivo rabbit ileum. Clin. Res., 31, 284A.

9. Brody, M. J. and Kadowitz, P. J. (1974). Prostaglandins as modulators of the autonomic nervous system. Fed. Proceed., 33, 48-60

10. Hemker, D. P. and Aiken, J. W. (1981). Effects of prostaglandins on autonomic function in vivo, with special emphasis on PGD_2 and PGD_3. Prog. Lipid Res., 20, 511-4

11. Ehrenpreis, S. (1981). Prostaglandin as a modulator of acetyl-choline release in guinea pig myenteric plexus. Prog. Lipid Res., 20, 505-9

61

Electrical Activity of Cat Intestine Following Defunctionalization

A. BORTOFF and L. F. SILLIN

INTRODUCTION

Chronically recorded electrical activity of cat intestine consists
of slow waves (SW's), spike potentials (SP's), and migrating spike
complexes (MSC's). SW's and SP's are similar to those occurring in
other species. MSC's, although unique to the cat in some respects,
exhibit certain properties of migrating myoelectric complexes (MMC's).
For example, the MSC migrates caudally at a velocity of ca 1 mm/sec
(1). Furthermore, it occurs primarily during the fasted state, and it
can traverse a region of transection and anastomosis (2).

The purpose of these experiments was to determine what changes
occur in the chronically recorded electrical activity, and in the
structure and intercellular electrical coupling of circular muscle in
the functional and defunctionalized portions of the intestine following surgical bypass of its middle third.

METHODS

Chronic Electrical Recording. Six bipolar electrodes, equally spaced
from duodenum to distal ileum, were implanted in each of 6 cats.

Beginning 10 days later, control recordings were obtained during at least seven 3 hr periods, each following a fast of 18-20 hrs. The middle 50 cm of intestine, containing electrodes 3 and 4, was then resected and defunctionalized by closing the proximal end and attaching the distal end to the ileum beyond electrode 6. Recording sessions commenced 10 days later and continued for several months thereafter.

Measurement of Intercellular Electrical Coupling. The degree of intercellular coupling in circular muscle was determined by measuring the specific tissue impedance of strips of circular muscle taken from mid-jejunum of 4 control cats, and from the functional and defunctionalized regions of jejunum in 4 experimental animals. Measurements were based on a method originally devised by Tomita (3,4).

Histological studies. Prior to the removal of tissue from the animal the circumference of the intestine was determined in each of the areas under study. Strips of intestinal wall were fixed at their in situ length with phosphate-formalin fixative, stained with hematoxylin-eosin, and examined under a light microscope.

RESULTS

Chronic Electrical Activity. Chronically recorded electrical activity consisted of SW's, SP's and MSC's (FIGS 1 and 2). Prior to by-pass surgery MSC's occurred sporadically, but always migrated in the caudal direction, sometimes traversing the entire length of the small intestine (FIG 1). As reported previously, however, (2) the frequency of MSC's was lowest in the duodenum and gradually increased to mid-jejunum where it reached a plateau that tended to be maintained over the remainder of the small intestine (FIG 4). Following bypass surgery the frequency of occurrence of MSC's was essentially unchanged at the

recording positions on the functional intestine, but dropped significantly in the bypassed segment (FIG 3). In 6 cats the average frequency at electrodes 3 and 4 of the bypassed segment dropped from a
control value of 1.25/hr to 0.56/hr following surgery. The difference
is significant (p<.01).

During the first 4 weeks following bypass surgery no MSC's were
observed to traverse the anastomosis between electrodes 2 and 5. Over
the next 2-3 weeks, however, such traversal became more and more
apparent. An example of this is shown in the tracings of Fig. 2,
taken 47 (A) and 73 (B) days after surgery. Similar traversals of the
anastomosis between electrodes 2 and 5 were evident in all 6 animals.
In contrast, slow waves did not propagate across the anastomosis, as
is evident by the sustained drop in SW frequency occurring below the
anastomosis (FIG 4).

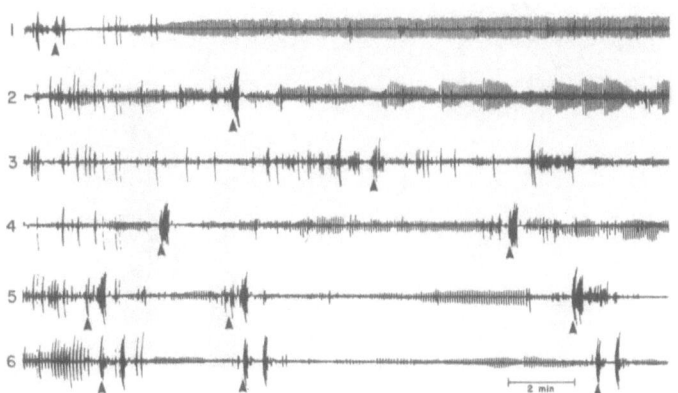

FIGURE 1. Example of chronically recorded electrical activity during
control period prior to bypass surgery. Onset of MSC at each electrode position is indicated by arrow. Although 3 MSC's occurred in
the ileum during this period, the first originated in the lower ileum,
the second originated in the upper ileum or lower jejunum, and only the
third originated in the duodenum and migrated the entire length of the
small intestine. Note that in the ileum the MSC tends to occur as a
double spike burst. The first 5 electrode pairs were each separated
by 25 cm, the 5th and 6th, by 10 cm.

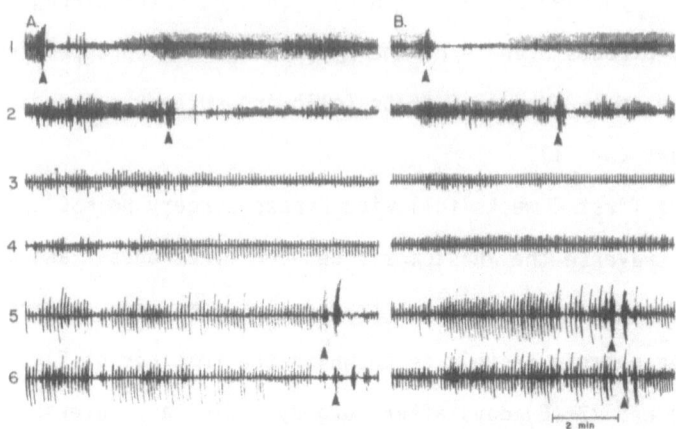

FIGURE 2. Chronically recorded electrical activity 47 days (A) and 73 days (B) after bypass. Same animal as in FIGURE 1. Note that MSC traversed anastomosis between electrode 2 and electrode 5. Migration velocity from 2 to 5 appears to increase between days 47 and 73.

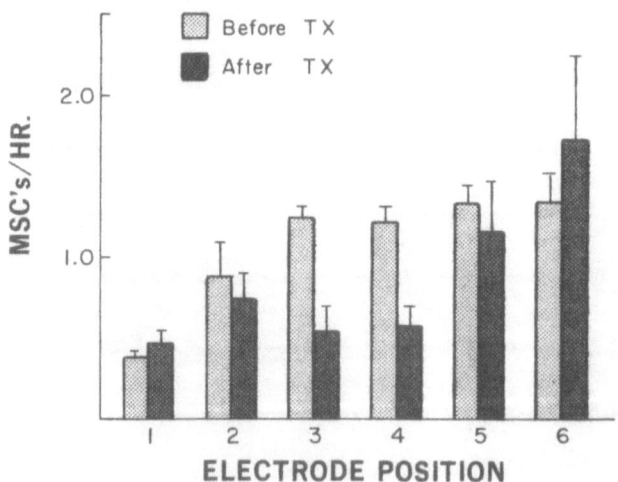

FIGURE 3. Average frequency (+SE) of MSC's at each electrode position in 6 cats prior to and following intestinal bypass (TX). Total recording hours: control, 200; bypass, 250. (See FIGURE 1).

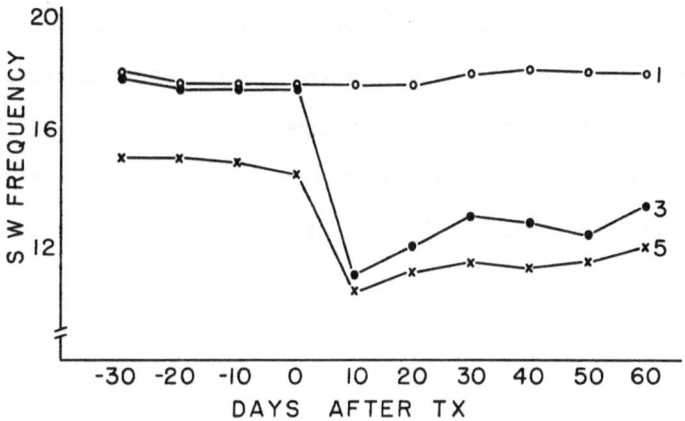

FIGURE 4. Slow wave frequency at electrode positions 1 (duodenum), 3 (mid-jejunum which forms part of the bypassed segment) and 5 (distal ileum) prior to and following intestinal bypass (TX).

Intercellular Electrical Coupling. The difference in specific impedance between the values obtained at low (30 Hz) and at high (30 KHz) current frequencies was taken as the specific junctional impedance, while that at the high frequency was taken to represent specific myoplasmic impedance (2,3). Values for normal control were determined for 14 strips of circular muscle taken from jejunums of 4 cats which did not undergo bypass surgery. Values were also determined for 13 similar strips taken from the proximal ends of the defunctionalized segments, and from 6 strips taken from the functional jejunums of 4 cats which had undergone bypass surgery at least 2 months previously. The mean values ($\pm$SE) of the junctional (Rj) and myoplasmic (Rm) specific impedances are given in Fig. 5. The mean values for myoplasmic impedance of all 3 groups of tissue is essentially the same, ca 115 ohm-cm. In contrast, the mean values for junctional impedance are significantly different from one another: normal control, 117

ohm-cm; bypassed, 243 ohm-cm; functional, 59 ohm-cm.

Histological Studies. Histological measurements revealed no differ-

ence in circular muscle thickness between bypassed and functional

jejunum. Average circumference of bypassed jejunum was 3.0+.3 (SD)

cm, while that of the functional jejunum of the bypassed animals was

3.9+.3 cm. The difference is significant (p<.05).

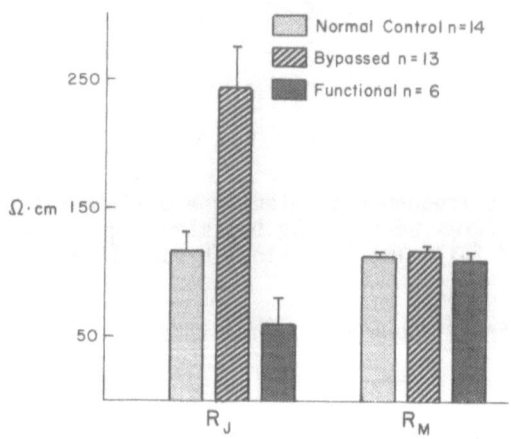

FIGURE 5. Specific tissue impedance of strips of circular muscle from
4 normal cats and from 4 cats which had undergone bypass surgery 2-6
months earlier. Rj represents the specific junctional impedance, which
is the difference between the impedance calculated at 30 Hz and 30 KHz,
while Rm represents the specific myoplasmic impedance, or that value
calculated at 30 KHz. Rj of the bypassed segment is significantly
higher than that of the normal controls (p<.01), while Rj of the functional segment is significantly lower (p<.02).

DISCUSSION

    These studies indicate that following defunctionalization of a

segment of cat jejuno-ileum the frequency of MSC's in that segment is

significantly reduced. This is apparently in contrast to the MMC,

the frequency of which is unchanged or even slightly increased in

similarly defunctionalized loops of intestine (5,6). This difference between MMC's and MSC's may reflect different mechanisms for their initiation. The decrease in MSC frequency after defunctionalization may be accounted for, at least in part, by the absence in the defunctionalized segment of those MSC's which originate more proximally and normally migrate past the electrodes now on the bypassed segment. This would imply that the number of MSC's recorded from the bypassed segment is equal to the number which normally originate there, although this remains to be determined.

In previous studies (2) it was shown that the MSC, like the MMC, can readily traverse an anastomosis which bridges a simple transection. In these studies it was shown that the MSC can also, after a period of several weeks, traverse an anastomosis which replaces 50 cm of resected intestine. In neither case did SW's cross the anastomosis, and in no case was there any histological evidence of smooth muscle bridging the anastomosis. Because of the apparent involvement of the myenteric plexus in propagation of MMC's (5,7), it would be of interest to determine if the traversal of MSC's is associated with nerve regeneration in the anastomotic tissue.

An increase in specific junctional impedance of circular muscle from bypassed jejunum is not surprising in view of the fact that the circumference of the bypassed segment is some 30% less than that of the functional jejunum. Since specific junctional impedance is a measure of the lumped impedance of the junctions in a cubic cm of tissue there should be some 30% more junctions in series, giving a specific junctional impedance which is 30% greater in the bypassed, as compared to the functional tissue. However, the junctional impedance of bypassed tissue appears to be approximately 4 times greater than its functional counterpart. This implies that there may be fewer nexuses or gap junctions per cell in the bypassed muscle, and that there may be more

nexuses per cell in the functional muscle as compared to normal con-

trols. Also, since the thickness of circular muscle in the bypassed

segment was not significantly different from that of the functional

intestine, it appears that cell atrophy in the bypassed muscle occurs

primarily along the major axis, the diameter of the cells being essen-

tially unchanged.

(Supported in part by NIH Grant #AM-06958.)

REFERENCES

1. Weisbrodt, N. W. and Christensen, J. (1972). Electrical activity
in the cat duodenum in fasting and vomiting. Gastroenterology, 63,
1004-1010.

2. Bortoff, A., Sillin, L. F. and Sterns, A. (1983). Chronic electrical activity of cat intestine. (Submitted to Amer. J. Physiol.)

3. Tomita, T. (1969). The longitudinal tissue impedance of the
smooth muscle of guinea-pig taenia-coli. J. Physiol. Lond., 201,
145-159.

4. Bortoff, A. and Gilloteauz, J. (1980). Specific tissue impedances of estrogen- and progesterone-treated rabbit myometrium.
Amer. J. Physiol., 238, (Cell Physiol. 7), C34-C42.

5. Aeberhard, P. F., Magnenat, L. D. and Zimmerman, W. A. (1980).
Nervous control of migratory myoelectric complex of the small bowel.
Amer. J. Physiol. (Gastrointest. Liver Physiol. 1), G102-G108.

6. Eeckhout, C., De Wever, I., Vantrappen, G. and Janssens, J.
(1980). Local disorganization of interdigestive migrating complex by
perfusion of a Thiry-Vella loop. Amer. J. Physiol. 238 (Gastrointest. Liver Physiol. 1), G509-G513.

7. Sarna, S., Stoddard, C., Belbeck, L. and McWade, D. (1981). Intrinsic nervous control of migrating myoelectric complexes. Amer. J.
Physiol., 241 (Gastrointest. Liver Physiol.), G16-G23.

62

Vagal and Splanchnic Influences on Small Intestinal Motility in the Anaesthetized Ferret

P. I. COLLMAN, D. GRUNDY and T. SCRATCHERD

INTRODUCTION

The extrinsic nervous system has the ability to initiate, terminate or alter the patterns of motility in the gastrointestinal tract. Classically, the parasympathetic nerves have a dominant role in regulating motility to the needs of digestion although more recent studies have revealed an increasingly complex organisation of both the parasympathetic and sympathetic nervous systems regulating GI function.

The urethane anaesthetized ferret shows well developed intestinal motility. In the jejunum, this is characterised by a bursting type of motility similar to the "minute rhythm" seen in other animals (1). More caudal regions of intestine (distal ileum) exhibit a relatively continuous pattern of motility. The present paper deals with the extent of the vagal and splanchnic influences on the patterns of motility in these two regions of small intestine.

METHODS

Details of the methods are available elsewhere (2). Briefly, ferrets were anaesthetized with urethane (1.5 g kg^{-1} i.p.) after an overnight fast. Two saline filled cannulae were inserted into the intestine (one in the jejunum and the other in distal ileum) in an oral direction taking care not to introduce fluid into the loop of intestine. The cannulae were connected to pressure transducers and intraluminal pressure was recorded. The pylorus was ligated and the abdomen closed. Electrical stimulation (20V, 0.5 msec, 1-50 Hz) of the cervical or thoracic vagi was performed after bilateral cervical vagotomy. In vagal cooling experiments, both cervical vagi were placed intact on cooling thermodes perfused with a cold alcohol-water mixture. The temperature of each thermode was monitored by a thermocouple and maintained at 38°C except during periods of cooling when the nerves were held at $2-4^\circ$C. Splanchnic nerve section was achieved by dissecting free the nerves at the crus of the diaphragm and placing a ligature beneath each one. The ligatures were fed into plastic tubes and then led out through the mid-line incision. Pulling sharply on the ligatures severed the nerves without disturbing the position of the viscera. These experiments were performed after ligating both adrenal glands.

RESULTS

Spontaneous motility in the jejunum and ileum

The jejunal motility showed a "bursting" pattern similar to the "minute rhythm" seen in other species (1). This consisted of bursts of contraction of approximately 50 sec duration separated by periods of similar duration in which little or no motility occurred (Fig. 1A). During the bursts, the contractions occurred at· 29.4 ± 0.15 min^{-1} whilst during the quiescent phase, slower contractions of $7-10$ min^{-1} were apparent. In the ileum, the contractions occurred continuously in most (12/14) animals although the larger amplitude contractions tended to group together (Fig. 1B). The contractions occurred at a lower frequency than in the jejunum (18.7 ± 0.44 min^{-1}). In two animals, the ileal motility showed discrete bursts of activity as in the jejunum. However, the duration of the inactive periods was less than in the jejunum and they occurred less often. Peak contraction amplitude was similar in both jejunum and ileum at about 0.85 kPa.

Cooling both cervical vagal trunks to below 4°C prevents the conduction of impulses (3) and provides a reversible vagotomy. In all experiments, "bursting" jejunal motility was abolished on vagal cooling and there was a small fall in tone (Fig. 2). The motility which persisted during vagal cooling was of the $7-10$ min^{-1} type normally seen during the interburst period. On rewarming the nerves, cyclical activity returned and often showed a transient increase in contraction amplitude. The ileal response to cooling was much less consistent. In the majority of cases (75%) vagal cooling had no effect on spontaneous motility. In the remaining animals, ileal motility was reduced or abolished by vagal cooling and returned on rewarming.

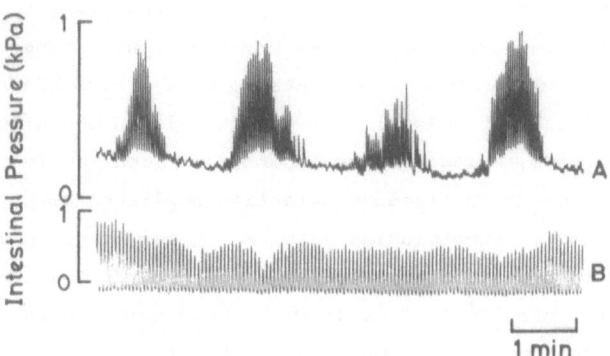

FIGURE 1   Spontaneous motility in the jejunum (A) and ileum (B) of the anaesthetized ferret

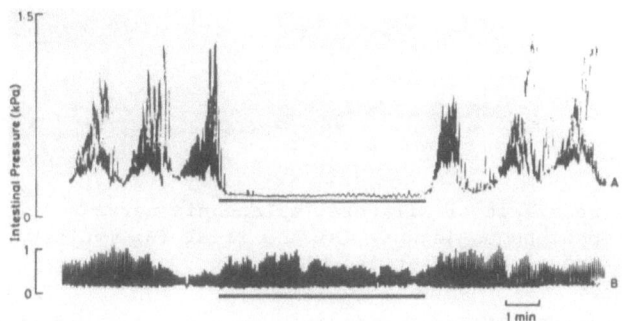

FIGURE 2   The effect of cooling the cervical vagi to $2^{\circ}C$ on spontaneous jejunal (A) and ileal (B) motility. The duration of the cool is shown by the black bars

The different sensitivity to vagal cooling in the two regions of intestine was reflected in the effect of atropine (1 mg kg^{-1}) on jejunal and ileal motility. All jejunal motility was abolished by atropine and there was an accompanying fall in tone. In the ileum, the response was more varied varying from complete abolition in 20% of animals to no change in 40% with the remainder showing either a reduction in contraction amplitude or a transient period of inhibition.

Unfortunately, it was not possible to cool the splanchnic nerves.

Bilateral splanchnic section resulted in a biphasic change in jejunal
motility. Immediately following section, there was a transient
abolition of cyclical activity in the jejunum lasting 3.2 ± 0.83 min
(N=7) presumably due to an efferent volley of splanchnic activity
resulting from injury to the nerves (Fig. 3). Following this
inhibition, the peak amplitude of the bursting contractions was
increased slightly from 0.62 ± 0.22 kPa to 0.75 ± 0.22 kPa although
not significant at the 5% level. In two animals in which jejunal
motility was absent, splanchnectomy induced cyclical activity. The
ileum did not show an increased contraction amplitude after
splanchnic section. Phentolamine (2 mg kg) given after splanchnectomy
markedly increased peak contraction amplitude in the jejunum from
0.52 ± 0.25 kPa to $1.2 \pm .72$ kPa (N=6) but had only a slight and not
significant effect on spontaneous ileal motility.

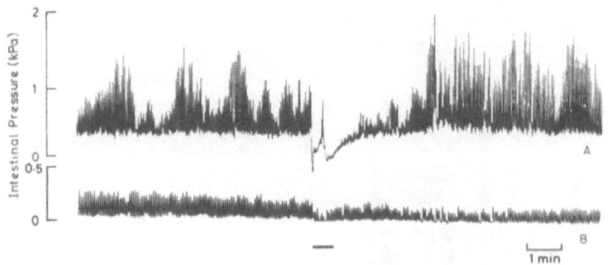

FIGURE 3   The effect of bilateral splanchnic nerve section on
spontaneous jejunal (A) and ileal (B) motility. The nerves
were sectioned at the black bar

Effect of electrical vagal stimulation on jejunal and ileal motility

Electrical stimulation of the peripheral end of either the cervical or
thoracic vagi for 1 min always stimulated, in a frequency dependent
manner, jejunal motility. The maximum response occurred at 20 Hz and
motility ceased abruptly when stimulation ended. Longer periods of
stimulation (5-10 min) applied to the thoracic trunks gave rise to
bursts of contractions followed by periods of quiescence, despite the
stimulation being continuous (Fig. 4B). The ileal responses were much
more variable showing a mixture of excitation and inhibition with the
latter being the dominant response especially at higher stimulation
frequencies ($>$ 5 Hz). The inhibition occurred after a short latency

as both a fall in tone and an inhibition of spontaneous contractions
(Fig. 4D) and persisted beyond the stimulation period for 78 $\pm$ 16.2
sec. Only one animal showed an entirely excitatory response over the
whole frequency range (Fig. 4C). The jejunal response to vagal
stimulation was changed by atropinization. The latency was longer,
the amplitude was lower, higher stimulus frequencies were required to
elicit a response and the response persisted beyond the period of
stimulation. Long periods of stimulation still evoked bursts of
contraction separated by periods of quiescence. Neither the
inhibitory nor the excitatory ileal responses to vagal stimulation
were abolished by atropine, although the excitatory responses were
reduced. In three animals, the jejunal response to electrical vagal
stimulation was enhanced by splanchnic section although the ileal
responses were unaffected.

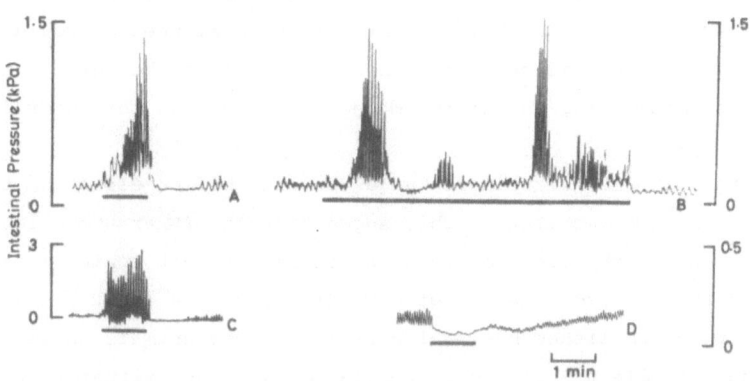

FIGURE 4   The effect of electrical stimulation of the vagus (A):
           Jejunal response to cervical vagal stimulation at 5 Hz,(B):
           Jejunal response to thoracic vagal stimulation at 5 Hz for a
           period (C) and (D) ileal response to cervical vagal
           stimulation at 5 Hz and 20 Hz respectively. All responses
           are from different animals and were given at 25V, 0.5 msec.
           Length of stimulation is given by the bar.

DISCUSSION

The anaesthetized ferret has two main types of spontaneous motility in
the small intestine. In the ileum, motility is mainly continuous but
in the jejunum, bursts of contractions alternate with periods of
greatly reduced, or absent, motility. This type of activity is

similar to the "minute rhythm" seen in other animals. In conscious animals, minute rhythm is seen during phase II (the irregular contraction phase) of the MMC and also in the fed state (1). However, in the anaesthetized ferret, neither jejunal minute rhythm nor ileal motility follows the established MMC pattern of the conscious ferret (4).

The bursting pattern of contractions in the jejunum is abolished by vagal cooling, a procedure which prevents the conduction of action potentials in nerve fibres (3). Indirectly acting cardiovascular or respiratory effects caused by vagal cooling are not responsible for the abolition of motility (2). This suggests that the minute rhythm is dependent on a tonic vagal discharge. Vagal stimulation confirms this possibility as long periods of stimulation ($>$ 1 min) caused bursts of contractions interspersed with periods of quiescence, despite the continuous stimulus. The vagal discharge producing the bursts could occur just before contractions commenced or could be continuous, with some other mechanism controlling the periodicity. A likely candidate for the timing mechanisms would be the enteric nervous system.

In the majority of animals, vagal cooling had no effect on the continuous ileal motility. This suggests that either there is little vagal input to the ileum or that the fibres are not tonically active. Clearly there is some degree of a vagal excitatory input since ileal motility was abolished by vagal cooling in some animals while others responded to electrical vagal stimulation with an excitatory response. The main effect of vagal stimulation however, was either a relaxation and/or an inhibition of ileal motility, presumably due to activation of a vagal inhibitory pathway.

Both areas of gut responded differently to atropine. Spontaneous jejunal motility seems to be entirely controlled by cholinergic excitatory fibres while ileal motility was largely resistant to atropine. Similar atropine resistant motility has been reported in the colon of the ferret (5). After atropine, vagal stimulation still evoked contractions in the jejunum although the response was of lower amplitude and longer latency. Ileal excitatory or inhibitory responses were still present after atropine although the excitatory responses were reduced in amplitude. These findings suggest that both areas receive a cholinergic and non-cholinergic excitatory supply which is vagally controlled. Additionally, the ileum received a non-cholinergic inhibitory supply.

The splanchnic supply to the intestines exerts a tonic inhibitory influence on motility. In the cat, the ileum receives a greater amount of inhibition than the jejunum (6). In our experiments, the jejunum seemed to be more influenced by the sympathetic system than the ileum. Both spontaneous and vagally induced jejunal motility were increased by splanchnectomy while the ileum was little affected. Although the distal intestine may receive its sympathetic supply via an alternative pathway, the observation that phentolamine also had little effect would indicate less tonic nor-adrenergic input to the ileum than jejunum. The finding that phentolamine resulted in further enhancement of jejunal motility may indicate reflex pathways via the pre-ventebral ganglia as reported in the colon (7).

In the anaesthetized ferret, therefore, the level of spontaneous contraction activity in the jejunum is dependent upon the balance between tonic activity in the vagal and splanchnic supply. In the ileum, on the other hand, spontaneous motility is largely uninfluenced by the extrinsic supply.

REFERENCES

1. Fleckenstein, P., Bueno, L., Fioramonti, J. and Ruckebusch, Y. (1982). Minute rhythm of electrical spike bursts of the small intestine in different species. Am.J.Physiol., 242, 9654-9659

2. Collman, P.I., Grundy, D. and Scratcherd, T. (1983). Vagal influences on the jejunal "minute rhythm" in the anaesthetized ferret. J. Physiol. (in press)

3. Linden, R.J., Mary, D.A.S.G. and Weatherill, D. (1981). The effect of cooling on transmission of impulses in vagal nerve fibres attached to atrial receptors in the dog. Q.J. exp Physiol. 66, 321-332

4. Bueno, L., Fioramonti, J. and More, J. (1981). Is there a functional large intestine in the ferret? Experientia, 37, 275-277

5. Collman, P.I., Grundy, D. and Scratcherd, T. (1983). Vagal control of colonic motility: Evidence for a non-cholinergic

excitatory innervation. J. Physiol. (in press)

6. Kewenter, J. (1965). The vagal control of the jejunal and ileal motility and blood flow. Acta Physiol. Scand., 65, Suppl. 251, 1-68

7. Kreulen, D.L., and Szurszewski, J.H. (1979). Reflex pathways in the abdominal pre-vertebral ganglia: evidence for a colo-colonic inhibitory pathway. J. Physiol., 295, 21-32

The M.R.C. is thanked for support. *M.R.C. Research Studentship.

Section 5
Lower Digestive
Tract

63

Relationship between Contractile and Intracellular Electrical Activities in Canine Colon Muscle Layers

Y. J. KINGMA, M. M. CHAMBERS and K. L. BOWES

INTRODUCTION

The coordination and the mechanisms underlying the coordination of the mechanical activity of muscle layers of the large bowel are poorly understood (1). During mass movement, coordination between the circular and longitudinal muscle coats is required; at other times such synchronism may not be necessary.

Since electrical cell potentials and mechanical activity are closely related, it is essential that simultaneous measurements of these two parameters be made in order to understand the mechanisms involved in this organ. Measurements must be made in isolated muscle layers (both proximal circular and longitudinal) and in specimens of intact muscle wall. In isolated muscle samples the typical properties of the separate layers can be studied and in intact samples it may be possible to recognize the summation of these signals in addition to signals arising from an interaction of the two muscle layers.

There is evidence that electrical spike bursts recorded form the colon originate in the longitudinal muscle layer, in which they coincide with contractions (2), but uncertainty remains concerning spike generation in circular muscle. Slow waves have been shown to be present continually in circular muscle and to be synchronous with contractile activity when the latter is seen. However, it has not been shown that this contractile activity is always present.

The hypotheses which we tested were the following:

383

1.   There is an inherent relationship between the contractile activities of the two muscle layers of the colon.

2.   Contractions in the circular muscle require spikes.

3.   Cyclic contractile activity in circular muscle is always present, synchronous with the continuously present electrical slow waves.

METHODS

Proximal colon samples were surgically removed from healthy mongrel dogs anaesthesized with sodium pentobarbital. The colon segments were cut open along the mesenteric border and the mucosa was removed by sharp dissection. T-shaped specimens (10 mm x 10 mm) with one axis in each of the circular and longitudinal directions were prepared for simultaneous measurements of contraction in both directions as well as intracellular measurements in circular muscle cells. Strips (2 mm x 10 mm) of intact and isolated circular and longitudinal muscle were prepared to perform similar measurements.

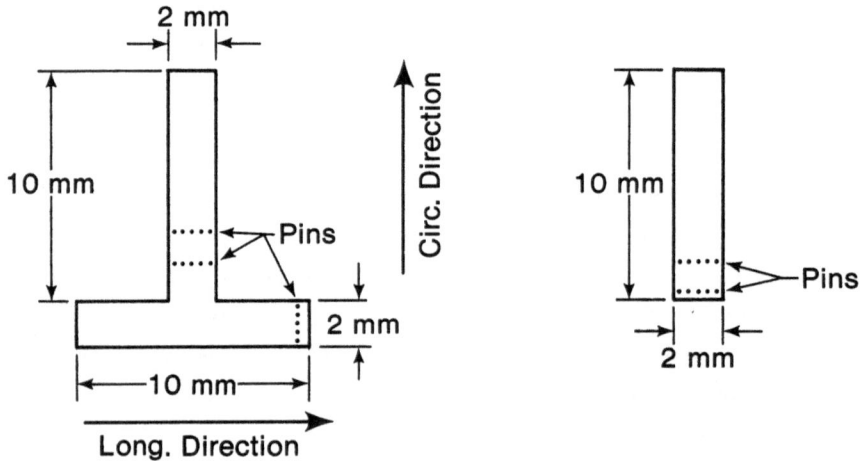

Fig. 1   Dimensions of the Specimens

All specimens were mounted in an organ bath perfused with oxygenated Krebs' at 37.5°C.   The contractile forces were measured with Grass
force transducers (type FT03) and the intracellular potentials were
measured with KCl-filled micropipettes.   Al measured signals were recorded on a Beckman (type 611) polygraph.

RESULTS

The contractile activity of intact and isolated longitudinal muscle
showed a variety of patterns.

1.   Large (1 g) of a repetitive nature (1.20 ± 0.27 cpm).   These
large contractions were modulated by a ripple of 21.8 ± 4.9 cpm.   The
frequency of the ripple was the same as the cyclic changes of the
membrane potential.

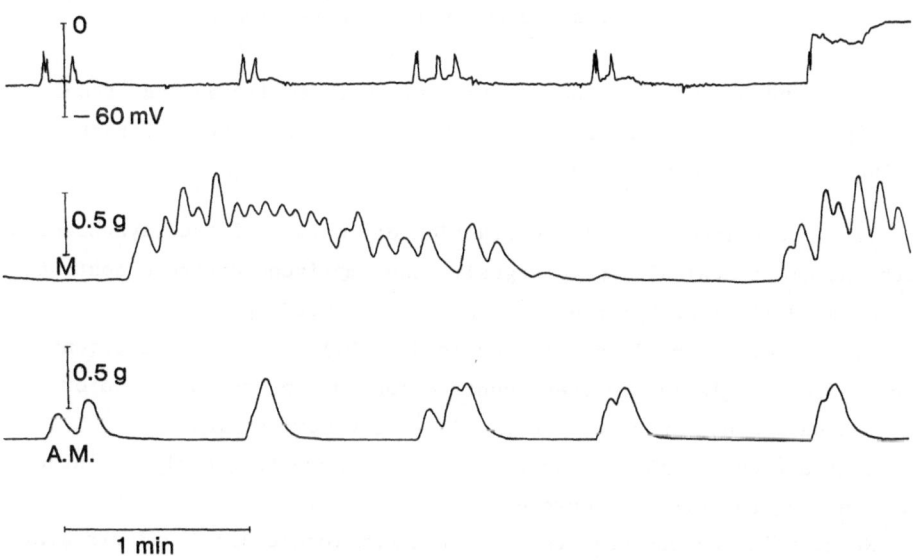

Fig. 2   Isolated longitudinal muscle; top and bottom
            channels are electrical intracellular and
            mechanical signals from the same specimen.

2.   Prolonged contractions (1 g) with duration varying from 1 to 5 minutes; these contractions occurred intermittently and invariably had a ripple component superimposed on them (21.8 ± 4.9 cpm)

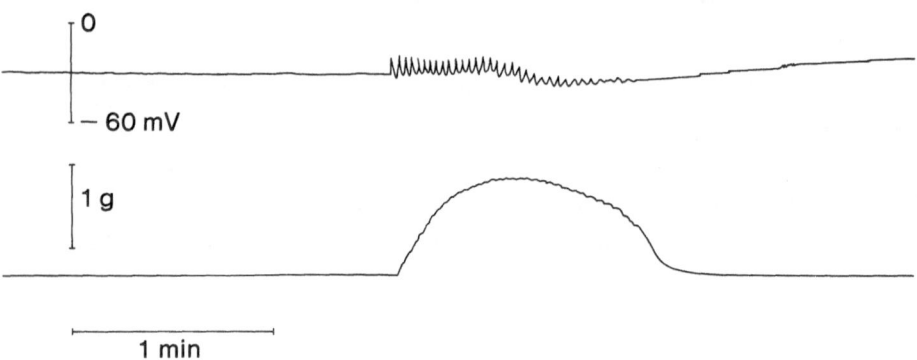

Fig. 3   Isolated longitudinal muscle; electrical,
          intracellular and mechanical; channels
          shows continuous cyclic contractions.

3.   Randomly varying contractions (in both amplitude and frequency; figure 2, middle channel). The contractile activity of intact and isolated circular muscle was of two types:

1.   A continuous cyclic contraction of small amplitude,synchronous with the electrical slow wave signal. The amplitude of these contractions was 0.11 ± 0.08g; the frequency 5.60 ± 0.89 cpm.

2.   Intermittent large contractions (0.8g). These contractions occurred as single intermittent contractions or in groups of two or more, always synchronous with electrical slow wave cycles.

Contractions of the second type occurred more frequently in intact than in isolated circular muscle (79% vs 37.5%).

No correlation was seen to exist between longitudinal and circular contractions.

The intracellular electrical slow wave activity from isolated and intact circular muscle was always present in all samples. One or more spikes appeared on the slow wave plateau when the intermittent large contractions occurred. If a minimum time of 1 second elapsed between the initial peak of the slow wave and the first spike, a secondary

component was observed superimposed on the primary contractile component. A lesser time lapse resulted in the two components fusing
together.

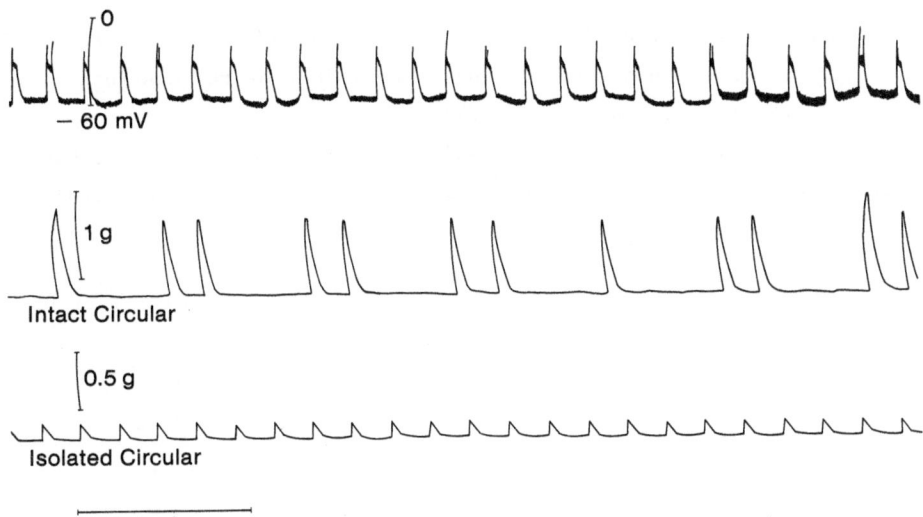

Fig. 4   Isolated and intact circular muscle; channels
1 and 2 are electrical intracellular and
mechanical; channel 3 shows continuous cyclic
contractions.

The large repetitive and the prolonged contractions in isolated
and intact longitudinal muscle coincided with rapid depolarizations of
the cell membrane. The frequency of these depolarizations was identical to that of the ripple superimposed on the contractions. The depolarizations were triangular in form, in some cases the top of the triangle had a sharp spike on it.

CONCLUSIONS

1. Hypothesis 1 is rejected: we could not show that contractile
activity in one muscle layer is correlated with contractile activity
in the other.

2. Hypothesis 2 is partially accepted: large amplitude contractions
in circular muscle are associated with spikes; ripple contractions are
not.

3. Hypothesis 3 is accepted: ripple contractions are always present in circular muscle, associated with continuously present slow waves.

REFERENCES

1. Szurszewski, J. H. (1981). Electrical basis for gastrointestinal Motility. In: Johnson, L. R. (ed). Physiology of the Gastrointestinal Tract. 58. (Raven Press N.Y.)
2. Debski, L. et al. Longitudinal and Circular Muscle of the Canine Colon Have Different and Characteristic Electrical and Mechanical Activities. These proceedings.

64

Modulation of the Pacemaker Activity in Circular Muscle of the Canine Colon

J. D. HUIZINGA, N. E. DIAMANT and T. Y. EL-SHARKAWY

INTRODUCTION

The smooth muscle cells of the circular muscle layer of the canine colon exhibit periodic waves of depolarization (slow waves) which serve a pacemaker function similar to that of their counterparts in the small intestine (1). Slow waves bring the membrane potential periodically close to or above threshold for spiking activity. Slow waves with spiking activity on their peak depolarizations are associated with phasic contractions (1,2). In addition to these rhythmic contractions, the circular muscle is capable of generating prolonged forceful contractions for periods which would normally span several slow wave cycles (3,4). These contractions are most noticeable under stimulated conditions, i.e. with neostigmine, and appear to perform a propulsive function. Such contractions cannot easily be explained in the framework of the control function of the slow waves (3). Therefore the possibility was examined that endogenous excitatory substances of either neural or hormonal origin could alter the regular pacemaker activity to allow such prolonged contractions to occur. The present paper deals with the effects of two excitatory substances, the acetylcholine analog carbachol and substance P, on the electrical and mechanical activities of circular muscle of the dog colon.

METHODS

A segment of proximal colon was removed from anesthetized dogs. Transverse strips (about 1x25 mm) were cut and the mucosa, submucosa and longitudinal muscle layer were removed by sharp dissection. The sucrose gap method was used at 37° C as described previously (5). The duration of the slow wave and the relative amount of time the membrane potential was in the depolarized (plateau) state were measured at half maximal amplitude. Data are expressed as mean $\pm$ SEM.

RESULTS

The spontaneous electrical activity of circular muscle consisted of regular slow wave activity with a mean frequency of 4.7 ± 0.4 cycles/min (cpm), an amplitude of 14.9 ± 1.4 mV and a duration ranging from 2.0 - 4.0 sec (n=17, figs. 1-4). In some preparations spikes occurred, superimposed on the slow waves, with an estimated amplitude of 17.4 ± 3.2 mV. Only the slow waves with spikes generated phasic contractions, each lasting about 4 sec.

Carbachol (n=11) and substance P (n=8) depolarized the smooth muscle cells, prolonged the slow wave plateau, occasionally decreased the slow wave frequency and enhanced spiking activity. These electrophysiological effects were associated with enhancement of the motor activity and alteration of the contraction pattern.

Effect on "resting" membrane potential

Carbachol and substance P depolarized the muscle in a dose dependent manner. The depolarization amounted to 7.5 ± 2.1 and 12.6 ± 7.7 mV in carbachol ($5x10^{-9}$M and 10^{-7}M), and 2.9 ± 1.8 and 8.7 ± 2.8 mV in substance P (10^{-10}M and $3x10^{-8}$M). It should be mentioned however, that membrane potential changes in response to excitatory substances may be influenced by potential drifts due to muscle contraction.

Effect on slow wave activity

Carbachol and substance P increased the duration of the slow wave plateaus in a highly characteristic manner. A regular pattern of electrical activity emerged in the presence of low doses of carbachol (10^{-8}M) and substance P (10^{-10}M) such that one prolonged slow wave, with a duration of 28 to 42 sec, alternated with a rather constant number (3 to 8) of slow waves of "normal" duration (figs. 1,2,3). Slow waves were marked as "normal" when their duration was < 5 sec and

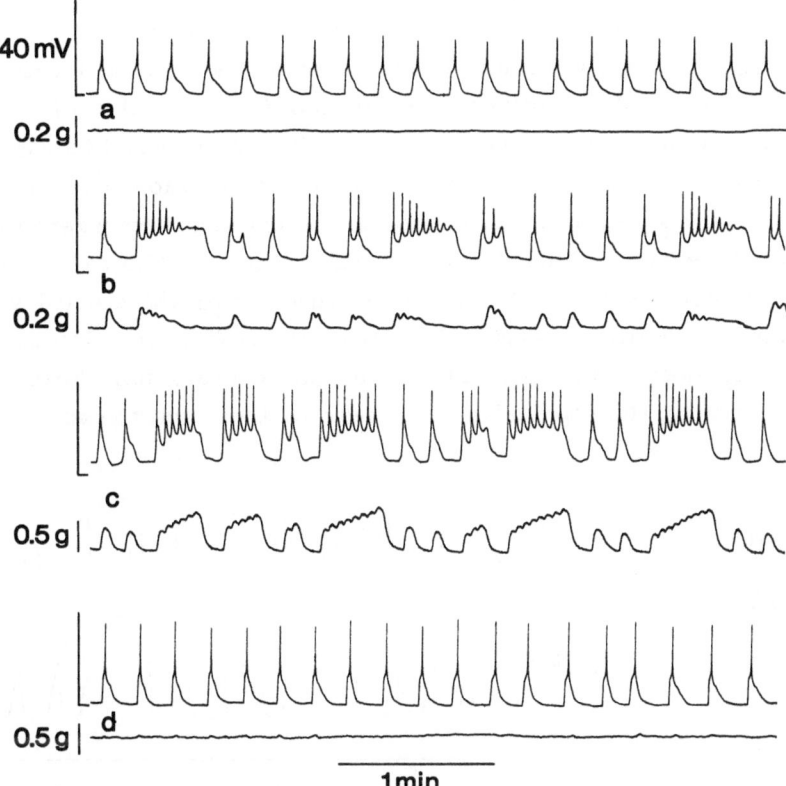

FIGURE 1   Effect of carbachol on pacemaker, spiking and contractile
activity. In each panel, upper and bottom tracings represent
the electrical and mechanical activities respectively. a and
d: Spontaneous activity in normal Krebs solution before
addition and after washout of carbachol respectively. b and
c: Activity in the presence of carbachol (2×10^{-8}M and 10^{-7}M
respectively). Note the regularity in the pattern of
electrical activity. The frequency of the contractions is
related to the slow wave frequency and the duration and
amplitude of each contraction is related to the spiking
activity superimposed on the slow wave plateau. Note the
depolarization as the deviation from the horizontal line in
the calibration bar.

"prolonged" when their duration exceeded 5 sec, since the slow wave

duration in normal Krebs solution at 37° C did not exceed 5 sec.

With increasing concentrations, the prevalence of prolonged slow waves

increased while their maximum duration often decreased. Prolongation

of the slow wave duration always led to an increase in the amount of time the membrane potential was in the depolarized state (plateau phase) and usually but not neccesarily led to a decrease in the slow wave frequency. The membrane potential was at the plateau level 58 ± 6 % of the time in the presence of carbachol (10^{-7}M) and 88 ± 5 % of the time in the presence of substance P (10^{-8}M), as opposed to 24 ± 4 % of the time in normal Krebs solution. The prolonged slow waves recorded in the presence of both carbachol and substance P consisted of an initial potential followed by a plateau potential. The amplitudes of both potentials did not deviate significantly from the control values. However, the membrane potential level at the peak of the slow wave did increase, most noticeably at higher concentrations. This was a consequence of the depolarization caused by these substances.

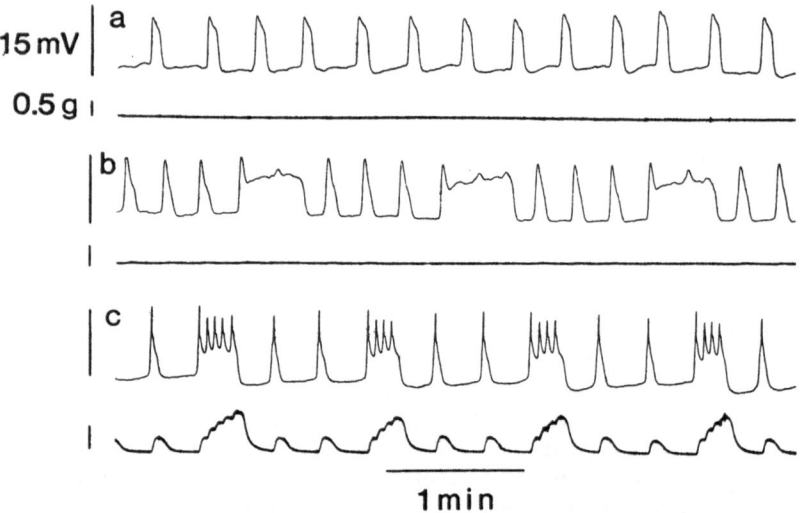

15 mV

0.5 g

a

b

c

1 min

FIGURE 2   Spiking rather than prolongation of the slow wave plateau is associated with the contractile response to carbachol. a: Normal Krebs solution: regular slow wave activity. This particular experiment was performed at 34° C, hence the decreased spontaneous slow wave frequency. b: Carbachol (10^{-7}M) dramatically prolonged the plateau of some slow waves. Neither the normal nor the prolonged slow waves were associated with contractile activity. c: A higher concentration (2×10^{-7}M) induced spiking activity on the slow wave plateau. Each slow wave had superimposed spikes and was associated with a contraction.

In the presence of substance P, the frequency of the normal slow waves was occasionally increased (to 8.2±0.5 cpm; n=3) in addition to the appearance of prolonged slow waves (fig. 4).

Effect on spiking activity

Following the application of carbachol ($>10^{-8}$M) or substance P (10^{-9}M) spiking activity was introduced when absent or increased when present. A prepotential-like oscillation always preceeded each spike potential. In most experiments, the first prepotential-spike complex to appear on top of a slow wave had the highest amplitude and the amplitudes of subsequent ones declined progressively. The prepotential (spike) frequency of the slow waves was 26.0±3.1 cpm for carbachol (n=9), and 18.0±2.2 cpm for substance P (n=8). The occurrence of prepotentials and spikes was limited to the plateau phase of the slow waves, i.e. no spikes were observed to occur during the inter-slow wave periods.

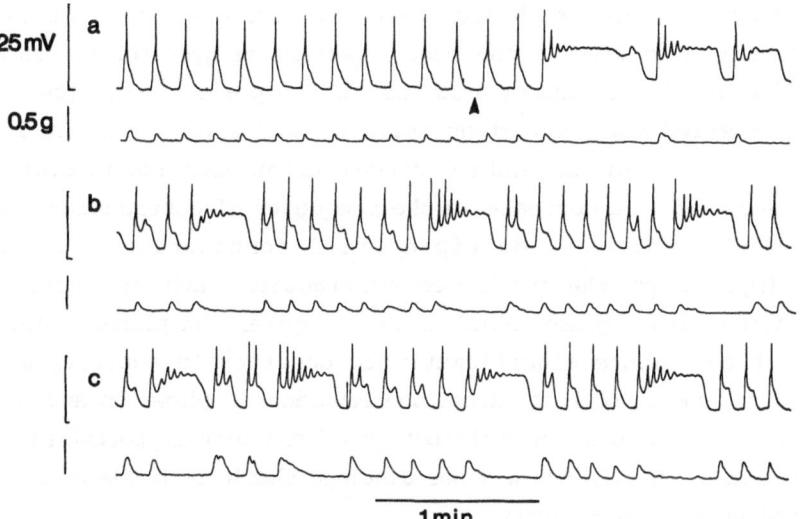

FIGURE 3   Effect of substance P on pacemaker, spiking and contractile activity. a: Spontaneous activity, substance P (10^{-9}M) was added at arrow. Note that the first prolonged slow wave has the longest duration. b: A regular pattern of electrical activity follows in which prolonged slow waves alternate with slow waves of about normal duration. c: Activity in the presence of substance P (2×10^{-9}M).

Effect on contractile activity

Phasic contractions occurred in tissues in which the slow waves had superimposed spiking activity with each slow wave–spike complex being associated with a contraction. The enhancement of spiking activity by carbachol and substance P was clearly related to enhancement of contractile activity when present or its initiation when absent. In some experiments, the appearance of prepotential-like oscillations was associated with enhancement of contractile activity without the appearance of spikes. In such cases, it was difficult to determine if the oscillations superimposed on the slow wave plateau were prepotentials or "aborted" spikes. The duration of the individual contractions was dependent on the duration of spiking or prepotential activity, the maximum duration of spiking activity being equal to the duration of the slow wave. A regular slow wave with one spike and a prolonged slow wave with a single spike at the onset of the depolarizing phase (fig. 3) induced similar contractions indicating that among the electrophysiological effects described above, the initiation of spiking is the most important trigger for contraction. In addition, the prolongation of the plateau phase of the slow waves, if accompanied with persistant spike or oscillatory activity led to prolonged contractions and the concomittant decrease in slow wave frequency led to a decrease in the frequency of contractions (figs. 1,2,3). On occasions, multiple brief contractions were seen superimposed on the prolonged contraction each of which was associated with a prepotential and/or a spike. The plateau potential did not contribute significantly to contractile activity at low concentrations of both carbachol and substance P (figs. 2b and 3a). At higher concentrations, a contribution of the plateau potential might be present (fig. 1c), but was not distinguishable from the contraction induced by spiking activity.

The actions of both carbachol and substance P were similar in the absence and presence of tetrodotoxin (2×10^{-7}M). Atropine (2×10^{-6}M) abolished the action of carbachol without altering the effect of substance P.

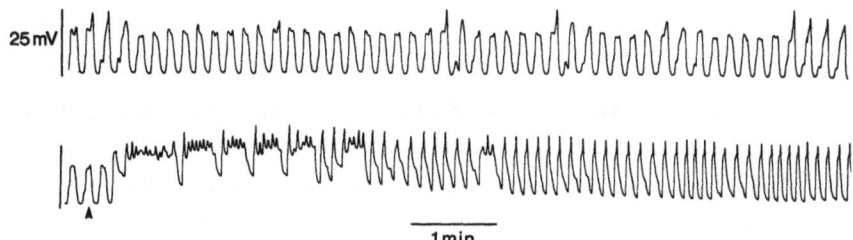

25 mV

1 min

Figure 4   Effect of substance P (10^{-8}M), added at arrow, on the electrical activity. A period of prolonged slow waves was superimposed on a depolarization and was followed by a period of slow waves at an increased frequency. This experiment was performed in the presence of TTX ($2x10^{-7}$M), but similar effects occurred in its absence.

DISCUSSION

In the small intestine, it is generally accepted that excitatory agents of physiological importance act by enhancing the ability of the pacemaker potentials (slow waves) to generate spiking activity without appreciably altering their frequency or duration. Thus their effect on motor activity is to increase the force of contractions without altering their frequency or duration (6). The present study indicates that although the slow waves of the canine colonic circular muscle serve a pacemaker function similar to that of the small intestine (1,2,6), they are highly responsive to carbachol and substance P. These two excitatory substances depolarized the membrane and enhanced the prepotential and spiking activity on the peak depolarizations of the slow waves but also dramatically prolonged the slow wave plateau and often decreased the slow wave frequency. The enhancement of spiking and prepotential activity rather than the prolongation of the slow wave plateau appeared to be directly responsible for the enhancement of contractile activity. However the prolongation of the slow wave plateau when associated with a prolonged spike burst superimposed on it led to a prolonged contraction. In addition, the plateau potential may directly contribute to motor activity particularly at higher concentration of the excitatory substances. Often, brief contractions, each being associated with a spike or prepotential, were superimposed on the prolonged contractions. Such a contraction pattern could not be predicted from the slow wave activity in non-excited tissue (1,2,3).

The findings of this study provide the electrophysiological mechanisms by which prolonged contractions and prolonged spike bursts can occur in the circular muscle of the colon. Prolonged contractions were routinely observed by us in acute in vivo studies and were also recorded in ex vivo (3) experiments from the canine colon. The results of the present study further suggest that the fast electrical oscillations and long spike bursts recorded from the colon in vivo (2,4) may arise not only from the longitudinal (1,2,5) but also from the circular layer. Finally the dramatic effects of the excitatory agonists on the slow wave activity reported in this study suggest that in addition to altering the ability of the slow waves to generate spike discharges, drugs, neurotransmitters and hormones may act to alter the slow wave activity resulting in a significant alteration of the contraction pattern.

REFERENCES

1. El-Sharkawy, T.Y. (1983). Electrical activities of the muscle layers of the canine colon. J. Physiol., in press.

2. El-Sharkawy, T.Y., Bardakjian, B.L., MacDonald, W.M. and Diamant, N.E. (1982). Origins of the multiple patterns of electrical control activity in the colon. In: Motility of the Digestive Tract, ed. M. Wienbeck, pp. 491-497, Raven Press, New York.

3. Kocylowski, M., Bowes, K.L. and Kingma, Y.J. (1979). Electrical and mechanical activity in the ex vivo perfused total canine colon. Gastroenterology 77: 1021-1026.

4. Fioramonti, J., Garcia-villar, G., Bueno, L. and Ruckebusch, Y. (1980). Colonic myoelectrical activity and propulsion in the dog. Dig. Dis. Sci. 25: 641-646.

5. Huizinga, J.D., Diamant, N.E. and El-Sharkawy, T.Y. (1983). Electrical basis of contractions in the muscle layers of the pig colon. Am. J. Physiol. 245, in press.

6. Daniel, E.E. (1973). A conceptual analysis of the pharmacology of gastrointestinal motility. In: International Encyclopedia of Pharmacology and Therapeutics, Sec. 39a, Pharmacology of Gastrointestinal Motility and Secretion. Ed. P. Holton, pp. 457-545, Pergamon Press, Oxford.

65

Longitudinal and Circular Muscle of the Canine Colon have Different and Characteristic Electrical and Mechanical Activities

L. DEBSKI, K. L. BOWES, Y. J. KINGMA and R. GILL

INTRODUCTION

Although electrical and mechanical activities of the colon have been extensively studied in recent years, the relationships between them as well as their characteristics still remain to be adequately defined (1-9). This study was undertaken to determine the patterns of electrical and mechanical activities occurring in longitudinal and circular muscle layers of the canine colon. Distinctive and different electrical and mechanical activity patterns were observed in the two muscle layers.

METHODS

Short segments of different parts of the colon were removed from dogs at laparotomy under general (sodium pentobarbitol) anesthesia. After the mucosa was removed, seven types of muscle sample (0.7 x 4 cm) were prepared by sharp and blunt dissection in oxygenated (95% O_2, 5% CO_2) Krebs' solution:

1. Intact muscle with longitudinal orientation
2. Intact muscle with circular orientation
3. Isolated longitudinal muscle
4. Isolated circular muscle
5. Isolated circular muscle with submucosa removed
6. Intact muscle with longitudinal orientation and submucosa removed
7. Intact muscle with circular orientation and submucosa removed

397

The specimens were mounted in a tissue chamber and bathed continuously with oxygenated Krebs solution. Electrical activities were monitored with two pressure electrodes placed on the appropriate surface (serosal for longitudinal muscle; submucosal for circular muscle). Mechanical activity was monitored by a strain gauge attached to the end of each strip.

RESULTS

A. Electrical Activity

Four different patterns of electrical activity were observed:

1. A low frequency continuous regular oscillation (LFO) (slow wave) with a range of 4-8 cpm and an average frequency of 5.57 $\pm$ 1.2 cpm (mean $\pm$ SD). The frequency was not different in different parts of the colon. This was observed in isolated circular (Fig.1) and both circularly and longitudinally orientated intact muscles (Fig.2,3,7). LFO amplitudes recorded on the submucosal side of intact muscle preparations appeared to be bigger by 30-50% than those seen on the serosal side of strips. LFO was not seen in isolated longitudinal muscle (Fig.4,4a) or after removal of submucosa from isolated circular muscle and intact muscles (Fig.5,6).

2. A high frequency usually continuous oscillation with a range of 15-30 cpm and a mean frequency of 19.03 $\pm$ 2.5 cpm (HFO). This was seen in isolated longitudinal muscle (Fig.4,4a) and less commonly in intact longitudinally orientated muscles.

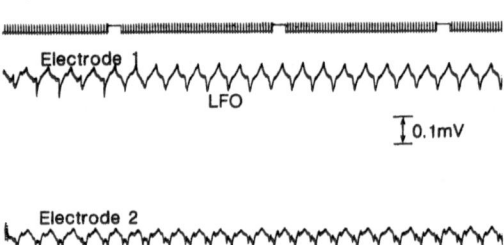

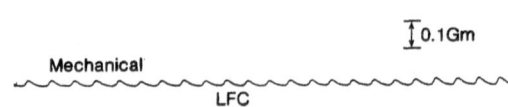

FIGURE 1   ISOLATED CIRCULAR MUSCLE (with Submucosa)

3. Spike or spindle bursts (SB). A high frequency oscillation that resembled either classical continuous spiking or bursts of increased amplitude of HFQ. These were seen in intact muscle specimens with submucosa attached (Fig.3) or removed (Fig.5) as well as in isolated longitudinal muscle (Fig.4,4a). They were not seen in isolated circular muscle (Fig.1).

4. Single spikes (SS). These were seen in isolated longitudinal and intact muscle specimens with submucosa attached or removed. They were not seen in isolated circular muscle (Fig.1).

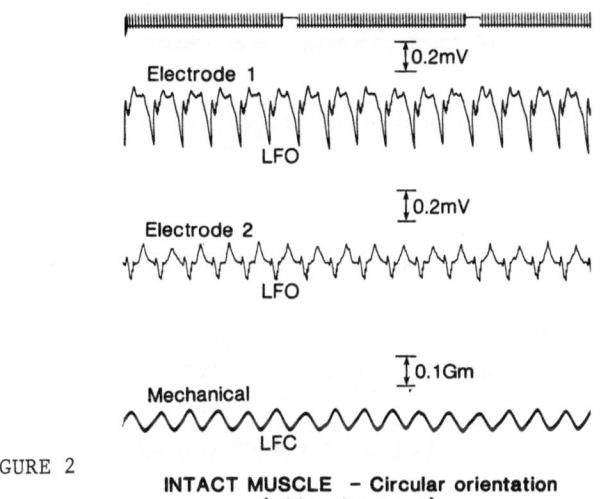

FIGURE 2

INTACT MUSCLE – Circular orientation
(with submucosa)

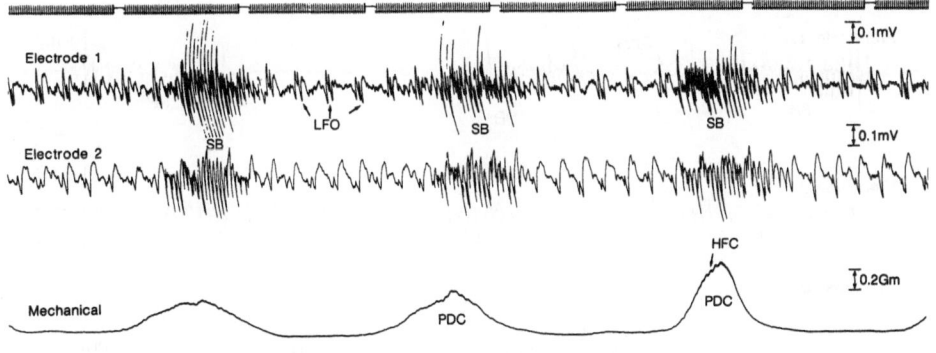

FIGURE 3   **INTACT MUSCLE – Longitudinal orientation (with submucosa)**

B. Mechanical Activity

Four patterns of mechanical activity were observed:

1. A repetitive low frequency low amplitude contraction (LFC) with
a range of 4-8 cpm and a mean frequency of 5.76 ± 1.3.
LFC coincided with LFO electrical activity and there was no significant
difference in frequency between them. It was seen in isolated circular
muscle (Fig.1) and circularly orientated intact muscles (Fig.2,7).
It was not seen in isolated longitudinal muscle (Fig.4,4a) and after
removal of submucosa from isolated circular and intact muscles (Fig.6).

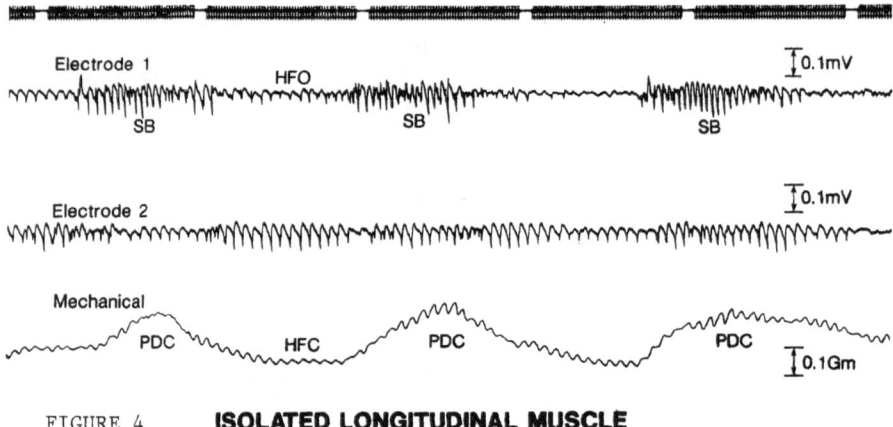

FIGURE 4   **ISOLATED LONGITUDINAL MUSCLE**

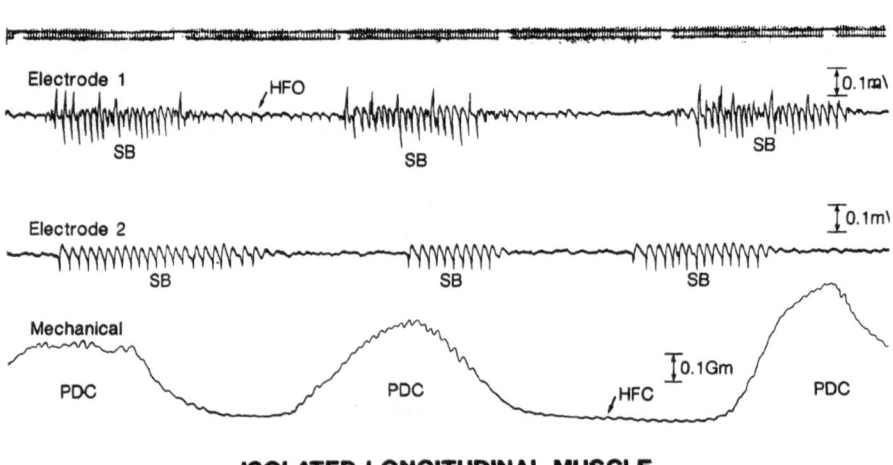

FIGURE 4a   **ISOLATED LONGITUDINAL MUSCLE**

2. A repetitive high frequency low amplitude contraction (HFC) with a range of 15-30 cpm and a mean frequency of 18.5 $\pm$ 2.67. This usually coexisted with HFO electrical activity and there was no significant difference in frequency between them. It was seen in isolated longitudinal muscle (Fig.4,4a) and less commonly in intact longitudinal muscles. It was not seen in circular muscle preparations (Fig.1,2,7).

Electrode 1
0.1mV
SB
SB
Mechanical
0.4Gm
PDC
PDC

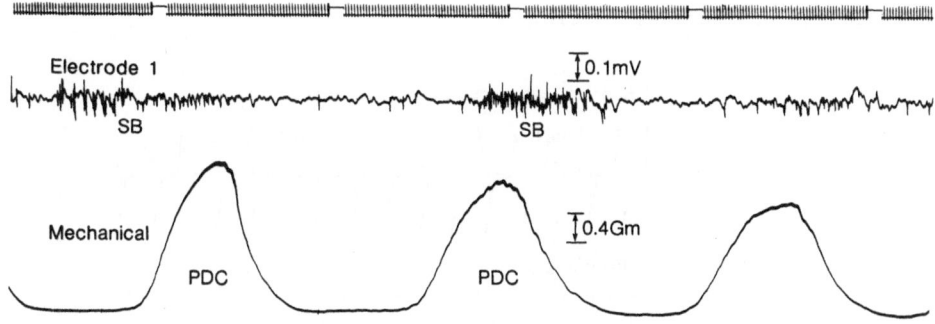

INTACT WALL - Longitudinal orientation - Submucosa removed

FIGURE 5

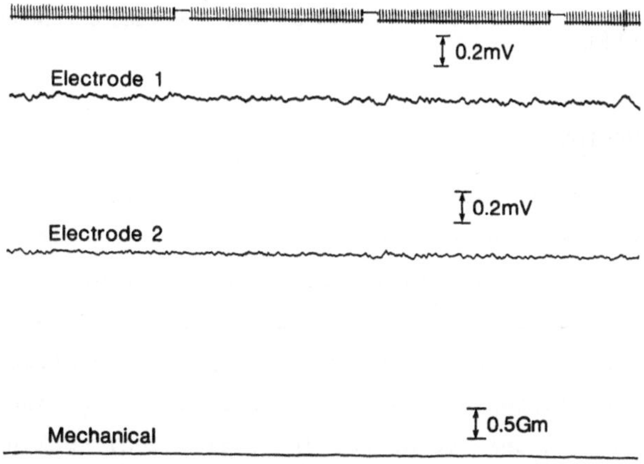

0.2mV
Electrode 1
0.2mV
Electrode 2
Mechanical
0.5Gm

FIGURE 6 **INTACT WALL - Circular orientation (submucosa removed)**

3.   A large amplitude prolonged duration contraction (PDC).   This
was seen in isolated longitudinal muscle (Fig.4,4a), intact longitudinal muscle (Fig.4,4a), intact longitudinally orientated with submucosa attached (Fig.3) or removed (Fig.5) and rarely in intact
circularly orientated muscles.   It was not seen in isolated circular
muscle (Fig.1).   It appeared in association with SB.

4.   An increase in muscle tone.   This was seen in intact circularly
orientated muscles with submucosa attached (Fig.7) and less commonly
in isolated longitudinal muscle.

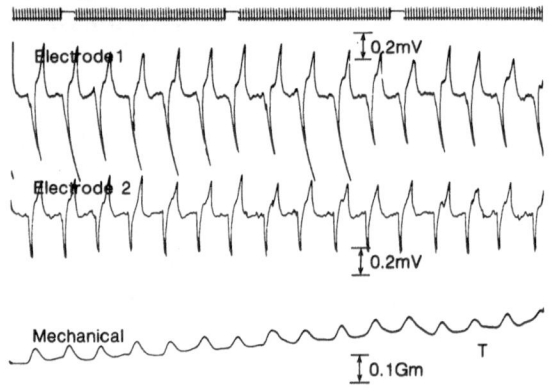

INTACT WALL – Circular orientation (with submucosa)

FIGURE 7

DISCUSSION

In this study distinctive and different electrical and mechanical
activities have been observed in the two muscle layers of the canine
colon.   In longitudinal muscle a high frequency electrical oscillation
is observed in association with a low amplitude mechanical ripple at
the same frequency.   When large amplitude contractions are present, the
HFO oscillation alters to either a pattern of increased amplitude
(often in a spindle shape) or to classical spiking.

In circular muscle the predominant electrical activity is a low
frequency oscillation that is usually termed "slow wave".   This
activity is associated with a mechanical ripple at the same frequency.
As previously described, this electrical activity can be abolished by
removal of tissue at the circular muscle submucosal interphase (5).

Classical spikes were not observed in isolated circular muscle. They were observed in tissues that did not exhibit slow waves. They were not observed in association with either the high or low frequency mechanical ripple. Spikes are therefore not dependant upon the presence of slow waves and are not necessary for the low amplitude contractions of both muscle layers. Whether spikes are generated in longitudinal muscle or in the myenteric plexus has not been defined by this study. The latter could have been damaged or removed in preparing the isolated circular muscle preparations.

REFERENCES

1. Bowes, K. L., Shearin, N. L., Kingma, Y. J., Koles, Z. F. (1978). Frequency analysis of electrical activity in dog colon. In: Duthie, H. L. (ed). Gastrointestinal Motility in Health and Disease. London: MTP. pp. 251-8.

2. Caprilli, R., Vernia, P., Frieri, G., Melchiorri, P. (1975). Two electric rhythms in the colon. Rendic. Gastroenterol. 7, 65-6.

3. Chambers, M. M., Bowes, K. L., Kingma, Y. J., Bannister, C., Cote, K. R: (1981). In vitro electrical activity in human colon. Gastroenterology. 81, 502-8.

4. Christensen, J., Caprilli, R., Lund, G. F. (1969) Electric slow waves in circular muscle of cat colon. Am. J. Physiol. 217, 771-6.

5. Durdle, N. G., Kingma, Y. J., Bowes, K. L., Chambers, M. M. (1983) Origin of slow waves in the canine colon. Gastroenterology. 56, 317-22.

6. El-Sharkawy, T. Y., Bardakjian, B. L., MacDonald, W. M., Diamant, N. E. (1982). Origins of the multiple patterns of electrical control activity in the colon. In: Wienbeck, M. (ed). Motility of the Digestive Tract. 491. (New York: Raven Press)

7. Sarna, S. K., Bardakjian, B. L., Waterfall, W. E., Lind, J. F. (1980). Human colonic electrical control activity (ECA). Gastroenterology. 78, 1526-36.

8. Shearin, N. L., Bowes, K. L., Kingma, Y. J. (1978). In Vitro electrical activity in canine colon. Gut. 20, 780-6.

9. Van Merwyk, A. J., Duthie, H. L. (1980). Characteristics of human colonic smooth muscle in vitro. In: Christensen, J, (ed). Gastrointestinal Motility. 473-8. (New York: Raven Press)

66

The Relationship between Extracellular and Intracellular Slow Waves

N. G. DURDLE, Y. J. KINGMA and K. L. BOWES

INTRODUCTION

Intracellular microelectrode measurements from smooth muscle cells are
very difficult to obtain and simultaneous multicell intracellular
measurements have never been reported. For these reasons, the majority
of in vitro slow wave studies have used extracellular pressure
electrodes of the type described by Bortoff (1). An understanding of
the relationship between extracellular pressure electrode slow wave
signals and their related intracellular potential variations is
necessary to obtain maximum information from extracellular studies.

   In 1946 Graham and Gerrard (2) demonstrated that the impalement of
muscle cells by large microelectrodes resulted in the measurement of an
intracellular potential that was far less than the expected membrane
potential. It was thought that an injury to the cell caused a drop in
the intracellular potential and thus the measured potential was
referred to as an "injury potential". Gillespie (3) demonstrated that
an injury potential resulted from the deformation of smooth muscle
cells of the rabbit colon. Bortoff (1) proposed that an injury
potential was responsible for the extracellular signal obtained from
pressure electrodes. He stated that deformation of cells by the
pressure electrode resulted in a reduction in membrane impedance of
cells under the electrode. This in turn would result in a proportional
reduction in both the cells' resting potentials and the amplitudes of
any time varying components such as slow waves or spikes.

405

The objectives of this work were:

1. To determine if the pressure electrode theory as described by
   Bortoff is the mechanism responsible for the generation of the
   slow wave signals recorded extracellularly from the canine colon.
2. To determine the relationship between the extracellular slow wave
   signal and the intracellular variations in cells surrounding the
   pressure electrode.

METHODS

Specimens of proximal colon were obtained at operation under general
anaesthesia from healthy mongrel dogs. The mucosa was removed using
sharp dissection. Circularly oriented strips (0.2cm by 2.5cm) were
mounted horizontally with the mucosal side up, in a constant
temperature tissue chamber and superfused with oxygenated Krebs-
Ringer solution.

Two groups of experiment were conducted:

Group I. In three experiments simultaneous recordings were obtained
to compare extracellular and intracellular potentials. A 2mm glass
encapsulated silver-silverchloride pressure electrode (Kingma, et al.
(4)) (Figure 1) was applied to the muscle strip with a force of 6gm.
Intracellular microelectrode measurements were then obtained from cells
in the region around the extracellular electrode. The microelectrodes
were pulled from 1.2mm borosilicate glass tubing and had tip diameters
in the range from 0.1 to 0.5 microns. The extracellular and intracellular electrode holders caused the two measurement sites to be
separated by 5mm.

Group II: Eight experiments were conducted to determine if an
injury potential was associated with pressure electrode recordings.
The pressure electrode was replaced by the apparatus shown in Figure
2. This apparatus, designed to simulate the pressure electrode, was
constructed from the 2mm diameter glass used to construct the extracellular electrodes. This simulated pressure electrode was first
applied to the mucosal side of the tissue with a known force of 0.5 to
5 grams. Then the microelectrode was positioned in the center of the
cylinder (Figure 2) and gradually advanced until cell penetration was
obtained.

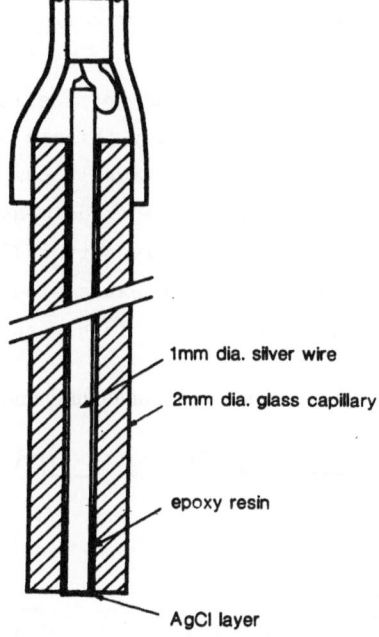

1mm dia. silver wire

2mm dia. glass capillary

epoxy resin

AgCl layer

Figure 1. Pressure Electrode Details

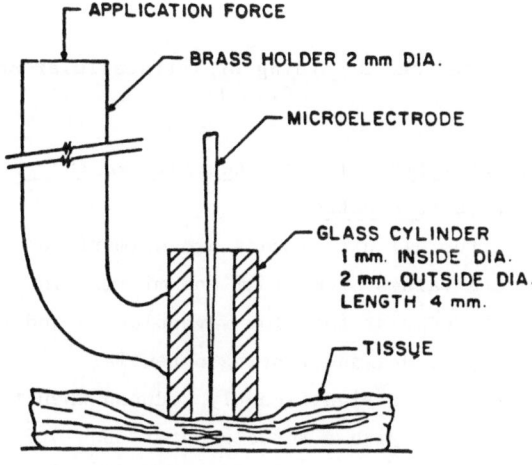

APPLICATION FORCE

BRASS HOLDER 2 mm DIA.

MICROELECTRODE

GLASS CYLINDER
1 mm. INSIDE DIA.
2 mm. OUTSIDE DIA.
LENGTH 4 mm.

TISSUE

Figure 2. Apparatus Simulating The Application Of The Pressure
Electrode To An Intact Muscle Specimen.

RESULTS

A. Simultaneous measurement of extracellular and intracellular
   potentials:

Simultaneous extracellular and intracellular waveforms were similar
in shape and of the same frequency (Figure 3). The size of the tissue
specimen was minimized to reduce muscle contractions and thus
facilitate obtaining the microelectrode measurement. This resulted in
the tissue specimen not completely surrounding the pressure electrode
and as a consequence of this the extracellular waveform shape was not
as regular and noise free as from larger specimens.

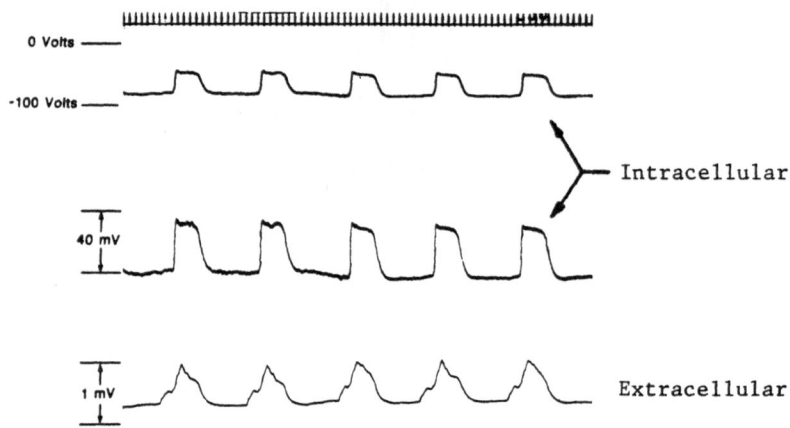

Figure 3. Simultaneous Recording Of Intracellular And Extracellular
Signals.

B. Measurement of intracellular potentials in the region under the
   simulated pressure electrode:

The results from all experiments are summarized in Table 1. V_{max}
and V_{min} indicate values of maximum and minimum intracellular
potentials which occur at the slow wave plateau and trough respectively.
The slow wave amplitudes and resting potentials of cells under the
pressure electrode were significantly reduced when the extracellular
electrode was applied with a force greater than 0.5 grams (Figure 4).

A summary of the data resulting from the application of the
simulated pressure electrode is as follows:

(a)   The mean slow wave amplitude was reduced from 28.9 ± 4.0mV to

Table 1. Summary of results arranged in order
of increasing electrode force.

FORCE (GM)	NO. OF PENETRATIONS	V_{max} (mV)	V_{min} (mV)	S.W. AMPLITUDE (mV)
0.0	83	−47.9±7.9	−76.4±6.8	28.9±4.0
0.5	12	−44.8±5.2	−63.6±13.1	19.6±8.4
1.0	20	−45.7±3.8	−58.6±3.9	12.7±2.5
2.0	10	−46.2±2.8	−59.9±4.6	15.6±1.6
3.0	5	−46.1±3.2	−58.01±1.3	13.5±.9
4.0	7	−47.8±2.6	−60.4±5.6	12.0±2.6
5.0	4	−43.8±2.5	−53.8±2.5	10.0±0.0

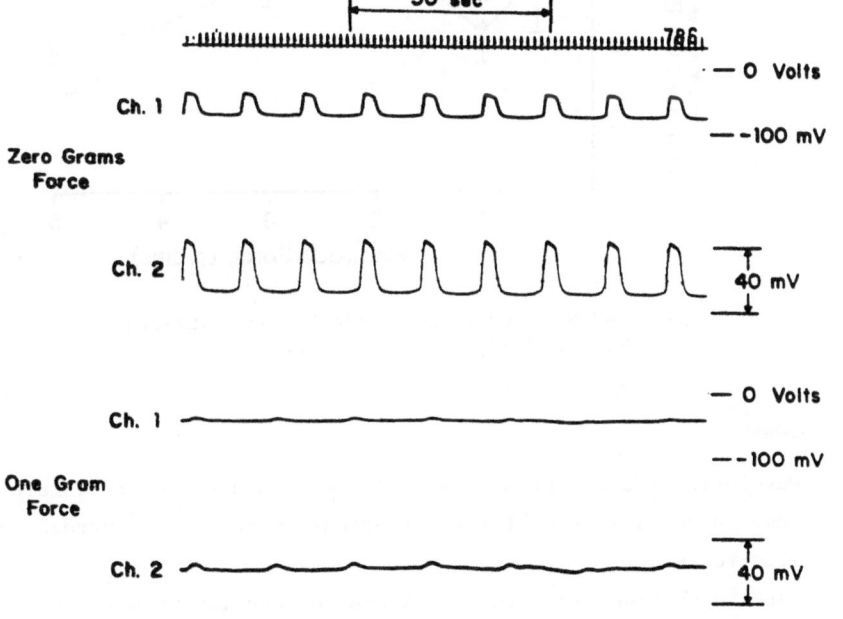

Figure 4. Intracellular Potentials In The Presence Of An
Extracellular Pressure Electrode.
Channel 1 is calibrated for DC potentials and
Channel 2 has the DC component removed.

14.43 ± 4.3mV.

(b)   The mean cellular resting potential increased from −76.4 ± 6.8mV to −59.7 ± 7.0mV.

(c)   The mean value of the slow wave plateau increased a very small amount from −47.9 ± 7.9mV to −43.8 ± 3.8mV. This increase was not in proportion to changes in slow wave amplitude and resting potential.

The relationship between the reduction in slow wave amplitude and the magnitude of the electrode application force was nonlinear as shown in Figure 5. For application forces greater than 1 gram the slow wave amplitude is reduced to less than 60 percent of its basal value.

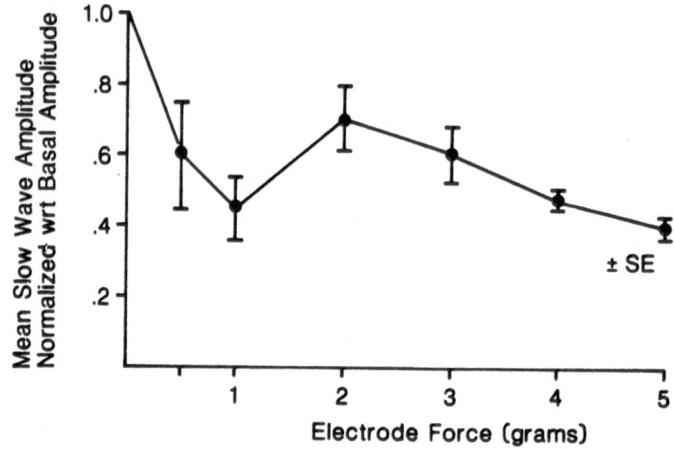

Figure 5. Normalized Slow Wave Amplitude Versus Extracellular
Electrode Application Force.

CONCLUSIONS

1. The waveforms recorded from extracellular pressure electrodes are of the same shape as intracellular variations in the cells surrounding the electrodes.

2. The results obtained from this work are not consistent with the pressure electrode theory as proposed by Bortoff. This theory predicts a proportional reduction in the slow wave plateau and the cellular resting potential. This was not observed in the results.

The electrical models proposed by both Gillespie (2) and Bortoff (1) represent the cell membrane with a single membrane resistance which is reduced to zero by cell distortion. The results from this work are consistent with the concept that the membrane must be represented by two components of resistance. These two components are a constant resistance primarily responsible for the resting potential and a variable component which causes the membrane potential variations called slow waves.

REFERENCES

1. Bortoff, A. (1967). Configuration of intestinal slow waves obtained by monopolar recording techniques. Am. J. Physiol., 213(1): 157-162.
2. Graham, J. and Gerrard, R.W. (1946). Membrane potentials and excitation of impaired single muscle fibres. J. Coll. and Comp. Physiol., 28:99 - 116.
3. Gillespie, J.S. (1962). Spontaneous mechanical and electrical activity of stretched and unstretched intestinal smooth muscle cells and their response to sympathetic nerve stimulation. J. Physiol., 162:54 - 92.
4. Kingma, Y.J., Durdle, N.G., Lenhard, J., Bowes, K.L., and Chambers, M.M. (1983). Improved Ag/AgCl pressure electrodes Med. and Biol. Eng. and Comput., 21:351 - 357.

67

The Electrical Basis for the Inhibitory Response of the Guinea Pig Internal Anal Sphincter to Nerve Stimulation and Drugs

S. P. LIM and T. C. MUIR

INTRODUCTION

The guinea pig internal anal sphincter (gpIAS) is innervated by three
types of efferent nerves, cholinergic excitatory, adrenergic excitatory and non-adrenergic, non-cholinergic (NANC) inhibitory nerves, the
transmitter for which is unknown (1).

The effects of stimulation of NANC nerves differs in different
tissues and species both quantitatively, in the extent of the hyperpolarization which accompanies the mechanical relaxation and in the
response to drugs (2). For example, the hyperpolarization underlying
the mechanical inhibition produced by NANC nerve stimulation in the
rat anococcygeus (AC) (3) and bovine retractor penis (BRP) (4) muscles
is significantly smaller than that found in either the rabbit anococcygeus (5) or the guinea pig taenia coli (TC) (6). Pharmacologically,
the bee venom, apamin, which blocks relaxations of the TC to NANC
nerve stimulation (7) is ineffective in the AC and BRP to stimulation
of these nerves (8). Conversely, oxyhaemoglobin blocks relaxations in
both the BRP and AC muscles to stimulation of their NANC nerves but is
ineffective in the TC (8).

These observations invited the question as to whether the responses
to NANC nerves in the gpIAS resembled those in the TC or those in the
AC and BRP. Accordingly, in the present investigation, the electrical
and mechanical responses of the gpIAS to NANC nerve stimulation, to
apamin and oxyhaemoglobin have been determined. The electrical and

413

mechanical responses to a number of adenine nucleotides and peptides - transmitter candidates in other NANC nerve containing tissues - have also been compared with those to NANC nerve stimulation.

METHODS

Adult guinea pigs (200-300 g) were killed by stunning then bled. The IAS was dissected out (1), set up in an organ bath and perfused (6 ml/min) with oxygenated (95% O_2/5% CO_2) Krebs solution at 36 $\pm$ 0.5°C pH 7.4. One end of the sphincter was attached to a stainless steel hook and the other, passed through Ag/AgCl ring electrodes to permit field stimulation, was connected to an isometric transducer to record tension. Intracellular electrical recordings were made with glass microelectrodes (resistances 15-40 megaohms) filled with 3 M KCl. The effect of displacement of membrane potential on the responses to field stimulation was investigated by the method of Abe & Tomita, 1968 (9).

RESULTS

The gpIAS showed a spontaneous discharge of action potentials some 30-40 mV in amplitude often superimposed on a membrane depolarization and accompanied by oscillations in mechanical activity. The resting membrane potential was -44 $\pm$ 3 mV, S.D., n = 214.

In the absence of drugs, field stimulation (single pulse or trains at 5-20 Hz) inhibited spontaneous activity, hyperpolarized the membrane producing inhibitory junction potentials (ijps) and relaxed the muscle. Excitatory responses to field stimulation were rarely seen; on the other hand noradrenaline invariably depolarized the membrane, increased the rate of spike discharge and contracted the muscle. These effects were abolished by phentolamine (5 x 10^{-6}M) indicating the presence of α adrenoceptors. To eliminate effects of stimulating either cholinergic or adrenergic nerves, phentolamine (5 x 10^{-6}M) and atropine (10^{-6}M) were used routinely. In their presence, the ijps - up to 40 mV - and mechanical responses to field stimulation were unaffected but were abolished by tetrodotoxin (5 x 10^{-6}M) confirming their mediation by NANC nerves (1). They resembled in amplitude ijps of the TC and contrasted with the very slight change in membrane potential which accompanied the inhibition of tone in the AC (Fig. 1). The ijps were enhanced by halving and reduced by doubling the external $[K_o^+]$. Measurement of the effects of membrane displacement on the

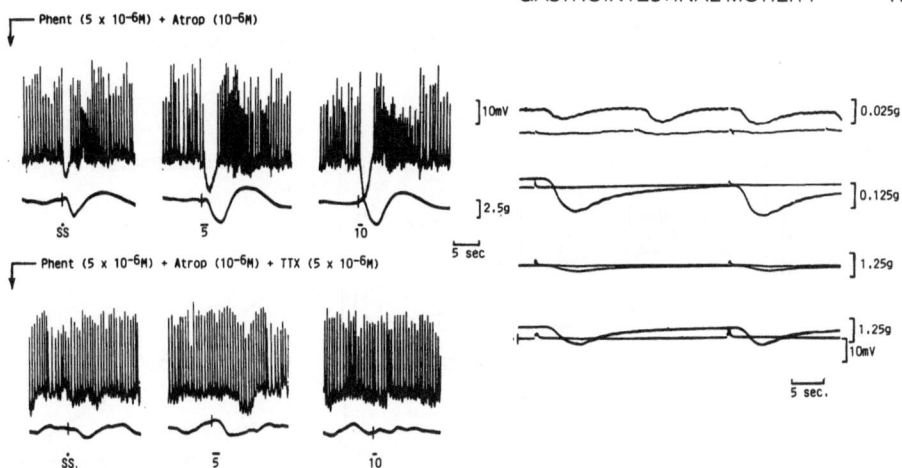

FIGURE 1   Stimulation of NANC nerves (single (SS), 5 pulses at 5 and
10 Hz) in the gpIAS (a) in the presence of phentolamine
(Phent 5 x 10^{-6}M) and atropine (ATR 10^{-6}M) inhibits
spontaneous activity, hyperpolarizes the membrane potential
and relaxes tone. These effects are abolished by tetrodotoxin (TTX 5 x 10^{-6}M). In the AC stimulation of NANC
nerves (8 Hz) in the presence of guanethidine (5 x 10^{-6}M)
relaxes tone without any significant membrane potential
change. From J.Physiol. (1975) 245, p. 40 with permission.

ijps revealed a linear relationship, with a reversal potential of -98 $\pm$
6 mV, S.D., n = 4. This confirms the role of K^+ in the ijp (Fig. 2).

Apamin (5 x 10^{-8} - 5 x 10^{-7}M), inhibited or abolished the response
of the gpIAS to field stimulation (Fig. 3). In contrast, oxyhaemoglobin (up to 8 x 10^{-6}M) was without effect but was effective in the
BRP (Byrne & Muir, unpublished).

Adenosine triphosphate, ATP (10^{-6} - 10^{-4}M) and adenosine (1.5 - 2.5
x 10^{-4}M) each abolished spike discharge, hyperpolarized the membrane
and relaxed the sphincter. ATP was the more effective and produced
membrane changes comparable in magnitude and duration with those
produced by stimulation of NANC nerves (Fig. 4). Like the responses to
inhibitory nerve stimulation, the effects of ATP were abolished by
apamin and unaffected by oxyhaemoglobin.

Vasoactive intestinal polypeptide, VIP (1.25 - 5 x 10^{-7}M) and
bradykinin (1.25 - 5 x 10^{-6}M) each abolished spike discharge, hyperpolarized the membrane and relaxed tone (Fig. 4). Substance P on the
other hand depolarized the membrane, increased spike frequency and
contracted the sphincter (Fig. 4). Bombesin (10^{-9} - 10^{-7}M) and

somatostatin $(10^{-9} - 10^{-7}M)$ were ineffective in this respect.

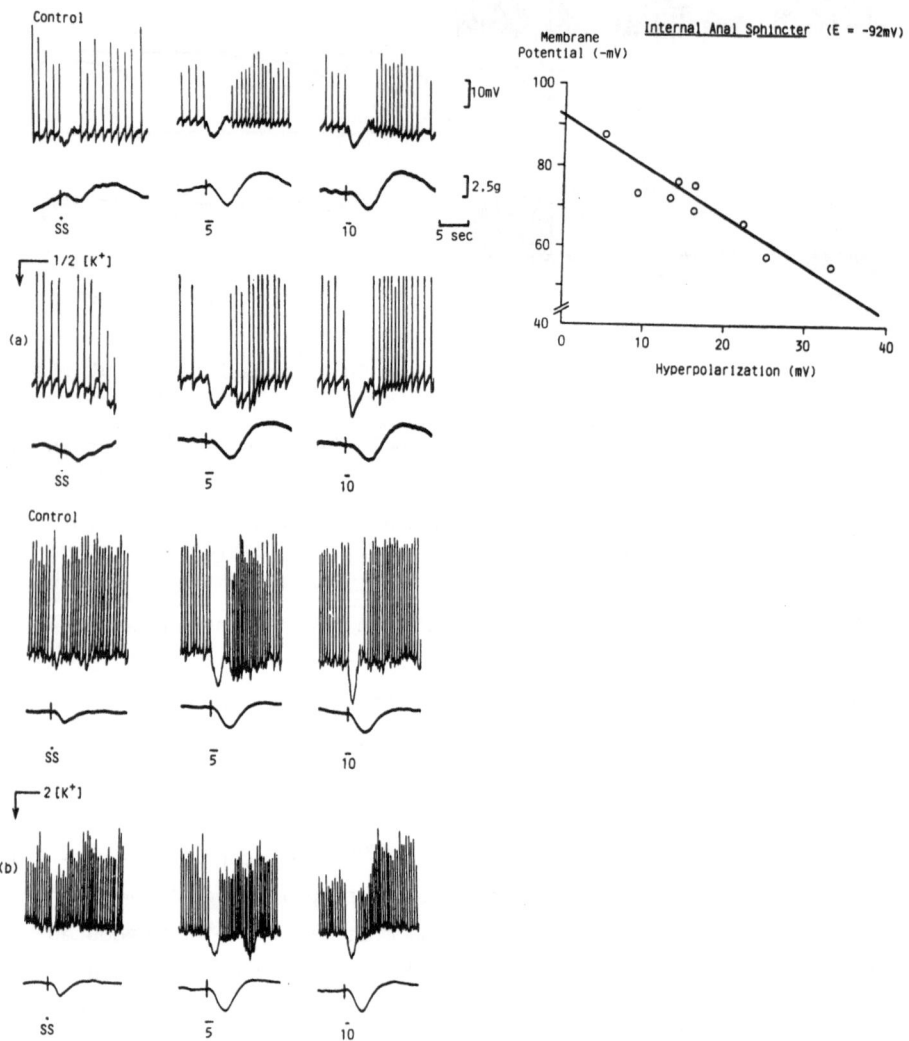

FIGURE 2 Halving (a) the $[K_o]$ increases, while doubling the $[K_o]$
decreases the response to stimulation of NANC nerves
(single SS 5 pulses at 5 and 10 Hz) in the gpIAS.
Reversal potential (-92 mV) suggests the response is
mediated by an increased K conductance.

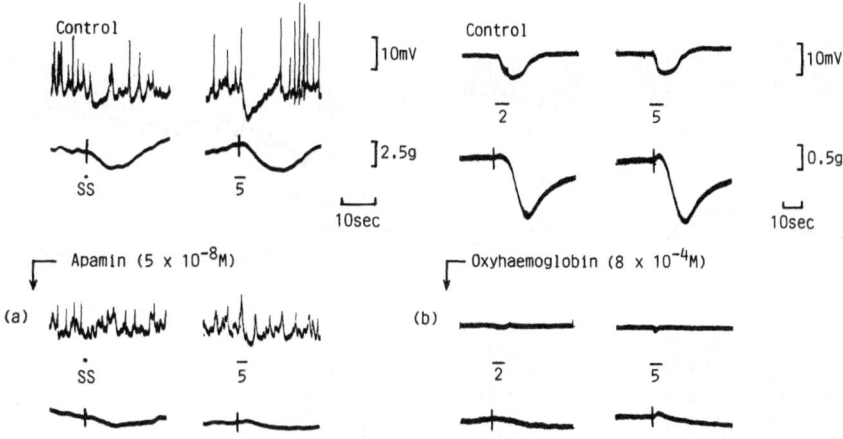

FIGURE 3   In the gpIAS (a) apamin (5 x 10⁻⁸M) and in the BRP (b)
oxyhaemoglobin (4 x 10⁻⁶M) antagonised the inhibitory
response to NANC nerve stimulation.

DISCUSSION

The gpIAS is spontaneously active.   In the absence of drugs, the
response to field stimulation is predominantly inhibitory; spontaneous
activity is abolished, the membrane hyperpolarized and the muscle
relaxed.   The frequent absence of any excitatory response to nerve
stimulation contrasts with the phentolamine-sensitive membrane depolarization, increased spike discharge and muscle contraction found
routinely in cat anal sphincter (Lim & Muir, unpublished).

The present results indicate that the responses to NANC nerve
stimulation in the gpIAS resemble closely those of the TC of the same
species.   Both are spontaneously active, discharge spike potentials
and respond to NANC nerve stimulation with a significant, frequency-
dependent membrane hyperpolarization and relaxation which are blocked
by apamin but not by oxyhaemoglobin.   In contrast, neither the BRP nor
AC are spontaneously active and respond to NANC nerve stimulation with
a relaxation of tone which is accompanied by much smaller changes in
membrane potential.   Apamin is relatively ineffective while oxyhaemoglobin antagonizes the response to NANC nerve stimulation on
these tissues.   The reasons for these differences in response to nerve
stimulation are unclear.   They may reflect differences in the transmitter concerned or, if the same transmitter is involved, in the

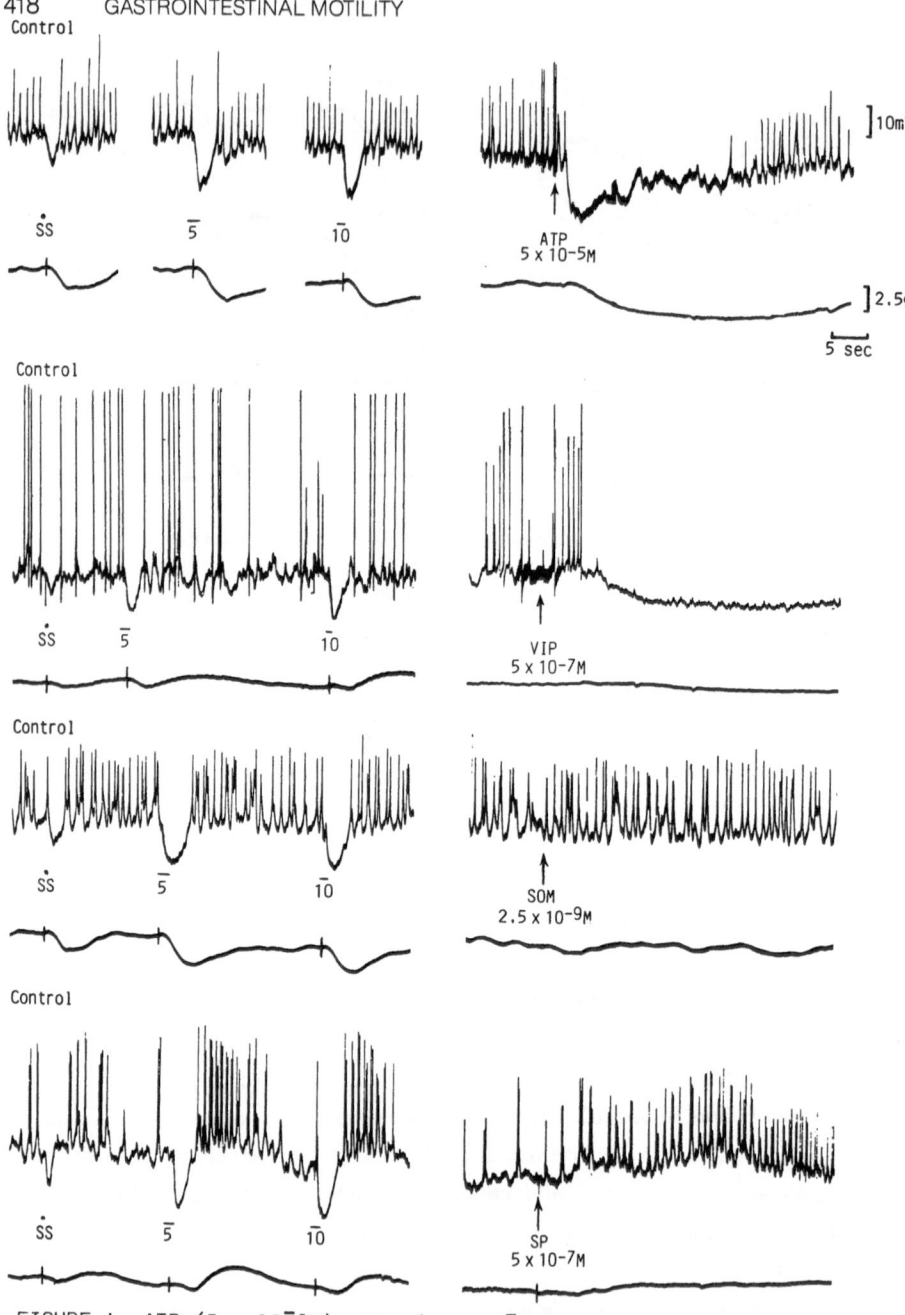

FIGURE 4   ATP (5×10^{-5}M), VIP (5×10^{-7}M) and nerve stimulation (single SS, 5 pulses at 5 and 10 Hz) but neither somato-statin (SOM 2.5×10^{-9}M) nor Substance P (SP 5×10^{-7}M) inhibit spontaneous activity, hyperpolarize the membrane and relax the gpIAS.

underlying receptor mechanisms. Significantly in gpIAS, TC (11), and BRP (Byrne & Muir, unpublished), the NANC response appears to be mediated by an increase in K conductance (5). However, differences in the response to apamin among these tissues may indicate that the K channels which operate during the inhibitory potential may differ and account for the differences observed in the NANC responses (12). Alternatively, the conductance change responsible for the inhibitory potential, at least in BRP (4), may be sensitive to membrane voltage as reported for amphibian ganglion neurones (13). In consequence, at a membrane potential around -50-60 mV, the inhibitory potential decreases as the membrane potential becomes depolarized. This could account for the comparatively small hyperpolarization observed in response to NANC nerve stimulation in this tissue in which the development of tone necessary to demonstrate the inhibitory potential, is accompanied by a significant depolarization of the membrane (4).

The problem of the identity of the NANC transmitter in the gpIAS remains. The present investigation indicates that adenosine, ATP, VIP and bradykinin inhibit spontaneous activity, hyperpolarize the membrane and relax the muscle. On the other hand, bombesin, somato-statin and substance P appear unlikely candidates. Clearly, in terms of the membrane potential changes produced, several substances resemble the response produced by NANC nerves. However, this does not imply that the mechanisms underlying the production of such responses are identical.

REFERENCES

1. Costa, M. and Furness, J.B. (1973). The innervation of the internal anal sphincter of the guinea-pig. In: The Proceedings of the 4th International Symposium on Gastrointestinal Motility, 681-90

2. Gillespie, J.S. (1982). Non-adrenergic non-cholinergic inhibitory control of gastrointestinal motility. In: Weinbeck, M. (ed). Motility of the Digestive Tract. pp. 51-66. (New York: Raven Press

3. Creed, K.E., Gillespie, J.S. and Muir, T.C. (1975). The electric-al basis of excitation and inhibition in the rat anococcygeus muscle. J. Physiol., 245, 33-47

4. Byrne, N.G. and Muir, T.C. (1982). The electrical basis of the bovine retractor penis to field stimulation and an inhibitory extract. J. Physiol., 328, 53P

5. Creed, K.E. and Gillespie, J.S. (1977). Some electrical properties of the rabbit anococcygeus muscle and a comparison of the effects of inhibitory nerve stimulation in the rat and rabbit. J. Physiol., 273, 137-53

6. Bennett, M.R., Burnstock, G. and Holman, M.E. (1966). Transmission from intramural inhibitory nerves to the smooth muscle of the guinea-pig taenia coli. J. Physiol., 182, 541-58

7. Baidan, L.V., Vladimirova, I.A., Miroshnikov, A.I. and Taran, G.A. (1978). Effects of apamin upon synaptic transmission in various types of synapses. Dokl. Akad. Nauk. SSSR., 241, 1224-7

8. Bowman, A. and Gillespie, J.S. (1982). Block of some non-adrenergic inhibitory responses of smooth muscle by a substance from haemolysed erythrocytes. J. Physiol., 328, 11-25

9. Abe, Y. and Tomita, T. (1968). Cable properties of smooth muscle. J. Physiol., 196, 87-100

10. Bowman, A., Gillespie, J.S. and Pollock, D. (1982). Oxyhaemoglobin blocks non-adrenergic non-cholinergic inhibition in the bovine retractor penis muscle. Eur. J. Pharmac., 85(2), 221-4

11. Den Hertog, A. and Jager, L.P. (1975). Ion fluxes during the inhibitory junction potential in the guinea-pig taenia coli. J. Physiol., 250, 681-91

12. Jenkinson, D.H. (1981). Peripheral actions of apamin. In: Trends in Pharmacological Sciences, December, pp. 318-20. Elsevier

13. Hartzell, H.C., Kuffler, S.W., Stickgold, R. and Yoshikami, D. (1977). Synaptic excitation and inhibition resulting from direct action on acetylcholine on two types of chemoreceptors on individual amphibian parasympathetic neurones. J. Physiol., 271, 817-46

ACKNOWLEDGEMENTS

The authors acknowledge the Churchill Trust for a travel grant to SPL, the Lee Foundation and the Medical Research Funds of Glasgow University.

68

Effects of Salicylic Acid (SA) and Aspirin (ASA) on Met-Enkephalin (FK) and Acetylcholine (ACH) Stimulated Motility of the Isolated Rat Colon

U. SCHEURER, E. DRACK and F. HALTER

Prostaglandins (PG) have been suggested to modulate morphine-induced motor actions of the canine intestine. Effects of SA and ASA on the motility of the isolated rat colon, stimulated with the met-enkephalin analogue FK 33-824 (FK) and ACH, were investigated. Intraluminal colonic pressure changes were measured by perfusion manometry in organ preparations, maintained in a standard organ bath.

RESULTS

FK and ACH dose-dependently increased integrated tonic colonic pressure with a response of 42 ± 0.6 AU (arbitrary units, $\bar{x} \pm$ SEM, n=12) at 10^{-6}M FK and 51.2 ± 0.8 AU at 10^{-4}M ACH. Pre-treatment of animals with ASA (300 mg/kg b.i.d. for 3 days and 1 h before removal of the colon, with and without addition of 1 g ASA/1 nutrient) suppressed the stimulatory effect of 10^{-8} to 10^{-5}M FK but did not affect the ACH stimulated colonic tone. Inhibition of the FK stimulated colonic tone was observed when only .1, .5 or 1 g ASA/1 nutrient were given. A 2 hour washout of organ preparations was unable to completely abolish the inhibitory effects of ASA.

In contrast, SA pre-treatement of animals (100 mg/kg b.i.d. and 1 h before removal of the colon) neither

421

influenced FK nor ACH stimulated colonic tone
significantly. The subsequent addition of .5 or 1 g SA/l
nutrient was followed by a similar inhibtion of the FK
effect as obtained with ASA but did not affect ACH
stimulation. A one hour-washout completely abolished the
inhibitory effects of SA.

CONCLUSION

FK stimulated colonic tone of rat preparations seems to
be PG dependent. Similar inhibitory effects of ASA
pre-treatment or ASA and SA in the nutrient on FK
stimulated motility are suggestive for potent action on
cyclooxygenase. The inability of SA pre-treatment to
counteract FK stimulation is suggested to be caused by
its quick washout.

69

Effect of Leu-Enkephalin on Synaptic Transmission in the Inferior Mesenteric Ganglion

J. H. SZURSZEWSKI and H. SHU

Enkephalin immunoreactive fibers are present in the guinea pig inferior mesenteric ganglion (IMG). The purpose of this study was to determine if leu-enkephalin (L-enk) inhibits natural synaptic activity from cholinergic, colonic mechanosensory afferents. Preparations consisted of a segment of the colon attached to the IMG via the lumbar colonic nerve. In a two-compartment organ bath, the IMG was placed in one compartment and the colon in the other. Intraluminal pressure recording techniques were used to study colonic motility and intra-cellular recording techniques were used to study synaptic transmission in the IMG. Administration of L-enk (10^{-6} M - 10^{-5} M) to only the colon decreased colonic motility and decreased mechanoreceptor synaptic input to neurons in the IMG as evidenced by a decrease in the frequency of action potentials and in the frequency and amplitude of e.p.s.p.s. These effects were antagonized by naloxone (10^{-6} M). When L-enk was added to only the ganglion compartment, the resting membrane potential hyperpolarized from -61.7 ± 3.2 mV to -66.3 ± 3.4 mV (mean $\pm$ SEM; p < 0.01). L-enk converted mechanoreceptor, synaptic input from threshold action potentials to subthreshold e.p.s.p.s and decreased

the amplitude and frequency of e.p.s.p.s. The inhibitory effect of

L-enk was antagonized by naloxone (10^{-6} M). In preparations of IMG

without attached colon, L-enk converted synchronous action potentials,

in response to electrical stimulation of lumbar colonic nerves, to

subthreshold e.p.s.p.s. However, the resting membrane potential and

the cell input resistance were not changed. Action potentials

initiated by passing intracellular depolarizing current pulses

(50 msec) at suprathreshold intensity were not altered by L-enk.

These data indicate that L-enk inhibits colonic motility. In the IMG,

L-enk depresses transmission by acting at specific opiate receptors

located on cholinergic terminals of mechanosensory afferents.

(Supported by NIH Grant AM 17632.)

70

Effects of Trimebutine (TMB) on Spontaneous Electrical Activity and on Junction Potentials Evoked by Parasympathetic Nerve Stimulation in Cat and Rabbit Colon

F. BLANQUET, M. BOUVIER and J. GONELLA

Most of the drugs which affect intestinal motility increase the activity of excitatory or inhibitory nerves controlling smooth muscle contractions (i.e. cholinergic or adrenergic nerves). TMB being a drug which modulates colonic motility, we have attempted to determine the modifications of electrical activity underlying the motor effects of this drug. The experiments have been carried out on cat colon and on rabbit proximal colon, on anaesthetized animals and in vitro. Electrical activity was recorded with extracellular pressure electrodes. Parasympathetic efferent nerve fibres were excited by stimulation of the pelvic nerves in the cat, and the vagus nerves in the rabbit. The effects of TMB remained unaffected by adrenergic blocking agents (phentolamine, propranolol, guanethidine) excluding any participation of sympathetic nerves. The action of TMB (0.5 to 2mg/kg in vivo ; 10^{-6} to 10^{-5}M in vitro) consisted in vivo as well as in vitro of an initiation or of an increase of spike potential activity lasting 10-20 minutes (8 animals). Spike activity was potentialized by atropine (0.1mg/kg for the cat ; 2 to 3mg/kg for the rabbit ; 10^{-6}M in vitro for both species). Moreover, in the cat under atropine, spike activity became cyclical, i.e. bursts of spikes were interrupted by periods of electrical silence. In the cat, TMB induced a significant decrease in the excitatory junction potential (EJP) amplitude (9 animals). In order to record inhibitory junction potentials (IJPs) without EJPs, experiments were performed under atropine. Under these

425

conditions, TMB induced rhythmic variations in the amplitude of IJPs for 30 to 40 minutes (2 animals). In the rabbit under TMB, EJPs were enhanced (7 animals), whereas IJP amplitude was decreased (6 animals). These variations were statistically significant. All the effects of TMB on spontaneous activity as well as on junction potentials are very similar to those observed, in a previous work, with morphine and enkephalins (1). The effects of TMB were antagonized by naloxone (2mg/kg in vivo, 10^{-6}M in vitro). These results strongly suggest that the action of TMB would be mediated through opiate receptors presumably located on intramural neurones (1). Thus it can be hypothesized that the atropine-resistant excitatory effects of TMB on spike activity would be due to an activation of intramural non-cholinergic excitatory neurones.

1. Blanquet, F., Bouvier, M. and Gonella, J. (1982). Effects of enkephalins and morphine on spontaneous electrical activity and on junction potentials elicited by parasympathetic nerve stimulation in cat and rabbit colon. Br.J.Pharmac., 77, 419-429.

71

Food Increases the Propagating Myoelectric Spiking Activity in the Human Colon

J. C. SCHANG and G. DEVROEDE

The present study was designed to describe the myoelectrical activity of the sigmoid and left colon with contact electrodes, in normal man, in fasting and postprandial conditions.

MATERIAL AND METHODS

Ten healthy volunteers were studied. Age ranged from 19 to 65. There were 5 males and 5 females. They had not complained of gastrointestinal symptoms, and had not taken laxatives or other medication for at least 5 years. Stool frequency ranged from 4 to 8 per week. The absence of colonic lesion was confirmed by endoscopy, when the probe was set into the colon. The probe used for recording colonic electrical activity was made of a polyethylene tube, 0.5cm in diameter and 100cm in length. Four bipolar electrodes were fixed at 10cm intervals on the upper end of the tube. Each bipolar electrode was composed of two rings of 0.5mm silver-silver chloride wire which were sewn around the tube 4mm apart. The wires leading from the electrodes to the recorder were introduced into the lumen of the tube and came out at its lower end, where they were soldered into a connector. The probe was introduced into the colon by means of a flexible sigmoidoscope and all four electrodes were located at 50,40,30 and 20cm from the anal verge. A.C. coupled amplifiers with a time constant of 0.03 sec were used (BECKMAN R 611 Dynograph Recorder) for recording the

1.

myoelectrical signals. Subjects were fasting for at least 10 hours before recordings. On the day before the study, they received a saline enema to clear the distal colon. No colonic preparation was used on the day of the recordings. Recording session began 45 minutes after the end of endoscopy. A two hour period of tracings was obtained in the fasting state at the end of which the subjects took an 800 kcal mixed meal. Recording was continued for two hours after the meal. The tracings were analysed by visual reading. The spike potentials were characterized by their number, duration, presence at the level of one or more electrode, time-lag between electrodes and number per minute. The number of bursts of spike potentials per unit of time for the four electrodes was also averaged. Each parameter was expressed for each consecutive 10 minute interval over the 4 hour recording session. Statistic analysis of the results was made by means of the

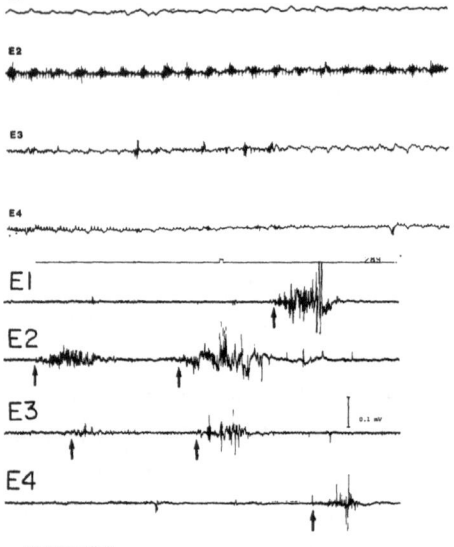

Fig. 1: type I potentials

Fig. 2: type II potentials

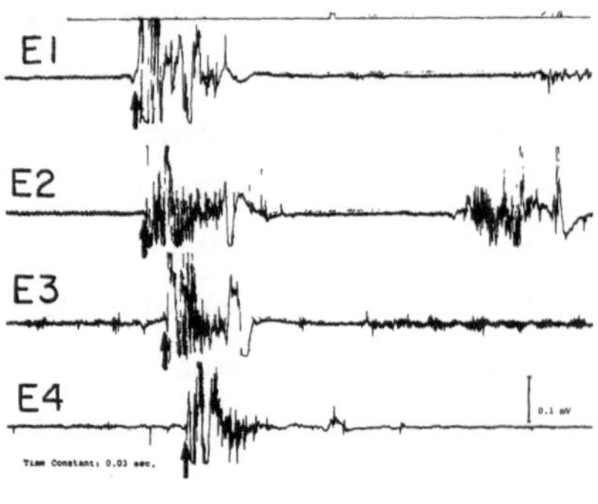

Fig. 3: type III potentials
(for comments, see text)

2.

Student t-test.

RESULTS

1)- Qualitative Analysis

Three different types of spike potentials were obtained:

A- Type I spike potentials   (figure 1)

These occurred in bursts that were fairly regularly spaced in a rhythmical pattern, at an average rate of 10.0 ± 0.1 (mean$\pm$S.D.) bursts per minute. The mean duration of each type I burst was 3.0 ± 0.2 sec. (mean$\pm$S.D.). The duration of the periods during which this type of spiking was observed ranged from 1.4 to 17 minutes. Type I bursts were made of spikes which amplitude was about 100-200 microvolts and frequency of about 10-40 Herz. These spike bursts occurred at the level of only one electrode at a time, and were not seen to propagate along the colon. Type I spike potentials were observed in 5 out of the 10 subjects during fasting, and only in 3 subjects during the postprandial period.

B- Type II spike potentials   (figure 2)

The individual duration of these bursts was much more variable, ranging from 1 to 180 seconds (mean$\pm$S.D.: 12.1 ± 4.0 sec.). The amplitude of the spikes was about 100-500 microvolts and frequency about 1 to 20 Herz. The bursts showed up in an irregular, sporadic and unpredictable pattern. Most of them were seen at the level of only one electrode, suggesting a local, non propagating contraction. However, many occurred simultaneously at the level of two, three or even four electrodes. In some cases the lag between the electrodes was regularly oriented orally or aborally. In other cases, the lag was irregularly oriented and all possible combinations were observed. Therefore, it is impossible to tell from these observations whether these spike potentials are propagating along the bowel wall.

C- Type III spike potentials   (figure 3)

This type of potentials, whose amplitude and frequency were similar to that of type II potentials, was characterized by its propagation along the colon. Namely the signal was successively observed at the level of consecutive electrodes with a near constant time-lag between each electrode and the next. The velocity of propagation ranged

3.

from 1 to 16 cm/sec. (mean±S.D.: 8.4±2.5 cm/sec.) and was oriented
aborally in 79.6% of the cases and orally in 20.4%.

2)- Quantitative Analysis

   The three types of spiking activity were observed in the fasting
and in the postprandial state. Total duration of spiking (cumulation
of the duration of the bursts) was about 31.30% of recording time during fasting, while after a meal this increased to 44.53%. Much of
this increase was due to more frequent type II activity which occupied
34.83% of the recording time after the meal, as opposed to 15.86% before. The difference is highly significant (p 0.005). The duration
of each individual burst of potential showed no significant change
after (12.2±3.9 sec.), as compared to before (12.0±4.3 sec.) the meal.
The postprandial increase in type II activity occurred in two distinct phases. The first phase began within 5 minutes of the beginning
of the meal and peaked within 10-20 minutes. The level of activity
then decreased slightly before increasing again. Another peak occurred at about 70-80 minutes. Whereas the first peak was of high amplitude and short duration, the second was of lower amplitude but much
more prolonged, lasting well beyond two hours.

   Type III activity also significantly increased after a meal, the
total time of spiking activity rising from 2.65 to 7.70% of the recording time (p 0.005). Here again, this increase was due to a greater
frequency of the bursts rather than to any change in their duration
(22.9±3.7 sec. before versus 25.5±4.5 after the meal). No significant
difference was observed in the direction of propagation, the ratio of
orally to aborally propagated potentials being 24.0% to 76.0% before
and 18.7% to 81.3% after the meal. Finally, there was only one peak
of type III activity, occurring at about 60-70 minutes. Thus, this
peak did not quite correspond to that of the type II activity. Finally, type I activity decreased after the meal. The total duration
of type I activity dropped from 10.0% of the recording time to 2.0%.
Since these bursts are seen in 5 out of 10 subjects in the fasting
state and only in 3 subjects after feeding, this difference was not
significant. When present, this activity did not significantly

4.

change in frequency within each spiking period (9.93 bursts per minute versus 10.25 after the meal).

CONCLUSION

Our findings confirm the observation that there is a general increase in spiking activity after a meal. We found the mean postprandial level of spiking activity to increase 2.2 times for sporadically occurring potentials, while rhythmical spiking activity was decreased 4.9 times. These changes should result in a decrease in segmental activity and an increase in propulsive activity. Another observation is the double peak of postprandial response in type II activity whose timing is different from that of the single peaked type III activity. The timing of the first peak of type II activity, occurring 10-20 minutes after food intake, corresponds to that of the so-called gastrocolic reflex. However, the second peak of activity associated with maximal Type III activity is poorly documented, probably because the duration of the recording sessions has generally been too short in previous studies. Also, this second peak does not appear as clearly as the first one because of its lower amplitude and longer duration. This second peak of activity may actually be considered as the proper colonic response to the meal.

72

Effects of Pancreatic Polypeptide, NPY and PYY in Relation to Sympathetic Influence on Colonic Motility and Blood Flow

P. M. HELLSTRÖM, O. OLERUP and K. TATEMOTO

INTRODUCTION

The neuropeptide Y (NPY) and the peptide YY (PYY) have been isolated from the brain and intestine, respectively (1,2). NPY and PYY have 36 amino acid residues and possess structural similarities with pancreatic polypeptide (PP) (1). Sympathetic noradrenergic neurons contain NPY-like immunoreactivity (3). Recently, it has been shown that NPY may be responsible for the sympathetic vasoconstriction resistant to α-adreno-ceptor blockade (4). Thus, it is suggested that NPY may act as a sympathetic neurotransmitter. PYY-like immunoreactivity is localized to endocrine cells in the mucosa of mammalian distal intestine. PYY causes vasoconstriction and inhibition of colonic motility (5).

The effects of NPY on colonic motility and blood flow have been analyzed in relation to the effects of noradrenaline and sympathetic nerve stimulations. As a further analysis, the effects of porcine PP, NPY and PYY on colonic motility and blood flow were compared.

MATERIAL AND METHODS

Experiments were performed on 30 cats, anesthetized with chloralose-urethane. Systemic arterial blood pressure was continuously recorded. The greater omentum, spleen and small intestine were exstirpated and the caudal mesenteric artery was ligated. A branch of the cranial mesenteric artery was cannulated for administration of close i.a. infusions. The colonic venous effluxes of the proximal and distal colon were separately monitored by drop recorder units. The volume changes of

the corresponding proximal and distal colon were registered by water-
filled flaccid balloons connected to reservoirs at a hydrostatic pressure of 15 cm H_2O. The reservoirs were suspended on force displacement
transducers. The preganglionic splanchnic and postganglionic lumbar
colonic nerves were dissected free and cut. The peripheral ends were
stimulated with a square-wave pulse generator.

Noradrenaline, porcine PP (gift from Dr. R.E. Chance, Eli Lilly
Research Lab., Indianapolis), PYY, NPY and synthetic NPY (Bachem Inc.)
were dissolved in 0.9 % NaCl solution containing 0.5 % bovine serum
albumin and infused i.a. PYY was also infused i.v. Guanethidine, 3 mg
x kg^{-1}, phentolamine, 3 mg x kg^{-1}, propranolol, 0.5 mg x kg^{-1}, and
hexamethonium, 10 mg x kg^{-1}, were administered i.v. For statistical
analysis the two-tailed sign test for two matched samples was used.

RESULTS
Electrical stimulation of the splanchnic nerves reduced blood flow in
the proximal colon ($p<0.01$) and increased proximal and distal colonic
volumes ($p<0.01$) (Fig. 1). Electrical stimulation of the lumbar colonic
nerves reduced blood flow in the distal colon ($p<0.01$) and increased
proximal and distal colonic volumes ($p<0.01$) (Fig. 1). Upon cessation
of both nerve stimulations a rapidly developing vasodilatation was
registered ($p<0.01$) (Fig. 1). After propranolol the colonic relaxation during nerve stimulation was reduced compared to controls ($p<0.05$).
However, the vasoconstrictor responses were unaltered (Fig. 1).
Phentolamine induced an intense motility. Upon splanchnic nerve stimulation increase of colonic volume ($p<0.05$) and reduction in proximal
blood flow was still present, i.e. 43.2±30.2 % of that registered
during control stimulations ($p<0.01$) (Fig. 1). No post-stimulatory
vasodilatation was seen ($p<0.01$). Similarly, stimulation of the lumbar
colonic nerves reduced the distal blood flow to 64.0±24.8 % of that
obtained at control stimulations ($p<0.01$) with no post-stimulatory
vascular escape ($p<0.01$). Increase of colonic volume was also registered ($p<0.01$) (Fig. 1). After guanethidine the motility ($p<0.05$)
and blood flow ($p<0.05$) responses to splanchnic nerve stimulation
were abolished. However, lumbar colonic nerve stimulation now produced a contraction of the colon ($p<0.05$) that was readily blocked by
atropine ($p<0.05$), but no change in blood flow was registered ($p<0.05$)

(Table 1). After hexamethonium the responses to splanchnic nerve stimulation on motility and blood flow were abolished (p<0.05).

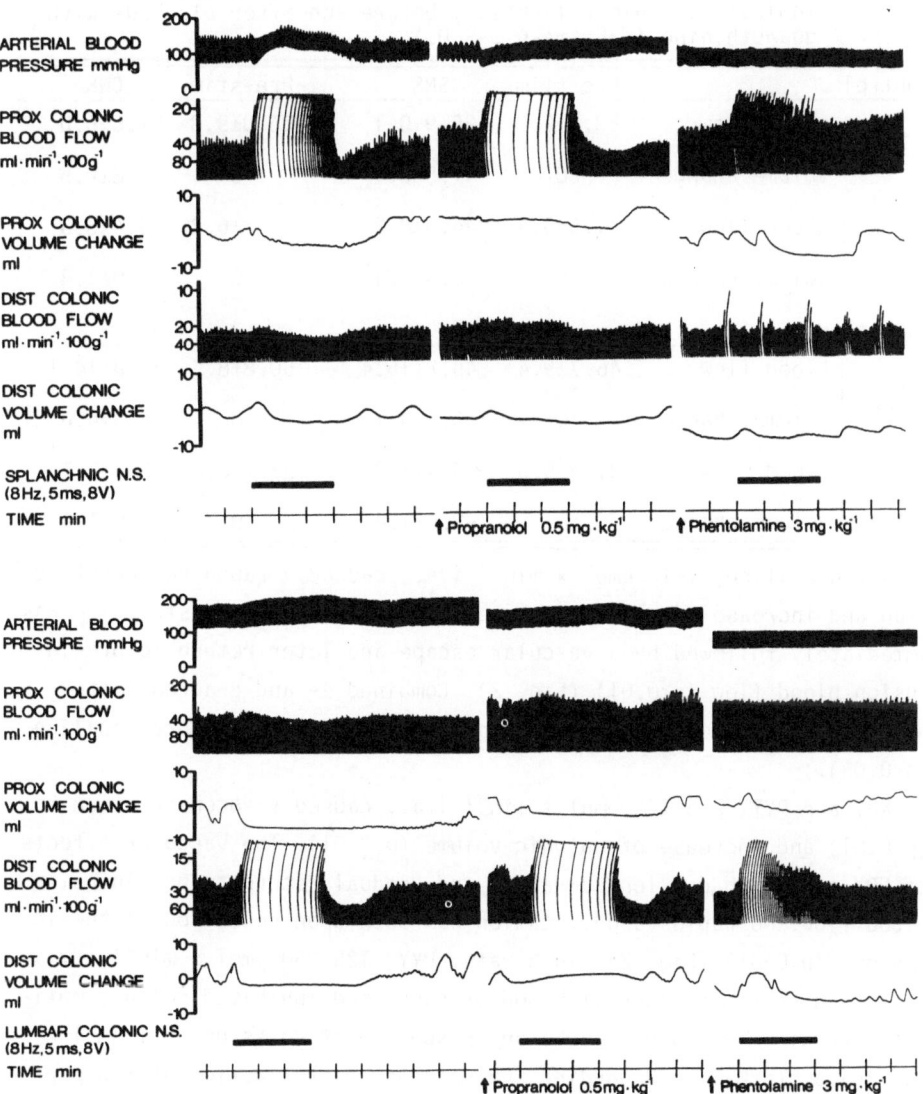

Figure 1. The effects of splanchnic nerve stimulation (upper panel) and lumbar colonic nerve stimulation (lower panel) on systemic arterial blood pressure, proximal and distal colonic blood flow and volume change. Nerve stimulations were performed before and after consecutive adrenoceptor blockades with propranolol and phentolamine. Note the absence of post-stimulatory vascular escape after α- and β-adrenoceptor blockade.

Table 1. The effects of splanchnic (SNS) and lumbar colonic (LCNS) nerve stimulation on proximal and distal colonic blood flow ($ml \times min^{-1} \times 100 \ g^{-1}$) and volume change (ml; negative values indicate colonic relaxation) before and after blockade with guanethidine (n=5; mean ± S.D.)

Control		Pre-stim.	SNS	Pre-stim.	LCNS
Prox. colon	blood flow	53.2±2.8	25.9±0.1	55.0±9.8	51.6±5.0
	volume change	0	-1.5±0.7	0	-4.8±2.5
Dist. colon	blood flow	41.9±5.4	44.5±8.2	50.2±6.3	9.4±8.3
	volume change	0	-2.0±1.4	0	-4.0±1.4
Guanethidine					
Prox. colon	blood flow	46.7±9.4	45.2±16.4	50.8±8.5	46.8±14.1
	volume change	0	-0.5±0.7	0	4.8±4.6
Dist. colon	blood flow	31.3±5.5	26.4±4.9	33.1±8.0	33.1±7.1
	volume change	0	-2.0±1.4	0	7.0±1.4

Noradrenaline, 1-10 nmol $\times min^{-1}$ i.a., caused a rapid vasoconstriction and increase of colonic volume (p<0.01). The vasoconstriction was immediately followed by a vascular escape and later return to pre-infusion blood flow (p<0.01) (Fig. 2). Combined α- and β-adrenoceptor blockade abolished the vascular and motility effects of noradrenaline (p<0.05).

NPY and PYY, 2.5-125 pmol $\times min^{-1}$ i.a., caused vasoconstriction (p<0.01) and increase of colonic volume (p<0.01). The vascular effects of NPY and PYY had a long duration and gradual return to pre-infusion blood flow. No rapid vasodilatation was seen upon cessation of the infusions (p<0.01) (Fig. 2). In 3 cats, PYY, 125-250 pmol $\times min^{-1}$ i.v., increased systemic arterial blood pressure and inhibited colonic motility. Porcine PP did not evoke any responses at doses up to 1 nmol $\times min^{-1}$ i.a. (p<0.01). Regarding the vasoconstrictor action of the peptides, PYY was 4 times as potent as NPY. A 50 % reduction of the blood flow was obtained at 100 pmol $\times min^{-1}$ of NPY and at 25 pmol $\times min^{-1}$ of PYY (Fig. 3). Denervation of the colon or administration of guanethidine, phentolamine or propranolol did not change the responses of NPY and PYY (p<0.05). In 3 cats, synthetic NPY, 125 pmol $\times min^{-1}$, was administered. The responses were of equal magnitude as those seen with natural NPY, indicating that synthetic NPY had a similar potency as natural NPY.

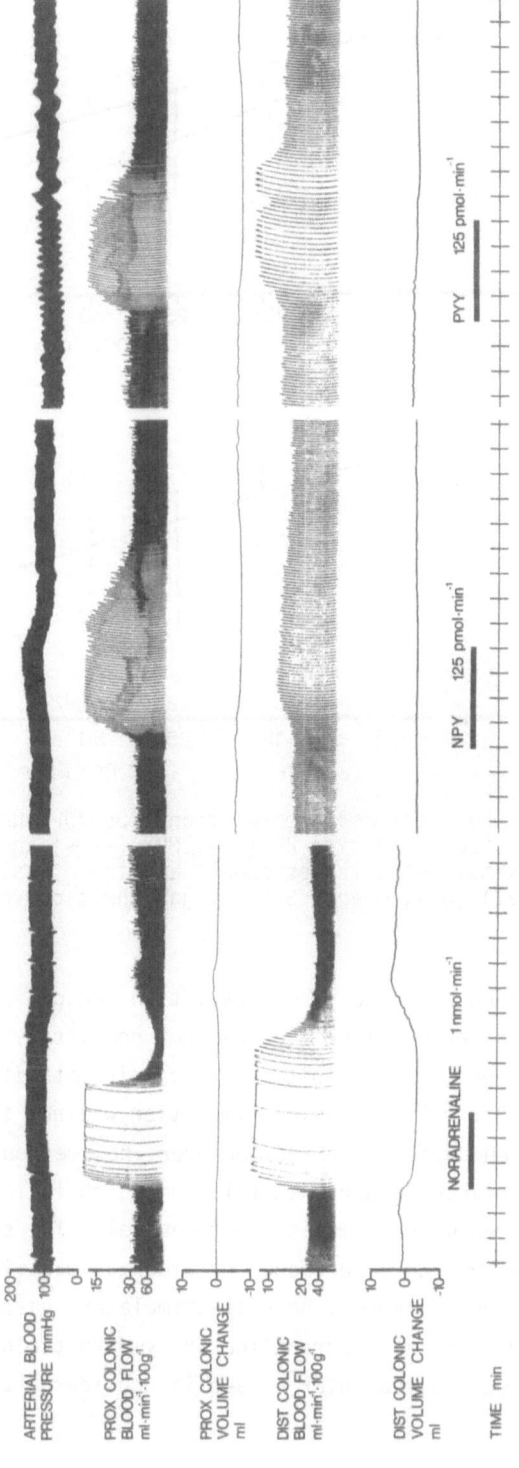

Figure 2. The effects of noradrenaline, NPY and PYY on systemic arterial blood pressure, proximal and distal colonic blood flow and volume change. Note the absence of vascular escape upon cessation of the infusions of NPY and PYY.

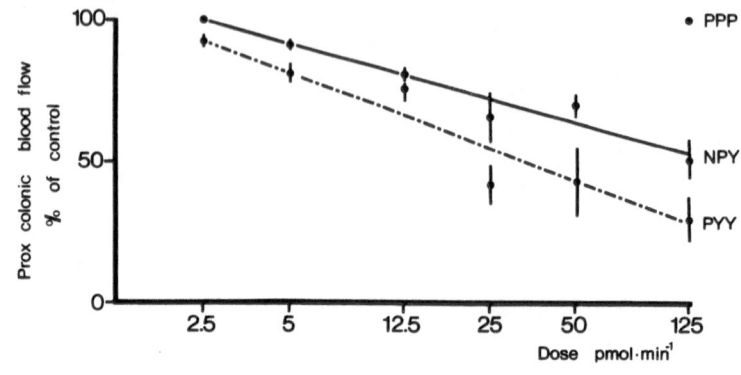

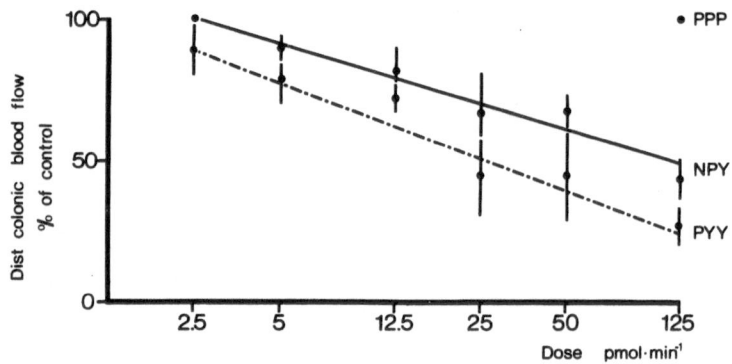

Figure 4. Summary of the dose-response relationships for the vasoconstrictor action of porcine PP (•), NPY (•——•) and PYY (•-•-•)
of the proximal colon (upper panel) and the distal colon
(lower panel) (n=4; mean ± S.D.; logarithmic curve fit).

DISCUSSION

The present results show that the vasoconstriction induced by splanchnic and lumbar colonic nerve stimulation was not completely blocked by
phentolamine. Furthermore, the inhibition of colonic motility induced
by splanchnic and lumbar colonic nerve stimulation was not inhibited by
combined α- and β-adrenoceptor blockade. However, hexamethonium blocked the responses to splanchnic nerve stimulation which indicates that
no afferent nerve fibres were stimulated retrogradely. The sympathetic
vasoconstriction resistant to α-adrenoceptor blockade was slow in onset and of long duration. Moreover, no post-stimulatory vascular escape similar to that seen after noradrenaline or sympathetic nerve stimulation was registered. The vascular escape is considered to be due

to an α-adrenoceptor mediated release of vasodilatory purine metabolites such as adenosine from the effector cells (6,7). Guanethidine abolished all vascular and motility responses to splanchnic nerve stimulation. However, during lumbar colonic nerve stimulation a colonic contraction was elicited, but vascular responses were abolished. Since the motility and vasoconstrictor responses to sympathetic nerve stimulation remaining after α- and β-adrenoceptor blockade were abolished by guanethidine, another substance than noradrenaline may be released during sympathetic nerve stimulation.

NPY antisera have been shown to react with noradrenergic sympathetic neurons. In the cat, sympathetic cells of the coeliac ganglion as well as submucous plexus and nerve fibres in the small intestine have been visualized by NPY antisera (3). Recently, in rats, the presence of NPY-immunoreactive cell bodies in the submucosal and myenteric ganglia indicates an intrinsic origin of NPY fibres. Additional extrinsic NPY fibres are suggested around blood vessels (8). The distribution of NPY-immunoreactive fibres in all layers of the gut wall suggests the possibility of a local sympathetic regulation of both motility and blood flow mediated by NPY. Our findings that NPY induces vasoconstriction and inhibition of colonic motility resistant to denervation and adrenergic blocing agents are in agreement with such a hypothesis.

In this study, PYY was 4 times more potent than NPY regarding vasoconstriction. The vascular response of PYY was similar to that of NPY but quite different from that of noradrenaline. Likewise, colonic motility was inhibited. Both the motility and vascular effects of PYY were unaffected by denervation or adrenergic blocking agents. PYY is exclusively localized to endocrine cells mainly in the distal intestine (5). PYY is active upon i.v. administration and more potent than NPY. PYY may be released from endocrine cells of the gastrointestinal mucosa upon stimulation by intraluminal contents to exert its action.

The present data show that the inhibition of motility and vasoconstriction of the colon during sympathetic nerve stimulation may in part be mediated by a non-adrenergic component. NPY may be released from noradrenergic neurons and exert vasoconstriction and inhibition of colonic motility during sympathetic nerve activity. PYY may have similar effects via an endocrine or paracrine action.

ACKNOWLEDGEMENTS
The present study was supported by grants from the Swedish Medical Research Council (3518), Ruth and Rickard Julins fond and Karolinska Institutets fonder.

REFERENCES
1. Tatemoto, K. (1982). Isolation and characterization of peptide YY (PYY) a candidate gut hormone that inhibits pancreatic exocrine secretion. Proc. Natl. Acad. Sci., 79, 2514-2518
2. Tatemoto, K., Carlquist, M. and Mutt, V. (1982). Discovery and isolation of neuropeptide Y (NPY), a brain peptide that has structural similarities to intestinal PYY and the pancreatic polypeptide. Nature, 296, 659-660
3. Lundberg, J.M., Terenius, L., Hökfelt, T., Martling, C.R., Tatemoto, K., Mutt, V., Polak, J., Bloom, S.R. and Goldstein, M. (1982). Neuropeptide Y (NPY)-like immunoreactivity in peripheral noradrenergic neurons and effects of NPY on sympathetic function. Acta Physiol. Scand., 116, 477-480
4. Lundberg, J.M. and Tatemoto, K. (1982). Pancreatic polypeptide family (APP, BPP, NPY and PYY) in relation to sympathetic vasoconstriction resistant to α-adrenoceptor blockade. Acta Physiol. Scand. 116, 393-402
5. Lundberg, J.M., Tatemoto, K., Terenius, L., Hellström, P.M., Mutt, V., Hökfelt, T. and Hamberger, B. (1982). Localization of peptide YY (PYY) in gastrointestinal endocrine cells and effects on intestinal blood flow and motility. Proc. Natl. Acad. Sci., 79, 4471-4475
6. Fredholm, B.B. (1976). Release of adenosine-like material from isolated perfused dog adipose tissue following sympathetic nerve stimulation and its inhibition by adrenergic α-receptor blockade. Acta Physiol. Scand. 96, 422-430
7. Fredholm, B.B. and Hedqvist, P. (1978). Release of (^{3}H)-purines from (^{3}H)-adenine labelled rabbit kidney following sympathetic nerve stimulation and its inhibition by α-adrenoceptor blockade. Br. J. Pharmacol., 64, 239-245
8. Sundler, F., Moghimzadeh, E., Håkanson, R., Ekelund, M. and Emson, P. (1983). Nerve fibres in the gut and pancreas of the rat displaying neuropeptide-Y immunoreactivity. Cell Tissue Res., 230, 487-493

73

Ultrasound Used to Measure the Response of Colonic Motility to Essential Oils

B. A. TAYLOR, H. L. DUTHIE, R. B. OLIVEIRA and J. RHODES

INTRODUCTION

Some essential oils, including peppermint oil (PO) and citral, have been shown to antagonise the 'in vitro' stimulation of carbachol on the guinea pig ileum, the magnitude of this effect being directly related to the solubility of the oil.[1] Further studies have shown that the same oils reduce spontaneous 'motility' of the proximal colon in the intact dog.[2] Also, in patients with Irritable Bowel Syndrome (IBS), PO significantly reduced abdominal symptoms in a double-blind cross over trial[3], while anecdotal reports suggest a use for PO in reducing colon spasm during colonoscopy and in reducing colic during whole bowel irrigation.

The Doppler principle has been used in the past to investigate gut motility, both in dogs using isolated small gut loops, and in humans in an entirely non-specific, non-localised way.[4]

The aim of the present study was to investigate the effects of oral and topically administered essential oils in normal controls and in patients with IBS. A combination of intraluminal pressure recordings and 'localised' Doppler shift signals was used to investigate motility, and a 'real-time' scanner to localise the recto-sigmoid colon more accurately and to obtain intraluminal Doppler shift signals.

441

MATERIALS

(a) Oral citral capsules: 11 patients with IBS were included in a double-blind cross over trial of citral versus placebo (polysorbate vehicle alone). Specially prepared capsules, designed to release their contents - in the distal small gut and colon[5], were administered 3 times a day for 1 week, and 'motility indices' calculated using intraluminal pressure recordings and Doppler shift signals as described below. At the end of the first week each patient was 'crossed over' and the procedure repeated. Colon motility was stimulated prior to each recording using neostigmine, 0.5 mg I.M.

(b) Topical instillation of oil: 14 healthy subjects were each twice subjected to intraluminal recto-sigmoid pressure recordings after topical instillation of either an essential oil or placebo in random order. 6 subjects received 0.2 ml of PO, while 8 received 0.1 ml of citral, the active agents being suspended in 50 ml normal saline with polysorbate (1:10,000). Colon motility was stimulated prior to each recording using neostigmine, 0.5 mg I.M.

(c) Real-time ultrasound recordings: 4 healthy volunteers, who had not voided urine for approximately 2 hours, were investigated in the fasting state using a combination 'real-time' and Doppler frequency shift ultrasound scanner, in order to assess (i) the feasability of accurate non-invasive localisation of bowel loops, and (ii) the extent to which intraluminal gas interferes with these recordings.

METHODS

(a) Intraluminal pressure recordings: A triple-lumen tube was placed into the recto-sigmoid via a sigmoidoscope, with the most proximal opening about 20 cm from the anal verge.   The lumens were perfused using a low compliance system connected via pressure transducers to a multi-channel pen recorder. After allowing 20 minutes for the effects of placement of the tube to pass, 'motility indices' were calculated for 3 successive 10 minute periods following instillation of either oil or placebo.

(b) Doppler frequency shift recordings: An ultrasonic foetal heart monitor, focussing at approximately 8 cm, was placed in the left iliac fossa to obtain maximum deflection when a balloon attached to the tip of the intra-luminal pressure recording tube was inflated (Fig. 1). Subsequent recordings were made with the monitor fixed in this position, and duration of activity was calculated as a percentage of each 10 minute period.

(c) 'Real-time' ultrasound recordings: A 'Duplex' scanner (Advanced Technology Laboratories, Seattle, USA) was used to localise the recto-sigmoid and sigmoid colon in each case. This was made easier by instilling between 200 and 300 ml of normal saline into the lumen of the bowel through a rectal tube in order to displace intraluminal gas. After locating a bowel loop, a Doppler frequency shift signal was obtained from within the bowel lumen.

RESULTS

(a) Oral citral: In contrast to previously reported results with PO[3], no significant improvement was demonstrated with citral. Similarly, neither the 'motility indices', calculated from manometric recordings, nor the duration of activity, calculated from ultrasonic recordings, showed a significant difference after citral when compared with placebo. However, in 7 of the 11 cases, good correlation was demonstrated between ultrasonic and manometric recordings (Fig. 2), while in the remaining 4 cases, no such correlation existed. In all 7 cases demonstrating good correlation, it had been possible to localise the balloon at the tip of the pressure recording tube, while in the remaining four this had been impossible.

(b) Topical instillation of oil: Both topical citral and PO demonstrated significant inhibition of motor activity, this effect being maximal during the first 10 minute period after instillation, and decreasing thereafter (Figs. 3 & 4). Complete inhibition of motor activity was seen with both oils, and lasted for periods varying up to 20 minutes. This effect was not seen with placebo. There was no apparent difference between

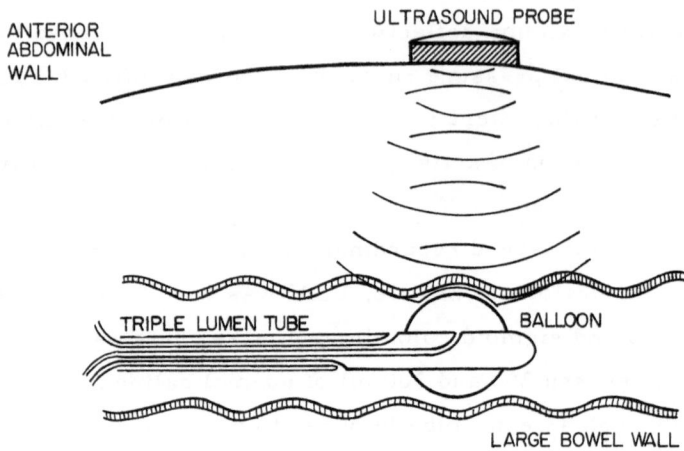

Figure 1:   Foetal heart monitor on abdominal wall, localising segment of large bowel from which intraluminal pressure recording is being made.

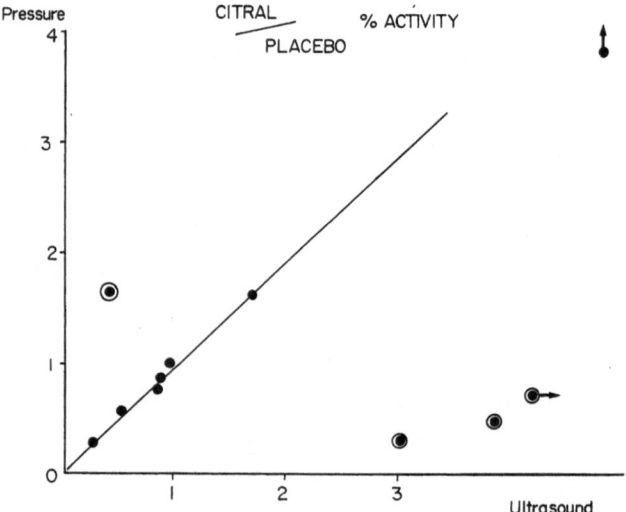

Figure 2:   Correlation between ultrasonic and manometric recordings (◉ indicates recording in which it was impossible to locate intraluminal balloon).

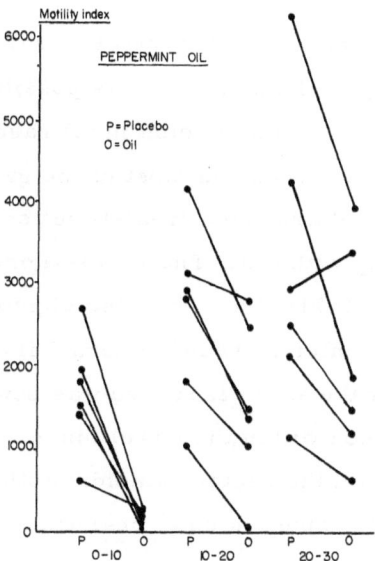

Fig 3: Motility indices for three consecutive 10 minute periods following instillation of either peppermint oil or placebo.

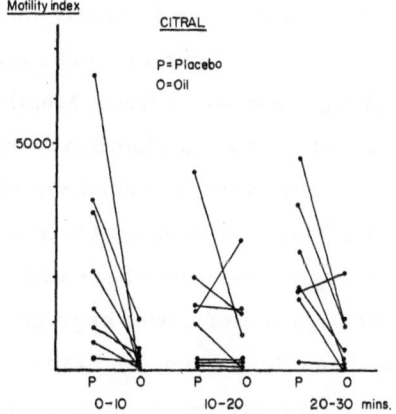

Figure 4: Motility indices for three consecutive 10 minute periods following instillation of either citral or placebo.

citral and PO.

(c) 'Real-time' recordings: Although intraluminal gas considerably interfered with imaging of the bowel, it was possible to localise both the recto-sigmoid and the sigmoid colon in all cases. Filling the bowel segment with liquid displaced most of the gas, and the lumen appeared as an 'echo free' area on a 'real-time' scan, with small echogenic areas moving within it. The recto-sigmoid could be located immediately behind a full bladder, while the sigmoid colon could be similarly located lying anterior to left external iliac vessels (Figs. 5 &6). Confirmation that the area visualised was bowel was obtained both by inflating a balloon within the bowel lumen, and by increasing the volume of fluid within the recto-sigmoid. Both manoeuvres produce characteristic responses on a 'real-time' image.

DISCUSSION

The consistent inhibitory effect of topical PO on distal colon motility perhaps explains the previously shown symptomatic improvement following oral PO in patients with IBS. The combination of the failure of oral citral to produce a symptomatic improvement in IBS, and its reproducible inhibition of motility when topically instilled into the distal colon presumably indicates either that oral citral is metabolised or absorbed before reaching the distal colon. Menthol, which is thought to be the active agent in PO, is chemically distinct from citral, and may therefore be metabolised or absorbed via different pathways. In either case, citral would seem at present to have little to offer in the treatment of IBS, although patient numbers are small.

Accurate ultrasonic localisation of bowel segments is a technique which has not previously been described, and close correlation between ultrasonic and manometric recordings is demonstrated when such localisation is possible. A 'real-time' scanner may provide a refinement to the technique, and the 'Duplex' Scanner has demonstrated that Doppler frequency shift signals are generated by the fluid content of the bowel lumen rather than by the bowel wall itself. Ultrasound

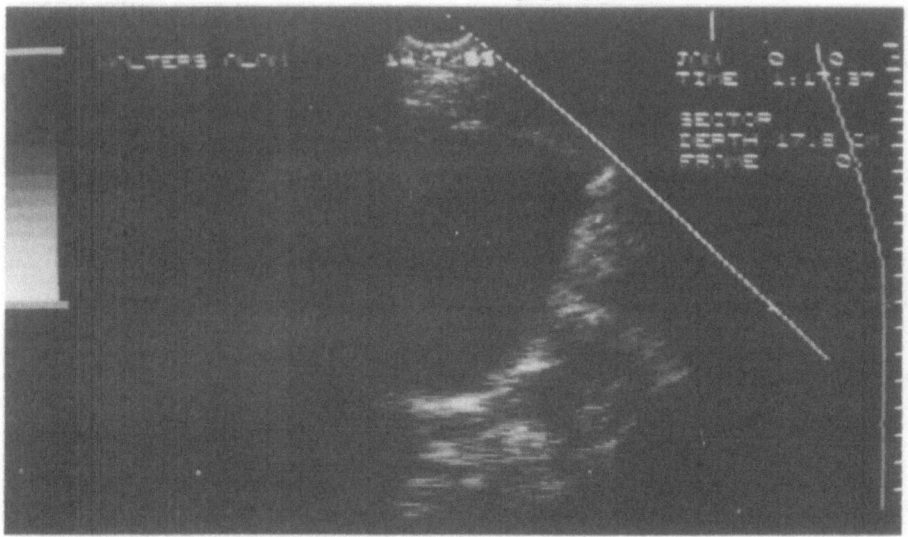

Figure 5: 'Real-time' ultrasound scan demonstrating the recto-sigmoid colon in longitudinal section, lying immediately behind a full bladder.

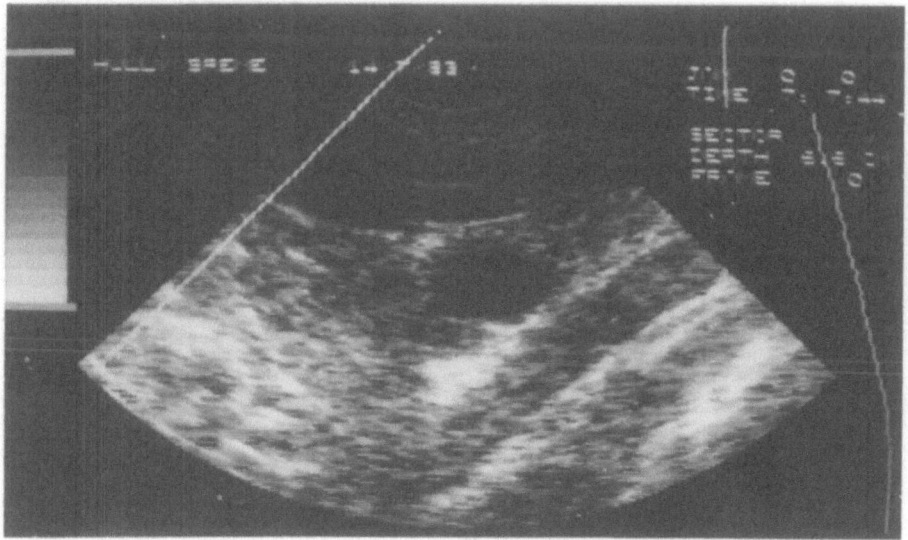

Figure 6: 'Real-time' ultrasound scan demonstrating the sigmoid colon in transverse section, lying immediately anterior to the external iliac vessels.

may have a part to play in the future investigation of gut motility, although quantitative analysis has not yet been attempted.

ACKNOWLEDGEMENTS

B.A.T. was supported by a grant from the Welsh Scheme for the Development of Health and Social Research. R.B.O. was supported by a grant from Fundacao de Amparo a Pesquisa do Estado de Sao Paulo. We would like to thank Prof. J.P. Woodcock for his assistance.

REFERENCES

1.   Evans, B.K., James, K.C. and Luscombe, D.K. (1972). A correlation between solubility and carminative activity. J. Pharm. Pharmac., 24 (Suppl), 173P.

2.   Evans, B.K., Heatley, R.V., James, K.C. and Luscombe, D.K. (1975). Further studies on the correlation between biological activity and solubility of some carminatives. J. Pharm. Pharmac., 27 (Suppl), 66P.

3.   Rees, W.D.W., Evans, B.K. and Rhodes, J. (1979). Treating irritable bowel syndrome with peppermint oil. Br. Med. J., 2, 835.

4.   Barrett, G.D. and Sheiner, H.J. (1982). The ultrasonic motilo-gram. In: Weinbeck, M. (ed). Motility of the Digestive Tract, p. 219.

5.   Dew, M.J., Hughes, P.J., Lee, M.G., Evans, B.K. and Rhodes, J. (1982). An oral preparation to release drugs in the human colon. Br. J. Clin. Pharmac., 14, 405.

74

Nervous Reflexes Involved in the Co-ordination of the Motility of Internal Anal Sphincter and Urinary Bladder

M. BOUVIER, J. C. GRIMAUD, J. SALDUCCI and J. GONELLA

Relationships between motility of urinary bladder and internal anal sphincter (IAS) were studied by recording changes of the electromyographic activity of the IAS during stimulation of vesical afferent nerve fibers in anaesthetized spinal cats.

Vesical afferent nerve fibers were activated either by electrical stimulation of nerves running on the urinary bladder near the junction with the ureters, or by vesical distension within physiological ranges (from 10 to 20ml). Both types of stimuli induced : 1) IAS excitation consisting of an increase of the discharge frequency of the action potentials associated in some cases with an increase of their amplitude. This excitation was abolished by phentolamine and thus mediated through alpha adrenergic receptors ; 2) the inhibition of the excitatory response evoked in the IAS by stimulation of the distal end of one divided hypogastric nerve. This inhibition was blocked by naloxone, indicating that enkephalinergic neurones are involved. The disappearance of both reflexes under hexamethonium shows that at least one cholinergic synapse is activated. Both reflexes remained unaffected by section of sacral spinal roots, this excludes any participation of the parasympathetic nervous system, thus all the vesical afferent nerve fibers follow sympathetic nervous pathways. Both excitatory and inhibitory reflexes were decreased by section of lumbar spinal roots (between 2nd and 5th), they were completely abolished after section of the remaining hypogastric nerve. These reflexes are therefore achieved partly at the lumbar level of spinal cord and partly at the level of inferior mesenteric ganglia (IMG).

These results evidence crossed reflexes between urinary bladder and IAS.From the physiological standpoint, it is demonstrated that : 1) afferent nerve fibers running along sympathetic nerves do not only convey noxious information, indicating that the sympathetic nervous system is involved in regulatory mechanisms ; 2) the IMG behaves as a reflex nervous centre that co-ordinates urinary bladder and IAS motility.From the functional standpoint, these results indicate that these reflexes are presumably responsible for the alternating occurrence of micturition and defecation.

75

Relaxations of the Internal Anal Sphincter Elicited by Rectal and Extrarectal Distensions in Man

B. NAUDY, D. PLANCHE, B. MONGES and J. SALDUCCI

INTRODUCTION

The high pressure zone of the anal canal is mainly dependant at rest on the activity of the internal anal sphincter (IAS). This sphincter is reflexly relaxed when the rectal wall is distented. This phenomenon provoked by the stimulation of stretch receptors occurs in defecation or in experimental conditions after inflation of a balloon in the lumen. Such experimental distension is also effective in sigmoid (1). The present study was designed to investigate the responses obtained after distension of different parts of the lower digestive tract and to compare them to the response after rectal stimulation. It was attempted to define place of these reflex activities during defecation and among mechanisms of continence.

METHODS

Pressure in the anal canal was measured by means of a polyethylene catheter (internal diameter : 1mm) with side hole opening and constantly perfused (6 ml/h). The probe was positionned in the maximal pressure zone after 2/3 pull through. EMG of rectum and external anal sphincter (EAS) was recorded by bipolar stainless steel wires electrodes 0, 125 mm in diameter implanted in the muscular coat and easily removed at the end of experiment (2). Distensions were realised by inflation with air of a latex balloon secured to a catheter. The diameter of balloon varied with the amount of air inflated (2 cm : 15 ml − 3 cm : 30 ml − 5 cm : 70 ml − 7 cm : 130 ml).

451

Ten subjects of both sexes were studied. They were in a lateral or a supine position. They were exempt of colorectal disease and had received neither anaesthetics nor drugs which modify intestinal motility during the two preceding days. Three patients having a total colostomy (two after volvulus, one for carcinoma) with the two orifices separately fixed to the skin were included in the study. Inferior limit of sectioning was between 30 cm and 40 cm from the anal margin and two patients had a short bowel resection above.

RESULTS

1 - <u>Distensions of rectum</u>. The distensions were effected in subjects having stimulations in other areas for comparison and control. Rapid distension above threshold of about 10/15 ml of air induced constant response preceded by EAS guarding reflex and accompanied by rectal contraction. It occured after a delay varying from 1.8 to 2.5 seconds. The depth of relaxation increased with intensity of stimulation : complete opening (anal pressure similar to rectal pressure) occured beyond 40/50 ml of air. The duration of the response was between 7 to 20 seconds. Sphincteric tonic activity resumed always up to 130 ml of air. The response increased after vesical emptying (3 - 4).

2 - <u>Distensions of superior part of anal canal (Fig. 1)</u>. The balloon was inflated in the mid rectum with 20/30 ml of air and drawn against the superior orifice ; it was then pulled down suddendly upon 1 cm to open only the superior part of anal canal. The mechanical effect of traction appeared as a brief fall in pressure preceding the true relaxation which occured in 70 per cent of cases. The latency time was short : 1.6 to 1.8 s. Repetitive relaxations could frequently be obtained as soon as

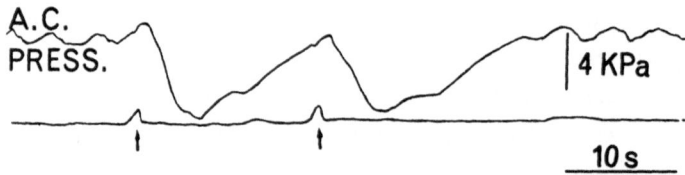

Figure 1 - IAS relaxations after distensions of the superior part of anal canal. (A.C. Press.: anal canal pressure).
Successive stretchs (arrows) of the superior part of anal canal by a balloon (diameter 2 cm) initially inflated in the rectum induce IAS relaxations after a short latency time (1.8 s.). Response is repetitive as soon as sphincteric tone is resuming.

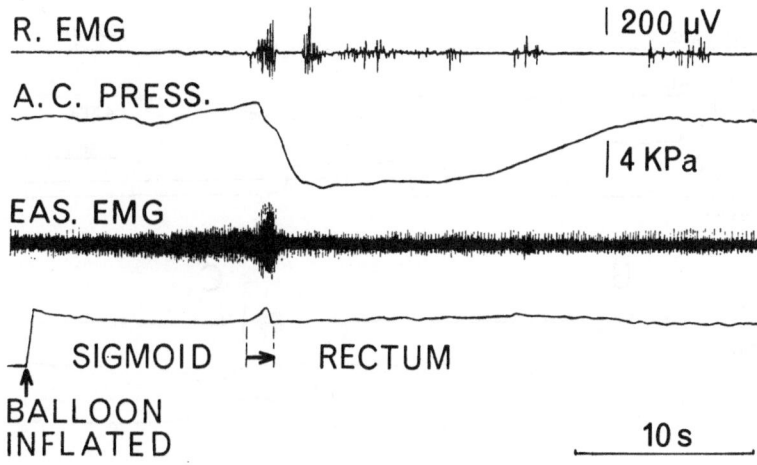

R. EMG | 200 µV

A.C. PRESS.

| 4 KPa

EAS. EMG

⌐ SIGMOID ⊢→ RECTUM
↑
BALLOON
INFLATED   10 s

Figure 2 - Effects of distension of the recto sigmoid junction.
After a balloon (20 mℓ of air - diameter 2.5 cm) was inflated into the
inferior part of sigmoid no IAS relaxation appeared. Then the balloon
is pulled down. As it distends the junction (peak of pressure - hori-
zontal arrow) large IAS relaxation is induced. Simultaneously a brief
reflex EAS contraction occurs. A sustained rectal EMG activity (R. EMG)
is recorded during IAS opening, beginning before the balloon enters the
rectum.

the sphincteric tone was resuming. Although depth of relaxation might
vary a strict relationship with the intensity of stimulation was not
observed.

3 - Distensions of rectosigmoid junction. The balloon initially inflated
in the sigmoid with an amount of air insufficient to provoke IAS relaxation (see further) was pulled down against the rectosigmoid junction.
A continuous force was then exerted : at the time of the opening of the
junction an IAS relaxation appeared and was frequently deep. A reflex
contraction of EAS (guarding reflex) and a rectal contraction were recorded before the balloon entered the rectum. The IAS relaxation was
practically constant beyond 40 ml of air and occured in these circum-
tances without straightening of the sigmoid. The response was not stric-
ly adapted to stimulation as in the preceding case. (Fig. 2).

4 - Distensions of sigmoid (Fig. 3). IAS relaxation was not constant
particularly for low volume of inflation (up to 40 ml). In some subjects
such distensions were ineffective during several minutes (Fig. 3 A).
The response when present often had a low amplitude and a variable latency time (1.8 to 3 seconds in some cases - Fig. 3 B ; several seconds

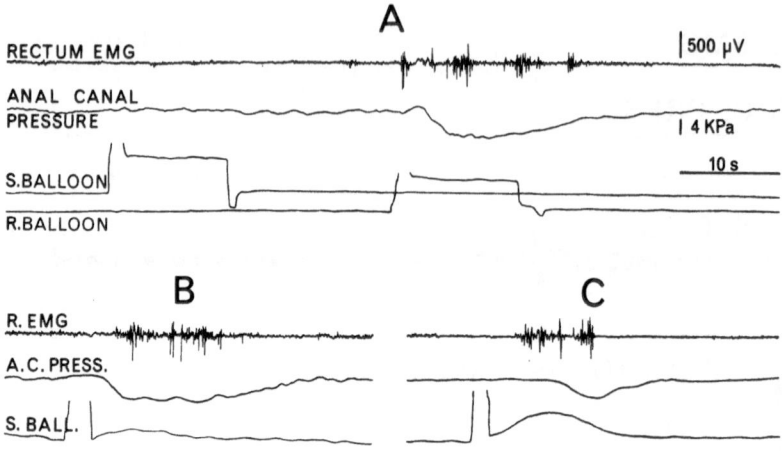

Figure 3 - Effects of distension of the sigmoid (S. = Sigmoid ;
R. = Rectum).
Patterns of responses recorded in different subjects after inflation
with 30 mℓ of air.
A - No response, although the same stimulation is effective in the rec-
   tum. Motor activity was previously low in this case.
B - IAS relaxation induced in a short time. Recording effected two mi-
   nutes before the onset of a propulsive activity.
C - IAS relaxation occuring several seconds after distension following
   sigmoid and rectal contractions.

in others cases - Fig. 3 C). In all cases rectal contraction occured simultaneously with IAS relaxation. The distal part of sigmoid was more
sensitive to stimulation. Responses after light stimulations or of short
latency time were chiefly induced before (for 5/10 minutes) and during
a special period of propulsive activity in the lower digestive tract
(see further).

5 - Periods of propulsive activity (Fig. 4). During some recordings a
special pattern of motor activity was observed. It consisted of large
bursts of spikes which were propagating from the rectosigmoid junction
to the lower rectum. Deep IAS relaxations occured as the upper rectum
was contracting and before the bursts reached the lower rectum. These
contractions recurred on an average of 10 minutes, and were pseudo-
rythmic 1.5 to 3/minute. The occurence of this periods seemed to be
either spontaneous or in several cases provoked by the repetitive distensions of the lower sigmoid effected to elicit IAS relaxations.

6 - Distensions of afferent and efferent loops in colostomised patients
(Fig. 5). IAS relaxations could be constantly obtained after distension

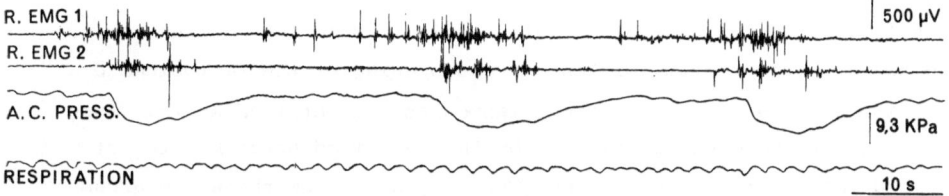

R. EMG 1   500 μV

R. EMG 2

A.C. PRESS.

                                                                     9,3 KPa

RESPIRATION   10 s

*Figure 4 - Rectum and IAS activities during propulsive period.
Rectum EMG was recorded at 18 cm (1) and 10 cm (2) from the anal margin. Recording was made during a long period of moderate awareness of
defecation (without issue of stool). Pseudo rythmic contractions propagated aborally from the recto sigmoid junction through the rectum
during ten minutes. Each of them was coupled with IAS relaxation which
began when the upper part of the rectum was contracting.*

of the efferent loop beyond 20/30 ml of air. Relaxations often where
deep with short latency time (mean duration 2.2 sec.). Rectal contraction was recorded as IAS relaxed. Enhanced reflex activities could be
elicited in the entire lower segment. They were not provoked by an ac-
cidental noxious stimulation which consists of a short IAS relaxation
preceded by strong EAS contraction. Responses from the afferent loop
were frequently of lower amplitude and sometimes absent. But the few
subjects 'studied with variable experimental conditions does not allow
to conclude.

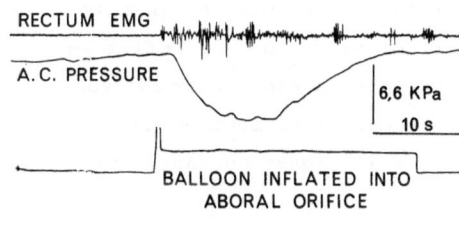

RECTUM EMG

A.C. PRESSURE
                              6,6 KPa
                              10 s

BALLOON INFLATED INTO
ABORAL ORIFICE

*Fig. 5 - Distension of efferent
loop after colostomy in sigmoid.
The balloon was inflated with 20ml
of air. The distension effected in
the inferior orifice at about 35cm
of the anal margin provokes a deep
IAS relaxation after a short latency. Sustained rectal contraction
is simultaneously recorded.*

DISCUSSION

        Distensions of different parts of the lower digestive tract
can induce IAS relaxations. The more constant and adapted responses are
obtained after such stimulations of the rectal wall. This has long been
used for the study of the reflex relaxation of IAS with well settled
results (1 - 5). Distensions of the two near narrowed areas are also

effective. Responses from the superior part of the anal canal although less frequent occur in a brief latency time, among the shortest observed above in the rectum. Distension and opening of the rectosigmoid junction produce almost constant responses. If obtained at rest they are then not preceded or followed by the sustained straightening of sigmoid that share in defecation. The responses from these two areas cannot be graded so accurately as from rectum by varying intensity of stimulation probably owing to a larger influence of their initial activity. Distension of sigmoid also elicit IAS reflex relaxation (1), the lower part being more sensitive. The response is not constant particularly for low stimulations known to be effective in the rectum. It appears in this case mostly related to the initial motility of sigmoid as shown by the enhanced responses observed before and during periods of propulsive activity. Sigmoid peristaltic contractions induced by some local distensions have been already evoked (6). A such activity has been reported in the rectum with manometric recordings (7). In this investigation EMG recording provides an evident pattern of propulsive activity in the rectum which can be expected to involve sigmoid considering the facilitation of its reflex activities at the same time. However this motor pattern is not always accompanied by issue of stools or even awareness of defecation.

After sectioning of sigmoid for colostomy the major feature is an increased reflex activity in the efferent loop. Previous pathological state could interfere but the deep relaxations obtained in this condition show that normal pathways exist for producing the reflex in this region although the response is frequently lacking in normal subjects. In vitro CHRISTENSEN (8) has found in cat after sectioning a rise in slow waves frequencies but a decrease in migrating fast activities.

Contraction of rectum coupled with IAS relaxation appeared constant on EMG recordings (2) although discussed on manometric recordings (1 - 9). After distension of other areas a rectal contraction accompanies also IAS relaxation. It appears mediated by extrinsic nerves considering the same delay in its occurence.

The multiple and high areas in which reflex can originate suggest that during defecation IAS relaxation can be induced when the stools are still in sigmoid and is successively reinforced as they move

distally. A decisive phenomenon seems to be the passage of the recto-
sigmoid junction. Distensions of rectum and of superior part of anal
canal appear as additionnal events becoming important if reflex is not
elicited above and if stools stay temporarily in the rectal ampulla
with variations in their volume. An important function of the propulsive activity is certainly the preparation of defecation.

        Large relaxations obtained in some circonstances from sig-
moid (after colostomy - propulsive activity) could be an indirect
evidence that inhibitory imputs impede them at rest. The role of parasympathetic pathways has been outlined in this function for sigmoid in
pathological observations (10) and in experimental conditions (11) ;
it appears more intricate for IAS (12). The drop of tone of the muscular coat allows the sigmoid to accomodate stools without stimulation
of propulsive activity. In this condition and in the absence of chronic retention of stools inside the rectum, responses after passage of
rectosigmoid junction and rectal distension are partially preserved
from these influences. Place of reflex and voluntary contraction of
EAS in the maintain of continence is not discussed here. However it
may be outlined the constant apparition in normal subjects of EAS
guarding reflex by passage of the rectosigmoid junction and distention of the rectum as the IAS relaxation is elicited.

REFERENCES

1. Schuster, M.M., Hendrix, T.R. and Mendeloff, A.J. (1963). The internal anal sphincter response : manometric studies on its normal physiology, neural pathways, and alterations in bowel disorders. J. of
Clinical Investigation, 42, 196-207

2. Monges, H., Salducci, J., Naudy, B., Ranieri, F., Gonella, J. and
Bouvier, M. (1980). The electrical activity of the internal anal
sphincter : a comparative study in man and in cat. In : Christensen, J.
(ed). Gastrointestinal Motility. pp. 487-493. (New York : Raven Press)

3 - Salducci, J., Planche, D. and Naudy, B. (1982). Physiological role
of the internal anal sphincter and the external anal sphincter during
miction. In : Wienbeck, M. (ed). Motility of the Digestive Tract.
pp. 513-521.(New York : Raven Press)

4 - Planche, D., Salducci, J. and Naudy, B. (1982). Corrélations vé-
sico anales durant la miction chez l'homme. J. Physiol. (Paris), 78,
235-239

5. Duthie, H.L. (1971). Anal continence. Gut, 12, 844-852

6. Connell, A.M. (1968). Motor action of large bowel. In : Code, C.F. (ed). Handbook of Physiology. Section 6 : Alimentary Canal. Volume 4 : Motility. pp. 2075-2091. (Washington D.C. : American Physiological Society)

7. Scharli, A.F. and Keiseweiter, W.B. (1970). Defecation and continence : some new concepts. Dis. Col. Rect., 13, 81-107

8. Christensen, J., Anuras, S. and Hauser, R.L. (1974). Migrating spike bursts and electrical slow waves in the cat colon : effect of sectioning. Gastroenterology, 66, 240-247

9. Haynes, W.G. and Read, N.W. (1982). Ano rectal activity in man during rectal infusion of saline : a dynamic assessment of the anal continence mechanism. J. Physiol., 330, 45-56

10. Connel, A.M., Frankel, H. and Guttman, L. (1963). The motility of the pelvic colon following complete lesion of spinal cord. Paraplegia, 1, 98-115.

11. Gonella, J. and Gardette, B. (1974). Etude in vivo de la commande nerveuse extrinsèque parasympathique du côlon. J. Physiol. (Paris), 68, 393-415

12. Bouvier, M. and Gonella, J. (1981). Nervous control of the internal anal sphincter in the cat. J. Physiol., 310, 457-469

76

Rectal Function in Patients with Idiopathic Chronic Constipation

J. BEHAR and P. BIANCANI

INTRODUCTION

Idiopathic chronic constipation is a common but poorly understood syndrome. It is thought that its causes are multifactorial with disordered colonic or rectosigmoid motor function as important patho-genetic factors (1, 2). The rectum plays a crucial role in the production of a normal stool. Distension of the rectal ampulla by a fecal bolus causes the urge to defecate and triggers the defecation reflex which ultimately leads to the evacuation of its content (3, 4).

In the present investigation, we examined both rectal perception and motor function in patients with idiopathic chronic constipation and in control subjects.

MATERIALS AND METHODS

These studies were performed in 15 subjects with normal bowel movements defined as 1-2 formed stools per day and in 56 consecutive patients referred to the Gastrointestinal Motility Laboratory for rectal function studies because of idiopathic chronic constipation of at least one year duration. All these patients suffered from constipation defined by 2 stools a week or less and were unresponsive to convention-al treatment for constipation consisting of increased fiber in their diet and mild laxatives. Most of these patients frequently resorted to the use of enemas for the evacuation of stools. Detailed history revealed that most patients had constipation for many years and that

459

lack of urge to defecate was a major complaint. Bloating, abdominal distension, and cramps were common complaints. Those patients were ambulatory and had no evidence of any systemic disease, back trauma, neuropathies, or any other gastrointestinal disease. They were not taking any medication that could affect the motor function of the gastrointestinal tract such as anticholinergic, ganglionic blockers, or muscle relaxants. Both control and constipated subjects had normal sigmoidoscopy and barium enema. Barium enema did not reveal any dilatation of the colon or rectosigmoid.

All subjects received enemas the night and morning before the rectal motility studies. Rectal exam prior to the motility study revealed that the ampulla was empty of stool. Rectal studies were carried out with a four lumen tube, three of which had side openings 2 cm apart and the fourth lumen was connected to a balloon placed 2 cm orad to the most distal opening. The triple lumen tube was constantly perfused using a low compliance pneumohydraulic pump. Pressures were recorded by Statham pressure transducers connected to a 6-channel Beckman polygraph. The four lumen tube with the balloon was introduced in the rectum and advanced to about 25 cm and was gradually pulled back until the initial side opening detected the beginning of the high pressure zone of the internal anal sphincter (IAS). Rectal pressures were recorded for 10 minutes and then the balloon was randomly inflated with air to volumes of 10, 20, 30, 40, 50, 60, 70, and 80 cc. Prior to the inflation with a given volume, the balloon was completely deflated by aspirating the air from the balloon. To avoid rectal accomodation (5), the balloon was rapidly inflated to the desired volume with a 100 cc syringe. The patient was then asked to describe the rectal sensation felt with each balloon distension. Patients were also asked to describe any sensation while the balloon remained deflated. Patients were told that they should expect to perceive pressure or urge to defecate. Rectal perception was scored as follows: 0=no sensation; 1=barely noticed pressure; 2=clear sensation to fullness; and, 3=urge to defecate. Each volume was used twice in a random fashion.

After assessing rectal perception, we proceeded with a gradual pull through at 1 cm steps to determine resting pressures and per cent relaxation of the IAS. The high pressure zone was recorded with all three side openings. The highest pressure recorded in any of the three side openings was taken as indicative of IAS pressures. At each point of the high pressure zone of the IAS, the balloon was inflated with volumes between 50 and 80 cc of air to elicit relaxation. In small groups of 4 control subjects and 5 patients with chronic constipation, relaxation was induced at the highest pressure point with balloon volumes of 10, 30, 50, and 70 cc of air (P>0.05).

RESULTS

Patients with idiopathic chronic constipation had a marked decrease in rectal perception (Fig. 1). Perception was significantly reduced with all balloon volumes when compared to control subjects (P<0.01). Only 5 patients had perception curves similar to the mean rectal perception of control subjects. Abnormal perception was more evident with small volumes. Fourty-seven (91%) of the remaining 51 patients with impaired rectal perception had complete absence of perception with balloon volumes from 10 to 40 cc's. Resting IAS pressures and percent relaxation during rectal distension with maximal balloon volumes were not different in patients and in controls. IAS pressure (Fig. 2) was 59 ± 1.6 (mean ± SE) in control subjects and 67 ± 3.9 mm in patients with chronic constipation (P<0.2). In 8 patients, however, the pressure was greater than 83 mm Hg and thus was more than 2 SD greater than the mean pressure of normal subjects. Likewise, the percent relaxation of the IAS (Fig. 3) was 88% ± 2.6 in controls and was 79% ± 3.2 (P<0.3) in patients with chronic constipation.   In 11 patients, however, the IAS relaxation was 60% or less. This was more than 2 SD below the mean of control subjects. Of these 11 patients with abnormal IAS relaxation (Fig. 4), 5 had normal perception curves with 4 patients having extremely low per cent IAS relaxation (37% or less). The remaining 6 patients who had IAS relaxation from 40 to 60% also had impaired rectal perception.

IAS relaxation as function of increased balloon volumes also was investigated. Fig. 5 shows that the per cent relaxation induced by balloon volumes of 10, 30, 50, and 70 cc's was the same in control subjects and patients with chronic constipation.

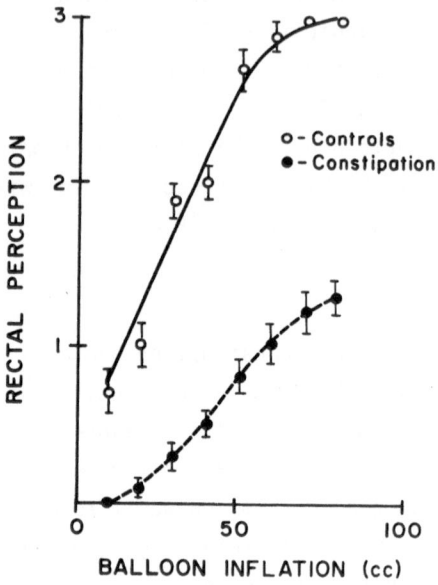

Fig. 1: Rectal perception of increasing balloon volumes in 15 control
subjects and in 56 patients with idiopathic chronic constipation. Values are means ± SE. Rectal perception in
patients with chronic constipation is markedly reduced when
compared to control subjects (P<0.01).

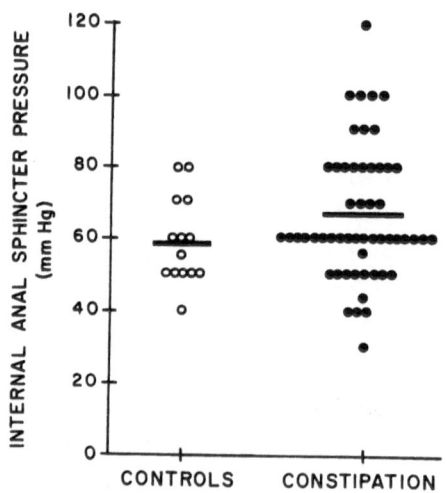

Fig. 2: Internal anal sphincter pressure in control subjects and in
patients with idiopathic chronic constipation. Points are
pressures of individual subjects. Lines indicate the mean
values.

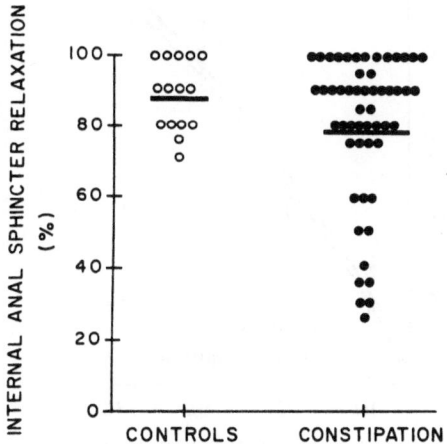

Fig. 3: Internal anal sphincter relaxation in control subjects and in patients with idiopathic chronic constipation. Points represent the per cent relaxation of each individual subject. The mean values are expressed as lines.

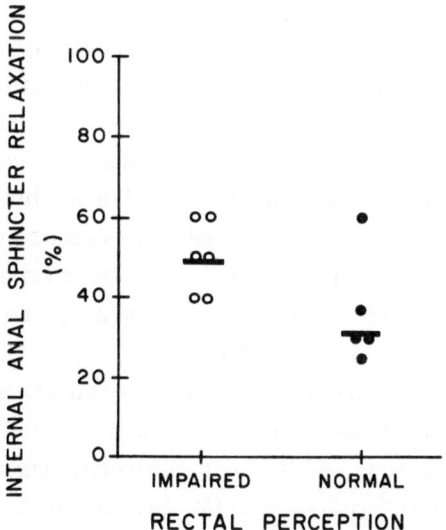

Fig. 4: Rectal perception in a subgroup of patients with impaired internal anal sphincter relaxation. Points represent in-dividual values and lines mean values. Patients with normal perception tended to have greater impairment of relaxation.

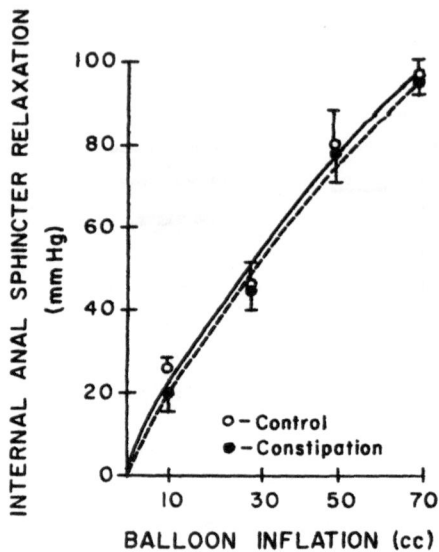

Fig. 5:   Internal anal sphincter relaxation as a function of rectal
           balloon volumes in 4 control subjects and in 5 patients with
           idiopathic chronic constipation. Values are means ± SE.

DISCUSSION

Patients with idiopathic chronic constipation frequently complain of
lack of urge to defecate. The results of the present study explain
this symptom with the finding of impaired perception to rectal distension with balloon volumes from 10-80 cc's. Most of these patients
had complete absence of rectal perception to balloons inflated with
volumes between 10 and 40 cc's and impaired but present sensation with
volumes of 50-80 cc's. The smaller balloon volumes mimick the normal
caliber, and suggest that lack of urge to defecate may be an important
factor in the pathogenesis of constipation.

   While most patients with chronic constipation had abnormal perception, their IAS exhibited normal pressures and relaxed fully in
response to rectal distension. A distinct subgroup, however, comprising 20% of the patients studied had IAS relaxation 2 SD lower than
the mean values of control subjects. In about half of these patients,
who also had the most abnormal IAS relaxation, rectal perception to
balloon distension was normal. In this small group of patients, the
failure of the IAS to fully relax may be of clinical significance and

could have contributed to the pathogenesis of patient's constipation. (6).

Although rectal perception of the stool appears to be an important factor in the physiology of normal defecation, complete absence of perception did not affect IAS relaxation in response to rectal distension. The per cent relaxation in normal subjects and in patients with chronic constipation, most of whom had abnormal perception, was the same at all volumes of rectal distension.

These studies suggest that absence of perception of rectal distension may be a major contributing factor in patients with idiopathic chronic constipation confirming the patient's history of lack of urge to defecate. This abnormal rectal perception does not appear to be related to the diameter of the rectum since the rectal diameter as determined by barium enema was not different in patients with chronic constipation and in control subjects. Impairment of rectal perception could be the result of the chronic constipation itself. Continuous presence of a large fecal bolus in the rectum could desensitize its sensory receptors. This perception, however, should be corrected after prolonged and successful therapy of the constipation. Rectal perception remained abnormal in 5 constipated patients who responded well to treatment with normal bowel movements, one stool per 1-2 days for at least a year (Behar J., Unpublished Observations). The sample is too small, however, to completely exclude this possibility. The effect of rectal perception on normal bowel habits also has been demonstrated in other diseased states. Increased sensitivity to rectal balloon distension has been shown in patients with active ulcerative colitis (7). The inflamed rectum is unable to tolerate large volumes resulting in frequent stools. Reflex relaxation, however, was unaffected by the altered sensory response.

These findings suggest that voluntary training may be an important part in the management of patients with idiopathic chronic constipation.

REFERENCES

1. Mendeloff, A.L. (1968). Defecation. In: Code, C.F. (ed). Handbook of Physiology: Section 6: Alimentary Canal. Vol IV, pp. 2140-
2143. (Baltimore, Maryland: Waverly Press, Inc.).
2. Devroede, G. and Soffie, M. (1973). Colonic absorption in idiopathic constipation. Gastroenterology, 64, 552-561.
3. Schuster, M.M. (1968). Motor action of rectum and anal sphincters
in continence and defecation. In: Code, C.F. (ed). Handbook of
Physiology: Section 6: Alimentary Canal. Vol IV, pp.2121-2140.
(Baltimore, Maryland: Waverly Press, Inc.).
4. Ihre, T. (1974). Studies on anal function in continent and incontinent patients. Scand. J. Gastroenterol., Suppl. 25, 1-64.
5. Arhan, P., Faverdin, C., Persoz, B. et al. (1976). Relationship
between viscoelastic properties of the rectum and anal pressure in
man. J. Appl. Physiol., 41, 677-682.
6. Martelli, H., Devroede, G., Arhan, P., and Duguay, C. (1978).
Mechanisms of idiopathic constipation: Outlet obstruction. Gastroenterology, 75, 623-631.
7. Farthing, M.J.G. and Lennard-Jones, J.E. (1978). Sensibility of
the rectum to distension and the anorectal distension reflex in
ulcerative colitis. Gut, 19, 64-69.

77

Severe, Idiopathic Constipation is Caused by a Distinct Abnormality of the Colonic Myenteric Plexus (Abstract)

S. KRISHNAMURTHY, M. D. SCHUFFLER, C. E. POPE and C. A. ROHRMANN

We analyzed 26 patients, all women with severe constipation without obvious organic cause. Clinical: 24/26 were between 19-39 yrs. The duration of constipation was from ½-30 yrs. 7 had constipation from childhood and 7 from adolescence. Stool frequency was once every 5-30 days; 16/26 had stools once in 10-30 days. 25/26 had abdominal pain, bloating and distention; 22/26 had nausea and 4/26 occasional vomiting. 4 patients previously had anorexia nervosa and 3 had psychiatric problems. All 26 were on multiple laxatives. Radiography: One patient had gaseous distension of the stomach; but no patient had gaseous distention of small bowel or colon; 13/13 had normal UGI and small bowel series. Barium enemas were normal in 16/26; 10/26 had long redundant colons and 6/10 had increased colonic widths (8-15 cm). None had a narrowed rectal segment. Esophageal manometry: 12/22 were normal. 10/22 had high amplitude (180-240 mm) peristalsis, 3/22 had long duration waves. Solid meal gastric emptying studies were normal in 23/23. Pathology: Mucosal rectal biopsies showed normal submucosal neurons in 26/26 and melanosis coli in 6/26. 12 had subtotal colectomies because of severe constipation. H&E stains of the resected colons showed normal circular and longitudinal muscles in 11/12, and thin muscle layers in 1/12. By this technique we saw no definite abnormalities of the myenteric plexus (MP); quantitative neuron counts were normal in 12/12. In contrast, silver stains of longitudinal sections of the MP showed a) decreased numbers of argyrophilic neurons, b) predominance of active, variably sized nuclei in the ganglia, some with associated faintly staining cytoplasm and c) decrease in axons. The patients with constipation could be differentiated from normal controls on coded review. Conclusions: 1) Severe idiopathic constipation may cause significant clinical disability in young women; 2) barium enemas and rectal biopsies are helpful in excluding Hirschsprung's disease; 3) Esophageal manometric abnormalities, usually high amplitude contractions, are present in 50% of tested patients; 4) some patients have a distinctive abnormality of the myenteric plexus distinguishable from controls, and different from those previously encountered in pseudo-obstruction syndromes; 5) although total neurons are quantitatively normal, argyrophilic neurons are decreased in number.

78

Physiological Study of the Lower Digestive Tract in Primary Constipation

P. MEUNIER

Since the classical study by Connell (1) it is a common believe that, in constipation, the major motor disorder consists in oversegmentation of the sigmoid colon providing a pressure barrier for the transit of stools. Although often confirmed by others (2-5), this opinion might be well disputable since a single digital examination of the rectum proves high incidence of stool retention in the rectum of constipated patients. Moreover, in a previous study of sigmoid motility in primary idiopathic constipation, we observed that sigmoid motor functions were normal in most of cases (6). Furthermore, frequent anorectal motility disorders were found, recently, in constipated patients (7-10). The present study was therefore undertaken to establish which motility disorder is primarily involved in chronic idiopathic constipation. To this aim, manometric studies of the sigmoid colon and of the anorectum were carried out ; a compliance study of the rectum was added to the manometric investigation.

MATERIAL AND METHODS

Subjects. This investigation was carried out on
healthy volunteers and on chronically constipated
patients. The control population consisted of 20 subjects
(6 F, 14 M) aged 19-26 yr (mean age = 21 $\pm$ 1 yr) ;
these subjects considering themselves healthy were
selected using a standardized questionnaire, they passed
at least 3 normal stools in a week.
The constipated patients consisted of 56 subjects (40 F,
16 M) aged 18-63 yr (mean age = 38 $\pm$ 11.2 yr). They
were selected on well defined clinical criteria, among
them notably : longlife constipation, longlasting
laxative abuse and a recent failure to bran and/or
lactulose therapy. However, patients with objective
proofs of true laxative disease (absent haustration on
barium enema and hypokaliemia) were excluded of this
study. All constipated patients of this series were
thoroughly investigated to exclude any other
gastrointestinal disease and neurologic, endocrine or
drug induced constipation.

Methods. The manometric and compliance studies were
successively performed during a single test period which
followed a 18-20 hr fast. A cleansing enema was adminis-
tred 4 to 6 hr before each study. The total investigation
included the following three steps ; 1) sigmoid motility
study, 2) rectoanal manometric study, 3) rectal
compliance study.
    1. Sigmoid motility study : a double lumen catheter
with side-openings spaced at 10 cm interval was introduced into the sigmoid colon through a rigid rectoscope, so
that the openings were approximatively at 25 and 15 cm
from the anal margin. The 2 lumens (ID = 2 mm) were
perfused with water by means of a constant infusion pump
(flow rate = 0.13 ml/min). Each lumen was connected to a

pressure transducer, the output of which was amplified
and recorded on a multichannel galvanometer recorder.
During the motility study, the patient rested in the left
supine position. Motor activity was recorded 30 min while
the subjects were fasted ; then a test meal of between
2300 and 2500 kJ was eated in less than 10 min : finally
30 min of postprandial motor activity was recorded. The
quantitative study analysis described elesewhere in
details (6) was limited here to the postprandial motility
index (MI), that is the product of the mean amplitude of
waves and the percentage of activity. Only the recordings
obtained at 25 cm (in the sigmoid colon) were analyzed
here.

2. Rectoanal manometric study : details of the methods
have been reported previously (10), thus only the
essential will be reported presently. This step of the
study was done using a tandem system of 2 perfused catheters (flow rate = 0.24 ml/min) inserted respectively in
the rectal ampula and the anal canal. A latex balloon was
inserted in the rectum and allowed transient distension
of the rectal wall. The rectoanal inhibitory reflex (that
is an anal relaxation after rectal distension) was found
in each subject, ruling out constipation due to aganglionosis (11). The conscious rectal sensitivity threshold
(CRST), that is the first sensation after a transient
rectal distension was studied an expressed in ml. Then, a
single perfused catheter (flow rate : 4.4 ml/min) was
used to perform a rectoanal pressure profile and to
record the maximal anal resting closure pressure (MARCP)
expressed in kPa.

3. Rectal compliance study : at this last step of the
investigation, a pressure-volume curve of the rectum was
recorded using a double lumen catheter on which a disten-
ding balloon was mounted. One lumen of the catheter was
water filled and used to record the intraballoon
pressure. The second lumen was used to distend the

balloon (a simple condom) with air in incremental
fashion. This device was introduced in the rectum without
the help of a rectoscope. Filling of the rectum was
stopped immediately after the subject experienced a
painful reaction ; at this step, according to Ihre (12),
the maximal rectal tolerable volume was reached, the
corresponding pressure (maximal tolerable pressure) was
checked from the recording. The ratio of the maximal
rectal volume and the maximal rectal pressure provided
the maximal rectal compliance (MRC) expressed in ml/kPa.

RESULTS

Results founded in both populations are presented on
table 1.

Table 1 : Mean results ($\pm$ 1 SD) observed in control
subjects and constipated patients

	Controls	Patients
MI	488 $\pm$ 174.7	658 $\pm$ 558.7
MARCP	7.6 $\pm$ 2.66	11.2 $\pm$ 3.81
CRST	17.5 $\pm$ 9.80	32.2 $\pm$ 71.84
MRC	42.9 $\pm$ 9.31	57.4 $\pm$ 53.36

The comparisons, using "t" tests, of these mean values
proved that only the mean MARCP was significantly
different (higher) in the constipated patients. Nevertheless, considering that the normal range of the parameters
was the mean value $\pm$ 2 SD found in the controls   .
(table 2), a classification of the constipated patients
was undertaken.

Table 2 : Normal range (mean $\pm$ 2 SD) of
each parameter

	Lower limit	Upper limit
MI	138	798
MARCP	5.3	9.9
CRST		37
MRC	24.5	61.5

Thus, it appeared that constipation was related to a
pure sigmoid motility disorder (that is with normal
MARCP, CRST, and MRC) in 10 patients (18 %), 7 of whom
exhibited an increased MI ("hypermotor" patients) and 3
others had a decreased MI ("hypomotor" patients).
Twentyfour patients (43 %) presented pure rectoanal
disorders (with normal sigmoid motility) ; with notably :
increased MARCP (anal hypertonia) in 8 subjects,
increased CRST (decreased rectal sensitivity) in 8
patients, and increased MRC (high rectal compliance) in
12 patients. In 17 other patients, the motility disorders
were both colonic and rectoanal. Only 5 constipated
patients (9 %) had all parameters of the study normal.

DISCUSSION

In many cases, constipation is only a symptom related
to a primary cause (metabolic, neurologic, anal lesion,
or use of various drugs) and, when such a primary cause
is ruled out, the more often, constipation is considered
as "psychogenic". Obviously, very often, chronically
constipated patients do have an impaired personality, but
it has never been proved that psychogenic disorders alter
defecation mechanisms. To the contrary, some recent
studies (7-10) clearly demonstrated that patients with

idiopathic constipation do have abnormal colorectal
motility, a cause for which must be found. This study is
a further demonstration that in most of cases, in idiopathic constipation, there are abnormality in muscular
functions of the lower digestive tract. Here, only 9 % of
the patients exhibited all the parameters of the study
normal. Therefore, the "normal" patients call to mind
constipation due to stool retention in the proximal colon
observed by Martelli et al. (9) in their pellets transit
study. It clearly appears that only physiopathologic
studies are able to unravel the various and complex
mechanisms of idiopathic constipation.

This work has been performed in part with a grant from
la Faculté de Biologie Humaine, Lyon, and the material
support of INSERM U 45.

REFERENCES

1. Connell, A.M. (1962). The motility of the pelvic colon
II. Paradoxical motility in diarrhoea and constipation.
Gut, 3, 342-8
2. Chaudary, N.A., and Truelove, S.C. (1961). Human
colonic motility : a comparative study of normal subjects
patients with ulcerative colitis, and patients with the
irritable colon syndrome. II. The effect of protigmin.
Gastroenterology, 40, 18-26
3. Chowdury, A.R., Dinoso, V.P., and Lorber, S.H. (1976).
Characterization of a hyperactive segment at the recto-
sigmoid junction. Gastroenterology, 71, 584-8
4. Kirwan, W.O., and Smith, A.N. (1977). Colonic propulsion in diverticular disease, idiopathic constipation,
and the irritable colon syndrome. Scand. J.
Gastroenterol., 12, 331-5

5. Waller, S.L., and Misiewicz, J.J. (1972). Colonic motility in constipation or diarrhoea. Scand. J. Gastroenterol., 7, 93-6

6. Meunier, P., Roohas, A., and Lambert, R. (1979). Motor activity of the sigmoid colon in chronic constipation : comparative study with normal subjects. Gut, 20, 1095-1101.

7. Arhan, P., Devroede, G., Jehannin, B. et al. (1983). Idiopathic disorders of fecal incontinence in children. Pediatrics, 71, 774-9

8. Loening-Baucke, V. and Younoszai, M.K. (1982). Abnormal anal sphincter response in chronically constipated children. J. Pediatr, 100, 213-8

9. Martelli, H., Devroede, G., Arhan, P., et al. (1978). Mechanisms of idiopathic constipation : outlet obstruction. Gastroenterology, 75 : 623-31.

10. Meunier, P., Maréchal, J.M., and Jaubert de Beaujeu, M. (1979). Rectoanal pressures and rectal sensitivity studies in chronic childhood constipation. Gastroenterology, 77, 330-6

11. Lawson, J.O.N., and Nixon, H.H. (1967). Anal canal pressures in the diagnosis of Hirschsprung's disease. J. Pediatr. Surg., 2, 544-52

12. Ihre, T. (1974). Studies on anal function in continent and incontinent patients. Scand. J. Gastroenterol., 9 (suppl. 25), 1-80

79

Intestinal Transit time is Related with Different Anorectal Motility Patterns in Chronic Non-Organic Constipation

G. A. LANFRANCHI, G. BAZZOCCHI, M. CAMPIERI, C. BRIGNOLA, F. FOIS, L. MARZIO and G. LABÒ

Constipation is a symptom common to many and different dis eases. It is due, at any rate, to an altered transit of intestinal contents, but it can be a secondary symptom in an organic intestinal and extraintestinal disease, or it can be caused by a primary motor disorder of the bowel. Also in this latter case constipation may be either the main or the only symptom, or it may belong to the wide range of the irritable bowel syndrome. On the other hand, even the definition of constipation is controversial: constipation may be defined as a reduced frequency of evacuations, as a difficulty in stools expulsion or as expulsion of too small stools. For all these reasons, the patients suffering from constipation do not make a homogeneous group. The studies aiming at investigating the intestinal motor alterations responsible for constipation, should consider this problem and should therefore be carried out for cases selected according to clear nosological criteria.

On the basis of these considerations, we studied a group of 25 patients affected by severe constipation: they re ported spontaneous evacuations only every 8-15 days or evacuations exclusively induced by the use of laxatives or by the administration of enemas. The symptom was considered as chronic because persisting for more than five years. The

477

negative results of barium enema, rectosigmoidoscopy, and
screening biochemical examinations allowed to exclude an or
ganic origin of the disease. Previous works (1,2,3) ques
tioned the reliability of history for a precise definition
of constipation; therefore we decided to assess the sever
ity of the symptom by studying the gastrointestinal transit
by means of radioopaque markers according to the method
defined by Arhan and coll. (4). According to this research,
the upper limit of the excretion of 80% of the markers was
found to be 96 h in the control population. The total tran
sit time was above 96 h only in 56% of patients i.e.
177 ± 6.3 h (range 136 and above 192 h), while it was with
in this limit in the remaining 44% of patients i.e.
68 ± 7.5 h (range 24 - 85 h) (Fig 1).

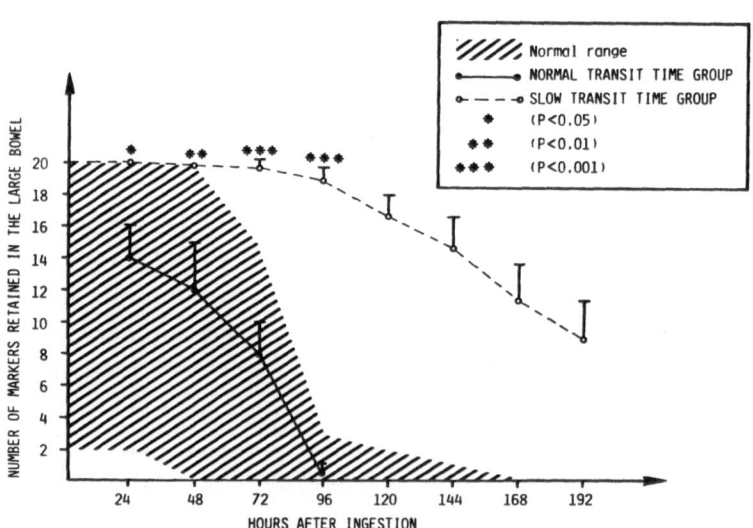

It can therefore be asserted that the severity of constipa
tion, deduced by the information given by patients, is not
related with the intestinal transit time.

All the patients were therefore submitted to an anorec
tal motility study by means of perfused catheters, follow
ing a method already reported (5). The parameters behaviour
was not uniform in all the patients, but it becomes uniform
if we take the transit time as reference point. In fact, in
patients presenting transit times above the normal level,
a resting pressure of the upper anal canal significantly
lower than that found in the group with normal transit time
was registered (Fig 2).

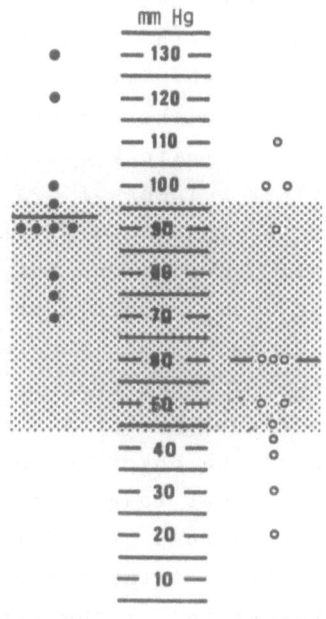

NORMAL TRANSIT   SLOW TRANSIT
TIME GROUP   TIME GROUP

MAXIMUM RESTING PRESSURE OF THE UPPER ANAL CANAL

Also the amplitude of the internal anal sphincter relax
ation is reduced in the first group, compared with the
second group and this discrepancy, already remarkable at
50 ml (52 $\pm$ 7.5 versus 31.6 $\pm$ 4.1 mm Hg, p 0.05 with
Student's T test for unpaired data) becomes more and more
marked with progressively increasing values of rectal dis
tention up to 200 ml of air (76 $\pm$ 7.2 versus 42.5 $\pm$ 5.5 mm
Hg, p $<$ 0.01).

Also rectal sensitivity is different in the two groups;
in fact, the patients with normal transit experienced rec
tal distention at 26.0 $\pm$ 8.0 ml (values within the normal
range), whereas in the patients with slow transit, the sen
sitivity threshold was reached at values higher than
40 $\pm$ 8 ml. These differences become even more evident for
other sensitivity parameters: the need to evacuate was re
ported at 70 $\pm$ 17 ml air in the first group (values within
the normal range), whereas in the second group the recorded
values, 168 $\pm$ 27 ml, are definitely abnormal. Rectal disten
tion became painful at air volumes of 176 $\pm$ 13 ml in the
first group (values at the lower limits of the normal range)
while the pain threshold was high and definitely abnormal
in the group presenting slow transit (348 $\pm$ 26.2 ml). There
fore, the distinction of two groups according to the intes
tinal transit time allows to show two significantly differ
ent patterns of the anorectal motility and sensitivity,
even though an overlap may be observed for single values.

Intestinal transit time was found to be related with a
clinical parameter, the presence of abdominal pain. In fact,
it was not reported by 76.6% of the patients with slow tran
sit, whereas it was present in all the patients with normal
transit.

In conclusion, the results obtained seem to confirm that
patients suffering from chronic non organic constipation
may be divided into two homogeneous groups for which a uni
form behaviour of the investigated parameters was regis
tered. One group is characterized by slow intestinal tran

sit, reduced motility of the internal anal sphincter and re
duced rectal sensitivity to distention; in these patients
abdominal pain is mostly absent. The other group is charac
terized by normal intestinal transit, combined with a motor
hyperactivity of the internal anal sphincter, as well as
with an increased rectal sensitivity; abdominal pain was re
ported by all these patients. The identification,within the
population complaining of constipation, of groups with dif
ferent intestinal motor activity, seems to be important,
not only for the interpretation of the pathophysiological
mechanisms, but also for the different therapeutic implica
tion.

References

1. Corazziari, E. et al. (1982). Italian Cooperative Study
on Chronic Constipation. In: Wienbeck,M. (ed).Motility of
the digestive tract. pp. 523-526 (New York: Raven Press)
2. Devroede, G. (1978). Constipation: mechanisms and manage
ment. In: Sleisinger, M.H. and Fordtran, J.S. (eds). Gastro
intestinal Disease. pp. 368-383. (Philadelphia - London -
Toronto. WB Saunders Company).
3. Preston, D.M. and Lennard Jones, J.E. (1982). Does fail
ure of bisacodyl-induced colonic peristalsis indicate in
trinsic nerve damage? GUT, 23, A 891.
4. Arhan,P. et al. (1981). Segmental colonic transit time.
Dis. Col. e Rect.,24, 625-629.
5. Lanfranchi, G.A. et al. (1983).Motor function and dysfun
ctions of the large bowel and the rectum. Colo-proct., 1,
19-22.

80

Is Incontinence in Diabetes Mellitus due to Diabetic Autonomous Neuropathy?

J. F. ERCKENBRECHT, H. J. WINTER, I. CICMIR, H. BERGER,
W. BERGES and M. WIENBECK

Changes in bowel habits are frequent manifestations of diabetic enteropathy. In a prospective study we evaluated stool frequency and stool continence by a standardized questionnaire, basal and squeeze anal sphincter pressure (ASP) by manometry, and continence to rectally infused saline (1500 ml) in 18 diabetics with autonomous neuropathy (AN), 9 diabetics without AN, and 18 nondiabetic controls comparable in sex and age to the diabetic patients. AN was determined by pathologic heart rate variation and pupillary reflex response to light, peripheral neuropathy (PN) by pathologic sensitivity to vibration and nerve conduction velocity. 9 of the 18 diabetics with AN and 3 of the 9 diabetics without AN were incontinent. Results:

	Incontinent diabetics (n = 12)	Continent diabetics (n = 15)	Nondiabetic controls (n = 18)
Basal ASP	50 ± 24^a	74 ± 27	71 ± 24
Squeeze ASP	105 ± 44^b	148 ± 35	153 ± 45
Squeeze increment	53 ± 29^c	72 ± 31	83 ± 26
Saline continence	225 ± 183^d	1315 ± 258	1387 ± 135

$^a p < 0.05$, $^b p < 0.01$, $^d p < 0.001$ compared to continent diabetics and nondiabetic controls, $^c p < 0.01$ compared to nondiabetic controls

Basal and squeeze ASP did not correlate with the degree of diabetic AN or PN.

It is concluded that fecal incontinence in diabetes mellitus is due to a) a dysfunction of the autonomous nervous system as evidenced by a decreased basal ASP and in addition b) to a dysfunction of the peripheral nervous system as evidenced by a decreased squeeze ASP and squeeze increment in incontinent diabetics compared to the non-diabetic controls. Fecal incontinence in diabetes mellitus may occur as a manifestation of diabetic AN and PN unrelated to neurological manifestations at other organs.

Section 6
Smooth Muscle, Nervous and Hormonal Control

81

Correlation between the Electrical Properties and Morphological Characteristics in the Smooth Muscle Cells during Culture

T. MARUYAMA

INTRODUCTION

Electrophysiological properties of smooth muscle cells have been extensively studied in various smooth muscle tissues. These distinct membrane properties of smooth muscle cells are based on the studies of organic tissues. Studies on the electrical properties of the smooth muscle cells from intact tissues raise certain problems because of the neural elements within the tissues, and because of the low electrical coupling between the smooth muscle cells. Furthermore, the presence of diffusion barriers and the intercellular current make it impossible to measure accurately the electrical properties of a single smooth muscle cell. To overcome such problems, researchers have described electrophysiological measurements on the cultured smooth muscle cell in vitro (1, 2, 3, 4 and 5). We re-investigated the cultured smooth muscle cells from guinea-pig taenia coli to elucidate the electrical properties of cultured smooth muscle cells.

METHODS AND MATERIALS

The cell culture

The smooth muscle cells were removed from male guinea-pig taenia coli (weight 150 to 220 g). With a razor blade, the smooth muscle cells were cut into 0.5 mm^3 blocks, which were placed into 50 ml dispersed flask with 10 ml culture medium (75 % Ham's F12 + 25 % fetal calf serum) containing 2000 units/ml disperse (Godo Shusei Co., LTD) and

0.2 % collagenase (Sigma C2139), and then slowly stirred for 2 hr. After rinsing the cells twice in the medium, the cell suspension was passed through a 50 μm pore filter and then the residues were trans- ferred to dishes (Falcon dish, 3001). The cells were grown routinely in a humidified atmosphere 5 % CO_2, 5 % O_2 and 90 % air at 37.5°C. After 5 days, the cells were incubated with the culture medium (containing 1000 units/ml disperse) for 3 hr and gently mixed for 10 min. After rinsing the cells in the medium, the cell suspension was passed through a 50 μm pore filter and the residues were transferred to Falcon dishes. In one week, most of cells formed colonies. After two weeks in the culture, the cells were incubated with the culture medium (containing 1000 units/ml disperse) for 1 hr and mixed for 10 min. After rinsing the cells in the medium, the cell suspension was passed through a 12 μm Nuclepore (N 1200CR04700) and the residues were transferred to Falcon dishes. The cells gradually prolifereated in our culture system.

Electrical measurements

The smooth muscle cells which were attached to the surface of the petri dish in the control medium (Joklik-Mod, Gibco 410-1300, 10 mM Hepes buffer, pH 7.4) were observed under phase contrast microscope (Olympus IMT, Japan), and the glass microelectrode was inserted in these cells. The membrane potential and input resistance were measured with the glass microelectrode filled with 3M KCl plus 10 mM K-citrate. Electrode having the final resistance between 70-90 x 10^6 ohm were selected for use. A reference electrode (Ag-AgCl plate) was immersed in the medium. A current pulse, using a stimulator unit (Nihon Koden model MSD-3) was applied through the same glass microelectrode, and the potential of membrane was monitored with a preamplifier unit (W-P Instrument model KS and 710). The data were observed on a storage oscilloscope (Tektronix model 5111), photographed by a Kymograph camera (Grass model C4F), and recorded by Rectigraph (San-Ei., LTD). To avoid an underestimation of the membrane potential, the electrical properties of each cell were determined 3 min after the establishment of electrical stability and steady state. All experiments were conduc- ted at 37 ± 1°C.

RESULTS AND DISCUSSION

We maintained groups of cultured smooth muscle cells in the same

dishes for 12, 24, 48, 120, 168 and 336 hr. Cell morphology and
growth were controled by phase contrast microscope. Fig. 1 shows phase
contrast micrographs at 12 and 168 hr. 12 hr after seeding, the cells
had just attached and were spread out. 168 hr after, the cells proli-
ferated, became semiconfluent and lined up in linear parallel arrays.
The 336 hr confluent culture showed flat, spindle-and ribbon-shaped
cells that exhibited the typical formation of smooth muscle cells (6,
7 and 8).

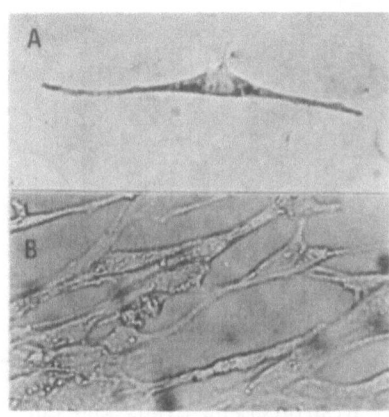

FIGURE 1 Phase contrast micrographs
of   cultured smooth
muscle cells. (A) after 12
hr in vitro, the cell is
just dividing and have two
nuclei. (B) after 168 hr in
vitro, semiconfluent cells.
x 220

The electrophysiological properties of cell membrane were performed in a single cell or a few smooth muscle cells in 12 and 168 hr
in culture since the cultured smooth muscle cells develop gap junctions (9, 10 and 11). Consequently electrical coupling were observed
between the cultured smooth muscle cells (3 and 4). Within 12 hr of
the culture, the cells were fragile. In most cases, the resting membrane potential in 1.8 mM Ca ions containing medium was - 24 $\pm$ 2.2 mV
(Mean $\pm$ SE, n = 26). When the extracellular Ca ions was increased to
10.8 mM, the membrane potential was increased to - 34.2 $\pm$ 1.6 mV
(N = 19). It appeared to be easier to obtain a successful impalement
in 10.8 mM Ca ions containing medium.

Fig. 2A shows the time course of the electrotonic potential change in response to rectangular hyperpolarizing current pulse of 500
msec duration. The rising phase of the electrotonic potential seems
adequately described by the equation for a simple RC circuit. Fig. 2B
shows a semilog plot of potential as a function of time and also demonstrates how the time constant was measured in these experiments.
The mean time constant in 168 hr   cultured cells in 1.8 mM Ca ions

containing medium was 78.2 msec. From the values of the electrical
time constant and input resistance, capacity was calculated as 1.3 nF.
The values of the resting membrane potential in cultured smooth muscle
cells in 1.8 mM Ca ions containing medium are in good agreement with
the early work of Robert D. Puves et al., (1), and the time constant
and capacity of cultured cells are qualitatively similar to those seen
in guinea-pig taenia coli (11).

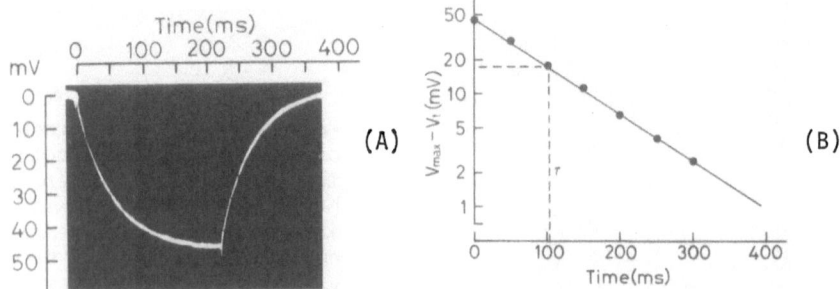

FIGURE 2 168 hr cultured smooth muscle cell. The time course of an
electrotonic potential and the method of calculating the
electrical time constant (τ). (A) The final potential displacement caused by the hyperpolarizing current pulse was 45.6
mV. (B) the maximal potential displacement minus the cur-
rent-evoked potential change at different times after the
start of current injection is plotted as a function of time
in a semilog diagram. The time constant (τ) is indicated.

Fig. 3 shows the typical example of membrane potential changes of
12 hr cultured cell caused by intracellular injection of depolarizing
or hyperpolarizing current pulses. The graded evoked spike was caused
by depolarizing current pulses, but, the delayed rectification was not
obvious in these cells.

The 168 hr cultured cells were capable of producing the action
potentials with overshoot when they were directly stimulated by depolarizing and hyperpolarizing current pulses applied through an intracellular recording electrode (Fig. 3B, 4A and 6B). The action potential
was followed by a hyperpolarization after-potential and similar action
potential was observed after the break of hyperpolarizing current pulse injection (Fig. 3B). Delayed rectification was seen in these cells.
The feature of these cultured cells was to present a spike followed
by a prolonged plateau phase (Fig. 4A and 6B). The prolonged plateau
phase was more prominent when the extracellular concentration of Ca
ions was raised from 1.8 mM to 10.8 mM. In these experiments, the

mechanisms of plateau phase are unclear, but it may involve a regenerative nature of membrane and may be caused by the voltage-dependent increase in permeability to certain ions whose flux maintained the membrane potential. The membrane potential at peak of the plateau varied widely from - 10 mV to - 40 mV.

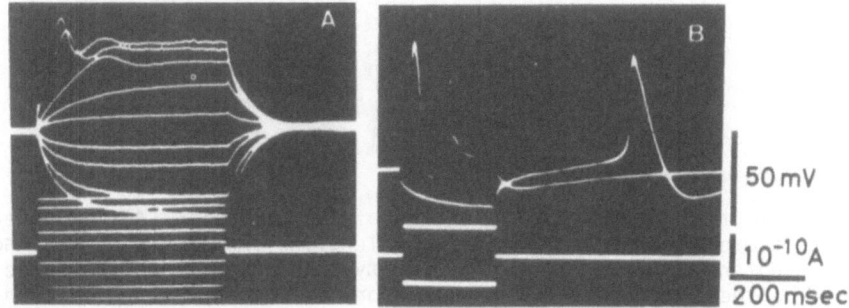

FIGURE 3 Electrophysiological responses of cultured smooth muscle cells. The upper trace of each figure shows the potential changes, while the lower shows the amplitude of applied depolarizing or hyperpolarizing currents. (A). 12 hr in vitro. (B) 168 hr in vitro.

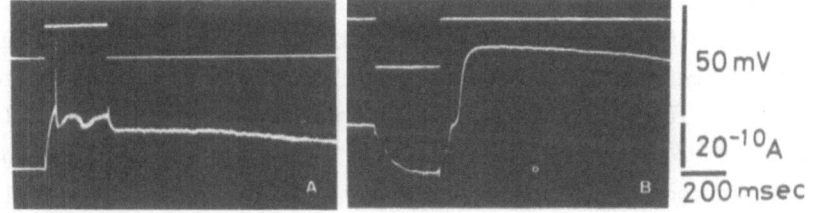

FIGURE 4 Electrophysiological responses of 168 hr cell. (A) and (B) are obtained from the same cell. The lower of each traces shows the evoked potential changes, while the upper of each traces shows the amplitude of applied depolarizing or hyperpolarizing currents.

The 168 hr cultured cells produce spontaneous action potentials (Fig. 5). These spontaneous electrical activities that are recorded in the cultured cells are similar to that observed from organ-bath preparation of guinea-pig taenia coli (12). Robert D. Purves (2) has shown that the electrical responses in the cultured cells are produced by application of ACh. In these experiments, ACh was applied to the cell by pressure injection from delivery pipette containing ACh, which was positioned about 20-30 μm from the cell. A typical potential change induced by ACh was the membrane depolarization associated with an increase of action potential frequency, as shown in Fig. 5A. The membrane depolarization lasted for about 77.8 msec. The ACh responses of the cell membrane was blocked by atropine (5 x 10^{-6} g/ml).

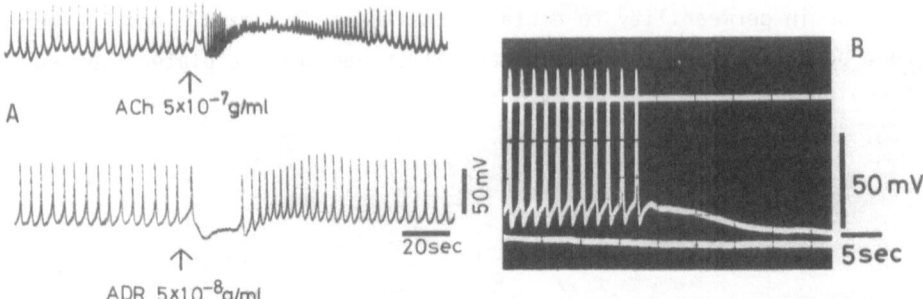

FIGURE 5 Electrophysiological responses of 168 hr cells. (A) The upper
trace shows the effects of acetylcholine (ACh) on the membrane
potential and electrical activity. The lower trace shows the
effects of noradrenaline (ADR) on the membrane potential and
electrical activity. (B) The effects of Co ions on the membrane activity.

In guinea-pig taenia coli, it was demonstrated that the mechanical inhibition by adrenaline was associated with abolition of the spontaneous spike discharge and membrane hyperpolarization (13 and 14).
When noradrenaline was applied to the cell membrane, the spontaneous
spike discharge was stopped and the membrane potential hyperpolarized
up to 15 mV (Fig. 5A). The actions of ACh and ADR on the 168 hr cultured cells showed a remarkable similarity to those recorded from organ-
bath preparations of guinea-pig taenia coli taken from adult animals
(13 and 14). However, the action of drugs were not obvious in 12 hr
cultured cells.

In general, the genesis of spikes in the smooth muscle cells are
caused by a rapid transient increase in Ca ions permeability and slowly
developing increase in K ions permeability (15 and 16). The membrane
response triggered by the applied current or the spontaneous action potentials were readily observed in TTX containing medium, however, when
Co ions were applied to the cell, the graded evoked spikes and the action potentials which were triggered by intracellular current injection
were suppressed (Fig. 5B and 6) ; the spontaneous action potentials
were also abolished by 9.8 mM Co ions (Fig. 5B). These results suggest
that part of regenerative responses in cultured smooth muscle cells
may involve a change in the permeability of Ca ions.

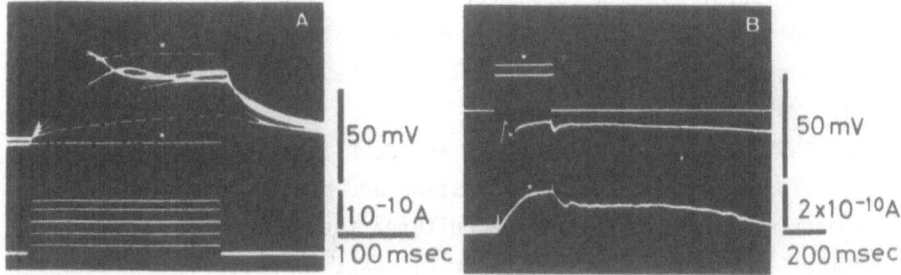

FIGURE 6 Electrophysiological responses of 12 hr (A) and 168 hr (B)
cells. (A) The upper traces show the evoked potential changes,
while the lower traces show the applied depolarizing currents.
✱ = addition of 5.4 mM Co ions. (B) the upper traces show the
applied currents, while the lower traces show the evoked membrane potential changes. ✱ = 5.4 mM Co ions.

The data indicate that the electrical properties of cultured
smooth muscle cells are in agreement with the results from studies of
organ-bath preparations of smooth muscle tissues. They also suggest
that the cultured smooth muscle cells resemble in some ways the smooth
muscle tissues and represents one useful method for research in smooth
cell physiology.

REFERENCES

1.   Purves, R.D., Mark, G.E. and Burnstock, G. (1973). The
      electrical activity of single isolated smooth muscle cells.
      Plügers Arch. ges. Physiol., 341, 325-330.

2.   Purves, R.D. (1974). Muscarinic excitation : a microelectro-
      phoretic study on cultured smooth muscle cells. Br. J. Pharmac.,
      52, 77-86.

3.   Mclean, M.J. and Speralakis, N.S. (1976). Electrophysiological
      recording from spontaneously contracting reaggregates of cultu-
      red vascular smooth muscle cells from chick embryos. Expl. Cell
      Res., 104, 309-318.

4.   Kimes, B.W. and Brandt, B.L. (1976). Characterization of two
      putative smooth muscle cell lines from rat thoracic aorta.
      Expl. Cell Res., 98, 336-347.

5.   Sinback, C.N. and Shain, W. (1979). Electrophysiological pro-
      perties of human oviduct smooth muscle cells in dissociated

cell culture. J. Cell Physiol., 98, 377-394.

6.   Campbell, G. R., Chamley, J. H. and Burnstock, G. (1974).
     Development of smooth muscle cells in tissue culture. J. Anat.,
     117, 295-312.

7.   Chamley, J. H., Campbell, G. R. and Burnstock, G. (1974).
     Dedifferentiation, redifferentiation and bundle formation of
     smooth muscle cells in tissue culture: the influence of cell
     number and nerve fibers. J. Embryol. exp. Morph., 32, 297-323.

8.   Chamley-Campbell, J., Campbell, G. R. and Ross, R. (1979).   The
     smooth muscle cell in culture. Physiol. Rev. 59, 1-61.

9.   Campbell, R. G., Uehara, Y., Mark, G. and Burnstock, G. (1971).
     Fine structure of smooth muscle cells grown in tissue culture.
     J. Cell Biol., 49, 21-34.

10. Ross, R. (1971).   The smooth muscle cell. II Growth of smooth
     muscle in culture and formation of elastic fibers. J. Cell Biol.,
     50, 172-186.

11. Tomita, T. (1966).   Membrane capacity and resistance in mammalian
     smooth muscle. J. theor. Biol., 12, 216-227.

12. Burnstock, G., Holman, M. E. and Prosser, C. L. (1963).
     Electrophysiology of smooth muscle. Physiol. Rev., 43. 482-527.

13. Bülbring, E. (1954).   Membrane potentials of smooth muscle fibres
     of the taenia coli of the guinea-pig. J. Physiol., 125, 302-315.

14. Bülbring, E. and Kuriyama, H. (1963).   Effect of changes in ionic
     environment on the action of ACh and adrenaline on smooth muscle
     cells of the guinea-pig taenia coli. J. Physiol., 166, 59-74.

15. Bülbring, E. and Kuriyama, H. (1963).   Effect of changes in the
     external sodium and calcium concentration on spontaneous
     electrical activity in smooth muscle of guinea-pig taenia coli.
     J. Physiol., 166, 29-58

16. Tomita, T. (1981).   Electrical activity (spikes and slow waves)
     in gastrointestinal smooth muscles.   In: Bülbring, E., Brading,
     A. F., Jones, A. W. and Tomita, T. Ed.   Smooth muscle: an
     assessment of current knowledge. pp. 127-156. (london: Edward
     Arnold)

82

Interstitial Cells of Cajal: Selective Uptake of Methylene Blue Inhibits Slow Wave Activity

L. THUNEBERG, V. JOHANSEN, J. J. RUMESSEN and B. G. ANDERSEN

INTRODUCTION

The cellular origin of intestinal slow waves is uncertain. It has been argued (2) that slow waves of small intestine originate in the longitudinal muscle layer, since the recordable activity follows this layer only, upon separation of the muscle layers. Slow-wave amplitudes, measured at various depths within the intact muscularis, reach a maximum at or near the boundary between the longitudinal and circular muscle layers (3, 5).

In a morphological study (6) of interstitial cells of Cajal (ICC) of mouse small intestine we divided ICC in four types, according to location in the muscularis. The network of ICC sandwiched between the muscle layers, we referred to as type I cells (ICC-I). A close, spatial correlation between ramifications of ICC-I and local contraction patterns suggested an active or passive (cf. 4) involvement of ICC-I in the excitation of intestinal muscle. Our studies of the ultrastructural organization and morphology, held together with the available electrophysiological data, led us to suggest an active role of ICC-I as intestinal pacemakers.

In the same report (6) it was demonstrated that lengths of mouse small intestine, when incubated in an oxygenated Krebs-bicarbonate solution with a low concentration of methylene blue, develop characteristic staining patterns, which cover areas of variable distribution and extension. A specific part of the intestine (A) may remain unstained

495

for hours; (B) may develop a selective staining of variable numbers of smooth muscle cells (always longitudinal muscle only); (C) may develop a selective staining of elements of Auerbach's plexus; or (D) may develop a selective staining of ICC-I. These specific patterns appear within 5-30 minutes of incubation, and most often all four staining patterns are represented along the length of a single incubated intestine.

The trapping of the oxidized dye in the selectively stained cells produces a high contrast, which allows the identification of patterns A-D at the magnification of a stereomicroscope (Figs. la, b).

To examine the hypothesis that ICC-I are intestinal pacemaker cells, we have looked for effects of a selective uptake of methylene blue on the recordable slow wave activity.

MATERIALS AND METHODS

Female albino mice were sacrificed by cervical dislocation and the intestines were quickly transferred to a modified Krebs-bicarbonate solution (NaCl 121.5; KCl 5.9; NaH_2PO_4 0.6; $NaHCO_3$ 7.7; histidine 10.0; glucose 12.6; $CaCl_2$ 5.0; $MgCl_2$ 2.4; methylene blue 0.075 (all mM); pH 7.15), which had been preequilibrated with a 95% O_2 / 5% CO_2 mixture, and warmed to 37^OC. In the reported experiments, the proximal 5 cm of the small intestine were carefully isolated and suspended in an incubation chamber by fixing the ends of the intestinal segment to the opposite walls of the chamber, whereafter a 1 mm glass capillary was introduced in the lumen to reduce sideward movements. Care was taken, not to stretch or distend the segment. The bath was perfused at 5-10 ml/min with the oxygenated medium, in most experiments at 32^OC. Oxygen concentrations were measured with an oxygen electrode (Radiometer, Copenhagen). For the identification of staining patterns (see INTRODUCTION) a Leitz stereomicroscope was used at a fixed magnification of 30x.

Electrical activities were initially recorded from the incubated tissue using extracellular (pressure or suction) electrodes. However, with these larger electrodes, it proved difficult to obtain stable records, probably due to the thinness and fragility of the muscle layers. For intracellular measurements microelectrodes of tip diameters 0.1-0.2 um were pulled (Narishige puller) from glass capillaries containing a luminal glass fibre (Clark Electromedical Instr., GC 100F-4) to allow

trouble-free backwards filling of the tip. They were filled with 3M KCL
or the incubation medium. Because of the vigorous contractions, a
floating microelectrode was used; this was suspended from a high input impedance preamplifier, which was mounted on a Leitz micromanipula-
tor. Signals were amplified and recorded by conventional techniques.

High intensity illumination was obtained from a 15V/150W halogen
lamp, connected with fibre optics and a focusing lens; or from a
1.5 mW He-Ne-laser (Siemens LGR 7621), wavelength 632.8 nm. For orientation purposes, illumination was restricted as much as possible.

RESULTS AND DISCUSSION

Under the incubation conditions used, a selective staining of the net-
work of ICC-I, extending over the surface of Peyer's patches (Figs. 1a,
b), was usually the first visible coloration of the tissue (appearing
within 10 minutes of incubation). A typical intracellular record from
a Peyer's patch with selectively stained ICC-I is in Fig. 2 compared
with a typical record from its unstained surroundings. From unstained
Peyer's patches normal records, similar to Fig. 2b, were obtained.

No consistent differences in electrical activity were observed between totally unstained areas and areas with scattered, stained muscle
cells (as in Fig. 1; cf. Figs. 3a, b). A complete staining of the longitudinal muscle layer was never observed in the living intestine, but
a heavy staining (with more than 50% of the longitudinal muscle cells
coloured) was seen (Fig. 3, lower trace).

The electrical activities shown in Fig. 2 were recorded from a preparation, which was incubated at a "low" oxygen tension (P_{O2} 300 mm Hg).
The maximal oxygen tension, which could be maintained in the incubation
medium, was about 600 mm Hg (Figs. 4 and 5). Only with this very high
oxygen level it was possible to demonstrate an initial, regular electrical activity of areas, in which ICC-I were visibly stained. The
rapid change with time of the electrogram is illustrated in Figs. 4b,
c, d and 5 c, d, e: Slow wave amplitudes decrease drastically and become more variable; a basic slow-wave frequency similar to control (unstained areas) usually persist, but with higher frequencies interfering.
The changes in slow wave activity is paralleled by changes in spike activity to produce a pattern (Figs. 5 f, g), which may show similarities
to the electrical activity, which is recordable from unstained, but
anoxic areas (Figs. 5 h, i).

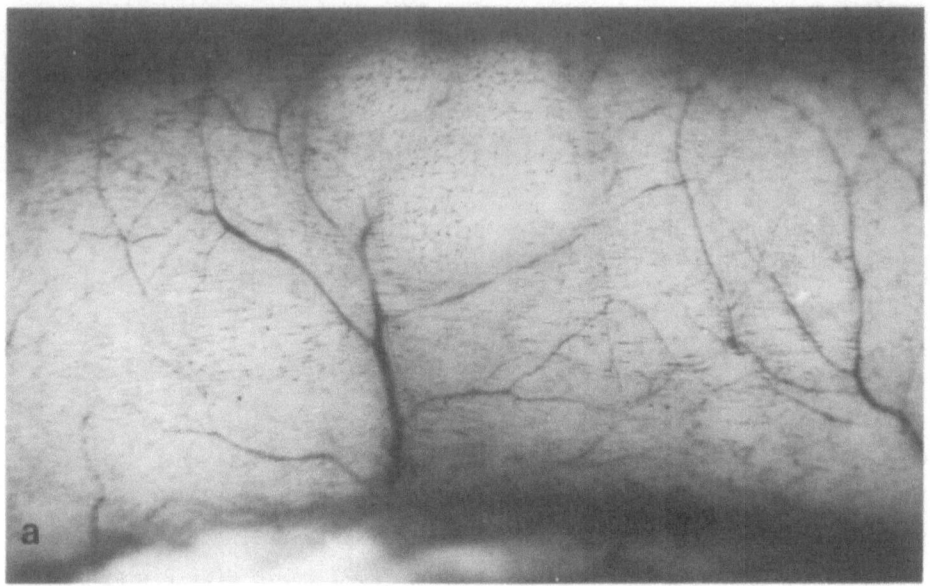

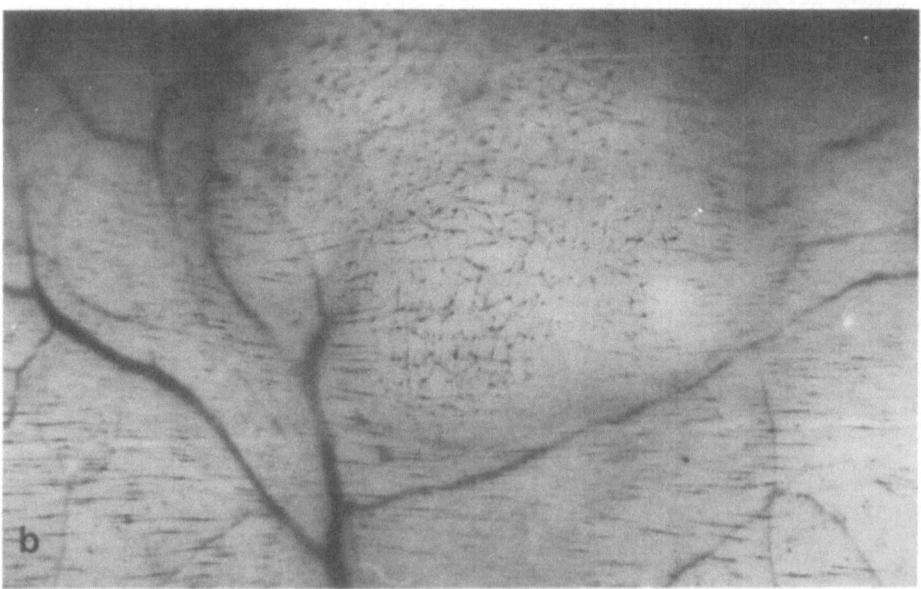

Fig. 1.   Duodenum, supravital methylene blue. The musculature overlying
a Peyer's patch shows selectively stained ICC-I, while the surrounding
musculature shows scattered, stained longitudinal muscle cells.
a: x22,   b: x42.

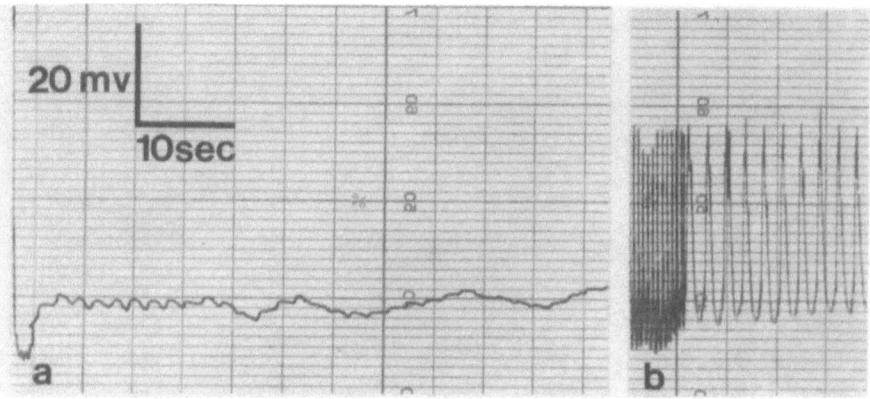

Fig. 2. Intracellular records of the electrical activity from <u>a</u>: an area with selectively stained ICC-I; <u>b</u>: an unstained neighbouring area (the first part recorded at one fourth of the indicated speed).

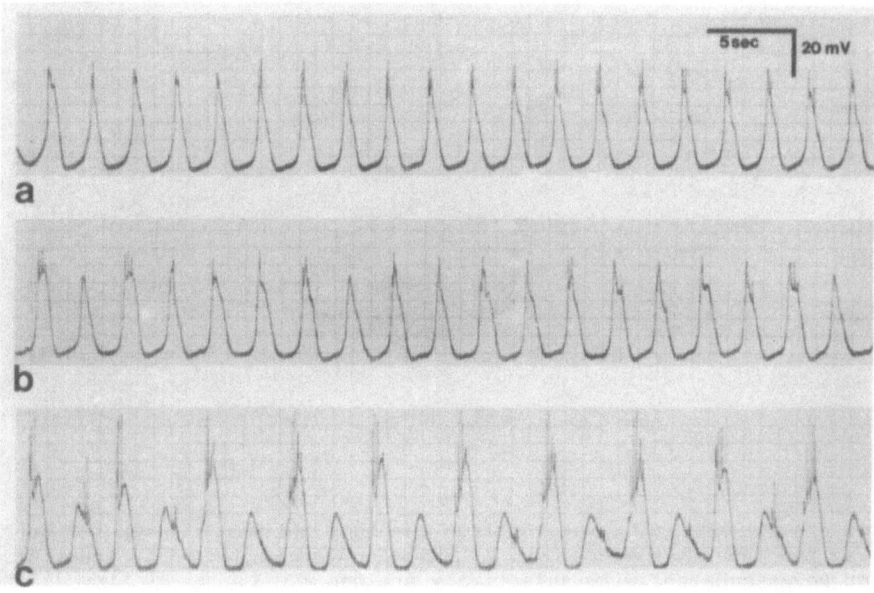

Fig. 3. Intracellular records of the electrical activity from <u>a</u>, <u>b</u>: Areas with scattered, stained smooth muscle cells of the longitudinal muscle layer; <u>c</u>: An area with a heavy staining of the longitudinal muscle layer (more than half of the muscle cells stained).

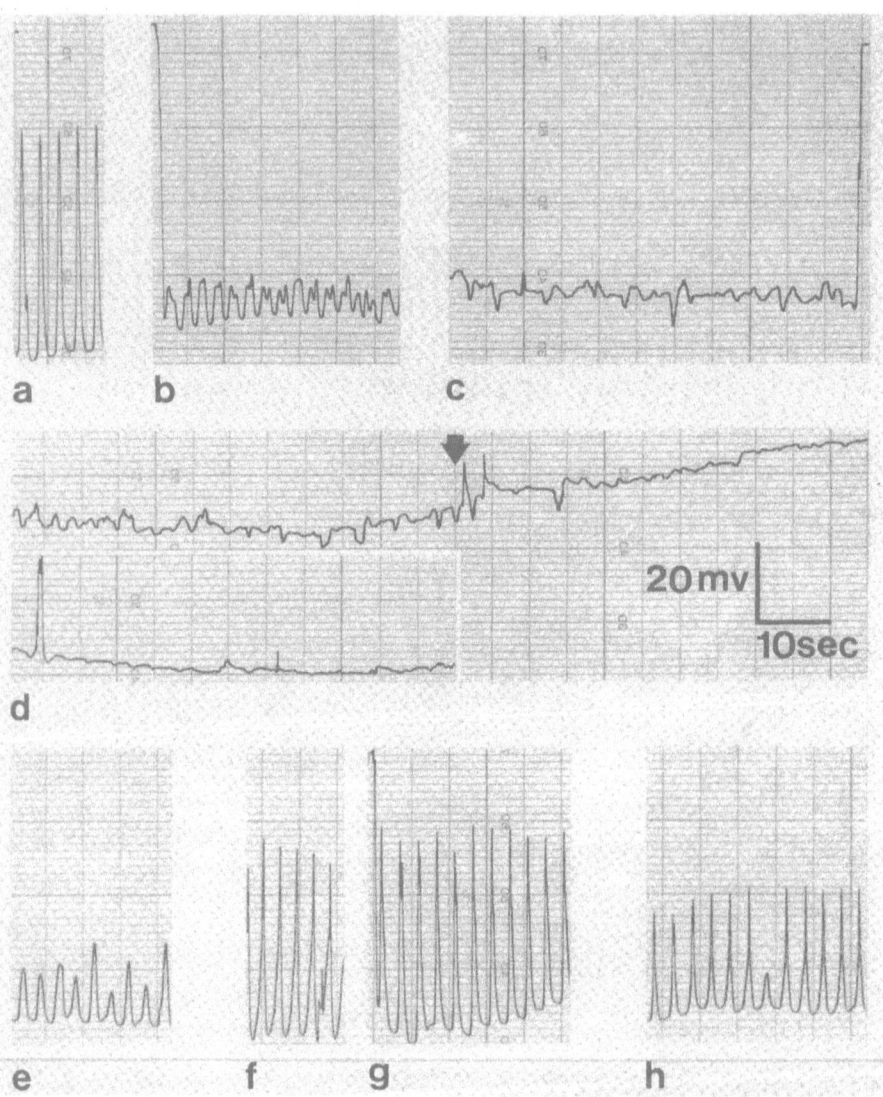

Fig. 4. Intracellular records from the same intestinal preparation and using the same microelectrode. a: Unstained area. b,c,d and inset:Area (not Peyer's patch) with selectively stained ICC-I; b: at time 0 (about 10 min after the sacrifice of the mouse); c time 17 min; d time 23 min. Arrow: He-Ne-laser on. Inset: Impalement of another cell after 2 min laser illumination. e: Unstained area close to the former area, and illuminated by laser. f,g: Unstained area after 30 and 40 min incubation, before and after 10 min laser illumination (not the same cell). h: Peyer's patch with Auerbach's plexus stained, after 3 min exposure to laser.

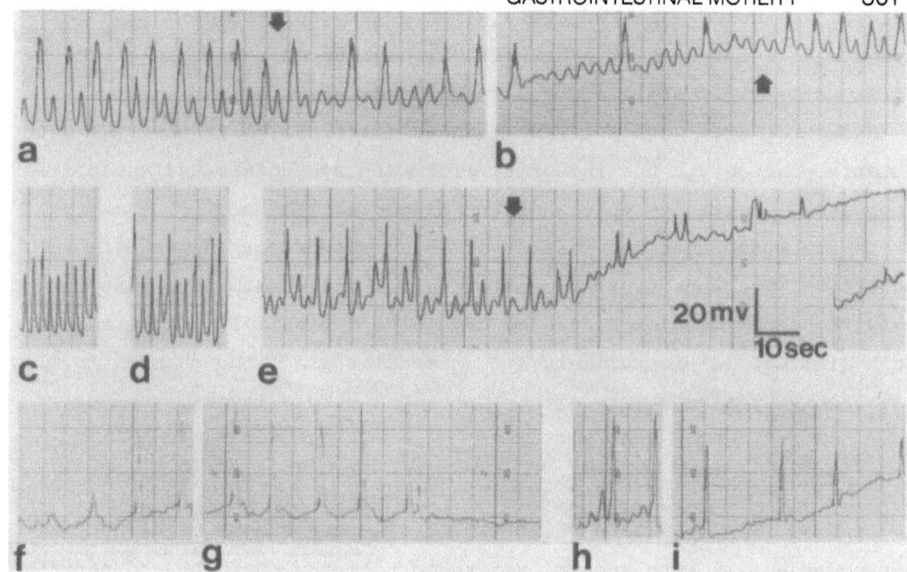

Fig. 5.   Intracellular records from three different preparations. a,b: Area with selectively stained ICC-I. Halogen lamp on between arrows. c,d,e: Area with selectively stained ICC-I (high oxygen, high flow), at 3 min, 5 min, and 16 min after start of recording. Arrow: laser on. Inset: Impalement of another cell in laser-exposed area. f,g: Area with selectively stained ICC-I; h,i: Unstained area of the same preparation, made anoxic by shift to nitrogen-equilibrated medium.

Figs. 4 and 5 also illustrate our preliminary observations of a photo-dynamic effect on the electrical activity of selectively stained (ICC-I) areas (Figs. 4d, 5a,b,e) with little or no effect of light on all other stained or unstained parts of the incubated intestinal segment (smooth muscle partially stained, Figs. 4 f,g; stained Auerbach's plexus, Fig. 4h). The effect on areas of stained ICC-I of illumination for a few minutes by the low-effect laser was striking, in that slow waves were barely seen in all subsequent records from the illuminated area. The wavelength of the laser source (632.8 nm) is fairly close to the absorption maximum of methylene blue (665 nm).

All the illustrated traces were obtained from cells, where the rapid, initial deflection upon impalement was not less than 60 mV.

This work is, to our best knowledge, the first study of ICC function. In which way cells that concentrate methylene blue are damaged, is uncertain. However, among the bewildering number of effects of exposure of cells to the dye, which are reported in the literature (for review, see 1), are noted a marked stimulation of oxygen uptake, and photo-dynamic effects, such as a drastic, light-induced reduction of the via-bility of vitally stained unicellular organisms.

Since the slow wave activity changes drastically in parallel with putative changes in the integrity of ICC-I (dye-uptake and associated increased sensitivity to changes in oxygen tension and illumination), it is concluded that the results strongly support our hypothesis (6), that ICC-I are intestinal pacemaker cells. The possibility that our ob-servations could be explained by damage to a passively conducting net-work of ICC-I (4) is unlikely, in particular since the changes in slow wave activity always were extended to both muscle layers.

REFERENCES

1. Barbosa, P. and Peters, T.M. (1971). The effects of vital dyes on living organisms with special reference to methylene blue and neutral red. Histochem. J., 3, 71-93
2. Bortoff, A. (1976). Myogenic control of intestinal motility. Physiol. Rev., 56, 418-434
3. Kobayashi, M., Prosser, C. L. and Nagai, T. (1967). Electrical pro-perties of intestinal muscle as measured intracellularly and extracel-lularly. Am. J. Physiol., 213, 275-286
4. Taylor, A. B., Kreulen, D. and Prosser, C. L. (1977). Electron mi-croscopy of the connective tissues between longitudinal and circular muscle of small intestine of cat. Am. J. Anat., 150, 427-442
5. Taylor, G.S., Daniel, E. E. and Tomita, T. (1976). Origin and mecha-nism of intestinal slow waves. In: Vantrappen, G. (ed). Proc. 5th int. symp. gastrointest. motil. pp. 31-36. (Herentals: Typoff)
6. Thuneberg, L. (1982). Interstitial cells of Cajal: Intestinal pace-maker cells? Adv. Anat. Embryol. Cell Biol., 71, 1-130

83

The Mechanism of Action of Pentagastrin on Circular Muscle from Canine Gastric Corpus

S. M. COLLINS

Gut peptides and neurotransmitters induce contraction of gastro-intestinal smooth muscle by interacting with specific receptors. Occupation of these receptors produces an increase in the concentration of cellular calcium, resulting in contraction of the smooth muscle cell (1). However, in most instances the mechanisms underlying peptide-induced contraction of gastrointestinal smooth muscle are poorly understood.

Examination of the excitation-contraction coupling process using intact tissue preparations, such as muscle strips, is limited by the presence of diffusion barriers and an extensive extracellular space (2). Such studies are constrained further by the potential of gut peptides to influence smooth muscle contractility indirectly by causing the release of active substances from neurons and mast cells present in muscle strips. These constraints may be overcome by using a homo-geneous suspension of single smooth muscle cells isolated by colla-genase digestion (3).

In the present study, such a preparation was used to study the mechanism by which pentagastrin, the biologically active C-terminal pentapeptide of gastrin, induces contraction of circular muscle from the canine gastric corpus. The purpose of this paper is to provide a short account of this study. A more detailed account is in preparation.

Smooth muscle cells were isolated by modification of a recently described technique involving collagenase digestion (3), and unless stated otherwise, cells were suspended in a Krebs-HEPES buffer containing 1.8mM $CaCl_2$, 1.2mM $MgCl_2$, and 4.7mM KCl at pH 7.4. Cell length was measured by image-splitting micrometry after fixing with acrolein, as previously described and validated by Bitar et al (4). Contraction was assessed by calculating the mean length of 50 randomly encountered cells exposed to a test agent and expressing it as a percentage of the mean length of 50 randomly encountered control cells (4).

In the presence of 1.8mM $[Ca^{++}]o$, pentagastrin, in concentrations as low as 10fM, caused contraction of the isolated cells and maximal contraction was induced by 10pM pentagastrin. The time course of pentagastrin-induced contraction was biphasic with a rapid peak component occurring at 30 seconds and declining subsequently by about 30% to a sustained component which persisted for at least 90 seconds. Pentagastrin-induced contraction was inhibited by the glutaramic acid derivative proglumide (IC_{50} 0.1mM), a specific competitive antagonist of gastrin and structurally-related peptides such as cholecystokinin (5). In contrast, low concentrations of atropine (0.5nM), which inhibited carbamylcholine-induced contraction, did not influence contraction induced by pentagastrin, thus illustrating the pharmacologic specificity of the action of pentagastrin on isolated smooth muscle cells from canine gastric corpus.

Occupancy of specific receptors by agonists such as pentagastrin brings about an increase in the myoplasmic concentration of calcium and results in contraction of the muscle cell. This may occur as a result of an influx of extracellular calcium through receptor-operated voltage-sensitive or voltage-insensitive channels, or by mobilizing intracellular stores of calcium (1,6). The influx of calcium through voltage-sensitive channels is accompanied by depolarization of the muscle cell membrane, and is believed generally to be the mechanism by which high extracellular concentrations of potassium induce contraction of smooth muscle (1). Calcium channel blockers such as verapamil and nitrendipine may selectively abolish the influx of calcium through voltage-sensitive channels, although in some instances their actions may be non-specific (7).

In the next part of the study, potassium-induced contraction of the isolated cells was characterized, and the action of the calcium channel blocker nitrendipine examined. In these experiments, potassium chloride

replaced sodium chloride in equimolar amounts to preserve the osmolarity of the buffer. In the presence of 1.8mM extracellular calcium,
potassium produced a dose-dependent contraction of isolated smooth
muscle cells over a concentration range of 20-40mM KCl and the maximal
contraction of 28% was comparable to that induced by pentagastrin.
Potassium-induced contraction was biphasic with rapid and sustained
components similar to those observed with pentagastrin. In the absence
of extracellular calcium and in the presence of 2mM EGTA, both the
rapid and sustained components of contraction induced by 40mM KCl were
abolished (see Table 1). However, in the presence of 1.8mM extracellular calcium, both components of potassium-induced contraction
could also be abolished by adding 10nM nitrendipine (see Table 1).

Table 1. Effects of nitrendipine and removal of extracellular calcium
on contraction induced by 40mM KCl

Contraction (percent decrease in mean cell length from control $\pm$ 1SD)		
	Rapid component (30 sec)	Sustained component (90 sec)
1.8mM Ca^{++}	26.0 $\pm$ 4.8	15.8 $\pm$ 2.5
Zero Ca^{++} plus 2mM EGTA	0.9 $\pm$ 0.9	1.1 $\pm$ 1.8
1.8mM Ca^{++} plus 10nM nitrendipine	1.7 $\pm$ 0.7	1.4 $\pm$ 0.8

These results indicate that potassium-induced contraction is critically
dependent on extracellular calcium and since high-potassium concentrations have been shown to cause depolarization of this tissue (8),
these results support the hypothesis that nitrendipine blocks calcium
influx through voltage-sensitive channels in smooth muscle cells
isolated from the circular layer of the canine gastric corpus.

The calcium dependence of pentagastrin-induced contraction was
examined next. As illustrated in Table 2, in the absence of added
extracellular calcium and in the presence of 2mM EGTA, the rapid and
sustained components of contraction induced by pentagastrin were sub-
stantially inhibited but not abolished. These results indicate that
both components of pentagastrin-induced contraction of the isolated
cells are dependent largely on the influx of extracellular calcium.
However, the persistence of a small degree of contraction in the
presence of a calcium free buffer with EGTA raises the possibility that
the occupation of the gastrin receptor may also stimulate the release

of calcium from intracellular stores.

To examine whether the pentagastrin-stimulated influx of calcium occurred through receptor-operated voltage-sensitive or voltage-insensitive channels, the effect of nitrendipine on pentagastrin-induced contraction was studied. As illustrated in Table 2, in the presence of 1.8mM extracellular calcium, 10nM nitrendipine selectively attenuated the rapid component of contraction but did not affect the sustained component.

Table 2. Effects of nitrendipine and removal of extracellular calcium
on contraction induced by 10pM pentagastrin

Contraction (percent decrease in mean cell length from control $\pm$ 150)		
	Rapid component (30 sec)	Sustained component (90 sec)
1.8mM Ca^{++}	30.3 $\pm$ 1.6	22.3 $\pm$ 2.9
Zero Ca^{++} plus 2mM EGTA	7.3 $\pm$ 2.2	4.4 $\pm$ 2.2
1.8mM Ca^{++} plus 10nM nitrendipine	13.3 $\pm$ 1.2	19.1 $\pm$ 9.6

These results indicate that at least two distinct mechanisms underly pentagastrin-induced contraction of isolated smooth muscle cells from the circular layer of canine gastric corpus. The nitrendipine-sensitive rapid contraction is mediated largely by the influx of calcium through voltage-sensitive channels, whereas the sustained nitrendipine-resistant component of contraction is mediated by the influx of calcium through voltage-insensitive channels. These results also support the findings of Morgan and Szurszewski (8), based on studies using simultaneous mechanical and intracellular electrode recordings on muscle strips, that pentagastrin induces contraction of circular muscle from canine gastric corpus by activating voltage-sensitive and voltage-insensitive channels. Although the ionic basis for these findings was not examined in that study, the results of the present study identify calcium as the important ion in the excitation-contraction coupling process induced by pentagastrin in this tissue.

In summary, the results of this study support the hypothesis that the gastrin receptor on smooth muscle cells from the circular layer of canine gastric corpus operates both voltage-dependent and voltage-independent channels, through which calcium enters the cell to induce contraction. In addition, this receptor may also stimulate the release of calcium from intracellular stores.

ACKNOWLEDGEMENTS

This study was supported by research grants to S.M. Collins from the Ontario Ministry of Health (MOH PR955E) and from the Medical Research Council of Canada (MA7637).

REFERENCES

1. Bolton, T. B. (1974). Mechanisms of action of transmitters and other substances on smooth muscle. Physiol.Rev. 59, 606-718

2. Gabella, G. (1979). Smooth muscle cell junctions and structural aspects of contraction. Br.Med.Bull. 35, 213-218

3. Collins, S. M. and Gardner, J.D. (1982). Cholecystokinin-induced contraction of dispersed smooth muscle cells. Am.J.Physiol. 243, G497-G504

4. Bitar, K. N., Zfass, A. M. and Makhlouf, G.M. (1979). Interaction of acetylcholine and cholecystokinin with dispersed smooth muscle cells. Am.J.Physiol. 237, E172-E176

5. Hahne, W. H., Jensen, R. T., Lemp, G. F. and Gardner, J.D. (1981). Proglumide and benzotript:members of a new class of cholecystokinin receptor antagonists. Proc.Natl.Acad.Sci. USA, 78, 6304-6308

6. Daniel, E. E., Crankshaw, D. and Kwan, C.Y. (1979). Intracellular sources of calcium for activation of smooth muscle. In:Kalsner, S. (ed). Trends in Autonomic Pharmacology. pp443-484. (Urban and Schwarzenberg Inc. Germany)

7. Triggle, D. J. and Swamy, C. F. (1980). Pharmacology of agents that affect calcium:agonists and antagonists. Chest 78 Suppl., 174-179

8. Morgan, K. G. and Szurszewski, J. H. (1980). Mechanisms of phasic and tonic actions of pentagastrin on canine gastric smooth muscle. J.Physiol. 301, 229-242

84

Role of Bombesin in Muscularis Mucosa of Canine Colon

F. ANGEL, V. L. W. GO and J. H. SZURSZEWSKI

We have shown previously the presence of a non-cholinergic, non-adrenergic excitatory innervation in the muscularis mucosa of the canine colon. Immunoreactive-like substance P was released in response to nerve stimulation. This release was reduced in the presence of tetrodotoxin and in a calcium-free solution. Bombesin, another peptide present in this muscle, was excitatory when applied exogenously. Excitation with bombesin was blocked by tetrodotoxin. The aims of this study therefore were to determine if bombesin is released during nerve stimulation and if bombesin causes contraction by releasing substance P. Strips of muscularis mucosa were placed in a superfusion apparatus to record contractile activity. Intramural nerves were stimulated by two platinum wire electrodes. The super-fusate which passed over each strip was collected and assayed for bombesin- and substance P-like immunoreactivity. Under control conditions, the concentration of bombesin was 6.0 ± 0.9 pg/ml (mean $\pm$ SEM). Following nerve stimulation (10 Hz, 10 V, 200 μs) the concen-tration of bombesin in the superfusate increased significantly ($p < 0.02$) to 9.41 ± 0.98 pg/ml (mean $\pm$ SEM). In the presence of tetrodotoxin (10^{-6} M) and in a calcium-free bathing solution, the increase in immunoreactive-like bombesin in the superfusate was no longer observed (respectively: 6.37 ± 1.07 pg/ml and 7.5 ± 1.4 pg/ml). Furthermore, applied bombesin (10^{-6} M) increased substance P levels (28 ± 1.7 pg/ml) in the superfusate. This increase was reduced significantly ($p < 0.05$) by tetrodotoxin (11.4 ± 6.5 pg/ml). Finally, with substance P-antiserum in the superfusate (dilution 1:75), the excitatory response induced by either nerve stimulation or exogenous bombesin was decreased. We conclude from these observations that transmural stimulation releases bombesin from intramural nerves and that bombesin acts on substance P-containing nerves to release substance P, thereby causing contraction. (Supported by NIH Grant AM 17238.)

85

Effect of Substance P on Non-Cholinergic Post-Stimulus Depolarization of the Circular Smooth Muscle of the Guinea Pig Ileum

J. P. NIEL, R. A. R. BYWATER and G. S. TAYLOR

The membrane potential of the cells of the circular layer of the guinea-pig ileum was recorded in vitro at 30°C in the presence of atropine (1.4×10^{-6} M) using intracellular microelectrodes. Following transmural (TM) nerve stimulation the inhibitory junction potential (i.j.p.) was followed by two separate depolarizing responses. The first of these (fast post-stimulus depolarization, FPSD) peaked 1.5 sec after the stimulus, whilst the second (slow post-stimulus depolarization, SPSD) peaked 3-4 sec after the stimulus (Bywater and Taylor, 1). After prolonged exposure (> 10 min) of the tissue to substance P (SP : 10^{-7} to 10^{-6} M), the circular muscle cells were depolarized by 6.4 $\pm$ 1.1 mV and their membrane resistance increased by 50 to 100 %. At this time, following TM nerve stimulation, the amplitude of the i.j.p. was increased by 20 to 50 %, FPSD was abolished whereas SPSD was generally unaffected. In some preparations however, the amplitude of SPSD was increased and it reached threshold for action potential generation. In the latter preparations and in the absence of stimulation, the membrane potential occasionally showed regular oscillations of approximately 10 mV in amplitude every 5 to 8 sec. Hyperpolarization did not restore FPSD indicating that its abolition was not a secondary effect due to the depolarization of the tissue by SP. Moreover, during an hyperpolarization of approximately 20 mV, a transient large depolarization was revealed during the phase of SPSD. Assuming that prolonged exposure to SP desensitizes the tissue to that substance, these results indicate that SP may be involved in the genesis of FPSD. SPSD probably results from a different mechanism and shows some similarities with slow waves.

Bywater, R.A.R. and Taylor, G.S. (1983) J. Physiol. (In press)

86

Gastrointestinal Motility Stimulating Properties of Cisapride, a Non-Antidopaminergic Non-Cholinergic Compound

J. M. Van NUETEN, P. G. H. Van DAELE, A. J. REYNTJENS,
P. A. J. JANSSEN and J. A. J. SCHUURKES

SUMMARY

Cisapride, a novel gastrokinetic compound, effectively improves electrically evoked contractions of the guinea pig ileum (ED_{50} = 9.2×10^{-9} M) most likely via facilitation of the release of acetylcholine. It also enhances spontaneous contractions of the stomach and induces contractions of colonic strips of the guinea pig. Furthermore, cisapride antagonizes gastric relaxations as induced by adrenergic, dopaminergic and serotonergic agonists or by sympathetic nerve stimulation. The enhanced contractions and reduced relaxations suggest a role for cisapride in gastrointestinal motor disorders.

INTRODUCTION

In order to test whether a drug devoid of dopamine antagonistic properties (as possessed by domperidone and metoclopramide) (1-3), but capable of enhancing electrically evoked contractions of the guinea pig ileum (as metoclopramide) (4), does possess gastrokinetic properties, cisapride [R 51 619: cis-4-amino-5-chloro- N-[1-[3-(4-fluorophenoxy)propyl]-3-methoxy-4-piperidinyl]-2-methoxy-benzamide monohydrate] (Fig. 1) was selected.

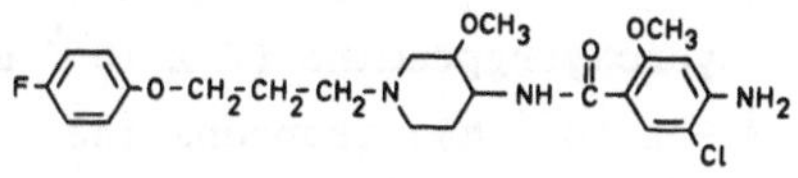

FIGURE 1 Chemical structure of cisapride.

The aim of this study was to quantify the motor effects of cisapride on gastrointestinal tissues and to unravel its mechanism of action.

513

METHODS

1. Transmural stimulation [1 msec, 0.1 Hz, submaximal (80 %) mA] of the guinea pig ileum (preload 1 g, isometric, 100 ml tyrode: KCl 2.7; $CaCl_2.2H_2O$ 1.8; $MgCl_2.6H_2O$ 1.04; $NaHCO_3$ 11.9; $NaH_2PO_4.H_2O$ 0.42; NaCl 136.9; glucose 5.55 mM; 37.5° C, 95 % O_2, 5 % CO_2) (5) induces contractions due to the release of acetylcholine from intramural nerves (6). Effects of cisapride (Janssen Pharmaceutica), clebopride (Almirall), alizapride (Delagrange) and metoclopramide (Delagrange) were expressed as % of maximal effect. Regression lines were calculated to determine the EC_{50} value.

2. Isotonic contractions of the guinea pig ileum (preload 0.75 g) were induced with logarithmically increasing doses of methacholine before and after exposure to cisapride or neostigmine.

3. The chick (50 $\pm$ 10 g) biventer cervicis nerve-muscle preparation (7) [optimal preload, isometric, 100 ml tyrode (glucose 11.1 mM)] was stimulated (rectangular pulses of 0.25 msec, 0.1 Hz, supramaximal intensity) to induce twitch contractions. The effects of cisapride were compared with those of neostigmine and nicotine.

4. The stomach-duodenal-bulb preparation of the guinea pig (2,8) filled wih 20 ml saline was suspended in 200 ml oxygenated Krebs-Henseleit solution (KCl 4.7; $CaCl_2.2H_2O$ 2.5; $MgSO_4.7H_2O$ 1.2; $NaHCO_3$ 25.0; KH_2PO_4 1.2; NaCl 118.1; glucose 5.55 mM). Changes in intraluminal volume at constant intraluminal pressure of 6 cm H_2O were recorded with an ultrasonic transit time transducer.

(a) The direct effect of a drug on frequency and amplitude of contractions and on antroduodenal coordination (= % of antral waves propagated to the duodenum) was expressed as ED_{50} value (9,10).

(b) Relaxations (8) before and in the presence of cisapride were induced by intraarterial administration (0.05 ml) of equiactive doses of phenylephrine (4.8 x 10^{-8} moles), dopamine (2.6 x 10^{-7} moles), 5-hydroxytryptamine (7 x 10^{-9} moles, in the presence of atropine 2.9 x 10^{-7} M), isoprenaline (3.2 x 10^{-9} moles), or by electrical stimulation (1 msec, 20 mA, 20 Hz, 10 sec/5 min) of the vagal nerves in the presence of atropine (2.9 x 10^{-7} M) or of the periarterial sympathetic nerves (11).

The relative inhibition of the induced relaxation was taken as a
measure of the effect of cisapride.

5. Segments of the colon ascendens of the guinea pig were suspended
for isotonic recording with a preload of 2 g in 100 ml De Jalon
solution (KCl 5.6 mM, $CaCl_2.2H_2O$ 0.54 mM; $NaHCO_3$ 5.9 mM; NaCl
154.1 mM; glucose 2.8 mM). Contractions induced by cisapride w
expressed relative to maximal contractions induced by methachc
(3.2×10^{-6} M). Reflex activity was evoked by connecting the
lumen of the segment to an ultrasonic transit time transducer to
record changes in volume at constant intraluminal pressure (5 cm
H_2O) (5).

RESULTS

Cisapride enhanced the contractile response to submaximal transmural
electrical stimulation of the guinea pig ileum (Fig. 2) from
concentrations as low as 1.4×10^{-9} M in a dose-dependent way.
Maximal effect (3.5 grams contraction) was reached at
3.4×10^{-7} M. To induce an equivalent increase in contractile
force with metoclopramide a concentration of 5×10^{-5} M was
needed. Figure 3 shows the difference in potency between cisapride,
clebopride, alizapride and metoclopramide.

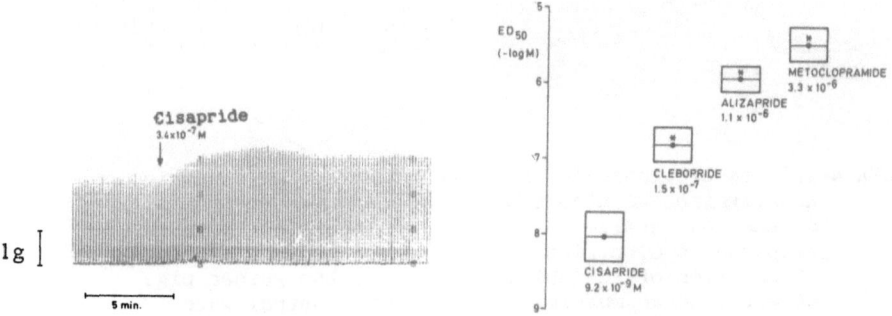

FIGURE 2 Cisapride enhances the
contractile response to
electrical stimulation
of the guinea pig ileum.

FIGURE 3 Potencies of cisapride,
clebopride, alizapride
and metoclopramide in
enhancing the contractile
response to electrical
stimulation of the guinea
pig ileum (* = different
from cisapride, p < 0.05).

At concentrations even up to 1.3×10^{-6} M, cisapride did not affect the responses of the guinea pig ileum to cumulative doses of methacholine. In contrast, neostigmine shifted the curve to the left.

Cisapride in concentrations up to 2.1×10^{-5} M had no effect on the twitch responses elicited by electrical stimulation of the chick biventer cervicis nerve-muscle preparation (Fig. 4). In contrast, neostigmine enhanced the twitch amplitude, whereas nicotine induced a tonic contraction.

Cisapride increased gastric peristaltic amplitude of the guinea pig at a concentration of 3.4×10^{-7} M (Fig. 5). From this concentration upwards cisapride also enhanced antroduodenal coordination. ED_{50} value for this effect was 4×10^{-7} M for cisapride and 2.5×10^{-5} M for metoclopramide (10).

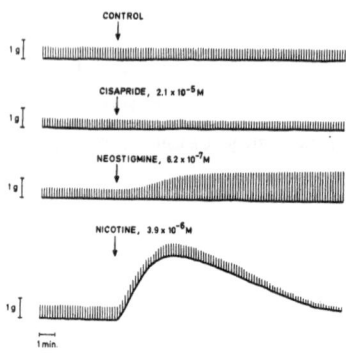

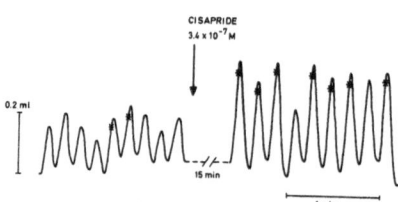

FIGURE 4 Effects of cisapride, neostigmine and nicotine on the contractile response to electrical stimulation of the chick biventer nerve-muscle preparation.

FIGURE 5 Effect of cisapride on spontaneous activity of the intact preparation of stomach and duodenum of the guinea pig. x = antral wave propagated to the duodenum.

On the same preparation cisapride antagonized, in order of effectiveness, IC_{50} values within brackets, relaxations induced by phenylephrine (7.1×10^{-7} M), dopamine (9.4×10^{-7} M), periarterial sympathetic nerve stimulation (1.4×10^{-6} M; Fig. 6), 5-hydroxytryptamine (2.8×10^{-6} M) and isoprenaline

(2.8×10^{-6} M). The relaxation induced by vagal stimulation in the presence of atropine was not affected by cisapride.

Cisapride induced dose-dependent direct contractions of the colon ascendens of the guinea pig (Fig. 7). The minimal effective concentration was 5.4×10^{-9} M. A maximal contraction equal to 45 % of the maximal methacholine-induced contraction was reached at

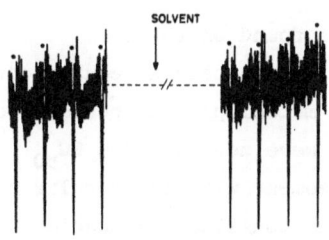

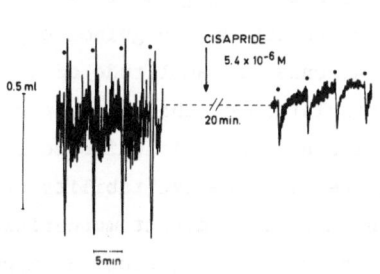

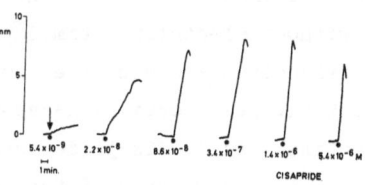

FIGURE 6 Effect of cisapride in reducing the gastric relaxation of the guinea pig, as induced by periarterial stimulation (●).

FIGURE 7 Effect of cisapride to induce contractions of the colon ascendens of the guinea pig.

3.4×10^{-7} M. ED_{50} value for this effect was 3.5×10^{-8} M.

In a different set up, the intraluminal pressure was raised to 5 cm H_2O to induce reflex activity. Cisapride increased the tone of the longitudinal muscle layer and emptied the colonic segment in a concentration range from 8.6×10^{-8} to 5.4×10^{-6} M.

DISCUSSION

Cisapride stimulates motor activity of the stomach (rhythmic activity), small intestine [duodenum: induction of coordinated contractions (10), ileum: enhanced contractile response to electrical stimulation] and large intestine (colon ascendens: direct contractile effect) of the guinea pig. The concentrations needed to obtain these direct stimulant effects were comparable for the different preparations.

The lowest ED_{50} value, 9.2×10^{-9} M was found on the transmurally stimulated guinea pig ileum. To obtain an equivalent response with clebopride, alizapride and metoclopramide respectively 16x, 120x and 350x higher concentrations were needed. The EC_{50} value for metoclopramide was in good agreement with the results of Kilbinger et al. (4) (3.4×10^{-6} M) on the longitudinal muscle preparation of the guinea pig.

An enhanced amplitude of the contractile response to electrical stimulation of the guinea pig ileum can be due to 1. an enhanced release of acetylcholine be it by a direct releasing effect or by increasing the excitability of the intramural cholinergic nerve endings; 2. a direct muscarinic agonism or a nicotine-like ganglionic stimulation; 3. a neostigmine-like inhibition of acetylcholinesterase activity or 4. a sensitization of the muscarinic receptor on the smooth muscle cells. Ad 2. Cisapride does not induce a direct contraction of the guinea pig ileum, with or without electrical stimulation, in contrast with both acetylcholine and nicotine, nor does it induce a contracture of the chick biventer cervicis nerve-muscle preparation as observed after nicotine. Ad 3. Cisapride does not induce irregularities in the contractile responses of the guinea pig ileum to electrical stimulation, as observed with neostigmine; it does not induce a leftwards shift of the dose-response curve to methacholine as neostigmine does. Furthermore, cisapride does not enhance the twitch response of the chick biventer preparation. Cisapride (up to 2×10^{-5} M) does not inhibit acetylcholine-esterase and pseudo-acetylcholine-esterase activity in in vitro test systems (H. Van Belle, unpublished). Ad 4. Cisapride does not potentiate the responses to exogenous acetylcholine on rabbit duodenum (unpublished) nor the responses to methacholine on the guinea pig

ileum. From these findings we propose that the action of cisapride
in enhancing the response to electrical stimulation of the guinea
pig ileum is due to an increased release of cholinergic
neurotransmitter. That indeed cisapride does affect the release of
acetylcholine was recently confirmed by Kilbinger (unpublished).

Cisapride combines motor stimulating properties with antagonism of
induced relaxation on the guinea pig stomach, being most effective
against relaxations induced by phenylephrine, dopamine and
periarterial stimulation and slightly less active against
relaxations induced by isoprenaline and 5-hydroxytryptamine (in the
presence of atropine). It is not effective against relaxations
induced by vagal stimulation in the presence of atropine.

On the rat tail artery and guinea pig ileum, cisapride also showed
5-hydroxytryptamine-antagonistic properties that appeared unrelated
to its effect on electrically stimulated guinea pig ileum
(unpublished). The lack of specificity to antagonize the effects of
dopamine in our experiments as well as the absence of a. binding
affinity to rat brain striatal dopamine receptors (Leysen,
unpublished); b. specific effects against apomorphine-induced
vomiting in dogs (Niemegeers, unpublished) and c. effects on
prolactin plasma levels in the human (Reyntjens, unpublished)
indicate that cisapride is not a dopamine antagonist.

The effects of cisapride on gastrointestinal motility suggest a
potential role for cisapride in motor disorders of the gut. In
particular its effects on gastroduodenal motility may explain its
effectiveness in enhancing gastric emptying of liquid and solid
meals (12).

The authors are indebted to Messrs E.C.R. Ghoos, L.F.M. Helsen,
J.G.M.G. Eelen and J.J.M.D. Kuyps for skilfull technical assistance,
and Mrs D. Verkuringen for typing the manuscript.

REFERENCES

1. Schuurkes, J.A.J. and Van Nueten, J.M. (1982). Domperidone
improves myogenically transmitted antroduodenal coordination by
blocking dopaminergic receptor sites. Scand. J. Gastroenterol. (in
press) (suppl. Seminar: "New Developments in Gut Motility", Belgium,
March 1983)
2. Van Nueten, J.M., Ennis, C., Helsen, L., Laduron, P.M. and
Janssen, P.A.J. (1978). Inhibition of dopamine receptors in the
stomach: an explanation of the gastrokinetic properties of
domperidone. Life Sci., 23, 453-8

3. Schulze-Delrieu, K. (1981). Drug therapy. Metoclopramide.
N. Engl. J. Med., 305, 28-33
4. Kilbinger, H., Kruel, R., Pfeuffer-Friederich, I. and Wessler,
I. (1982). The effects of metoclopramide on acetylcholine release
and on smooth muscle response in the isolated guinea-pig ileum.
Naunyn Schmiedebergs Arch. Pharmacol., 319, 231-8
5. Van Nueten, J.M., Janssen, P.A.J. and Fontaine, J. (1974).
Loperamide (R 18 553), a novel type of antidiarrheal agent. III. In
vitro studies on the peristaltic reflex and other experiments on
isolated tissues. Arzneim. Forsch., 24, 1641-5
6. Paton, W.D.M. (1957). The action of morphine and related
substances on concentration and on acetylcholine output of coaxially
stimulated guinea pig ileum. Brit. J. Pharmacol., 12, 119-27
7. Ginsborg, B.L. and Warriner, J. (1960). The isolated chick
biventer cervicis nerve-muscle preparation. Brit. J. Pharmacol.,
15, 410-1
8. Van Nueten, J.M. and Schuurkes, J.A.J. (1983). Studies on the
role of dopamine and dopamine blockers in gastroduodenal motility.
Scand. J. Gastroenterol. (in press) (suppl. Seminar: "New
Developments in Gut Motility", Belgium, March 1983)
9. Finney, D.J. (1962). Probit analysis. (Cambridge University
Press, Cambridge)
10. Schuurkes, J.A.J. and Van Nueten, J.M. (1983). Control of
gastroduodenal coordination: dopaminergic and cholinergic pathways.
Scand. J. Gastroenterol. (in press) (suppl. 2nd Int. Symp. on
Duodenogastric Reflux, Swiss, June 1983)
11. Schuurkes, J.A.J. and Van Nueten, J.M. (1982). Gastric
relaxation induced by peri-arterial (sympathetic ?) electrical
stimulation in vitro. Scand. J. Gastroenterol. (in press)
(suppl. 1st Int. Symp. on Sympathetic Influence on Gastric Function,
Denmark, March 1983)
12. Schuurkes, J.A.J., Akkermans, L.M.A. and Van Nueten, J.M.
(1983). Stimulating effects of cisapride on antroduodenal motility
in the conscious dog. This book, Chapter   , pp.

87

Characterization of ^{125}I-Trp^{11}-Neurotensin Binding to Rat Fundus Smooth Muscle Plasma Membranes

P. KITABGI, C.-Y. KWAN and J. E. T. FOX

INTRODUCTION

The brain-gastrointestinal tridecapeptide neurotensin (NT) has been shown to affect the contractility of a variety of gastrointestinal smooth muscle preparations in vitro [1]. In particular, it has been reported that NT contracts rat fundus smooth muscle strips [2]. Pharmacological experiments and structure activity studies have suggested that this effect was myogenic in nature and involved an interaction of NT with specific smooth muscle receptors [3]. In the present paper we provide direct evidence for the existence of such receptors from radioligand binding studies using ^{125}I-Trp^{11}-NT as the labelled ligand and highly purified rat fundus smooth muscle plasma membranes at the source of NT receptors.

METHODS

The preparation, purification and chemical characterization of biologically active monoiodo ^{125}I-Trp^{11}-NT (specific radioactivity, 2000 Ci/mmol) have been reported elsewhere [4]. Highly purified smooth muscle plasma membranes

from rat fundus were obtained as previously described [5].
The binding assay technique used here was essentially the
same as that reported previously for measuring the binding
of ^{125}I-Trp^{11}-NT to rat brain synaptic membranes [4]. All
experiments were carried out at 25°C in 50 mM Tris HCl,
pH 7.5, containing 0.2 % bovine serum albumin. Bound peptide was separated from free by filtration using cellulose acetate filters with a pore diameter of 0.2 μm. In
each experiment, the nonspecific binding was determined as
the amount of radioactivity bound in the presence of an
excess unlabelled NT(1 μM). In our standard assay conditions (25°C, 30 min of incubation, 0.1 nM ^{125}I-Trp^{11}-NT,
0.2 mg/ml of fundus membrane protein), the nonspecific
binding represented 15-20 % of total binding.

RESULTS

The specific binding of ^{125}I-Trp^{11}-NT in subcellular fractions from rat fundus smooth muscle showed a distribution
that paralleled that of several plasma marker enzymes such
as 5'-nucleotidase and phosphodiesterase I.

Kinetic experiments of association showed that the specific binding of ^{125}I-Trp^{11}-NT to fundus plasma membranes
increased with time and reached equilibrium by 20- 30 min.
At this point the binding was reversible as shown by
kinetic experiments of dissociation.

When the specific binding of ^{125}I-Trp^{11}-NT was measured
at equilibrium as a function of increasing labelled ligand
concentrations, it was found saturable. Scatchard analysis
of the data yielded a curvilinear plot, indicating the
existence of two classes of binding sites with Kd values
of 56 pM and 1.92 nM, and respective binding capacities of
6.6 fmol/mg and 11.4 fmol/mg of membrane protein. The Kd
value of the low affinity site (1.92 nM) was close to the
EC$_{50}$ for the NT-induced contraction in rat fundus which has

been reported to be in the nanomolar range [2,3].

Unlabelled NT competitively inhibited the binding of ^{125}I-Trp^{11}-NT to the high affinity binding sites with an IC_{50} of 0.25 nM. Fragments and analogues of NT competed for the binding of $^{125}Trp^{11}$-NT to high affinity sites with potencies similar to those previously reported for their contracting effect in rat fundus strips [3,6]. Biologically active peptides unrelated to NT such as Met-enkephalin, TRH and bradykinin had no effect on the binding of ^{125}I-Trp^{11}-NT binding to rat fundus membranes.

Cations like Ca^{++}, Mg^{++} and K^{+} at physiological and entraphysiological concentrations up to 25 mM did not affect the binding of the labelled ligand to fundus membranes. In contrast, Na^{+} in a concentration dependent manner decreased the binding of ^{125}I-Trp^{11}-NT to the high affinity smooth muscle binding sites. At 100 mM, the cation induced a 6-fold increase in the IC_{50} of NT for its ability to inhibit the binding of ^{125}I-Trp^{11}-NT. At this Na^{+} concentration the IC_{50} for NT was 1 nM, a value close to the Kd of the low affinity sites.

DISCUSSION

In the present paper we have demonstrated that ^{125}I-Trp^{11}-NT, a ligand of NT receptors, binds to rat fundus smooth muscle plasma membranes in a specific, time-dependent, reversible and saturable manner. The structural requirements for NT binding are similar to those for the NT-induced rat fundus contraction. Taken together our data suggest that 1) in the absence of Na^{+}, rat fundus smooth muscle binding sites exist in both high and low affinity states, 2) Na^{+} converts high affinity sites to low affinity sites and 3) the low affinity sites are the functional receptors involved in the contractile response of rat fundus smooth muscle to NT.

This is the first detailed biochemical characterization
of NT smooth muscle receptors. It was made possible by the
use of highly purified smooth muscle plasma membranes [5]
and of a well characterized biologically active ligand of
NT receptors, ^{125}I-Trp^{11}-NT, with high specific radioactivity [4]. The possibility in rat fundus smooth muscle
to study both NT-receptor binding interaction and NT-induced post receptor events (contraction) makes it a useful
model for investigating pharmacological or pathophysiological alterations of NT binding and their functional consequences.

ACKNOWLEDGEMENTS

The investigation was supported by the Centre National de
la Recherche Scientifique (CNRS) and the Ontario Heart
Foundation.

We would like to thank Dr.E.E. Daniel for helpful dis-
cussions. We also thank G. Clénet for excellent secretarial assistance.

REFERENCES

1. Kitabgi, P. (1982). Effect of neurotensin on intestinal smooth muscle : application to the study of structure-activity relationships. Ann. N.Y. Acad. Sci., 400,
37-55

2. Rökaeus, A., Burcher, E., Chang, D., Folkers, K.
and Rosell, S. (1977). Action of neurotensin and (Gln^4)-
neurotensin on isolated tissues. Acta Pharmacol. et Toxi-
col., 41, 141-147

3. Quirion, R., Regoli, D., Rioux, F. and St Pierre, S.
(1980). The stimulatory effects of neurotensin and related
peptides in rat stomach strips ans guinea-pig atria.
Br. J. Pharmacol., 68, 83-91

4.   Mazella, J., Poustis, C., Labbé, C., Checler, F.,
Kitabgi, P., Granier, C., Van Rietschoten, J. and Vincent,
J.P. (1983). Monoiodo-(Trp^{11})-neurotensin, a highly radio-
active ligand of neurotensin receptors. Preparation, biological activity, and binding properties to rat brain
synaptic membranes. J. Biol. Chem., 258, 3476-3481

5.   Kwan, C.Y., Sakai, Y., Grover, A.K. and Lee, R.M.
K.W. (1982). Isolation and characterization of plasma membrane fraction from gastric fundus smooth muscle of the
rat. Mol. Physiol,, 2, 107-120

6.   Quirion, R., Regoli, D., Rioux, F. and St Pierre, S.
(1980). Structure activity studies with neurotensin : analysis in positions 9, 10 and 11. Br. J. Pharmacol., 69,
698-692

88

Facilitation and Inhibition by 5-Hydroxytryptamine and R 51 619 of Acetylcholine Release from Guinea Pig Myenteric Neurones

I. PFEUFFER-FRIEDERICH and H. KILBINGER

INTRODUCTION

Electrophysiological (North et al., 1980) and neurochemical (Kilbinger and Pfeuffer-Friederich, 1982; Pfeuffer-Friederich and Kilbinger, 1983) experiments have shown that the cholinergic nerves of the guinea pig myenteric plexus are endowed with two types of 5-hydroxytryptamine (5-HT) receptors: 1. Exitatory receptors whose stimulation leads to an increased release of acetylcholine (ACh). This receptor is stimulated by 5-HT and by metoclopramide. It has been suggested that the increase by metoclopramide of smooth muscle contraction of the guinea pig ileum is related to the release of ACh (Kilbinger et al., 1982). 2. Inhibitory receptors whose activation by 5-HT or by LSD causes an inhibition of ACh release evoked by electrical stimulation of the myenteric plexus. The inhibitory receptor can be specifically blocked by methysergide and by methiothepine (Kilbinger and Pfeuffer-Friederich, 1982; Pfeuffer-Freiderich and Kilbinger, 1983).

The recently developed compound R 51 619 (Janssen, Beerse, Belgium) is chemically related to metoclopramide (Figure 1). The compound

R 51 619

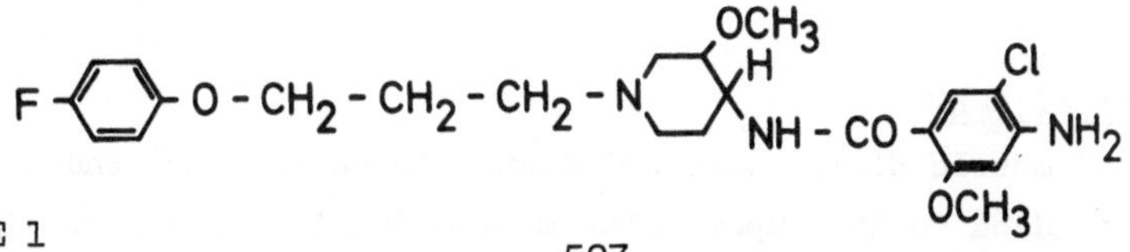

FIGURE 1

which is devoid of any dopamine blocking effects was found to stimulate gastrointestinal motility in vitro as well as in vivo (Schuurkes, personal communication). In the present experiments the effects of R 51 619 on spontaneous and evoked release of ACh from the guinea pig myenteric plexus were investigated and compared with those of metoclopramide and 5-HT.

METHODS

The method of measuring the release of ^{3}H-ACh from the guineapig myenteric plexus-longitudinal muscle preparation has been described in detail previously (Kilbinger and Wessler, 1980). Two strips (approximately 50 mg wet weight) were suspended isotonically under a tension of 1 g in a 2 ml organ bath in Tyrode's solution (composition in mM: NaCl 137; KCl 2.7; CaCl$_2$ 1.8: MgCl$_2$ 1.0; NaH$_2$PO$_4$ 0.4; NaHCO$_3$ 11.9; glucose 5.6; gassed with carbogen; 37 $^\circ$C) that contained in addition 1 μM choline. The strips were preincubated for 30 min with ^{3}H-choline (1 μM). During this labelling period the tissue was stimulated with square wave pulses (o.2 Hz; 1 ms). The strips were then superfused (1 ml/min) with Tyrode's solution containing 10 μM hemicholinium-3. After 60 min of superfusion collection of 3-min fractions of superfusate began. In most of the experiments the strips were stimulated once or twice by field stimulation (0.1 Hz; 10 min). Biphasic square wave pulses (1 ms) were applied by means of two platinum electrodes positioned parallel to the strips. The potential drop between the electrodes was 11 V/cm. Tritium was determined by liquid scintillation spectrometry and counting efficiency was determined with internal standards of ^{3}H-water. The outflow of tritium evoked by field stimulation or by drugs was obtained from the difference between the total outflow in the samples collected during and after stimulation, and the spontaneous outflow calculated by interpolation from the first 3 and the last 3 to 5 unstimulated samples as described previously (Kilbinger and Wessler, 1980). R 51 619 (10^{-3}M) was also dissolved in lactic acid (0.1 M).

RESULTS

1. Effects of 5-HT

Longitudinal muscle strips were stimulated twice (S1; S2) and 5-HT (10 μM) was added to the superfusion medium 30 min before S2. Figure 2

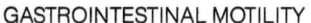
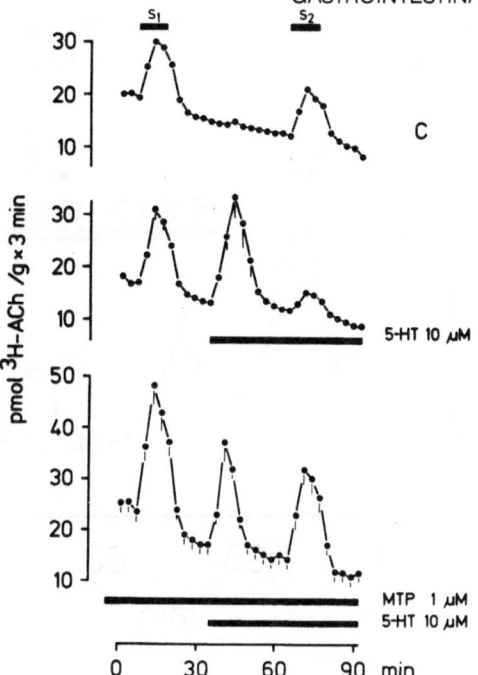

FIGURE 2   Effects of 5-hydroxytryptamine (5-HT) on spontaneous and
evoked outflow of ^{3}H-ACh.   Longitudinal muscle strips
were incubated with H-choline and then superfused with
Tyrode's solution.   After a 60 min washout period the
superfusate was collected in 3 min fractions.   Field
stimulation (0.1 Hz, 60 pulses, 1 ms) and superfusion with
drugs are indicated by the horizontal bars.   Methiothepine
(MTP) was added 30 min before S1.   Means $\pm$ SEM of 6
(control; C) 12 (5-HT) and 4 (5-HT plus MTP) experiments.

shows that 5-HT caused a transient increase in resting outflow of
^{3}H-ACh (68 $\pm$ 11 pmol/g) whereas the stimulation evoked outflow was
significantly inhibited (by 62 $\pm$ 2 %). Methiothepine (1 µM) which is
an antagonist at the 5-HT autoreceptor in rat brain (Göthert and
Weinheimer, 1979; Langer and Moret, 1982) was superfused from 30 min
before S1 until the end of the experiment. Figure 2 shows that methiothepine completely prevented the inhibitory action of 5-HT whereas the
facilitatory effect was not affected.

2. Effects of R 51 619

(a) Resting outflow of ^{3}H-ACh. Figure 3 shows that superfusion of the
strips with 10 µM R 51 619 elicited an increase in the outflow of
tritium. For comparison the strips had been stimulated electrically

before superfusion with R 51 619 was started. The outflow by field
stimulation was abolished by 300 nM tetrodotoxin (Figure 3). Previous

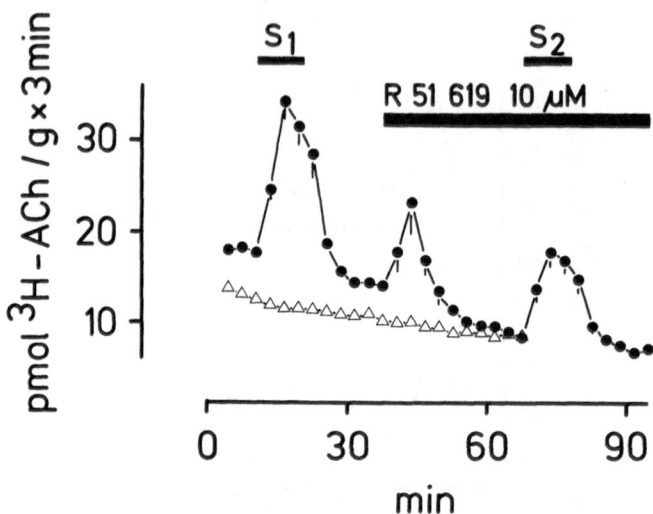

FIGURE 3   Effects of R 51 629 on outflow on ^{3}H-ACh in the absence
            (●) and presence (Δ) of tetrodotoxin. S$_1$, S$_1$, field
            stimulation of the strips (0.1 Hz, 10 min). Means ± SEM
            of 5 (●) and 2 (Δ) expts.

experiments have shown that the tetrodotoxin-sensitive outflow of
tritium from strips preincubated with ^{3}H-choline can be attributed to
the release of ^{3}H-ACh (Kilbinger and Wessler, 1980). We, therefore,
assume that the outflow caused by R 51 619 is due to depolarization-
induced release of ^{3}H-ACh.

In the presence of 0.1 μM 5-HT R 51 619 (10 μM) no longer elicited
an increase in ^{3}H-ACh release (Figure 4). Since desensitisation to
5-HT appears to be the most specific antagonist treatment available, it
is concluded that R 51 619 stimulates neuronal 5-HT receptors and
thereby releases ACh.

In two other experiments the strips were superfused first with
R 51 619 (1 μM) for 69 min and then, in addition, with 10 μM 5-HT.
Figure 5 shows that the facilitatory effect of 5-HT on ^{3}H-ACh release
was largely reduced in the presence of R 51 619. Thus, R 51 619 -
similar to 5-HT is assumed to have a dual action on 5-HT receptors,
namely first stimulation and subsequently desensitization.

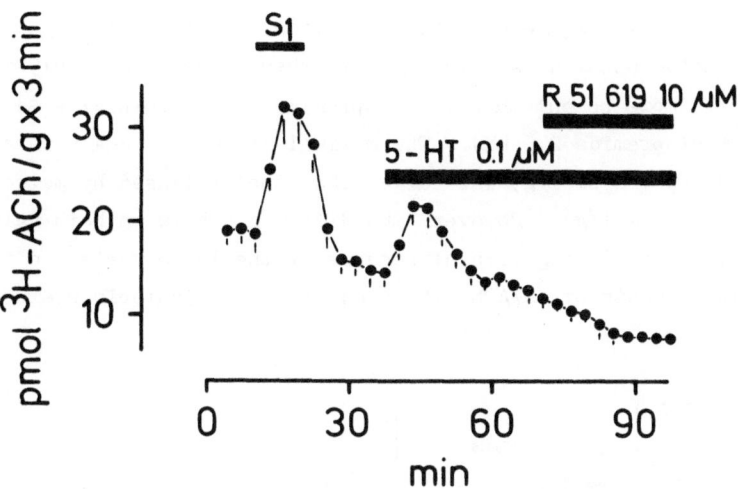

FIGURE 4   Effect of superfusion with 5-HT on ^{3}H-ACh outflow evoked
by R 51 619.   Means ± SEM of 4 expts.

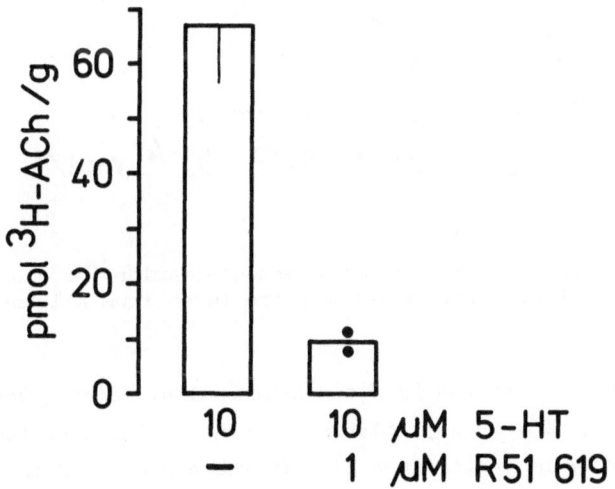

FIGURE 5   Effect of superfusion with R 51 619 on ^{3}H-ACh outflow
evoked by 5-HT. R 51 619 was added 69 min before 5-HT.

The effects of different concentrations of R 51 619 on outflow of ^{3}H-ACh are shown in Figure 6. For comparison the facilitatory actions of metoclopramide are included in this figure. R 51 619 is only slightly more potent than metoclopramide (EC 50 values: R 51 619 1.1 µM; metoclopramide 2.0 µM). The maximal amount of ^{3}H-ACh released by R 51 619 (23 ± 8 pmol/g) was larger than that released by metoclopramide (13 ± 2 pmol/g). However the difference between both values was not statistically significant because of the large variation in the absolute amounts of ^{3}H-ACh liberated from the myenteric plexus.

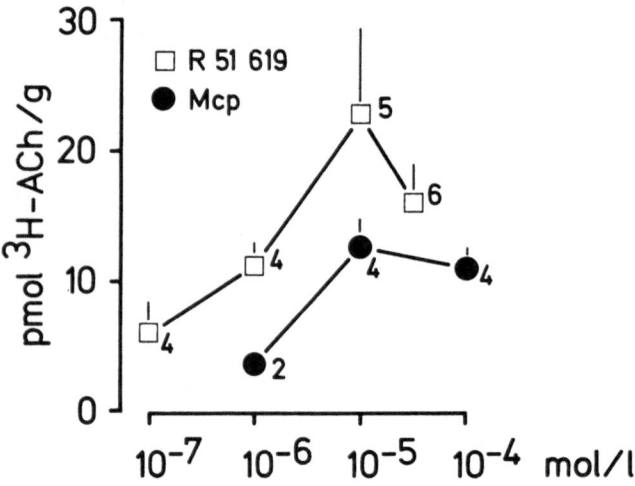

FIGURE 6   Increase by R 51 619 and metoclopramide (Mcp) of ^{3}H-ACh outflow.   Values for Mcp are taken from Kilbinger et al. (1982).

(b) ^{3}H-ACh outflow evoked by field stimulation. Strips were stimulated twice (S1; S2) and R 51 619 was present in the superfusate from 30 min before S2 on (cf. Figure 3). In the presence of 10 µM R 51 619 the evoked release of ^{3}H-ACh was significantly ($p < 0.05$) diminished (by 30 ± 4 %) (Figure 7). Methiothepin (1 µM) which is a specific antagonist on inhibitory 5-HT receptor of the guinea pig myenteric plexus (Kilbinger and Pfeuffer-Friederich, 1982) antagonized the inhibition of ^{3}H-ACh release by R 51 619 (Figure 7).

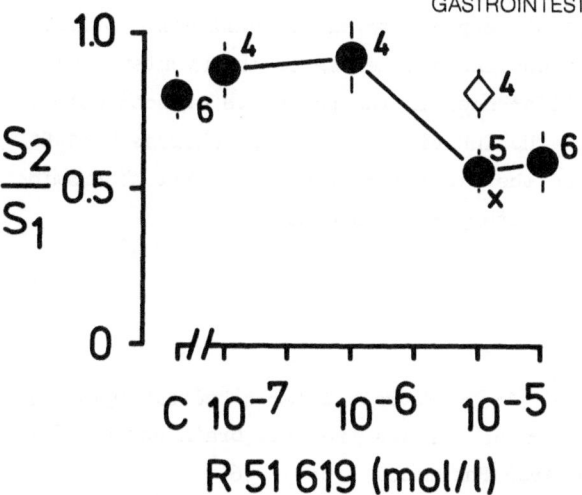

FIGURE 7   Inhibition by R 51 619 of stimulation-evoked outflow of
H-ACh.   Strips were stimulated in the absence (S) and
presence (S) of R 51 619.   R 51 619 was added 30 min
before S . x p 0.05 versus control (C)., effect of R 51
619 in the presence of 1 uM methiothepin which was added
to the superfusate 30 min before S .

DISCUSSION

R 51 619 is assumed to act on the excitatory 5-HT receptor for the
following reasons: (1) The increase of ACh release by R 51 619 was
abolished in the presence of a desensitizing concentration of 5-HT
(Figure 4). (2) R 51 619 elicited only a <u>transient</u> increase in ACh
release despite the continuous presence of the drug in the medium
(Figure 3).   (3) In the presence of R 51 619 the facilitatory effect
of 5-HT was reduced (Figure 5). Comparison of the maximal amounts of
ACh released by either 5-HT R 51 619 or metoclopramide suggests that
R 51 619 and metoclopramide have only weak agonistic effects; both
drugs probably act as partial agonists on the excitatory 5-HT receptor.

R 51 619, similar to 5-HT, also stimulates the inhibitory 5-HT
receptor and thus reduces the evoked release of ACh. Methiothepin
fully antagonizes the inhibitory action of R 51 619. Metoclopramide,
unlike R 51 619 or 5-HT, does not inhibit the stimulation-evoked outflow of ACh but, on the contrary, slightly enhances the evoked outflow (Kilbinger et al., 1982).

In conclusion, R 51 619 appears to exert qualitative similar effects as 5-HT on the cholinergic nerves of the myenteric plexus. There are, however differences in the potencies of both compounds. 5-HT is more potent on the inhibitory receptor whereas R 51 619 is somewhat more potent on the excitatory receptor. Metoclopramide only stimulates the excitatory 5-HT receptor.

REFERENCES

Göthert M, Weinheimer G (1979) Extracellular 5-hydroxytryptamine inhibits 5-hydroxytryptamine release from rat brain cortex slices. Naunyn-Schmiedeberg's Arch Pharmacol 310: 93-96

Kilbinger H, Wessler I (1980) Inhibition by acetylcholine of the stimulation-evoked release of ^{3}H-acetylcholine from the guineapig myenteric plexus. Neuroscience 5: 1331-1340

Kilbinger H, Kruel R, Pfeuffer-Friederich I, Wessler I (1982) The effects of metoclopramide on acetylcholine release and on smooth muscle response in the isolated guineapig ileum. Naunyn-Schmiedeberg's Arch Pharmacol 319: 231-238

Kilbinger H, Pfeuffer-Friederich I (1982) Facilitation and inhibition by serotonin of acetylcholine release from guineapig myenteric plexus: evidence for two types of neuronal serotonin receptors. Naunyn-Schmiedeberg's Arch Pharmacol 319: R 59

Langer SZ, Moret C (1982) Citalopram antagonizes the stimulation by LSD of presynaptic inhibitory serotonin autoreceptors in the rat hypothalamus. J Pharm Exp Therap 222: 220-226

North RA, Henderson G, Katajama Y, Johnson SM (1980) Electrophysiological evidence for presynaptic inhibition of acetylcholine release by 5-hydroxytryptamine in the enteric nervous system. Neuroscience 5: 581-586

Pfeuffer-Friederich I, Kilbinger H (1983) LSD induced inhibition of evoked acetylcholine release from guineapig myenteric plexus is mediated through serotonin (5-HT) receptors. Joint Meeting of the French and German Pharmacological and Toxicological Societies Freiburg i. Br., Sept. 20-23 1983

89

The Interaction of Adenosine with Isolated Myenteric Nerve Varicosities

M. A. COOK

INTRODUCTION

Adenosine and related compounds are presynaptic inhibitors of acetylcholine release from nerve endings in the myenteric plexus (1,2,3).
This inhibition is probably mediated by specific cell-surface receptors (4) and the possibility that they mediate physiological neuro-
modulation at nerves in the plexus has been suggested (5).

Previous studies (6,7) have demonstrated high-affinity binding
sites for adenosine on rat cortical synaptosomes and it thus appeared
useful to examine the nature of adenosine binding to the putative receptor sites on isolated myenteric varicosities (autonomic synaptosomes) prepared from guinea-pig ileum. The utility of this approach
is emphasized by the existence of considerable structure-activity data
for adenosine analogs as presynaptic inhibitors at the guinea-pig
ileum (8,9), and the possibility that isolated myenteric varicosities
may model the target system at which these data were established.

The feasibility of the approach was also of interest.

METHODS

Isolated myenteric varicosities were prepared from guinea-pig ileum
using established methods (10,11) with modifications (12). Occluded
lactate dehydrogenase (LDH), as a marker of cytoplasm enclosed within
a cell membrane, was determined on the purified varicosity fraction
(PV) as described in (12) and protein was determined by the method of
Hartree (13).

Adenosine binding to PV was measured using the rapid filtration method on Millipore HAWP filters with ~50 ug tissue protein per assay tube. The ligand used was 2,5', 8-[^{3}H]-adenosine (Amersham) and non-specific binding, in the presence of 10 mM unlabelled adenosine, was substracted from total binding to yield specific binding. Incubations were carried out at 22°C or 0°C for 90 mins and the incubation volume was 0.3 ml. Where appropriate, S^6-(4-nitrobenzyl)-6-thioinosine (NBMPR, Calbiochem, 10^{-7}M), an inhibitor of nucleoside transport and <u>erythro</u>-9-(2-hydroxy-3-nonyl)-adenine (EHNA, kind gift of Burroughs Wellcome, 25 μM), an inhibitor of adenosine deaminase, were present in the assay medium. Other experimental details are essentially as

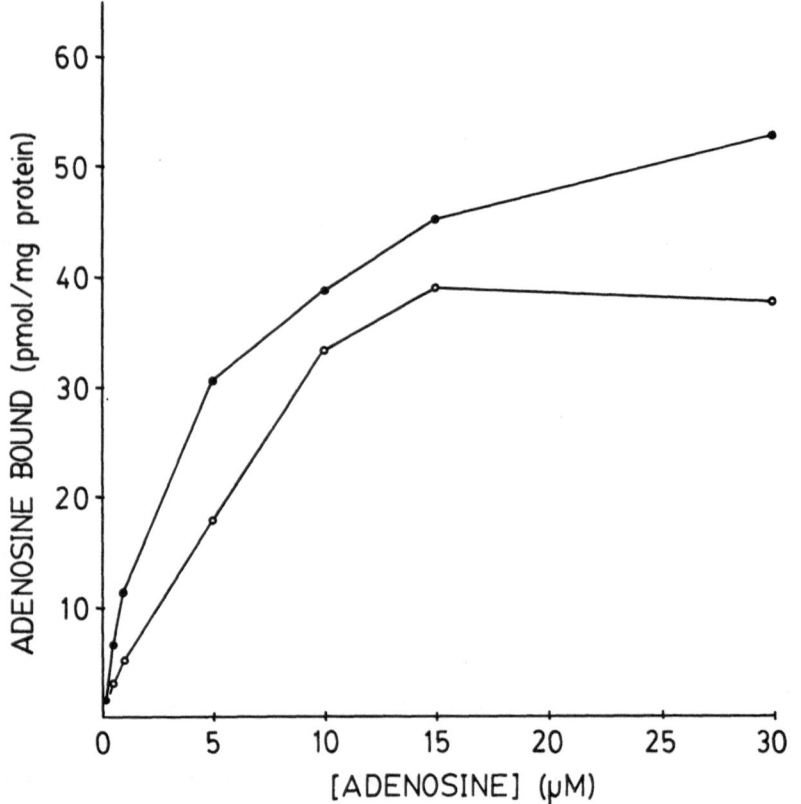

FIGURE 1   Specific binding of [^{3}H]-adenosine to myenteric varicosities in the absence (●) and presence (O) of NBMPR (10-^{7}M) at 22°C. Each point is mean of two experiments performed in duplicate.

in (6). Duplicate determinations were made at each point. Competi-
tion experiments between unlabelled analogs and 0.1 µM labelled
adenosine were performed in triplicate as described in (6). Analysis
of binding isotherms was as described in (14) and yielded corrected
values for the equilibrium dissociation constant (K_D) and maximal
binding capacity (Bmax).

RESULTS

Purified varicosities were prepared and their occluded LDH content
determined: typical values obtained were 531.2 ± 64.7 LDH units per
mg protein ($\bar{x}$ ± s.e.m., n=9) which compared favourably to those obtained by others (12). Examination of PV in the electron microscope
revealed that the most numerous profiles consisted of nerve terminals
with intact (resealed) cell membranes containing various types of

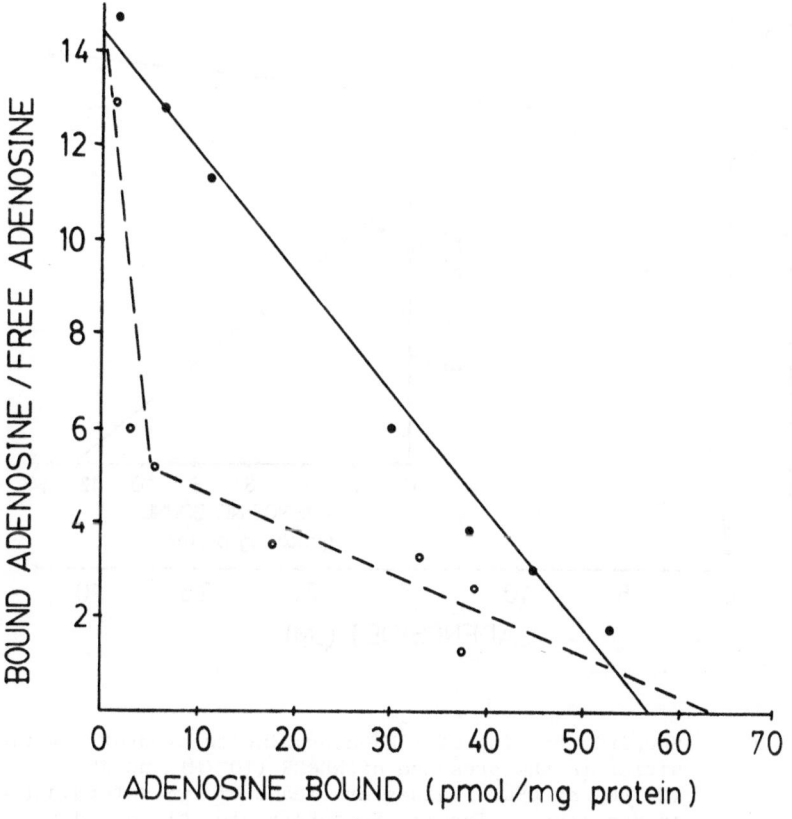

FIGURE 2   Scatchard plots of data from Fig. 1

vesicles. The dimensions of these varicosities ranged from

~ 0.5-1.8 µ in diameter. In addition, some free mitochondria and

membrane debris were seen. Some membranes had resealed to form

'ghosts'. Crude estimates suggested that approximately 80% of the

profiles in any given field were varicosities and ghosts.

The binding of [^{3}H]-adenosine to PV was examined at 22°C in the

presence and absence of NBMPR (Fig. 1). Scatchard analysis (Fig. 2)

revealed a single class of binding site with K_D=3.9 µM and Bmax=

56.5 pmoles/mg protein. Inclusion of the uptake inhibitor revealed

binding which could be resolved into that at a higher affinity site

with K_D=4.7x10^{-7} M and Bmax=7.07 pmoles/mg protein and a lower-affinity

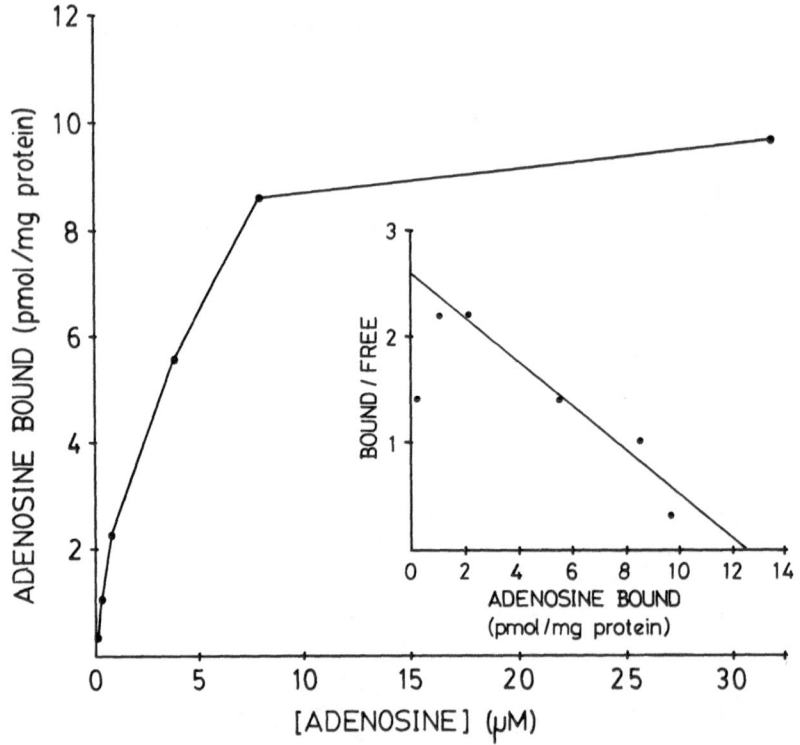

FIGURE 3   Specific binding of [^{3}H]-adenosine to myenteric varicosities in the presence of NBMPR (10^{-7}M) and EHNA
(25 µM) at 0°C. Values are means of two determinations
in duplicate. Inset: Scatchard plot of same data.

site with K_D=9.02 uM and Bmax=55.8 pmoles/mg protein. Performance of the assay at $0°C$ yielded binding parameters which were essentially similar to those obtained in the presence of NBMPR.

Inclusion of EHNA and incubation at $0°C$ revealed binding with K_D=4.5 μM and Bmax=12.1 pmoles/mg protein (Fig. 3).

Incubation of PV with 0.1 uM [³H]-adenosine and various concentrations of unlabelled structural analogs revealed a differential diminution in total binding as shown in Fig. 4.

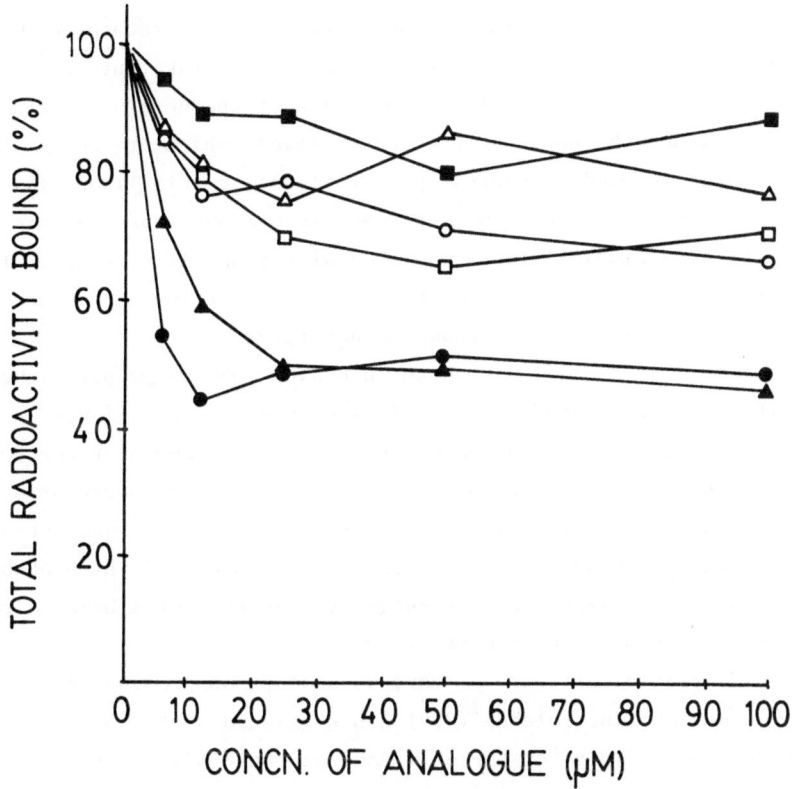

FIGURE 4   Diminution of [³H]-adenosine binding at 0.1 μM to myenteric varicosities by structural analogs of adenosine. Analogs and pD₂'s (from 9) are: 2-Cl-adenosine, 7.74 (▲); Adenosine, 5.91 (●); Nebularine, 4.63 (O); 8-Br-adenosine, 3.90 (☐); Inosine, 3.66 (■); Adenine, Inact. (△). Initial bound adenosine (100%): 2.7 pmol/mg protein (± 0.4 (2)). Assays performed at $0°C$. Each point is mean of three determinations

DISCUSSION

The preparation of purified myenteric varicosities proved relatively straightforward except that large quantities of tissue were required to yield sufficient PV for binding studies.

Saturation analysis of adenosine binding revealed, in the absence of inhibitors of metabolism and uptake, considerable binding to varicosities as evidenced by the large Bmax. The presence of NBMPR may have revealed a second, higher-affinity binding site. However, this is complicated by the virtual certainty of deamination of the ligand to inosine. Reduction of the incubation temperature to 0°C, which has been suggested to diminish nucleoside uptake into central synaptosomes by $\sim 70\%$, as well as inclusion of the deaminase inhibitor, EHNA, diminished the apparent binding to levels which are comparable to those demonstrated in central preparations for this ligand (6). It is clear, however, that these parameters are not those expected of a high-affinity binding site associated with a specific receptor for an endogenous ligand. Furthermore, the binding affinities measured may be at the limit of the method's capability.

Consideration of binding studies on brain membrane preparations using the non-metabolizable ligand (-)N^{6}-phenylisopropyl-[^{3}H]-adenosine (PIA) (15), which yielded K_{D}'s in the nanomolar range, suggest that this ligand may be more likely to reveal the postulated neuromodulator receptor on myenteric nerve endings. The demonstration in this study of an active nucleoside uptake system and the probable presence of metabolizing enzymes suggests that further studies with this target system may be fruitful.

The differential efficacy of various analogs as presynaptic inhibitors of acetylcholine release (8,9) has suggested that a parallel ranking of the affinity of these ligands at the binding site on PV might be obtained. The displacement study revealed that, in general, biological efficacy and ability to displace adenosine from its binding site are parallel and suggests that examination of this relationship using PIA will further illuminate the nature of the adenosine receptor.

The author thanks Ms. N. Huggins for technical assistance and Dr. R. Buck, Dept. of Anatomy, U.W.O. for assistance with electron microscopy. This work was supported by MRC Canada.

REFERENCES

1. Sawynok, J. and Jhamandas, K.H. (1976). Inhibition of acetylcho-
    line release from cholinergic nerves by adenosine, adenine nucleo-
    tides and morphine: Antagonism by theophylline. J. Pharmacol.
    Exp. Ther. 197, 379-390.

2. Vizi, E.S. and Knoll, J. (1976). The inhibitory effect of adeno-
    sine and related nucleotides on the release of acetylcholine.
    Neuroscience 1, 391-398.

3. Cook, M.A., Hamilton, J.T. and Okwuasaba, F.K. (1978). Coenzyme
    A is a purine nucleotide modulator of acetylcholine output.
    Nature (Lond.) 271, 768-771.

4. Okwuasaba, F.K., Hamilton, J.T. and Cook, M.A. (1978). Evidence
    for the Cell Surface Locus of Presynaptic Purine Nucleotide Re-
    ceptors in the Guinea-pig Ileum. J. Pharmacol. Exp. Ther. 207,
    779-786.

5. Fredholm, B.B., Gustafsson, L.E., Hedqvist, P. and Solleri, A.
    (1983). Adenosine in the regulation of neurotransmitter release
    in the peripheral nervous system. In: Berne, R.M., Rall, T.W.
    and Rubio, R. (eds.). Regulatory Function of Adenosine. pp. 479-
    495 (Boston: Martinus Nijhoff).

6. Newman, M.E., Patel, J. and McIlwain, H. (1981). The binding
    of [3H]-adenosine to synaptosomal and other preparations from
    the mammalian brain. Biochem. J. 194, 611-620.

7. Newman, M. and Levitzki, A. (1982). Characteristics of high-
    affinity [3H]-adenosine binding to rat brain synaptosomes and
    turkey erythrocyte membranes. Biochem. Biophys. Acta. 685.,
    129-136.

8. Cook, M.A., Hamilton, J.T. and Okwuasaba, F.K. (1979). Structure-
    Activity Relationship Studies of Purinergic Agonists: Some
    speculations on the Source and Identity of the Purinergic Mediator.
    In: Baer, H.P. and Drummond, G.I. (eds.). Physiological and
    Regulatory Functions of Adenosine and Adenine Nucleotides.
    pp. 103-113 (New York, Raven Press).

9. Paul, M.L., Miles, D.L. and Cook, M.A. (1982). The influence of
    glycosidic conformation and charge distribution on activity of
    adenine nucleosides as presynaptic inhibitors of acetylcholine
    release. J. Pharmacol. Exp. Ther. 222, 241-245.

10. Jonakait, G.M., Gintzler, A.R. and Gershon, M.D. (1979).
    Isolation of axonal varicosities (autonomic synaptosomes) from the
    enteric nervous system. J. Neurochem. 32, 1387-1400.

11. Briggs, C.A. and Cooper, J.R. (1981). A synaptosomal preparation
    from the guinea-pig ileum myenteric plexus. J. Neurochem. 36,
    1097-1108.

12. White, T.D. and Leslie, R.A. (1982). Depolarization-induced
     release of adenosine 5-triphosphate from isolated varicosities
     derived from the myenteric plexus of the guinea-pig small
     intestine. J. Neuroscience 2, 206-215.

13. Hartree, E.F. (1972). Determination of protein: A modifica-
     tion of the Lowry method that gives a linear photometric
     response. Anal. Biochem. 48, 422-427.

14. Zirin, J.A. and Waud, D.R. (1982). How to analyze binding,
     enzyme and uptake data: the simplest case, a single phase.
     Life Sci. 30, 1407-1422.

15. Schwabe, V. (1983). General aspects of binding of ligands to
     adenosine receptors. In: Berne, R.M., Rall, T.W. and Rubio, R.
     (eds.) Regulatory Function of Adenosine. pp. 77-96 (Boston:
     Martinus Nijhoff).

90

Effect of Peptide YY on Contractile Activity in the Stomach of Heidenhain Pouch Dogs

Z. ITOH, T. SUZUKI, M. NAKAYA, K. TATEMOTO and V. MUTT

INTRODUCTION

A new candidate regulatory peptide, peptide YY (PYY) has been isolated from extracts of the porcine upper small intestine (1), and its chemical structure has been determined (2). PYY has been found to inhibit both secretin- and cholecystokinin-induced pancreatic secretion in anesthetized cats (2). In the present study, the effect of this newly isolated peptide on gastric contractile activity in conscious Heidenhain pouch dogs.

MATERIALS AND METHODS

Preparation of animals

A Heidenhain-type gastric fundic pouch was constructed in 4 healthy adult mongrel dogs. The pouch was cannulated for spontaneous drainage of gastric secretion. Contractile activity of circular muscle contraction in the gastric antrum, in the gastric body and in a mid-portion of the pouch was measured by means of chronically implanted force transducers. A Silastic tube (602-205, Dow Corning Corp) was chronically introduced into the superior vena cava: this tube was used as a route for i.v. injection of test materials.

Contractile activity in the main stomach and the pouch was recorded with a recorder (EE13, Nihon Koden Kohgyo, Ltd., Tokyo). Test materials in 3.0 ml 0.9% saline or saline alone were given as a bolus injection through the indwelling silastic tube during the period of interdigestive migrating contractions (IMC) in the stomach.

Test materials

PYY was purified from extracts of the porcine small intestine at the Karolinska Institute by Tatemoto and Mutt. Pentapeptide of gastrin was purchased from ICI Japan. These peptide preparations were dissolved in 0.9% normal saline to a desired concentration immediately before experiment and administered through the chronically implanted tube.

RESULTS

Effect of PYY during the digestive state

PYY had no effect on the contractile pattern of the main stomach and the Heidenhain pouch during the digestive state. In this study PYY in doses less than 300 pmol/kg of body wt did not affect the digestive contractile pattern.

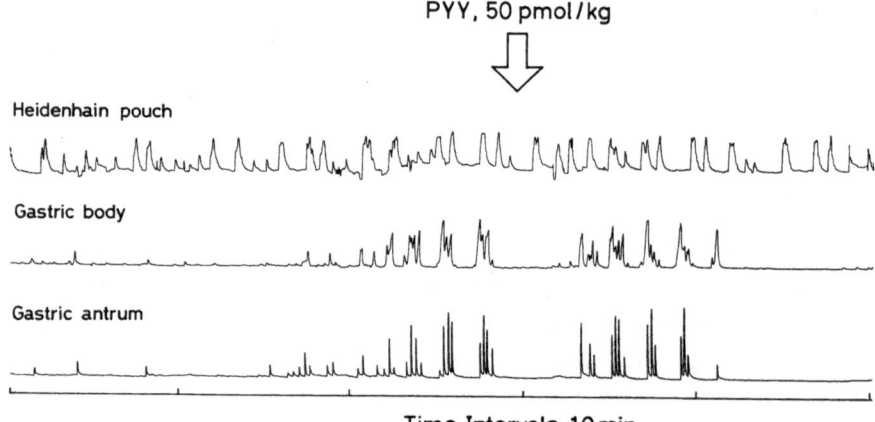

Figure 1. Effect of PYY (50 pmol/kg body wt) on the interdigestive migrating contractions in the Heidenhain pouch, gastric body and antrum in a conscious dog. Contractions in the gastric body and the antrum are completely suppressed for 4 min by PYY, but the pouch contractions are not affected at all.

Effect of PYY on interdigestive contractions

Figure 1 demonstrates the effect of PYY (50 pmol/kg body wt) on contractile activity in the Heidenhain pouch, the gastric body and antrum during the interdigestive state. Contractile activity in the gastric body and antrum is clearly inhibited for 4 min, but contractions in the Heidenhain pouch were not affected by PYY. A dose-response study between the mean inhibitory effect on the innervated stomach and doses of PYY from 12.5 to 100 pmol/kg body wt indicated that the inhibition is significant and dose-related from 1.2 ± 0.1 to 5.8 ± 0.3 min.

The cycle of the IMC was not affected by the injection of PYY, but the duration of the IMC was significantly prolonged by doses of 50 and 100 pmol/kg body wt in 3 dogs. PYY injection did not provoke any side effects such as restlessness, nausea, retching, and changes in respiration and pulse rate in each of 4 dogs.

Effect of pentagastrin on interdigestive contractions

Pentagastrin is known to inhibit the occurrence of the IMC in the stomach (3). However, with bolus doses less than 200 pmol/kg body wt, it did not influence contractile activity in either the main stomach or the vagally denervated pouch.

Effect of atropine

Atropine (0.05 mg/kg body wt) suppressed contractile activity in the Heidenhain pouch as well as the gastric body and antrum completely, but the IMC-like contractions recovered in all three sites 86 ± 5.2 min after atropine injection.

DISCUSSION

In the present study, it was found that postprandial contractile activity in the stomach is not affected by PYY in doses that inhibited pancreatic secretory response to secretin in cats (2), or gastric contractile activity during the interdigestive state in conscious dogs. During the interdigestive state, since the IMC-like strong contractions occur in the vagally denervated stomach in association with the main stomach (4), studies on the Heidenhain pouch dogs were carried out to eliminate the influence of vagal connection.

As demonstrated in the present study, it was revealed that contractile activity in the vagally denervated fundic pouch was not inhibited by PYY, and contractile activity in the normally innervated main stomach was dose-dependently inhibited by PYY, but the cycle of the IMC was not affected by PYY. This fact suggests that PYY does not act through the same site as motilin or atropine. Atropine acts through an intrinsic cholinergic pathway since its blocks the IMC in both the innervated and denervated stomach. The inhibitory effect of PYY is therefore considered to act at the preganglionic level of the vagus nerve. Another explanation for the dissociation of inhibition between the innervated and vagally denervated stomach is that the sensitivity of the pouch to PYY is diminished by vagal denervation as in the case of decreased sensitivity of the Heidenhain pouch to acid secretagogues.

In the present study, pentagastin abolished the IMC in the main stomach at doses more than 300 pmol/kg body wt, but contractions in the pouch were not inhibited by a bolus injection of 300 pmol/kg body wt. In our previous study (4), however, pentagastrin when infused intravenously in a dose of 1.0 μg (1302 pmol)/kg-hr, suppressed contractions in both the innervated and vagally denervated stomach. In this case, however, pouch contractions ceased in 11.6 ± 0.8 min after the initiation of the infusion. Consequently, it is concluded that contractile activity in the vagally denervated stomach is resistant to inhibitory activity of peptides, such as PYY and pentagastrin. Vagal denervation may elevate the threshold of sensitivity to these peptides, or contractile activity in the denervated pouch per se may differ in its control mechanism.

In conclusion, while the physiological role of PYY in the inhibitory activity of gastric motor activity is beyond specula-tion, this peptide inhibits the IMC in the stomach transiently, but dose dependently, probably through the extrinsic nerves, yet does not affect the regulation of IMC mechanism.

REFERENCES

1. Tatemoto, K. and Mutt, V. (1980). Isolation of two novel hormones using a chemical method for finding naturally occurring polypeptide. Nature **285**, 417–418.
2. Tatemoto, K. (1982). Isolation and characterization of peptide YY (PYY), a candidate gut hormone that inhibits pancreatic secretion. Proc. Natl. Acad. Sci. USA **79**, 2514–2518.
3. Itoh, Z., Takeuchi, S., Aizawa, I. and Couch, E.F. (1977). Inhibitory effect of pentagastrin and feeding on natural and motilin-induced interdigestive contractions in the stomach of conscious dogs. Gastroenterol. Jpn. **12**, 284–288.
4. Itoh, Z., Takayanagi, R., Takeuchi, S. and Isshiki, S. (1978). Interdigestive motor activity of Heidenhain pouches in relation to main stomach in conscious dogs. Am. J. Physiol. **234**, E333–338.

91

Alterations of Digestive Motility by *Escherichia coli* Endotoxin in Rabbits Mediated through Central Opiate Receptors

J. FIORAMONTI, L. BUENO and C. DU

INTRODUCTION

Disturbances of gastrointestinal motility are frequently associated
with infectious diseases. In the ileum of anaesthetized rabbits, ente-
rotoxigenic strains of *Escherichia coli* have induced a peculiar pattern
of motility with bursts of spikes rapidly propagated aborally (1).
Recently in rats it has been shown that migrating myoelectric complexes
are disrupted by administration of *E. coli* enterotoxin (2). Lipopolysa-
ccharide endotoxin of *E. coli* is known to induce fever with inhibition
of gastric motility and diarrhoea in several mammalian species (3).
Disturbances such as arterial hypotension and hypoglycaemia induced by
E. coli endotoxin in rats would involve opiate receptors since they are
blocked by naloxone (4,5). A central mediation of these effects may be
possible since small doses of endotoxin are able to increase the
secretion of β endorphin in sheep (6).
The aim of this study was to determine if the alterations of digestive
motility induced in rabbits by *E. coli* endotoxin can be mediated
through central opiate receptors. For that purpose, the effects of
E. coli endotoxin were compared to those produced by central and by
peripheral administration of morphine, and central and peripheral
injections of naloxone were used to block the effects of *E. coli*
endotoxin.

MATERIALS AND METHODS

Six New-Zealand rabbits, 2-3 kg in body weight, were used in these
experiments. Under halothane anaesthesia, groups of three electrodes
(insulated nichrome wire) were implanted at the following sites :
antrum (at 2 cm from the pylorus), duodenum and jejunum (at 10 cm, 1 m
and 2 m from the pylorus), ileum (at 15 cm from the ileo-caecal
junction), caecum (on the 5 th coil), and proximal colon (at 10 cm from
de caeco-colonic junction). In addition, a small polyethylene cannula
was inserted into a lateral cerebral ventricle. Six days after surgery,
the electrical activity was recorded with an electroencephalograph
(Mini-huit, Alvar, Paris). At 20-s intervals concurrent summation of
the spiking activity from three electrodes sites (antrum, jejunum and
caecum) was obtained by a linear integrator circuit connected to a four
channel potentiometric recorder with a paper speed of 6 cm/h. The fourth channel of the recorder was used to record variations of body temperature obtained from a thermistor probe placed subcutaneously at the
beginning of each recording session.

In each animal, after 2 h of control recordings, purified lipopoly-
saccharides (LPS) obtained from *E. coli* serotype 0127:B8 was injected
intravenously (IV) at a dose of 0.1 µg/kg alone or 20 min after administration of naloxone intravenously at a dose of 100 µg/kg or
intracerebroventricularly (ICV) at a dose of 10 µg/kg. The effects of
IV (1 mg/kg) and ICV (50 µg/kg) injection of morphine were also
determined.

RESULTS

- Control studies

The electromyogram of the antrum consisted of bursts of spikes lasting 3-5 s occurring at a mean frequency of 2.1 ± 0.4 /min (Fig. 1).
On the duodenum, groups of 2-4 spike bursts appeared coordinated with
antral spike bursts. Below Treitz's ligament, spike bursts were organized in migrating myoelectric complexes which recurred at very variable intervals (range 50 - 300 min). The electrical activity of the
caecum consisted of spike bursts lasting about 3 s occurring at a mean
frequency of 1.3 ± 0.3/min, that of the proximal colon was characterized by short spike bursts recorded for 60 % of the time.

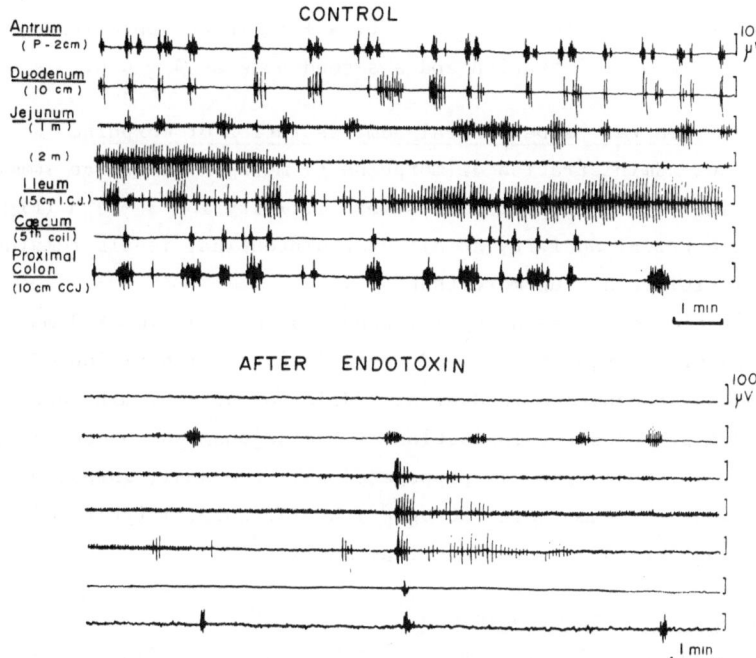

FIGURE 1 ' Gastrointestinal electromyogram in a rabbit before and two
hours after IV administration of *E. coli* endotoxin (0.1
µg/kg). Spiking activity of all the digestive sites was
strongly inhibited after endotoxin. Note the burst of
spikes rapidly propagated over the jejunum and the ileum,
and then on the caecum and the colon.

- Effects of endotoxin

Intravenous administration of endotoxin (0.1 µg/kg) induced after a
delay of 40-60 min, a total inhibition of stomach motility lasting
4 to 6 h. On the jejunum and the ileum the administration was followed
20 - 30 min later by a phase of regular spiking activity ; then the
spiking activity was strongly reduced for 4 - 6 hours. During this
period, bursts of spikes of large amplitude appeared, and propagated
to the jejunum, the ileum, the caecum and the proximal colon (Fig. 1).
Spiking activity of the caecum and the colon was also strongly inhibited during this period : the frequency of caecal spike bursts decreased
from 1.3 ± 0.3 to 0.1 ± 0.04 /min and spiking activity on the proximal

colon was present during 5 % of the time (vs 60 % in control studies).
After a delay of 20 - 30 min the body temperature increased biphasical-
ly from 37.8 $\pm$ 0.2 °C to 39.9 $\pm$ 0.3 °C, a first peak appearing 1,5 - 2h
after endotoxin administration and a second peak at 4 - 6 h.

- Effects of central vs peripheral administration of morphine

Intravenous administration of morphine (1 mg/kg) induced an immëdiate
and total inhibition of gastrointestinàl motility for 3 - 4 h (Fig. 3).
Then the electrical activity at all gastrointestinal levels remained
strongly inhibited during more than 4 h.

Administration of morphine by ICV route (50 μg/kg) mimicked most of
the effects of IV injection of endotoxin (Fig. 4). Inhibition of the
antrum and the caecum occurred after a delay of 40 - 60 min, and a
phase of RSA preceded the inhibition of the jejunum and of the ileum.
However, spike brusts rapidly propagated over the small intestine did
not appear. At the same dose (50 μg/kg) by IV route, morphine did not
affect the pattern of gastrointestinal motility.

- Antagonistic effects of naloxone

Previous (30 min) administration of ICV naloxone by (10 μg/kg) partially blocked the disturbances of gastrointestinal motility induced by
E. coli endotoxin. A 20 % and 30 % decrease in the frequency of antral
and caecal spike bursts was observed instead of the complete inhibition
which followed administration of endotoxin alone. Phase of RSA did not
appear on the jejunum and ileum where spiking activity was reduced by
40 % (vs 80 % after endotoxin alone). Moreover, the number of spike
bursts rapidly propagated aborally was significantly (P < 0.05)
reduced from 4.3 $\pm$ 0.7/h to 1.7 $\pm$ 0.5/h.

Naloxone given by IV route (100 μg/kg) did not block any of the effects of E. coli endotoxin. The increase in body temperature following
endotoxin injection was not modified by previous ICV or IV administration of naloxone.

DISCUSSION

Intravenous administration of E. coli endotoxin in conscious rabbits
induced nonpecific digestive motor disturbances. The bursts of spikes
rapidly propagated aborally resemble the migrating action potential
complexes (MAPC) caused by E. coli or cholera enterotoxin administered

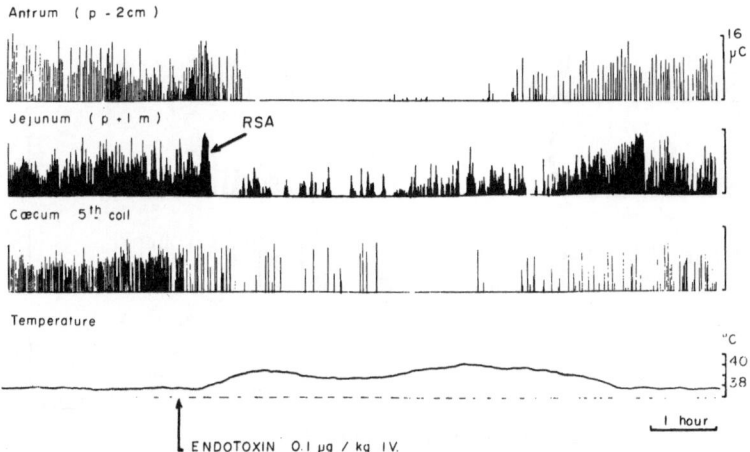

FIGURE 2   Effects of *E. coli* endotoxin on gastrointestinal motility
Integrated electromyograms obtained from the antrum the
jejunum (at 1 m from the pylorus), and the caecum. The
lower tracing indicates body temperature recorded from a
subcutaneous probe. The motility of the stomach and the
caecum was strongly inhibited after a delay of about 1 hour.
The inhibition of the jejunal motility was preceded by a
phase of regular spiking activity (RSA). Body temperature
was increased by 2°C after endotoxin administration.

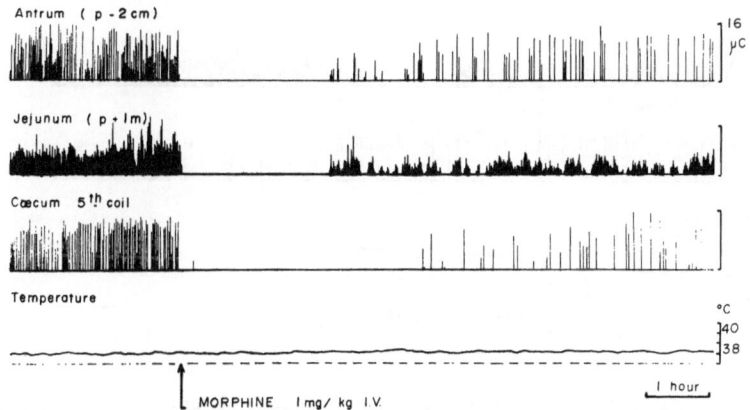

FIGURE 3   The intravenous injection of morphine was followed by an
immediate and complete inhibition of gastrointestinal
motility

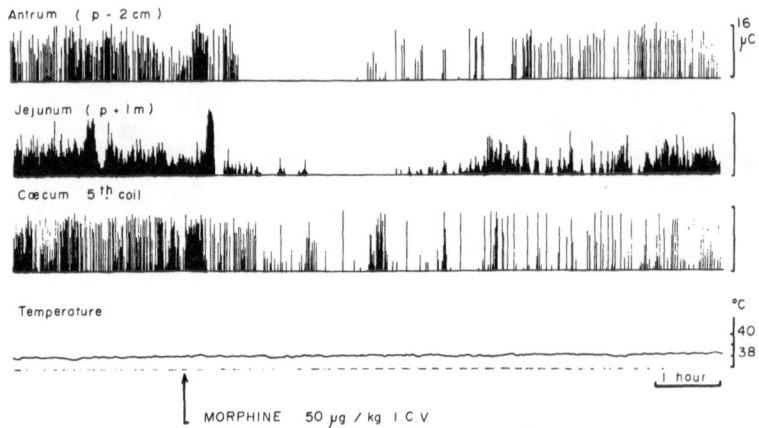

FIGURE 4   ICV injection of morphine almost mimicked that of IV
administration of endotoxin. The inhibition of the stomach
and the caecum appeared after a delay of about 1 h and that
of the jejunum was preceded by a phase of regular spiking
activity.

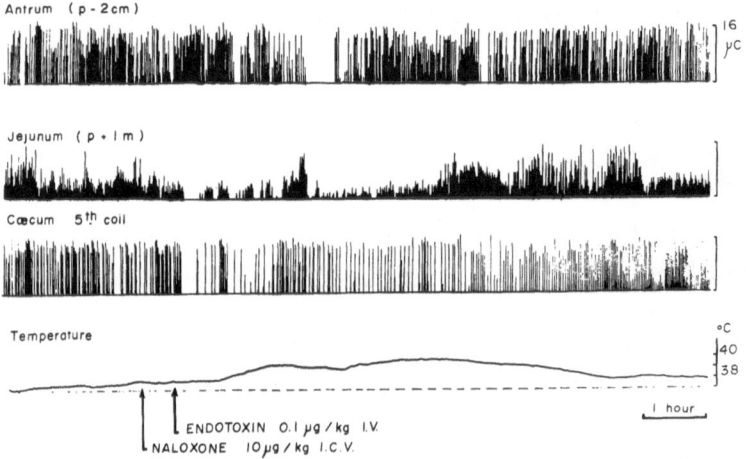

FIGURE 5   Naloxone administered by ICV route blocked the effects of
endotoxin. The inhibition of gastrointestinal motility was
strongly reduced by a previous ICV administration of
naloxone. The increase in body temperature persisted.

to anaesthetized rabbit (1,7). In experimental coccidiosis in rabbit strong inhibition of the small intestine motility has been also found (8). The effects of cholera enterotoxin may be mediated through a local mechanism, since MAPC have appeared *in vitro* in cholera-exposed rabbit ileum (7). Our results indicate that administration of *E. coli* endotoxin causes mainly the inhition of the gastrointestinal motility, an effect centrally mediated, since it is blocked by prior ICV administration of naloxone which is inactive when given by IV route at a dose 10 times higher. The involvement of central opiates receptors is suggested by ICV administration of naloxone which prevents the IV effects of *E. coli* endotoxin and by the similar effects of morphine ICV. As for endotoxin, morphine ICV induced an inhibition of gastrointestinal motility after a delay of 1 h and induced a phase of regular spiking activity on the small intestine. Such delay and activity phase failed to appear after IV administration of morphine. However, the mechanisms involved in the appearance of the peculiar spike bursts propagated aborally remain unclear since this activity was reduced after ICV administration of naloxone bu was not induced by ICV or IV injection of morphine. The effects of morphine observed herein in rabbit underline its diversity of action according to : the animal species, the site of the digestive tract considered (9) as well as the route of administration (10). The mechanisms and pathways for the centrally mediated effects of *E. coli* endotoxin and morphine are not known. The delay in the appearance of gastrointestinal disturbances observed herein suggests the involvement of an humoral mechanism rather than a neural pathway as already demonstrated for the inhibition of intestinal transit by ICV administration of morphine in the rat (11). Moreover, the lack of blockade by central administration of naloxone of the increase in body temperature confirms that the gastrointestinal disturbances induced by *E. coli* endotoxin are not related to hyperthermia, as already suggested in goats (12).

Our data suggest that gastrointestinal disturbances induced by endotoxin in rabbits are mainly mediated through central opiate receptors independently of the hyperthemia.

REFERENCES

1. Burns, T.W., Mathias, J.R., Carlson, G.M., Martin, J.L. and Sheilds, R.P. (1978). Effect of toxigenic *Escherichia coli* on myoelectric activity of small intestine. Am. J. Physiol., 235, E311-5.
2. Stahle, E., Gustavsson, S., Ronnberg, B., Wadstrom, T. and Wilen, T. (1982). Disorganization of the small bowel transport pattern by systemic administration of heat-stable enterotoxin in rats. 1st Eur. Symp. Gastrointestinal Motility, Bologna, Italy
3. Van Miert, A.S.P.J.A.M. and Frens, J. (1968). The reaction of different animal species to bacterial pyrogens. Zbl. Vet. Med. A., 15, 532-543
4. Faden, A.I. and Holaday, J.W. (1980). Naloxone treatment of endotoxin shock ; stereospecificity of physiologic and pharmacologic effects in the rat. J. Pharmacol. Exp. Ther., 212, 441-447
5. Adeleye, G.A., Furman, B.L. and Parrat, J.R. (1982). Possible involvement of opiate receptors in the response of conscious rats to *Escherichia coli* enterotoxin ; protective effect of naloxone. J. Physiol. (London), 329, 31P
6. Carr, D.B., Bergland, R., Hamilton, A., Blume, H., Kasting, N., Arnold, M., Martin, J.B. and Rosenblatt, M. (1982). Endotoxin-stimulated opioid peptide secretion : two secretory pools and feedback control in vivo. Science, 217, 865-6
7. Koch, K.L., Martin, J.L. and Mathias, J.R. (1983). Migrating action potential complexes in vitro in cholera-exposed rabbit ileum. Am. J. Physiol., 244, G291-294.
8. Fioramonti, J., Sorraing, J.M., Licois, D. and Buéno, L. (1981). The intestinal motor and transit disturbances associated with experimental coccidiosis (*Eimeria magna*) in the rabbit. Ann. Rech. Vét., 12, 413-420
9. Fioramonti, J., Niemegeers, C.J.E. and Awouters, F. (1983). Diarrhoea and antidiarrhoeal drugs. In : Ruckebusch, Y., Toutain, P.L. and Koritz, D. (eds). Veterinary Pharmacology and Therapeutics.(Lancaster ; MTP Press) in press
10. Weisbrodt, N.W., Thor, P.J., Anderson, J. and Copeland, E.M. (1982). Morphine's effect on intestinal motility is mediated via the central nervous system. In : Weinbeck, M. (ed). Motility of the Digestive Tract. pp. 462-466. (New York : Raven Press)
11. Stewart, J.J., Weisbrodt, N.W. and Burks, T.F. (1978). Central and peripheral actions of morphine on intestinal transit. J. Pharmacol. Exp. Ther., 205, 547-555

12. Van Miert, A.S.J.P.A.M., Van Der Wal-Komproe, L.E. and Van Duin, C.T.M. (1977). Effects of antipyretic agents on fever and ruminal stasis induced by endotoxins in conscious goats. Arch. Int. Pharmacodyn. 225, 39-50

92

Central Effects of Thyrotropin-Releasing Hormone on Gastrointestinal Motility in Fasted and Fed Rats

Y. RUCKEBUSCH, G. SOLDANI and J. P. FERRÉ

INTRODUCTION

Many actions on gastrointestinal functions[1-6] have been demonstrated for TRH since it has been located in the gastrointestinal tract[7]. Excitatory effects of TRH on duodenal and colonic motilities in anaesthetized rabbits[8,9] and rats[10] have been related to central administration of the peptide. Preliminary results have shown that small doses of TRH inactive under anaesthesia when given by intracerebroventricular (ICV) and intravenous (IV) routes, have induced an hyperactivity of the gastroduodenal junction at a dosage of 1 (ICV) to 5 (IV) in the conscious animal. We have examined, therefore, the effects on the patterns of small intestine electrical activity of an ICV vs. IV administration of TRH in conscious rats, either fasted or fed, under anaesthesia and after different pretreatments.

METHODS

Fourteen male Wistar rats (300-600 g) housed singly in wire-bottomed cages and fed UAR rat chow were used. Pairs of nichrome electrodes were implanted, under anaesthesia, in the duodeno-jejunum at 5, 15 and 25 cm from the pylorus, and polyethylene catheters were inserted into a lateral cerebral ventricle and the right jugular vein.

Recordings were started 5 days after surgery. The electrical activity was directly registered with an EEG machine (Reega VIII, Alvar, Paris) at a paper speed of 3 cm/min. The electrical spiking activity was summed

557

each 20 sec and automatically plotted on the "y" axis of a potentiometric recorder at a paper speed of 5 cm/h[11]. The rats, fed ad libitum
from 8:00 a.m. to 7:00 p.m., received TRH (Biodata, Milan, Italy) after
a 17-h fast (fasted state) or one hour after giving a 6 g lab chow meal
(fed state). The dosage varied from 2.6 nM to 0.26 μM for the IV route
and from 13 pM to 1.3 nM ICV in both fed and fasted states. The effects
of TRH (1.3 nM - ICV) were examined under anaesthesia and after atropine, naloxone, methylnaloxone, phenoxybenzamine (PBZ), promethazine,
cimetidine, bromocriptine, sulpiride and domperidone administered subcutaneously (SC). The total duration of the effects was calculated from
the integrated records. Statistical analysis was performed using the
paired "t" test and covariance analysis. Control rats received the same
volume (10 μl) of saline.

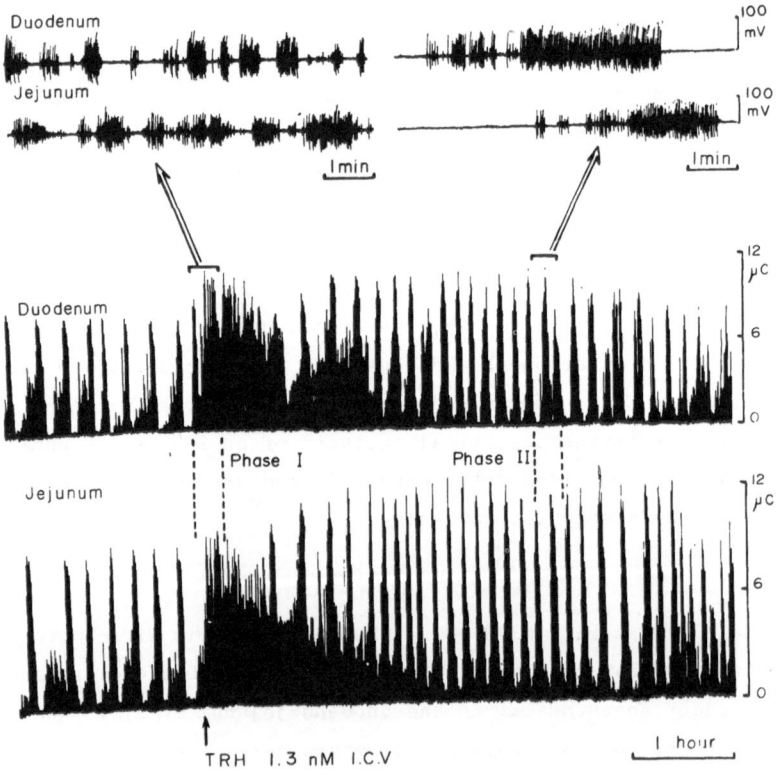

FIGURE 1   Direct and integrated record of duodenum and jejunum electro-
            myograms in the fasted rat. Disruption of the characteristic
            MMC pattern for about 40 min by TRH (phase I). Recurrence of
            the MMCs at a higher frequency and magnitude (phase II).

The electrical activity in fasted rats was organized into migrating myo-electric complex (MMC), recurring 4 to 5 times per hour. Each complex consisted of a phase of irregular and then regular spiking activity (ISA and RSA phases) lasting 10 to 11 min was followed by a short phase of quiescence of about 4 min. After the ingestion of 6 g lab chow, the pattern of activity was continuous for 5-7 hours.

Effects of ICV TRH in fasted versus fed conscious rats

The injection of TRH (13 pM, n = 5) in fasted rats failed to cause any increase in duodenal or jejunal motor activity. Erratic effects were obtained with a 0.13 nM TRH dosage. In contrast, in all animals, a 1.3 nM TRH dose disrupted the MMC pattern (phase I). The disruption of duodenal and jejunal cyclic motor activities lasted for 36.5 $\pm$ 13 min and 30.7 $\pm$ 11.7 min (n = 12) respectively. The spiking activity occupied approximately 60 % of the recording time on both duodenum and jejunum. In 72 % of treated rats, the MMC pattern recurred at a significant higher frequency than normally (5.6 $\pm$ 1.3 MMC/h vs. 4.17 $\pm$ 0.3 ; $P < 0.05$) during approximately 4-5 h in both duodenum and jejunum (phase II).

In fed rats, TRH injection (1.3 nM) caused an increased spiking activity for 53 $\pm$ 8.5 min (n = 4), which was followed within 2 h by a subsequent MMC pattern at a high frequency lasting 2 h for the duodenum and 4-5 h for the jejunum.

Influence of anaesthesia

In anaesthetized rats (pentobarbital Na, 50 mg/kg), the ICV infusion of TRH (1.3 nM) modified the motor profile, but the effects were nearly halved. Differences were not observed between fasted vs. fed states.

Effects of IV TRH in fasted versus fed rats

The injection of TRH (2.6 nM) did not modify the motor profile of either fasted or fed conscious rats. A period of increased activity for only 2-3 min and a disruption for 25-32 min of the fasted pattern was limited to the duodenum after an IV injection of 0.13 µM TRH in fasted rats (n = 3). At a higher dosage (0.26 µM), similar effects occurred also on the jejunum. The motor effects elicited by TRH (0.26 µM) under anaesthesia resembled as expected those recorded for a lower dosage (0.13 µM) in the conscious animals.

Receptor antagonists in conscious and fasted rats

Naloxone (5 and 10 mg/kg SC) 15 min before TRH (1.3 nM ICV) increased
the duration of phase I (n = 4, P < 0.01), meanwhile the MMC did not recur at a higher frequency during phase II (Fig. 2 & Table I). Lower dosage of naloxone (1 mg/kg SC) and methylnaloxone (30 mg/kg SC) were
inactive. Methylnaloxone (0.1 mg/kg) by ICV route prevented phase I from
appearing. Domperidone (5 mg/kg SC) had stimulatory effects per se,
hence disrupted the MMC pattern and, like bromocriptine (5 mg/kg IP),
enhanced the effects of TRH (1.3 nM ICV) without changing phase II
(Fig. 2). Sulpiride (5 mg/kg SC) did not modify the TRH effects. Either
atropine (0.25 mg/kg SC) or phenoxybenzamine (5 mg/kg SC) 30 min before
TRH (1.3 nM ICV) both prevented an increase in motility of the duodeno-
jejunum (Fig. 3). By the ICV route, atropine (0.1 mg/kg) blocked phases
I and II for 2-3 hours. Phenoxybenzamine (5 mg/kg) disrupted per se the
MMC pattern and prevented partially the phases I and II response to TRH.
Neither promethazine (10 mg/kg) nor cimetidine (50 mg/kg SC) premedication 30 min before TRH (1.3 nM) were able to modify significantly the
effects of the peptide. The effects of TRH were blocked by vagotomy.

TABLE 1 Motor effects induced by TRH (ICV) on the electrical activity
of the duodenum in fasted rats (n = 4) after naloxone (15 min)
or domperidone (30 min) pretreatments

	Duration of effects (min)	MMC frequency per h	Continuous spiking (min/15 min)	Quiescence (min/15 min)
Control saline ICV (5 μl)	−	4.17 ± 0.30	4.46 ± 2.27	3.92 ± 1.50
TRH ICV (1.3 nM)				
Phases I and II	36.5 ± 13.3 & + 310 ± 152	5.63** ± 1.18	9.50* ± 1.27 & + 2.37 ± 1.00	5.87 ± 1.56
TRH ICV after naloxone (10 mg/kg SC)				
Phases I and II	102* ± 28.7 & + 213 ± 114	5.66 ± 1.32	13.66* ± 0.88 & + 4.42 ± 1.01	2.84 ± 1.44
TRH ICV after domperidone (5 mg/kg SC)				
Phases I and II	93* ± 14.3 & + 273 ± 130	6.10 ± 1.10	9.10 ± 0.94 & + 3.05 ± 1.70	4.75 ± 0.95

Significantly different from saline or TRH alone at P < 0.01 (*) or
P < 0.001 (**)

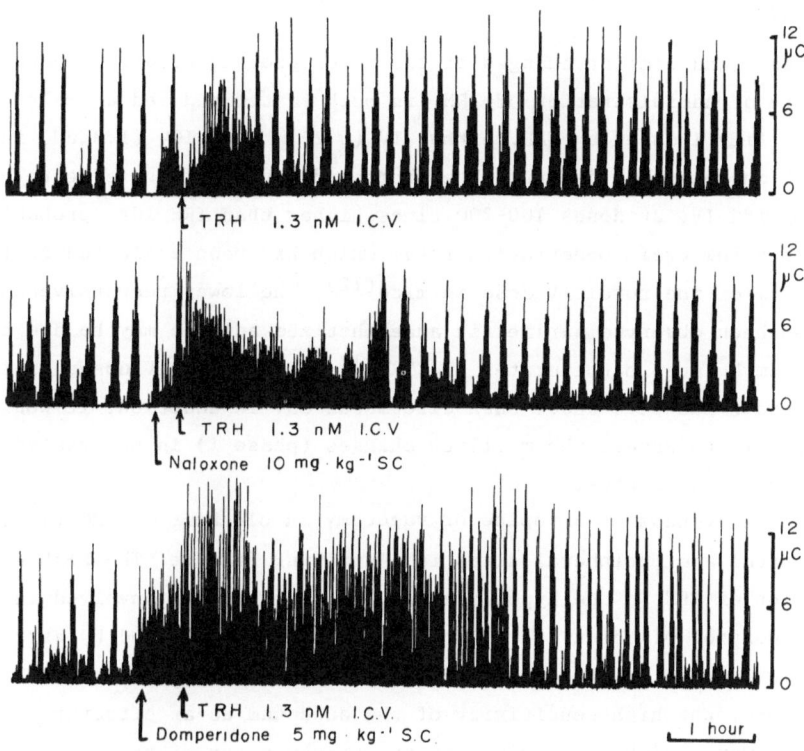

FIGURE 2   Enhancement of the TRH-induced motor effects on the duodenum
of a fasted rat by naloxone and by a dopamine antagonist,
domperidone.

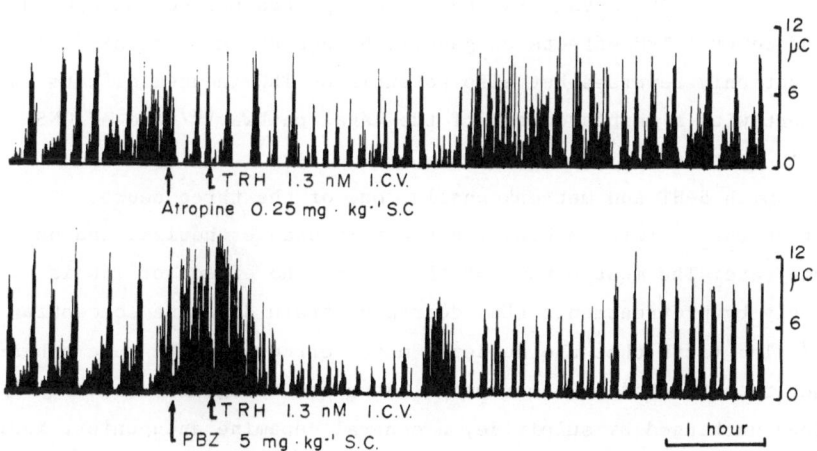

FIGURE 3   TRH-induced motor effects on the duodenum were totally prevented by atropine and partially prevented by phenoxybenzamine (PBZ).

DISCUSSION

Significant and similar changes of the motor profile occurred whatever the route of administration of TRH, in both fasted and fed animals. The hypermotility induced by TRH, either IV (0.26 µM) or ICV (1.3 nM, involved both duodenum and jejunum. The shorter duration of the effects elicited by TRH IV, at doses 100-200 times higher than TRH ICV, probably reflects a low brain penetration rate, which has been evaluated to less than 0.2 % of the total IV dose in mice[12]. The lower responsiveness that has been observed earlier in anaesthetized animals may be due to antagonism between barbiturates and TRH[13]. Even high IV doses of TRH would remain inactive under such circumstances. In addition, it would be difficult to assess the motility changes (phase I) in non-fasted animals under anaesthesia.

The effectiveness of atropine or vagotomy in blocking the TRH effects at both central and peripheral sites is a striking feature. The high concentration of TRH in the hypothalamus, an area which is involved in the central control of colonic activity[14] and that is blocked by atropine[9], may be the target of the inhibitory effects of ICV atropine. Furthermore, the high sensitivity of the duodenum as an effector of the vagal pathway, which is involved in the transmission of the neural inputs to peripheral sites[10], may explain the high responsiveness of this area to the effects of atropine. Another point of interest is the enhancement of the TRH effects by naloxone, and the blockade of phase I by methylnaloxone ICV. Antagonism has been reported between endogenous opiate and central TRH effects on gastric H^+ secretion in rats[2]. That naloxone not only reverses but also potentiates TRH-induced effects is in agreement with a reinforcement of the vagal pathway[5] and of CNS cholinergic neurones[15].

TRH is, with 5-HT and met-enkephalin, one of the three neurotransmitters that elicit shaking behaviour in unanaesthetized and unrestrained rats. The most potent of the three, the effect of TRH is reduced only by pretreatments that decreased brain dopamine concentrations[16]. The facts that the duodenal motor effects of TRH were enhanced rather than blocked by a peripheral dopamine antagonist (see Fig. 2), or remained unchanged by sulpiride, a central dopamine antagonist, indicate more subtle mechanisms. For example, TRH has been found able to lower serum calcium[17]. TRH also increases the plasma somatostatin-like

immunoreactivity in rabbits[18] and in the rat, the phase II elicited
by TRH resembles the central effect produced by somatostatin[19]. Furthermore, it is noteworthy that a central dopamine agonist, bromocriptine
(5 mg/kg) was able to nearly double the most characteristic TRH duodenal
motor effects, namely phase I. As already mentioned, phenoxybenzamine
was a strong antagonist of the TRH duodenal motor effects in the rat as
it is in rabbits[9]. This probable peripheral effect does not exclude
an effect on receptors of the CNS or the spinal cord[20]. In contrast
with some _in vitro_ findings[3], H_1 and H_2 receptors were not found involved in the duodenal motor effects of TRH.

To **summarize**, a central pathway involving the vagus nerves seems of
paramount importance for the action of TRH on gastrointestinal motility
in rats as confirmed by our results with atropine and vagotomy. This
vagal pathway seems to be strongly influenced by the opioid system and
to a lesser extent by the dopaminergic system.

References

1. Morley, J.E., Steinbach, J.H., Feldman, E.J. and Solomon, T.E. (1979).
The effects of thyrotropin-releasing hormone (TRH) on the gastrointestinal tract. Life Sci., 24, 1059-66.
2. Morley, J.E., Levine, A.S. and Silvis, S.E. (1981). Endogenous opiates inhibit gastric acid secretion induced by central administration of
thyrotropin-releasing hormone (TRH). Life Sci., 29, 293-7.
3. Bruce, L.A., Behsudi, F.M. and Fawcett, C.P. (1979). Histaminergic
involvement in thyrotropin-releasing hormone stimulation of antral tissue in the rat. Gastroenterology, 76, 908-12.
4. Dolva, L.D. and Hanssen, K.F. (1982). Thyrotropin-releasing hormone :
Distribution and actions in the gastrointestinal tract. Scand. J. Gastroenterol., 17, 705-7.
5. Soldani, G., Del Tacca, M., Martino, E., Bartelloni, A. and
Impicciatore, M. (1983). The involvement of the vagal pathway in the
antisecretory effect of thyrotropin-releasing hormone on gastric secretion in the dog. J. Pharm. Pharmacol., 35, 119-21.
6. Maeda-Hagiwara, M. and Watanabe, K. (1983). Influence of dopamine
receptor agonists on gastric acid secretion induced by intraventricular
administration of thyrotropin-releasing hormone in the perfused stomach

of anaesthetized rats. Br. J. Pharmacol., **79**, 297-303.

7. Martino, E., Lenmark, A., Seo, H., Steiner, D.F. and Refetoff, S. (1978). High concentration of thyrotropin-releasing hormone in pancreatic islets. Proc. Natl Acad. Sci USA, **75**, 4265-8.

8. Smith, J.R., La Hann, T.R., Chesnut, R.M., Carino, M.A. and Horita, A. (1977). Thyrotropin-releasing hormone : Stimulation of colonic activity following intracerebroventricular administration. Science, **196**, 660-2.

9. La Hann, T.R. and Horita, A. (1982). Thyrotropin-releasing hormone : Centrally mediated effects on gastrointestinal motor activity. J. Pharmacol. Exp. Ther., **222**, 66-70.

10. Tonoue, T. and Nomoto, T. (1979). Effect of intracerebroventricular administration of thyrotropin-releasing hormone upon the electroenteromyogram of rat duodenum. Eur. J. Pharmacol., **58**, 365-77.

11. Ferré, J.P. (1981). Motricité gastro-intestinale chez le rat. Nature et variations physio-pathologiques. Thèse Doct. 3e cycle, Toulouse.

12. Kalivas, P.W. and Horita, A. (1979). Thyrotropin-releasing hormone : Central site of action in antagonism of pentobarbital narcosis. Nature, **178**, 461-2.

13. Mitsuma, T. and Nogimori, K. (1983). Influence of the route of administration on TRH concentration in the mouse brain. Experientia, **39**, 620-2.

14. Rostad, H. (1973). Colonic motility in the cat. III. Influence of hypothalamic and mesencephalic stimulation. Acta Physiol. Scand., **89**, 104-15.

15. Yarbrough, G.G. (1983). Thyrotropin-releasing hormone and CNS cholinergic neurons. Life Sci., **33**, 111-8.

16. Drust, E. and Connor, J.D. (1983). Pharmacological analysis of shaking behavior induced by enkephalins, thyrotropin-releasing hormone or serotonin in rats : Evidence for different mechanisms. J. Pharmacol. Exp. Ther., **224**, 148-54.

17. Rojdmark, S., Andersson, D.E.H., Edstrom, E. and Lamminpaa, K. (1983). Serum calcium decline after intravenous administration of TRH in man. Horm. Metab. Res., **15**, 290-3.

18. Knudtzon, J. and Hanssen, L.E. (1983). TRH increases plasma somatostatin-like immunoreactivity in rabbits. Horm. Metab. Res., **15**, 309-10.

19. Buéno, L. and Ferré, J.P. (1982). Central regulation of intestinal motility by somatostatin and cholecystokinin octapeptide. Science, **216**, 1427-9.

20. Sharif, N.A. and Burt, D.R. (1983). Receptors for thyrotropin releasing hormone (TRH) in rabbit spinal cord. Brain Res., **270**, 259-64.

93

The Brain–Gut Axis: a Physiological Model

W. R. EWART and D. L. WINGATE

INTRODUCTION

Perhaps because normal gut movements are not consciously perceived, much emphasis has been placed on control by enteric nerves and 'gut hormones'; now that it is clear that the latter are common to both brain and gut, closer study of the 'brain–gut' axis is required and we have developed a model for this (1,2).

METHODS

In anaesthetised rats (Equithesin 0.27 ml/100 g body wt I/P), we have used glass multibarrel microelectrodes stereotaxically positioned in the region of the dorsal vagal nucleus and nucleus of the solitary tract to record extracellular neuronal activity. Physiological stimulation was by gastric distension produced by inflation of a small water-filled balloon placed in the stomach through a gastrostomy, or by duodenal perfusion of a 6 cm segment of duodenum with isotonic, isothermal D–glucose, using a single pass perfusion. The effects of cholecystokinin-octapeptide (CCK–OP) and leu-enkephalin on neuronal activity were tested, applied from the microelectrode by iontophoresis or pressure ejection.

RESULTS

137 single neurones were studied, over 50% of those studied showed changes in firing rate in response to gut stimulation. Responses to

intraduodenal glucose were an increase or decrease in firing rate
sustained during glucose perfusion. Gastric distension responses were
more varied including transient changes occurring only during
inflation or deflation of the balloon, consistent with the hypothesis
that this type of stimulus may activate both mucosal and muscle
tension receptors. Both resting and stimulated firing rates were
modulated by peptides, CCK–OP being predominantly excitatory and
opioids mainly inhibitory.

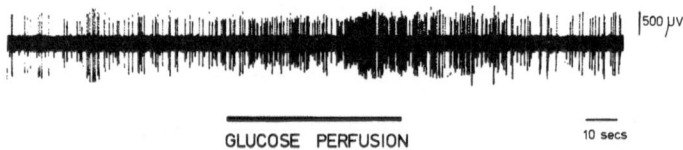

GLUCOSE PERFUSION   10 secs

FIGURE 1 Extracellular recording of a unit which was excited by
intraduodenal perfusion of isotonic, isothermal D–glucose. Horizontal
bar indicates period of glucose perfusion.

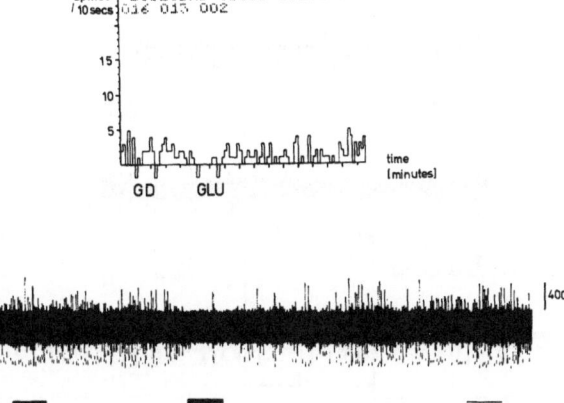

FIGURE 2 Shows an example of a neurone which was unaffected by gastric distension but which was inhibited by glucose perfusion. Upper trace shows computer generated spike frequency histogram, lower trace shows extracellular unitary acitvity.

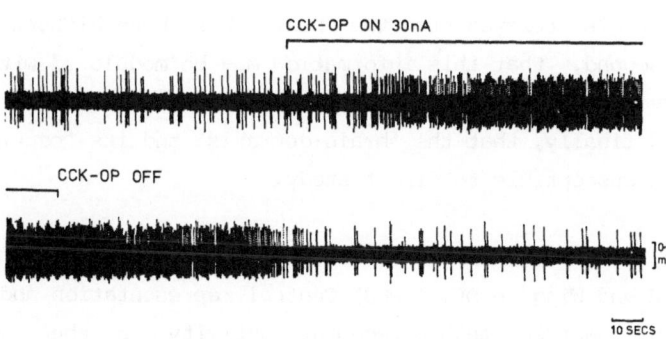

FIGURE 3 Shows a trace of extracellularly recorded action potentials showing the excitatory effect of CCK–OP on the firing rate of a DVN neurone.

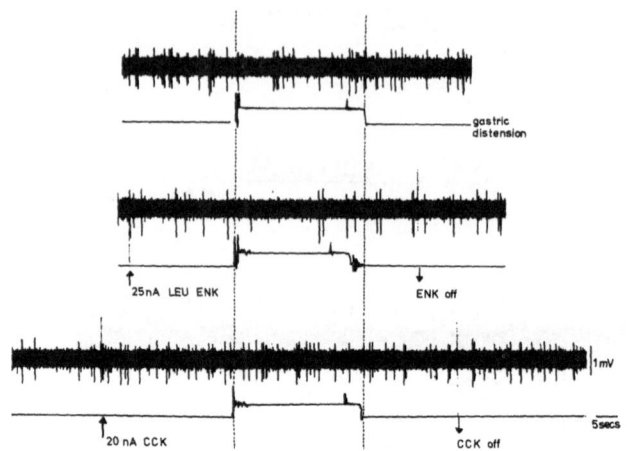

FIGURE 4 An example of a unit which showed a transient decrease in firing rate on inflation of the stomach. Leu-enkephalin had an inhibitory effect on the firing rate, whereas CCK-OP was excitatory. However, during either leu-enkephalin or CCK-OP application, the transient response to gastric distension was less marked.

CONCLUSION

We conclude that first, the extent and rapidity with which information from the gut is relayed to the brain has been hitherto underestimated, second, that this information may be modulated within the central nervous system by the local action of endogenous 'brain-gut peptides' and finally, that the 'brain-gut axis' and its 'peptidergic' modulation is susceptible to direct study.

REFERENCES

1   Ewart WR and Wingate DL. (1983) Central representation and opioid modulation of gastric mechanoreceptor activity in the rat. Am J Physiol 244 G27-G32

2   Ewart WR and Wingate DL. (1983) Cholecystokinin-octapeptide and gastric mechanoreceptor activity in the rat brain. Am J Physiol 244 G613-G619

94

Spinal, Supraspinal and Peripheral Sites of Opioid Intestinal Actions

T. F. BURKS, J. J. GALLIGAN, L. D. HIRNING and F. PORRECA

Opioid agonists, administered systemically, induce profound changes in gastrointestinal contractile and propulsive activity. It has now become apparent that opioids can exert effects at multiple sites within the body with different intestinal motility consequences. Also, the recognition of multiple subtypes of opioid receptors and the multiplicity of receptor actions of individual opioid agonists has recently provided new tools for the identification of sites and mechanisms of opioid actions affecting motility (1,2). It was our purpose to explore systematically the roles of brain, spinal cord, intramural neuron and smooth muscle components of opioid actions that influence gastrointestinal motility.

Morphine, D-Ala^2,MePhe^4,Gly-ol^5-enkephalin (DAGO) and morphiceptin were employed as selective mu opioid receptor agonists (3,4). U-50,488H was employed as the kappa opioid receptor agonist (5). Cyclic D-Pen^2,D-Pen^5-enkephalin (DPDPE) and met^5-enkephalin were employed as the delta opioid receptor agonists (2,6).

METHODS

Drug effects on small intestinal transit were evaluated using a method that has been described in detail previously (7). Female Sprague-Dawley rats (200-250 g) were anesthetized (ketamine HCl 100 mg/kg) and a silastic cannula was inserted into the duodenum with the distal end externalized through the skin of the back. Poly-

ethylene cannulas (PE-10) were also implanted in the right lateral
cerebral ventricle for intracerebroventricular (i.c.v.) administration
of drugs. Small intestinal transit in rats was determined 72 hr after
recovery from surgery by instilling 0.5 μCi of Na^{51}CrO$_4$ into the
duodenum via the previously implanted duodenal cannula. After 35 min
the rats were sacrificed and the distribution of radioactivity within
the small intestine was determined by gamma counting. Intestinal
transit was expressed as the geometric center (8). Gastrointestinal
transit was studied similarly in male ICR mice (20-30 g) by oral
administration of 0.5 μCi sodium chromate Na^{51}CrO$_4$. I.c.v. and
intrathecal (i.t.) injections were performed by standard techniques
(9,10).

Direct effects of opioids on intestinal contractile activity were
evaluated in the dog isolated, vascularly perfused canine small
intestine preparation previously described (11). Arterially perfused
small intestine segments were prepared from adult dogs of either sex
anesthetized with barbital sodium (250 mg/kg) and sodium thiopental
(15 mg/kg). Intraluminal pressure was measured from a small latex
balloon tied into the lumen of the segment. The vasculature was
perfused with warmed, Krebs bicarbonate solution bubbled with 95%
O_2-5% CO_2. Agonist drugs were injected i.a. in volumes of 0.01-0.1 ml
through the arterial cannula. Antagonist drugs were dissolved in the
perfusion solution. Excitatory responses were measured as increases
in intraluminal pressure.

Drugs used were morphine sulfate, DAGO (D-Ala^2,MePhe^4,Gly-ol^5-
enkephalin), U-50,488H (chloromethylpyrolidinylcyclohexylbenzene-
acetamide methane sulfonate), DPDPE (cyclo-D-Pen^2,D-Pen^5-enkephalin),
Met^5-enkephalin, morphiceptin (amide of β-casomorphin(1-4)), naloxone
HCl and tetrodotoxin (TTX).

RESULTS

The administration of morphine i.c.v. in rats and mice (Tables 1
and 2) dramatically inhibited intestinal transit of the radioisotope
marker indicated by decreases in geometric center. The highly

Table 1. Antitransit effects of opioid agonists administered i.c.v.
in rats. Data are expressed as geometric center (± S.E.M.).

Treatment	Dose (μg)	Transit
Saline		3.37 ± 0.25
Morphine	5	2.08 ± 0.18*
Morphine	20	1.65 ± 0.05*
Morphine	80	1.42 ± 0.10*
DAGO	0.4	1.95 ± 0.26*
DAGO	2	1.58 ± 0.21*
U-50,488H	5	3.45 ± 0.22
U-50,488H	25	4.05 ± 0.12
Vehicle[a]		2.76 ± 0.29
DPDPE	5	3.00 ± 0.30
DPDPE	25	3.14 ± 0.48

[a] Dimethylsulfoxide (1%) in saline was the vehicle for DPDPE.

* Different from saline, $P < 0.05$

Table 2. Antitransit effects of opioid agonists administered i.c.v.
in mice. Data are expressed as geometric center (± S.E.M.).

Treatment	Dose (μg)	Transit
Saline		5.06 ± 0.26
Morphine	1	3.09 ± 0.38*
Morphine	3	2.05 ± 0.24*
DAGO	0.3	2.13 ± 0.32*
DAGO	1	1.47 ± 0.06*
U-50,488H	10	5.39 ± 0.38
U-50,488H	30	5.05 ± 0.30
DPDPE	10	4.09 ± 0.60
DPDPE	20	5.06 ± 0.18

* Different from saline, $P < 0.05$

Table 3. Antitransit effects of opioid agonists administered i.t. in mice. Data are expressed as geometric center (± S.E.M.).

Treatment	Dose (µg)	Transit
Saline		5.31 ± 0.44
Morphine	3	2.71 ± 0.31*
Morphine	10	2.06 ± 0.22*
DAGO	1	1.40 ± 0.12*
U-50,488H	100	3.65 ± 0.57
DPDPE	10	1.87 ± 0.16*

* Different from saline, P < 0.05

Table 4. Contractions of dog intestine ex vivo induced by i.a. opioid agonists.

Treatment	Dose (µg)	Response (mmHg)
Morphine	0.2	26 ± 12*
Morphine	1	48 ± 11*
U-50,488H	100	3 ± 2
Met-enkephalin	25	39 ± 8*

* Significant increase, P < 0.05

Table 5. Effects of TTX (100 ng/ml) on opioid induced contractions of dog intestine ex vivo.

Treatment	Dose (µg)	Control	TTX
Morphiceptin	1	25 ± 8	7 ± 3*
Morphiceptin	5	40 ± 12	15 ± 7*
Met-enkephalin	1	21 ± 6	28 ± 7
Met-enkephalin	5	26 ± 6	31 ± 7

* Different from control, P < 0.05

selective mu agonist, DAGO, administered i.c.v. also decreased the geometric center of transit in rats and mice. In contrast, the selective kappa agonist, U-50,488H, did not inhibit intestinal transit. The delta receptor selective peptide, DPDPE, also did not reduce transit in rats or mice when given i.c.v. Effects of morphine and DAGO were antagonized by naloxone (2 mg/kg s.c.).

Spinal cord mediated opioid effects on intestinal transit were evaluated in mice by i.t. administration of opioid agonists. Morphine and DAGO, mu opioid receptor agonists, inhibited intestinal transit after i.t. injection (Table 3). As observed after i.c.v. injection in rats and mice, i.t. administration of the kappa opioid receptor agonist, U-50,488H, in mice had no significant effect on intestinal transit. In contrast to its effects in the brain, however, DPDPE, a selective delta receptor agonist, inhibited intestinal transit after i.t. administration in mice.

Direct intestinal effects of the selective opioid receptor agonists were evaluated in dog intestine ex vivo. The mu opioid receptor agonists, morphine and morphiceptin, induced contractions in dog isolated intestine (Tables 4 and 5). The delta receptor agonist, met-enkephalin, also induced contractions. U-50,488H, a kappa agonist, did not induce contractions (Table 4). Intestinal contractions induced by morphiceptin were abolished or reduced by TTX (Table 5), whereas contractions induced by met-enkephalin were not blocked by TTX. Inhibition of responses to morphine by TTX has been demonstrated in previous studies (12).

DISCUSSION

The ability of morphine to inhibit intestinal transit after i.c.v. administration has been observed previously (13,14). The present data reveal, however, that opioid agonists with differing selectivity for subclasses of opioid receptors exert differential effects on transit when administered into the brain. Agonists with selectivity for kappa and delta receptors did not produce inhibition of intestinal transit when administered i.c.v. However, the spinal cord appears to represent a site for intestinal regulation distinct from the brain in several respects. As with the brain, mu agonists inhibited intestinal transit by actions in the spinal cord. Also like the brain, the kappa agonists did not affect transit by actions in the spinal cord. In contrast to the brain, however, the delta agonist exerted significant antitransit effects at the level of the cord.

The direct intestinal effects of opioid receptor agonists also differed depending upon selectivity for individual opioid receptor subtypes. Agonists with activity at mu and delta opioid receptors increased contractions of dog isolated intestine whereas the kappa receptor agonist had no effect. Judged by insensitivity to blockade with tetrodotoxin, met-enkephalin and possibly other delta agonists may act directly on intestinal smooth muscle to induce contractions. Morphine and morphiceptin, mu receptor agonists, were inhibited by tetrodotoxin and evidently exert their intestinal stimulatory actions by effects on intramural nerves.

Our studies have thus shown that the brain, spinal cord, intramural neurons and intestinal smooth muscle represent distinct sites for opioid actions that affect gastrointestinal motility.

ACKNOWLEDGEMENTS

Supported by USPHS grant number DA 02163 from NIDA and by the Gibson-Stephens Institute (Tucson, AZ). J.J. Galligan is a PMAF Fellow. F. Porreca is a Merck Postdoctoral Fellow.

REFERENCES

1. Martin, W.R., Eades, C.G., Thompson, J.A., Huppler, R.E. and Gilbert, P.E. (1976). The effects of morphine and nalorphine-like drugs in the non-dependent and morphine-dependent chronic spinal dog. J. Pharmacol. Exp. Ther., 197, 517-523
2. Lord, J.A.H., Waterfield, A.A., Hughes, J. and Kosterlitz, H.W. (1977). Endogenous opioid peptides: multiple agonists and antagonists. Nature, 267: 495-499

3. Handa, B.K., Lane, A.C., Lord, J.A.H., Morgan, B.A., Rance, M.J. and Smith, C.F.C. (1981). Analogues of β-LPH$_{61-64}$ possessing selective agonist activity at μ-opiate receptors. Eur. J. Pharmacol., 70: 531-540

4. Chang, K.-J., Cuatrecasas, P., Wei. E.T. and Chang, J.-K (1982). Analgesic activity of intracerebroventricular administration of morphiceptin and β-casomorphins: correlation with the morphine (μ) receptor binding affinity. Life Sci., 30: 1547-1551

5. Von Voightlander, P.H., Lahti, R.A. and Ludens, J.H. (1983). A selective and structurally novel non-mu (kappa) opioid agonist. J. Pharmacol. Exp. Ther., 224, 7-12

6. Mosberg, H.I., Hurst, R., Hruby, V.J., Gee, K., Yamamura, H.I., Galligan, J.J. and Burks, T.F. (1983). Bis-penicillamine enkephalins possess highly improved specificity toward delta opioid receptors. Proc. Natl. Acad. Sci. USA, (In Press)

7. Galligan, J.J. and Burks, T.F. (1983). Centrally mediated inhibition of small intestinal transit and motility by morphine in the rat. J. Pharmacol. Exp. Ther., 226, 356-361

8. Miller, M.S., Galligan, J.J. and Burks, T.F. (1981). Accurate measurement of intestinal transit. J. Pharmacol. Methods, 6, 211-217

9. Haley, T.J. and McCormick, W.G. (1957). Pharmacological effects produced by intracerebral injection of drugs in the conscious mouse. Br. J. Pharmacol., 12, 12-15

10. Hylden, J.L.K. and Wilcox, G.L. (1980). Intrathecal morphine in mice: a new technique. Eur. J. Pharmacol., 67, 313-316

11. Burks, T.F. (1974). Vascularly perfused isolated intestine. Proc. Fourth Intl. Symp. Gastrointestinal Motility, pp. 649-656. (Vancouver: Mitchell Press)

12. Burks, T.F. (1973). Mediation by 5-hydroxytryptamine of morphine stimulant actions in dog intestine. J. Pharmacol. Exp. Ther., 185, 539-539

13. Parolaro, D., Sala, M. and Gori, E. (1977). Effect of intra-cerebroventricular administration of morphine upon intestinal motility in rat and its antagonism with naloxone. Eur. J. Pharmacol., 46, 329-338

14. Stewart, J.J., Weisbrodt, N.W. and Burks, T.F. (1978). Central and peripheral actions of morphine on intestinal transit. J. Pharmacol. Exp. Ther., 205, 547-555

95

Centrally-Administered Bombesin Delays Small Intestinal Transit but Stimulates Motility in the Rat

F. PORRECA, J. T. FULGINITI and T. F. BURKS

The concept of centrally-mediated effects on gastrointestinal motility has recently become established (1). Our laboratory has reported that bombesin, a neuropeptide localized in both the central nervous system and gastrointestinal tract of mammals (2,3), effectively reduces gastric emptying and small bowel transit after intracerebroventricular (i.c.v.) administration to rats (4). Similarly, morphine and the opioid peptides produce dramatic slowing effects on gastrointestinal transit after central administration (5).

The mechanism by which a slowing of intestinal transit might occur can vary with the species studied and with the drug. For example, morphine produces a stimulatory effect on intestinal motility in the dog (6,7) but has been found to inhibit motility in the rat (8). The present work attempts to determine whether bombesin and morphine produce their antitransit effects after i.c.v. administration to rats by similar motility patterns. We now report that while i.c.v. morphine inhibits small intestinal transit and motility in the rat (8), bombesin inhibits transit but stimulates motility in the small bowel of this species.

Determination of intestinal motility
in the conscious, unrestrained rat

Intestinal motility was measured as changes in small bowel intraluminal pressure. Female, Sprague-Dawley rats (180-220 g) were
anesthetized with ketamine HCl (100 mg/kg, i.p.) and prepared
surgically for recording of intestinal motility by implanting a piece
of silastic tubing (Dow Corning, 0.02 inch inside diameter x 0.037
inch outside diameter) in the proximal duodenum and in the jejunum,
respectively. Each piece of silastic tubing was secured in the lumen
of the small bowel by a suture tied around a small bulb of silicone
rubber (General Electric, RTV 112 silicone rubber). The other ends of
the silastic tubing were each fixed to a 23 gauge needle. The needles
were attached to a dental acrylic mold fashioned with the aid of the
top 2 cm of the barrel of a 6 cc syringe. The silastic cannulae were
brought from the acrylic mold subcutaneously for implantation in the
intestines. The dental acrylic mold (together with the needles and
silastic tubes) was then secured in the shoulder region of the rat.
At the same time, i.c.v. guide tubes were placed into the lateral
cerebral ventricles (4). Each animal was allowed to recover for 3
days prior to testing. The animals tolerated this procedure well and
ate after surgery. Each rat was fasted for 12-16 hr prior to testing
(see ref. 8 for complete details).

On the day of the test, each rat was placed into an empty box and
allowed to acclimate for 30 min. The cannulae were then connected via
the 23 gauge needles to an infusion pump (Harvard Apparatus) and a
pressure transducer (Statham P23Db) by way of a 3-way stopcock. The
cannulae were perfused with distilled water at a rate of 0.04 ml/min
and motility was recorded as alterations in pressure resulting from
changes in outflow resistance due to contractions of the intestine.
Pressure recordings were displayed on a Beckman R511 Dynograph.
Following a 30 min recording period, the rat was injected i.c.v. with
either saline or bombesin (5 µl given over 30 sec) and motility was
recorded for a further 60 min. Thus, motility was recorded over the
same time as that involved in the study of transit (4,8).

The motility recordings were analyzed by visual inspection. Contractions of amplitude greater than 2 cm of water were counted and the frequency of such contractions over each 30 min period was calculated. Data were analyzed using a t-test for paired values with significance established at the 95% confidence level. Effects of drug treatment are expressed as a percent of the frequency of contraction for each individual animal during the control period. Bombesin (Peninsula Laboratories) was diluted in distilled water and frozen in aliquots until immediately prior to use. Each aliquot was used only once. A minimum of 5 rats were studied per reported observation.

RESULTS

Records were analyzed for contractions of amplitude greater than 2 cm of water. The average frequency of contractions per min (and S.E.) when recorded over the 30 min pre-drug control period was found to be 5.8 ± 1.7 and 4.9 ± 0.9 in the duodenum and jejunem, respectively. This frequency was not significantly altered after the i.c.v. administration of saline (Table 1). The results of administration of saline or bombesin (0.1, 1 or 10 µg, i.c.v.) are expressed as a percent of each animal's individual control frequency and are shown in Table 2. Bombesin produced a dose-related stimulation of intestinal contractions with significant (t-test for paired data) increases in the frequency of contractions in both the duodenum and the jejunum at 1 and 10 µg. Surprisingly, a decrease in frequency of jejunal contractions was seen at the lowest dose. In all cases with doses of 1 or 10 µg, consistent increases in contractions were seen within the first 30 min and continued throughout the 60 min of study.

Table 1. Frequency of intestinal contractions before and after i.c.v.
saline (contractions greater than 2 cm of water per min)

	Presaline control	0–30 min	31–60 min
Duodenum	5.8 ± 1.7	4.5 ± 0.7	5.4 ± 0.6
Jejunum	4.9 ± 0.9	5.3 ± 1.2	4.6 ± 0.8

Table 2. Frequency of intestinal contractions (percent of control)

Bombesin Dose (µg, i.c.v.)	Duodenum		Jejunum	
	0–30 min	31–60 min	0–30 min	31–60 min
Saline	91.1 ± 9.9	108.8 ± 22.7	104.6 ± 10.9	109.4 ± 15.9
0.1	172.5 ± 77.9	137.2 ± 65.4	56.5 ± 11.7*	44.6 ± 12.1*
1.0	159.8 ± 17.3*	138.3 ± 12.7*	216.7 ± 42.2*	168.3 ± 37.8*
10.0	583.4 ±286.1*	393.9 ±151.4*	205.1 ± 64.5*	207.7 ± 52.3*

* Different from saline, $P < 0.05$, t-test for paired data.

DISCUSSION

The present work suggests that bombesin produces its antitransit
effects by stimulating non-propulsive contractions within the rat
small bowel. These results contrast sharply with those seen after
i.c.v. morphine. While morphine produced a dose-related decrease in
motility, bombesin showed a stimulation of the small intestine over

the same dose-range that effectively inhibited transit (4). Thus, while the two compounds produce the same qualitative result (i.e. inhibition of small intestinal transit), the mechanisms involved in the production of this effect are different. The correlation between transit and motility has always been particularly difficult. The present work indicates that this correlation is probably drug specific.

Interestingly, while morphine inhibited motility, this effect was not maximal until about 30 min after i.c.v. administration and was more marked in the jejunum. In contrast, bombesin produced an almost immediate (within 10 min) increase in intestinal contractions in both portions of the small intestine. This long-lasting bombesin effect occurred only at doses greater than 0.1 µg. Thus, while 0.1 µg of bombesin did not affect small bowel motility, this dose was also ineffective in slowing transit. The maximum inhibition of transit occurred within the first 20 min after bombesin, a time which corresponds well to the motility effects seen with this peptide. It is unclear why bombesin treatment resulted in a decreased frequency of contractions in the jejunum after administration of the lowest dose, however, central bombesin sites are known to increase release of adrenergic amines from the adrenal medulla, which could cause transient inhibition of contractions (9).

The maximum obtainable antitransit effect with bombesin occurred at 1 µg. While increasing the bombesin dose from 1 to 10 µg resulted in a further increase in the frequency of contractions (to approximately 300-500 and 200 percent of control in the duodenum and jejunum, respectively) no increased effect in slowing transit was observed. This suggests that the antipropulsive effect of intestinal contractions can result without maximal increases in frequency.

Our previous work has indicated a slowing of gastric emptying and a transient stimulatory effect on large bowel transit after i.c.v. bombesin. Whether these emptying/transit changes can be correlated with intragastric and intracolonic motility remains to be determined and is presently under study.

ACKNOWLEDGEMENTS

Supported by USPHS Grant Number DA 02163, a grant from Gibson-Stephens Institute, Tucson, Arizona, and a Merck Postdoctoral Fellowship to Dr. Porreca.

REFERENCES

1. Burks, T.F. (1978). Central sites of action of gastrointestinal drugs. Gastroenterology, 74, 332-324

2. Villarreal, J., Brown, M. (1978). Bombesin-like peptide in hypothalamus: chemical and immunological characterization. Life Sci., 23, 2729-2733

3. Brown, M.A., Allen, R., Villarreal, J., Rivier, J., Vale, W. (1978). Bombesin-like activity: radioimmunologic assessment in biological tissues. Life Sci, 23, 2721-2728

4. Porreca, F. and Burks, T.F. (1983). Centrally administered bombesin affects gastric emptying and small and large bowel transit in the rat. Gastroenterology, 85, 313-317

5. Galligan, J.J. and Burks, T.F. (1982). Opioid peptides inhibit intestinal transit in the rat by a central mechanism. Eur. J. Pharmacol., 85, 61-68

6. Bueno, L. and Fioramonti, J. (1982). A possible serotonergic mechanism involved in the effects of morphine on colonic motility in the dog. Eur. J. Pharmacol., 82, 147-153

7. Burks, T.F. (1973). Mediation by 5-hydroxytryptamine of morphine stimulant actions in the dog intestine. J. Pharmacol. Exp. Ther., 185, 530-539

8. Galligan, J.J. and Burks, T.F. (1983). Centrally mediated inhibition of small intestinal transit and motility by morphine in the rat. J. Pharmacol. Exp. Ther., 226, 356-361

9. Taché, Y. and Brown, M. (1982). On the role of bombesin in homeostasis. Trends Neurosci., 5, 431-433.

96

Effects of Hindbrain L-Glutamic Acid Application on Gastrointestinal Motor Function in the Cat

H. S. ORMSBEE, III, F. C. BARONE, D. M. LOMBARDI and L. C. McCARTNEY

INTRODUCTION

Electrical stimulation of the dorsal motor nucleus of the vagus nerve (DMV) generally increases circular muscle contractions in the stomach and small bowel [1,2]. The effect of DMV electrical stimulation on lower esophageal sphincter (LES) function recently has been determined [1]. A relatively large portion of the cat hindbrain, associated with the DMV, is involved in the control of LES pressure (LESP) [1].

The excitatory amino acid neurotransmitter L-glutamic acid (GLU) has a relatively high concentration and turnover in the DMV [3, 4]. In addition, the concentration of GLU in the DMV is dependent on intact glossopharyngeal and vagus cranial nerves [4]. GLU excites almost all cell bodies in the central nervous system [5], but does not activate axons [6].

The purpose of the present series of experiments was to test the hypothesis that GLU is a candidate hindbrain neurotransmitter which can modulate LES and upper GI motor function. GLU was administered either by topical application to the surface of the 4th ventricle or by direct microinjection into the DMV.

METHODS

Thirty-three cats of either sex (1.5 to 4.5 kg), were deprived of food for 24 hrs and anesthetized with α-chloralose (70 mg/kg

i.v.). A continuous infusion of isotonic saline (0.1 ml/min) and
supplemental doses of anesthesia were made via the jugular vein.
The carotid artery was also cannulated in order to continuously
measure arterial blood pressure. Heart rate was monitored from
subcutaneous electrodes. Animals were artificially respirated
through a tracheal cannula.

Strain gage force transducers [7] were sutured extraluminally to
the fundus and antrum of the stomach, on the pylorus, on the duodenum (3-5 cm from the pylorus), and/or on the jejunum (25 cm beyond
the ligament of Treitz). A gastric cannula was positioned at the
antral-corpus junction, and the duodenum was ligated 2 cm from the
pylorus. A manometric catheter system, including a Dent sleeve (8),
was positioned in the esophagus to continuously monitor intraluminal pressure from the esophageal body and the LES.

Cats were placed in a stereotaxic apparatus and the dorsal surface of the brainstem was exposed. Solutions were applied topically
to the floor of the 4th ventricle as a 10 µl drop by means of a 31
ga stainless steel cannula connected to a handheld syringe. The
drops contained 3.13, 6.25, 12.5 or 25 µmoles of GLU (monosodium
salt, pH = 7.0). Isotonic saline and hypertonic saline of equal
osmolality to GLU solutions were also tested for control purposes.
Microinjections of GLU were made directly into the DMV by means of a
31 ga stainless steel cannula connected to a calibrated infusion
pump or by means of a glass micropipette (tip diameter 10-15 µm)
connected to a Pneumatic Pressure System (Medical Systems Corp.).
Volumes of 0.06-1.0 µl containing 0.06-2.5 µmoles of GLU were
delivered into the DMV at a rate of 0.1-0.2 µl/min. Equivolume
isotonic and hypertonic saline solutions were injected similarly into
the DMV for control purposes. The cannula or micropipette was inserted stereotaxically into the DMV at an angle of 36°. Using obex
as a reference point, the DMV coordinates were A= 1.6 mm, L= 1.5-1.8
mm, and D= 1.0-2.0 mm from the hindbrain surface.

LES responses were analyzed in terms of maximum pressure changes
that occurred during or following hindbrain GLU stimulation. Changes
in heart rate, blood pressure and GI motility were determined during
maximum changes in LESP. GI circular muscle activity changes during

or following GLU stimulation were considered stimulus-induced if they differed by greater than 20% from prestimulation periods and were reproducible. Data are presented as individual examples and as means ± SEM. Statistical analyses were performed by two-tailed Student's t-tests.

RESULTS

The application of GLU onto the floor of the 4th ventricle of 20 animals always altered LESP, and resulted in an increase (N=1), decreases (N=10), or both an increase and decrease in LESP (N=9). For the 10 animals that exhibited GLU-induced increased LESP, mean LESP changed from 21.6±2.4 mmHg to 46.8±6.1 mmHg, for a maximum change of +228.2±25.3% (p<0.001). Bilateral cervical vagotomy completely eliminated GLU-induced LESP increases in 2 of 3 tests. For the 19 animals that exhibited GLU-induced decreased LESP, mean LESP changed from 26.6±2.6 mmHg to 6.7±1.5 mmHg, for a maximum change of -73.2±5.2% (p<0.0001). Bilateral cervical vagotomy (N=6) completely eliminated GLU-induced LESP decreases. Fourth ventricular GLU altered circular muscle activity of the esophagus (increased in 25% of animals tested), fundus (increased in 27% and decreased in 27% of animals tested), antrum (increased in 37% and decreased in 11% of animals tested), pylorus (increased in 70% and decreased in 15% of animals tested), duodenum (increased in 37% and decreased in 16% of animals tested), and jejunum (increased in 38% of animals tested). Changes in fundus motor activity consisted of increases or decreases in tone. Other upper GI area motor changes consisted of increases or decreases in phasic contractile activity. Bilateral cervical vagotomy eliminated these changes in circular muscle activity (N=5). The effects of 4th ventricular GLU on upper GI activity occurred immediately and lasted for several minutes to as long as 20 min. When biphasic responses occurred, initial increases or decreases in LESP occurred equally often. Fourth ventricular GLU decreased heart rate (p<0.02), and increased blood pressure (p<0.001).

Isotonic and hypertonic saline applied to the 4th ventricle did not alter LESP or upper GI motor activity. The 4th ventricular application of progressively larger GLU doses resulted in greater responses and/or responses of longer duration. In most cases, changes in fundus, antrum, pylorus and/or duodenum circular muscle activity occurred with changes in LESP (Fig. 1).

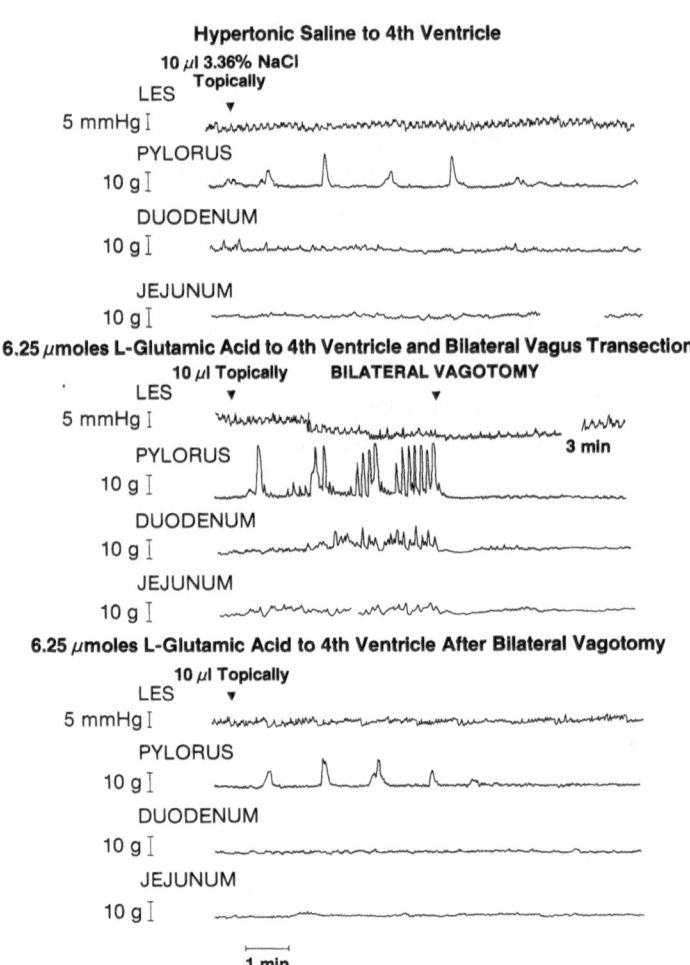

FIGURE 1. Effects of 4th ventricular application of GLU on LESP and upper GI circular muscle contractions in an individual animal. In the top panel, hypertonic saline, equiosmolar to 6.25 μmoles GLU, does not alter upper GI responses. In the middle panel, 4th ventricular application of 6.25 μmoles GLU decreases LESP and increases circular muscle contractions of the pylorus, duodenum and jejunum. Bilateral cervical vagotomy eliminates all responses to ventricular GLU as depicted in the middle and bottom panels.

The application of GLU directly into the DMV altered LESP in 24 of 26 tests and resulted in increases (N=8), decreases (N=6), or both an increase and decrease in LESP (N=10). For the 18 sites that resulted in GLU-induced increased LESP, mean LESP changed from 23.2+2.1 mmHg to 43.4+3.9 mmHg, for a maximum change of 199.2+17.7% (p<0.0001). Bilateral cervical vagotomy (N=4) completely eliminated GLU-induced LESP increases. For the 16 sites that resulted in GLU-induced decreased LESP, mean LESP changed from 24.7+2.1 mmHg to 9.6+1.4 mmHg, for a maximum change of -60.3+4.6% (p<0.0001). Bilateral cervical vagotomy (N=4) completely eliminated GLU-induced LESP decreases. The application of GLU into the DMV altered circular muscle activity of the esophagus (increased for 9% of the sites tested), fundus (increased for 27% and decreased for 55% of the sites tested), antrum (increased for 30% and decreased for 5% of the sites tested), pylorus (increased for 59% and decreased for 5% of the sites tested), duodenum (increased for 9% and decreased for 4% of the sites tested), and jejunum (decreased for 10% of the sites tested). These changes were similar to those described for the 4th ventricular GLU applications. Bilateral cervical vagotomy (N=5) eliminated GLU-induced changes in circular muscle activity. The effects of DMV GLU on upper GI activity occurred immediately and usually lasted from 1 to 10 min. Generally, effects had durations shorter than 4th ventricular GLU responses. Initial increases or decreases in biphasic LESP responses were equally probable and both right and left DMV GLU injections resulted in similar effects. DMV application of GLU decreased heart rate (p<0.003), and increased blood pressure (p<0.001).

Figure 2 depicts the effects of GLU injections into the DMV on LESP and pyloric contractions. Injections of isotonic or hypertonic saline into the DMV did not affect the LES or upper GI activity.

DISCUSSION

Hindbrain GLU application significantly alters upper GI motor function. Similar increases and/or decreases in LESP are observed when GLU is applied to the surface of the 4th ventricle or directly into the DMV. The fundus and pylorus are the next most responsive upper

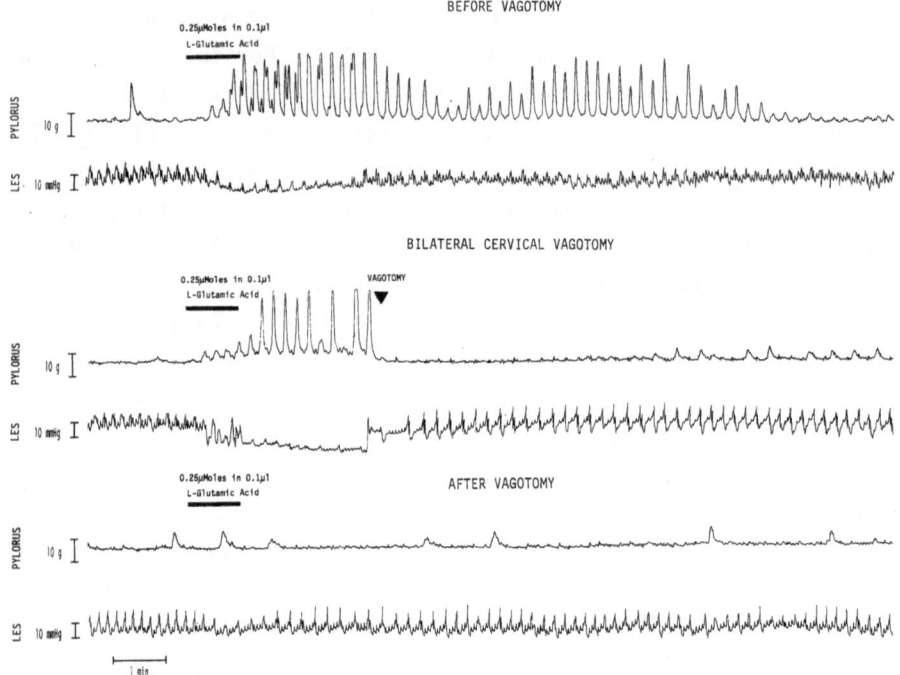

FIGURE 2. Effects of DMV application of GLU on circular muscle contractions of the pylorus and LESP. In the top panel, 0.25 μmoles
GLU in 0.1 μl injected into the DMV increases pyloric contractions and decreases LESP. Bilateral cervical vagotomy eliminates
all responses to GLU, as depicted in the middle and bottom panels.

GI areas to the hindbrain application of GLU. Non-specific effects
of GLU application (e.g. osmolality and volume) are unlikely in light
of the control experiments carried out.

All upper GI motor responses could be eliminated by cervical
vagotomy. Heart rate decreases were mediated by GLU-induced increases in vagal activity. Blood pressure increases were associated
with direct efferent sympathetic vascular mechanisms since they were
not eliminated by vagotomy. In addition, spontaneous respiratory
cessation was observed during hindbrain GLU stimulation that was not
eliminated by vagotomy. Based on the similar GI and cardiovascular
responses observed, 4th ventricular GLU-induced effects might be
mediated by GLU diffusion to and stimulation of the DMV area.

Although the specificity of action of compounds infused into the brain decreases with increasing concentration and volume [9, 10], similar results were obtained when small and larger volumes of GLU were delivered into the DMV. This suggests that the DMV was the primary area stimulated in our experiments. Small microinjections, 0.06-0.2 µl of 1.0 M GLU delivering 0.06-0.2 µmoles GLU into the DMV, resulted in more reproducible responses than larger, higher concentration GLU injections, probably because of glutamate neurotoxicity [11].

The fact that DMV GLU increased LESP more often than 4th ventricular GLU and that some upper GI areas were more often affected by 4th ventricular GLU indicates that the two types of GLU applications might be stimulating different, but overlapping populations of neurons that have their effects ultimately via vagal motor neurons. The larger doses of GLU applied to the 4th ventricle are probably responsible for the more prolonged upper GI responses that occurred under these conditions.

GLU application to the hindbrain produces upper GI motor effects similar to those that occur due to electrical stimulation of the hindbrain vagal motor nuclei [1]. However, GLU stimulation of the DMV produces more increases in LESP than electrical stimulation of the same area. The possibilities for this discrepancy are that GLU acts via inhibitory interneurons to decrease DMV vagal efferent output or that GLU selectively excites populations of neurons in the DMV which lead to muscle contraction and to muscle relaxation. Electrical stimulation of neural tissue results in a depolarization of both cell bodies and axons of passage [12]. Although GLU excitatory receptors appear to be restricted to the dendrites and soma of neurons [5] and not on fibers of passage [6], GLU can inhibit neurons directly by depolarization block [13] or indirectly by activating inhibitory interneurons [14]. It seems unlikely that such GLU-induced decreases in DMV neuronal activity can account for the differences between GLU and electrical stimulation of the DMV since electrical stimulation of the DMV can also less frequently result in increased LESP [1]. In addition, blocking vagal efferent activity by nerve transection [1] or by nerve cooling [15] has little or decreasing effects, respectively, on LESP. Activation of the vagus nerve decreases LESP [16, 17]. DMV electrical stimulation similarly appears to activate most vagal efferents simultaneously. GLU stimulation of the DMV, however, could activate vagal motor neurons that increase or decrease LESP at different times resulting in biphasic and more increased LESP responses. This interpretation is consistent with LES muscle recordings during vagal efferent stimulation. A mixed response of depolarization and hyperpolarization are observed under these conditions [18].

In conclusion, although complex, GLU fulfills some important criteria for a candidate neurotransmitter. It is localized in the DMV and mimics the vagally-mediated effects of electrical stimulation, but its release upon stimulation has not been demonstrated in the DMV. Whether GLU is an afferent neurotransmitter involved in DMV efferent control of upper GI motor function, as has been established for baroreceptor afferents to cardiovascular efferents [19], remains to be determined.

REFERENCES
1. Barone, F.C., Lombardi, D.M. and Ormsbee, H.S. III. (1983). Effects of hindbrain stimulation on lower esophageal sphincter pressure in the cat. Am. J. Physiol. Submitted.
2. Eliasson, S. (1953). Activation of gastric motility from the brainstem of the cat. Acta Physiol. Scand. 30: 199-214.
3. Siemers, E.M., Rea, M.A., Felten, D.L. and Aprison, M.H. (1982). Distribution and uptake of glycine, glutamate and γ-amino-butyric acid in the vagal nuclei and eight other regions of the rat medulla oblongata. Neurochem. Res. 7: 455-468.
4. Dietrich, W.D., Lowry, O.H. and Loewy, A.D. (1982). The distribution of glutamate, GABA and aspartate in the nucleus tractus solitarius of the cat. Brain Res. 237: 254-260.
5. Curtis, D.R. and Johnston, G.A.R. (1974). Amino acid transmitters in the mammalian central nervous system. In: Adrian, H. (ed.) Reviews of Physiology pp. 97-188 (Berlin: Springer).
6. Goodchild, A.K., Dampney, R.A.L. and Bandler, R. (1982). A method for evoking physiological responses by stimulation of cell bodies, but not axons of passage, within localized regions of the central nervous system. J. Neurosci. Meth. 6: 351-363.

7. Bass, P. and Wiley, J.N. (1972). Contractile force transducer for recording muscle activity in unanesthetized animals. J. Applied Physiol. 32: 567-570.

8. Dent, J. (1976). A new technique for continuous sphincter pressure measurement. Gastroenterology 71: 263-267.

9. Myers, R.D. (1971). Methods for chemical stimulation of the brain. In: Myers, R.D. (ed.) Methods in Psychobiology Vol. 1. pp. 247-280 (New York: Academic Press).

10. Myers, R.D. (1966). Injection of solutions into cerebral tissue: relation between volume and diffusion. Physiol. Behav. 1: 171-174.

11. Van Harreveld, A. and Fifkova, E. (1971). Light and electron microscope changes in central nervous tissue after electrophoretic injection of glutamate. Exp. Molec. Path. 14: 61-81.

12. Ranck, J.B. (1975). Which elements are excited in electrical stimulation of mammalian central nervous system: a review. Brain Res. 98: 417-440.

13. Eyzaguirre,, C. and Kuffler, S.W. (1955). Processes of excitation in the dendrites and in the soma or single isolated sensory cells of the lobster and crayfish. J. Gen. Physiol. 39: 87-119.

14. McLennon, H. (1971). The pharmacology of inhibition of mitral cells in the olfactory bulb. Brain Res. 29: 177-184.

15. Reynolds, R.P.E., El-Sharkawy, T.Y. and Diament, N.E. (1983). Role of central vagal innervation in feline lower esophageal sphincter function. Gastroenterology 84 (Part 2): 1285.

16. Clark, C.G. and Vane, J.R. (1961). The cardiac sphincter in the cat. Gut 2: 252-262.

17. Rattan, S. and Goyal, R.K. (1974). Neural control of the lower esophageal sphincter: Influence of the vagus nerves. J. Clin. Invest. 54: 899-906.

18. Gonella, J. Niel, J.P. and Roman, C. (1977). Vagal control of lower esophageal sphincter motility in the cat. J. Physiol. 273: 647-664.

19. Reis, D.J., Granata, A.R., Perrone, M.H. and Talman, W.T. (1981). Evidence that glutamic acid is the neurotransmitter of baroreceptor afferents terminating in the nucleus tractus solitarius. J. Auton. Nerv. Sys. 3: 321-334.

LECTURE

Gastrointestinal Hormones and Intestinal Motility

S. J. KONTUREK

CHARACTERISTICS OF GUT HORMONAL PEPTIDES AFFECTING INTESTINAL MOTILITY

In recent years, there has been a virtual explosion in discovery of various hormonal peptides isolated from the gastrointestinal tract and the pancreas. The truly remarkable development in digestive endocrinology could be attributed 1. to the successful isolation of what are generally regarded as the major gastrointestinal hormones (gastrin, CCK and secretin) – and since then, many peptides whose hormonal status has not yet been clarified and 2. to the application of highly sensitive methods of quantitative measurement of circulating hormones by radioimmunoassay and their tissue distribution by immunocytochemistry.

Sequence homologies permit classification of some of these peptides into "families" (Table 1); the best known are the gastrin-CCK family, sharing a carboxyterminal tetrapeptide, and the secretin-glucagon-VIP-GIP family, with numerous identical amino acids (1). Erspamer and coworkers succedeed in isolating a number of peptides from amphibian skin that have counterparts in mammalian gut and brain ("brain-gut-skin-peptides") such as substance P, gastrin releasing peptide, CCK, enkephalins etc. (2).

An important feature of gut peptides is their species and size heterogeneity. Prohormones or "big" peptides are less potent and more resistant to degradation than smaller hormonal peptides. Cleavage of prohormones to shorter forms increases biological activity in case of gastrin, CCK, glucagon and insulin. Another interesting pattern of such peptides as CCK, gastrin , GRP, PP, secretin, substance P, TRH and VIP is the C-terminal-amide structure, which is necessary for their full biological activity. The mechanism for amidation has not been established but it probably results from the enzymatic cleavage of the precursor extending at the C-terminal through a glycine residue (3).

Immunocytochemistry has provided an important clue about the possible role of several gut peptides by the demonstration of the localization and possible mode of release. Endocrine-type cells of APUD (Amine Precursor Uptake and Decarboxylation) series have been shown to contain CCK, gastrin, GRP, glucagon, enteroglucagon, motilin, neuro-

593

tensin, PP, secretin, somatostatin and substance P. Most of these
cells are of the "receptorsecretory" or "open" type i.e. hormone release can be elicited by mechanical and chemical stimuli acting on cell
receptors from the luminal side (4). Several gut peptides have been
located in the paracrine-type cells, in the nerve fibers or both. Bombesin-like peptides, enkephalins, TRH and VIP were found exclusively
in the nerves and appear to function primarily as neuropeptides to influence the structures adjacent to their release, although, a circulatory, neuroendocrine role cannot be excluded. Other peptides, such as
somatostatin and substance P, have been found in nerves and endocrine-
paracrine type cells and may be, therefore, released by axonal depolarization and luminal factors (5).

Table 1

STRUCTURE OF GUT PEPTIDES AFFECTING GASTRIC MOTILITY

Peptide	Structure
GASTRIN : hG 34	QLGPQGPPHLVADPSKKQGPWLEEEEEAYGWMDF #
hG 17	- - - - - - - - - - - - - - - - - - -
hG 14	- - - - - - - - - - - - - - - - -
CHOLECYSTOKININ : CCK 39	YIOOARKAPSGRVSMIKNLQSLDPSHRISDRDYMGWMDF #
CCK 33	- -
CCK 8	- - - - - - - - - - -
SECRETIN	HSDGTFTSELSRLRDSARLQRLLQFLV #
GASTRIC INHIBITORY PEPTIDE (GIP)	YAEGTFISDYSIAMDKIROODFVNWLLAQQKGKKSDWKHNITQ
VASOACTIVE INTESTINAL PEPTIDE (VIP)	HSDAVFTDNYTRLRKOMAVKKYLNSILN #
GLUCAGON	HSOGTFTSDYSKYLDSRRAQDFVQWLMDT
MOTILIN	FVPIFTYGELQRMQEKERNKGQ
PANCREATIC POLYPEPTIDE : pPP	ASLEPVYPGDDATPEQMAQYAAELRRYINMLTRPRY #
hPP	- P - - - - - - - BB - - - - - - - - - - - D - - - - - - - - - - - - -
BOMBESIN (frog)	QQRL - - - Q - - - - - - - -
GASTRIC RELEASING PEPTIDE (GRP)	APVSVGGGTVLAKMYPRGNHWAVGHLM #
SOMATOSTATIN : SS -28	SANSNPAMAPRERKAGCKNFFWKTFTSC
SS -14	- - - - - - - - - - - - - - -
NEUROTENSIN (hNT)	OLYENKPRRPYIL
SUBSTANCE P (equine)	RPKPQQFFGLM #
ENKEPHALINS : Leu	YGGFL
Met	- - - - M

Q, PCA (pyroglutamyl); #, carboxyl terminal amide; Y, tyrosine sulfate; h, human; p, porcine

The amounts of secreted hormone and its plasma levels depend on the
endocrine cell number and their responsiveness to secretory stimuli.
The release of some gut hormones in resting conditions exhibits intrinsic cyclic changes and this has been demonstrated with respect to motilin, PP and somatostatin (6,7,8). The release of others appears to be
relatively constant, resulting in relatively stable plasma levels. The
origin of the cyclic hormonal fluctuations in plasma is unknown but it
seems to result, at least in part, from the periodic changes in neural,
predominantly cholinergic, activity because blockage of cholinergic receptors eliminates these fluctuations (9). Feeding also abolished cyclic hormonal changes and resulted in the rise in plasma levels of some
hormones while reducing others (10). Among the factors influencing
hormonal response to food ingestion, the most important are 1. exogenous factors such as size of the load and chemical composotion of ingested food, 2. endogenous factors including the intraluminal pressure,
distention, pH, osmolarity etc., 3. functional changes such as transit
time (gastric emptying, intestinal passage), and responsiveness of en-

docrine cells (vagotomy, malabsorption, maldigestion) and 4. anatomical changes such as reduced number of endocrine cells (gastritis, coeliac disease, inflammatory bowel disease, stomach or gut resection, intestinal bypass etc.). If the absorption of food, but not merely its presence in the intestinal lumen, provides a trigger mechanism for hormone release (e.g. GIP), any means to impair absorption will decrease the hormonal response. Thus, an abnormal gut hormone profile may be either due to primary disorder in the release or secondary to gastrointestinal tract abnormalities, such as functional motility disorders, gut resection, intestinal bypass, altered transit time etc.(12). The alteration in the release may not be uniform for all hormones. Increased intestinal motility and shortened transit time or jejuno-ileal bypass usually diminish the response of the gut peptides located in the foregut (duodenum and upper jejunum) while increasing the response of peptides located in the ileum or colon (13).

Although there are many candidate hormones with new species continuously discovered, we will discuss here only those, whose hormonal status is well established, namely gastrin, CCK, secretin, motilin, neurotensin, somatostatin and pancreatic polypeptide (PP) (Table 2).

Table 2.   Site of production, cells of origin and major motor effect

Hormone	Site of release	Cell of origin	Motor action
Gastrin	Antrum, duodenum	G	↑Antral contractions
CCK	Duodenum, jejunum	I	↑Gallbladder contraction ↓Intestinal motility
Secretin	Duodenum, jejunum	S	↓Gastroduodenal motility
GIP	Duodenum, jejunum	K	unknown
PP	Pancreas	PP	unknown
Motilin	Small intestine	Mo	Regulation of MMC
Somato-statin	Antrum, small intestine, pancreas	D	↓Hormone release
Neurotensin	Jejunum, ileum	N	↑Intestinal motility

Gastrin is primarily a gastric hormone, while CCK, secretin, motilin, GIP, and somatostatin are mainly upper small bowel hormones, while neurotensin is a lower intestine hormone. PP is of pancreatic origin. The spectrum of biological action of each of these hormones includes multiple gastrointestinal target organs, such as exocrine and endocrine secretion, motility, circulation, absorption, metabolism and perhaps also food intake (11). Most of our informations about the effects of gut hormones on various digestive functions derive from the studies with systematic application of these hormones in the doses that usually are far beyond the physiological range. To accept any effect of a hormone as physiological, several criteria should be met. According to Grossman (14), the first criterion is the correlation between the phenomenon and fluctuations of endogenous hormone level. Second criterion is the reproduction of the same effects by exogenously administered hormone in amount and molecular form similar to those released by endogenous stimulus. Since the biological effects of the peptide hormones at the cellular level result from the binding to specific receptor sites at the cell membrane, the application of specific receptor antagonists may help to establish whether the postulated effect really results from the action of a given hormone and whether it is of physiological character. The list of such antagonists includes opiate receptor antagonists, such as naloxone for blocking the action of opiate peptides (15) or proglumide for gastrin (16). Another possibility of defining the physiological role of endogenous hormone is immunoneutralization of circulating hormone that has been applied successfully with respect to such hormones as secretin (17) and motilin (18).

It must be emphasized that under normal in vivo conditions one stimulus usually releases not one but several hormones and other transmitters, which may interact with each other at the effector organ or at the same receptor site resulting in the summation, potentiation or inhibition of their effects (19). The fact that certain gut peptides are present in nerve fibers and release during nerve activation in the periphery or in the brain adds to the complexity of endocrine and peptidergic control of the digestive functions.

INTERDIGESTIVE MOTILITY

Gastrointestinal functions exhibit major changes between the fasted and the fed state and the involvement of gut hormones in the control of these functions varies between these two conditions. The characteristic feature of fasting gastrointestinal motility is a cyclic pattern originally observed in dogs by Boldyreff in 1905 (20), and then rediscovered and carefully described by Szurszewski (21) in the dog and Vantrappen et al. (22) in man. Carlson et al. (23) and Code and Marlett (24) confirmed that fasting periodic motor activity usually originates in the foregut and is propagated to the terminal ileum. They divided it into four phases: phase I, representing a quiescent period with no spike activity and no contractions; phase II - the period of random spike activity or intermittent contractions; phase III - the period of regular spike bursts or regular contractions at the maximal frequency that migrate distally and phase IV - the transition period between phase III and I. Phase III has been called "activity front", "regular spike activity" or "interdigestive migrating myoelectric or motor complex" (MMC). The entire circle repeats every one to two hours and the propagation of MMC from upper gut to terminal ileum takes the same time. Some MMCs may arise distal to the stomach and duodenum and not all MMCs travel so far as the terminal ileum.

The physiological significance of MMCs has been related to cleaning the gut lumen from debris and secretion by means of a band of strong contractions in accordance to the concept of intestinal "housekeeper" proposed by Szurszewski (21) and Schlegel and Code (25). It continued for as long as 12 weeks in empty gut while the nutrition was supported by total parenteral alimentation but was disrupted after feeding, which initiated different pattern (26). Bueno and Ruckebush (27) indicated that the interruption of MMC by a meal is characteristic for carnivores (man, dog) and omnivores (pig) but not for herbivores (sheep, cattle).

The characteristic feature of cyclic motor activity is its association with the secretory gastrointestinal component. Boldyreff (28) observed in the dog that the increased gastric motor activity was accompanied by periodic increase in pancreatic secretion in the absence of any secretory stimulus. Hoelzel (29) described in man the coexistence of a cyclic increase in gastric secretion associated with the cyclic occurrence of gastric hunger contractions. Recently, Vantrappen et al. (30) confirmed the gastric, pancreatic and biliary secretory components of MMC in the human duodenum and indicated that the migrating motor and secretory activity constitute two aspects of the same periodic activity phenomena. Kaene et al. (31,32) identified similar increases in gastric, pancreatic and biliary secretions in close association with the duodenal MMCs in dogs and men. It may be, therefore, concluded that under fasting conditions both motor and secretory activity of the stomach, gut, pancreas and liver change periodically to provide both mechanical and chemical means of intestinal "housekeeping".

The factors controlling the initiation and migration of the cyclic motility pattern and accompanying gastrointestinal secretory component is understood incompletely. No doubt, the enthusiasm for finding various gastrointestinal hormones and seeking actions for them in physiology had much influence on the concept of the regulation of gastrointestinal motility particularly in the foregut, where most of these hormones have been localized. With the isolation and synthesis of motilin (33) and the findings that its intravenous administration triggers in the foregut a caudad moving series of strong contractions (34) or of intense action potential activity (35), similar to natural MMC, suggested that motilin is the "interdigestive hormone", which regulates the initiation of cyclic motor activity in the canine small intestine. The observations that motilin stimulates gastric and pancreatic secretion (36) suggested that this peptide may also be responsible for the secretory aspects of MMC in the foregut. Further findings of Itoh's (37) and Chey's (6) group that plasma motilin fluctuates during the interdigestive state and reaches the peaks that coincides with the activity front of MMC in the stomach and the duodenum strengthened motilin hypothesis of MMC.

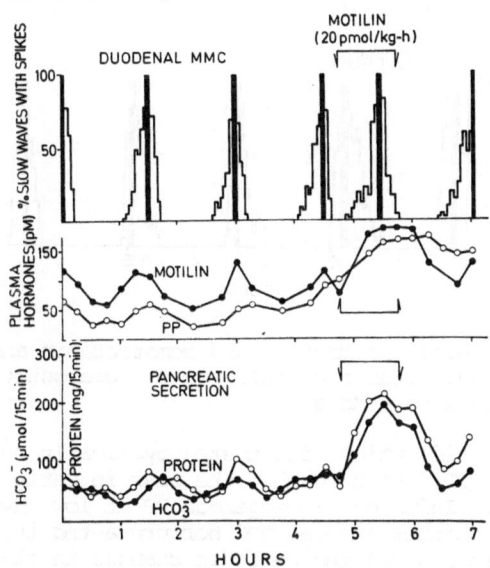

FIGURE 1   Duodenal MMCs, plasma motilin and PP levels and pancreatic HCO_3^- and protein secretion in fasted dogs before and after i.v. infusion of motilin. Mean ± SEM of 4 tests on 4 dogs.

Similar periodic increases in plasma motilin have been recently confirmed in fasted humans (6,8). The minimum dose of motilin that induced premature raised plasma hormone to the level comparable to that observed during spontaneous MMC (Fig. 1).

There are several arguments against motilin being the only initiator of MMC in the foregut. There was not always a one to one relation between phase III activities and the peaks of plasma motilin level. The immunoneutralization of motilin by specific antibodies reduced the background motilin levels for several days but MMCs in the foregut returned to normal conditions only after few hours (18). Several other peptides and drugs may trigger the premature MMCs. We reported that substance P (42), somatostatin (41), neurotensin (60) and morphine (15) infused in fasted dogs increased the occurrence rate of the MMCs. Sarna et al. (43) confirmed that morphine increases the frequency of MMCs.

Using dogs with monopolar electrods implanted along the small bowel and equipped with Thomas-type pancreatic fistulas, we confirmed that the occurrence of MMCs in the duodenum was accompanied by an increase in plasma levels of motilin and PP as well as by a rise in pancreatic secretion. Exogenous somatostatin infused i.v. in a dose of 50 pmol/kg-hr suppressed motilin fluctuations but failed to affect the initiation and propagation of MMCs (Fig. 2).

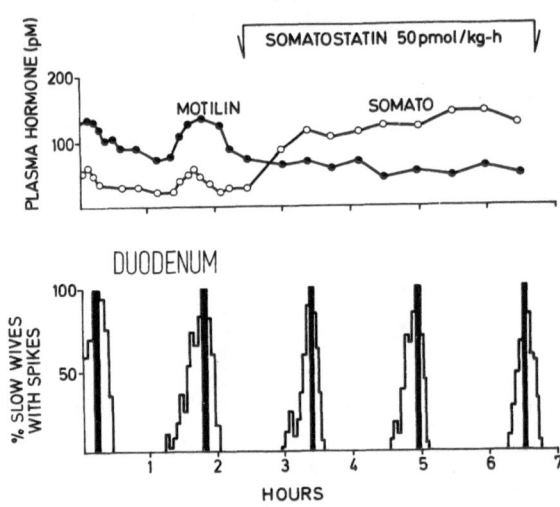

FIGURE 2   Plasma levels of motilin and somatostatin and duodenal MMCs before and after i.v. infusion of somatostatin. Mean ± SEM of 4 tests on 4 dogs.

Another gut peptide which fluctuates cyclically during the interdigestive period is PP, which reaches the peak in early phase III of MMC in duodenum (31). Infusion of exogenous PP at low physiological dose (100 pmol/kg-hr) neither induced MMC nor prevented its occurrence in the foregut but it reduced the periodic changes in plasma motilin. Larger doses of PP (200-400 pmol/kg-hr) strongly suppressed motilin release while causing only some delay in the appearance of MMCs in the foregut (38). Thus MMC in the canine foregut can be dissociated from the cyclic changes in plasma motilin.

Peeters et al. (8) reported that plasma somatostatin in humans exhibited cyclic fluctuations with peaks coinciding with the activity front in the upper duodenum. Intravenous infusion of exogenous somatostatin at a dose which raised plasma somatostatin to the physiological level inhibited gastric but stimulated duodenal phase III activity in spite of the fact that both motilin and PP levels were decreased. They suggested that somatostatin but not motilin has a physiological role in the regulation of the MMC in humans. In other species such as pigs, the MMCs in the foregut are not associated with increased motilin release (56).

The above findings in dogs and humans seem to undermine the motilin concept of the initiation of MMC but do not exclude the contribution of this and other peptides in modulating and influencing the timing of phase III of MMC that seems to be basically controlled by an enteric biological clock. As it was pointed out by Wingate et al. (39) and Sarna et al. (40) the control of initiation and propagation of MMCs in the foregut is built into the enteric nervous system and locally released paracrines or circulating hormones such as motilin or substance P (34,42) may advance but not reset the clock. They should be considered as triggering agents, rather than initiators of MMCs. The underlying mechanism responsible for the periodic activity of MMCs behaves as relaxation oscillators characterized by gradual increase in output until a threshold level is reached at which point oscillator output suddenly becomes maximal.   Then the output falls to its lowest level to start again gradual increase and repeat the cycle. When applied in the proper period after the last activity front and in the proper dose, an external stimulus like motilin, substance P or morphine (34,42,43) can drive the level of activity to the threshold level and hence precipitate a premature phase III. There is evidence for the regional variation in the organization of periodic activity. The foregut seems to be related to hormonal peptide release (motilin, substance P) whereas the rest of the gut is probably less dependent upon the hormonal factors but controlled by oscillatory mechanisms

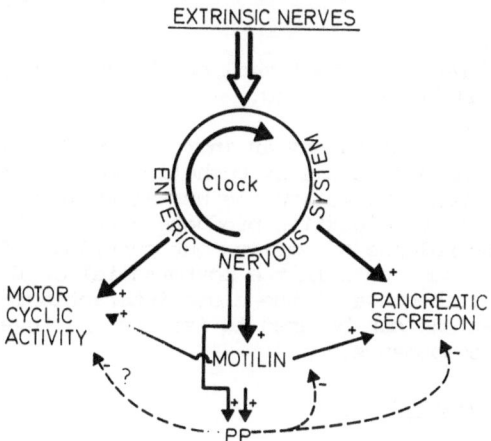

FIGURE 3   Model of the MMC in the canine foregut and accompanying exocrine and endocrine secretions.

Although there is little doubt that the biological clock which regulates periodic motor and secretory activities of the foregut, resides
in the bowel, extrinsic nerves may be important in turning "on" and
"off" the clock system. This biological clock in the foregut seems to
be responsible for both motor and secretory (exocrine and endocrine)
periodic activities. Motilin probably serves as a positive feedback
stimulant of MMC, PP release and exocrine pancreatic secretion whereas, PP plays an opposite role (Fig. 3).

POSTPRANDIAL MOTILITY

It now well established that feeding results in the interruption of the
interdigestive activity of the small bowel and in the appearance of the
characteristic fed-type pattern of spike potentials and contracttions.
The question arises what are the postprandial mechanisms inhibiting
MMC and transforming the fasted to fed pattern of intestinal motility.

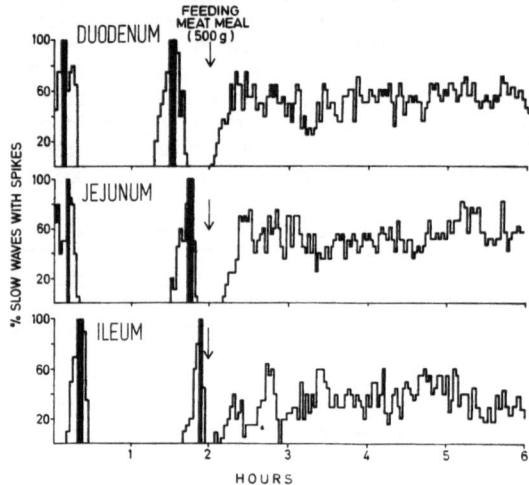

FIGURE 4   Effect of feeding a meat meal on the MMCs in the duodenum,
           jejunum and ileum in a dog.

It is known that feeding causes an increase in the gastrointestinal
exocrine and endocrine secretions by cephalic-vagal stimulation and
gastrointestinal distention, activating neural reflexes as well as by
chemical reactions of the digestive products with the intestinal mucosa, resulting in the release of various gut peptides. The analysis of
the role of various components in the postprandial or fed pattern of
motility is difficult because of the close interaction. Certain experimental manipulations can be used to isolate and investigate separately some of these components.

Cephalic-vagal stimulation

The effects of cephalic-vagal stimulation on the intestinal motility
has been little studied and the results are inconclusive. Lorber et al.
(45) found that sham-feeding resulted in the cessation of gastric peris-

taltic waves with increased fundal tonus and decreased antral tonus, lasting as long as the secretory response. Duodenal motor activity was not recorded. Preshaw and Knauf (46) reported that sham-feeding produced a sudden increase in motor activity of the vagally-innervated proximal duodenal pouch. In contrast, Steinbach and Code (47) noticed that vagal stimulation by sight or smell of food lengthened the period of the MMC even if the accompanying gastric secretion was drained to the outside via gastric fistula. In humans, sham-feeding was reported to disrupt the MMCs in the foregut (48) and to increase its secretory component but in these tests gastric acid was not emptied and not prevented from entering the duodenum. We reported (50) that 15 min sham-feeding of a meat meal in dogs with gastric fistula open to drain gastric secretion, resulted in a significant reduction in MMC interval by about 25% in most of animals tested. This reduction was not dependent upon the period of sham-feeding and was accompanied by a rise in plasma gastrin, PP and motilin levels.

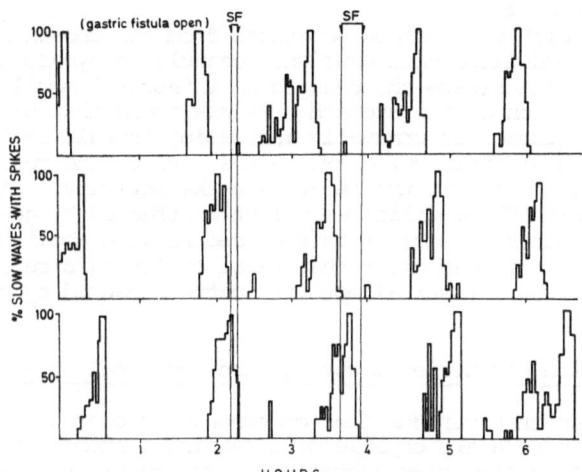

FIGURE 5   MMCs in duodenum (upper record), jejunum (middle record) and ileum (lower record) in fasted dogs with gastric fistula open before and after sham-feeding lasting 5 and 15 min.

Closing the gastric fistula and allowing gastric acid to enter the duodenum resulted in the typical fed pattern of activity accompanied by a smaller rise in serum gastrin and PP levels while decreasing plasma motilin levels. The pretreatment with antimuscarinic agents (atropine or pirenzepine) completely abolished MMCs induced by sham-feeding, suggesting an important role of cholinergic component in the cephalic-vagal modulation of MMCs. Whether gut peptides, particularly motilin and PP are also involved in the alteration of MMCs caused by vagal excitation remains to be established. The effect of sham-feeding on the MMC seems to be quite specific because pharmacological initiators of cephalic phase, such as insulin or 2-deoxy-D-glucose, which are known to interfere with the glucose supply to the brain, result in the interruption

of MMC and the appearance of fed-type motility pattern, whether or not
gastric acid was drained to the exterior to prevent duodenal acidification.

Gastrointestinal distention

Distention of the intact stomach and the duodenum is known to increase the rate of gastric acid and pancreatic enzyme secretion, probably via the activation of the short (intramural) and long (vago-vagal)
reflexes. Gut hormones appear to play a little role in the effects of
gastroduodenal distention as their plasma levels remain unchanged.
    Little information is available regarding the influence of control-
led gastric distention on intestinal motility pattern. Code and Marlett (24) observed that balloon distention of the stomach eliminated
the interdigestive cycles in the stomach and duodenum for the time of
distention but had little effect on the MMCs in distal part of the
small bowel. Gastric instillation of milk interrupted MMCs over the
entire small bowel and caused fed-type motility pattern. No attempts
were made to define the mechanism of these motility alterations caused
by gastric distention.
    Using dogs with the stomach separated from the duodenum by a double
mucosal bridge and large gastroduodenal cannula to bypass the pylorus,
we attempted to quantitate the changes in intestinal motility provoked
by saline distention of the stomach. It was found that saline distention of intact stomach at gradually increasing intraluminal pressures
(range 0-15 cm H_2O) interrupted MMC in the foregut and resulted in the
pressure dependent rise in the fed-type spike activity. Since plasma
hormones (gastrin, PP, motilin) were little affected by gastric distention and since motor effects of this procedure were abolished by vagotomy and atropine, it was clear that vagal cholinergic reflexes are
responsible for the intestinal motility pattern caused by gastric distention.

Chemical reaction of nutrients with gastrointestinal mucosa

It is well known that various food components in contact with gastric
and intestinal mucosa are capable of releasing a number of gut hormones
and of stimulating digestive secretions. The question remains whether
these hormones released postprandially contribute also to the transformation of fasted to fed-type motility.
    In general, the fed pattern in the dogs depends on the amount and
physico-chemical composition of food ingested. There is a minimum of
food (12 g/kg of canned food) which inhibits canine MMCs and increases
intestinal spike activity (51). When equicaloric canned food and ele-
mental diet were compared , the latter cause about one-half the number
of spike bursts of canned food suggesting that in addition to chemical
composition, the size of the meal plays an important role. Schang et
al. (52) compared specific food components, triglycerides, casein hydrolysate and glucose given single or in combination and found that all
of them disrupted the MMCs, but glucose caused the largest increase in
spike potentials, the peptides were next and lipids actually caused a
decrease below the fasting level. The duration of fed state and disruption of MMCs with equicaloric amounts of food components was longest
with lipids, followed by protein, and then carbohydrates. Since each
type of food component releases different gut hormones, the attractive
hypothesis will be hormonal mediation of fed pattern of intestinal motility. This hormone hypothesis is supported by several findings:

1. food is a potent releaser of several gut hormones such as gastrin, CCK, secretin and insulin, which have been reported to disrupt MMCs and to change the fasting pattern to one resembling the fed pattern (53-56); 2. feeding of animals with Thiry-Vella loops disrupts MMCs both in the isolated loops and the rest of the small bowel (39); 3. parenteral nutrition that does not affect gut hormone release, does not influence the generation or propagation of MMCs (26).

If hormones are involved in the postprandial change in intestinal motility, some kind of relationship is expected between this motility change and endogenous hormone release. Indeed, endogenous gastrin released by antral pouch irrigation with acetylcholine was reported by Thomas et al. (57) to abolish both gastric and duodenal cyclic motor activity and to produce intermittent spike activity in the duodenum. No attempts have been made to determine the effects of endogenous gastrin on motility pattern in the distal portion of the small bowel so it is unknown whether this hormone could produce the digestive pattern. Wingate et al. (59) who compared the intestinal motility pattern observed after feeding and after infusion of exogenous pentagastrin, CCK or secretin in different doses, reached the conclusion that none of these peptides reproduced the digestive pattern i.e. the abolition of MMCs at all levels of the small bowel and overall increase in spike activity of the gut. The striking difference between typical fed pattern and that induced by exogenous hormones e.g. CCK was the failure of the distal gut to respond to gut hormones. Effects of exogenous hormones resembling digestive pattern probably represented pharmacological rather than physiological action of these hormones.

To elucidate the possible role of endogenous hormones in digestive motility pattern, we used dogs with special gastroduodenal cannula that allowed complete separation and selective stimulation of the stomach and the duodenum by various test meals. Constant intragastric pressure (5 cm H_2O) was maintained by a barostat and a constant pH (2.5 or 5.0) was kept by means of intragastric titration. Monopolar electrodes spaced 25 cm apart in the small bowel served to examine the myoelectric activity of the gut. Liver extract (LE) meal kept in the stomach at pH 5.0 caused an increase in gastric acid secretion to about 80% of histamine maximum and it was accompanied by several fold increase in plasma gastrin while saline meal of pH 5.0 in the stomach stimulated acid output to about 30% of histamine maximum without affecting plasma hormone levels. With both LE and saline meals in the stomach, MMCs were disrupted in the duodenum and upper jejunum but occurred in the distal jejunum and ileum. The major difference between these meals was about twice higher increase in spike activity in the foregut in tests with LE than with saline. Acidification of gastric LE meal to pH 2.5 suppressed gastric acid output and plasma gastrin level and reduced the spike activity in the foregut, while MMCs remained interrupted and plasma levels of somatostatin significantly increased above control values (Figs 6-8).

These results could be interpreted that the distention of the stomach with peptone meal or saline immediately interrupts the MMCs in the foregut probably by a nervous pathway. Gastrin released by peptic digest (LE meal) but not by saline in the stomach probably did not contribute to the inhibition of MMCs but greatly increased spike activity of the gut. The combination of gastric saline distention and exogenous gastrin infusion (50 pmol/kg-hr) to raise plasma gastrin to the level observed after gastric LE meal fully restored the pattern of intestinal motility, which were identical to that recorded with a gastric LE meal. Note that exogenous gastrin alone at the dose used without saline distention of the stomach did not affect the generation and propagation of MMCs or intestinal spike activity. Thus we confirm previous findings of Wingate et al. (58) that gastrin at low physiological dose fails to affect intestinal motility pattern but increases intestinal spike activity when combined with gastric distention. The fall in the intestinal spike activity observed after acidification of gastric LE meal could be due either to the suppression of gastrin release or to the increase in somatostatin release or both (Fig. 6).

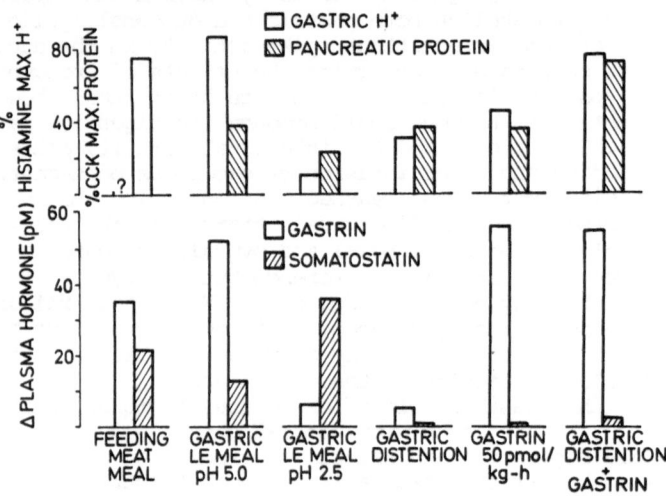

FIGURE 6   Gastric H^+ (expressed as % of histamine maximum), and pancreatic protein secretion as well as an increment in plasma gastrin and somatostatin levels in response to ordinary feeding, gastric LE meal of pH 5.0 or 2.5, gastric saline distention, gastrin infused i.v. (50 pmol/kg-hr) and the combination of gastric saline distention + gastrin infusion in dogs with chronic gastric and pancreatic fistulas and implanted monopolar electrodes along the gut.

The major changes in the intestinal motility pattern typical to the fed state were found when 5% LE meal was delivered to the duodenum while the stomach was kept empty by opening the gastric fistula. Intestinal perfusion with LE meal completely abolished MMCs at all levels of the small bowel and increased intestinal spike activity similarly as after a meat meal. Similar motility changes were observed when 10% protein hydrolysate was infused intraduodenally. Plasma gastrin was only slightly increased (so was also gastric H^+ secretion) while plasma CCK and PP were highly elevated. Instillation of saline into the gut at the same rate (20–150 ml/hr) as LE or protein hydrolysate meal did not affect intestinal motility by itself but when combined with a small dose of CCK (50 pmol/kg-hr) it reproduced fully the motility pattern induced by protein digest meal. Note that CCK alone also inhibited MMCs but only in the foregut and increased the spike activity of the small bowel. Thus, the combination of neural activity

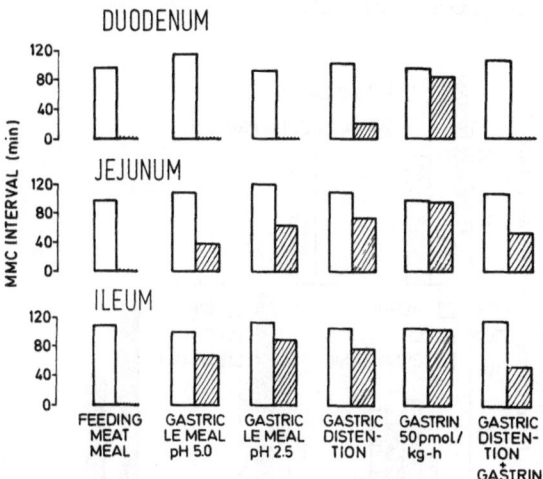

FIGURE 7   MMC intervals in the duodenum, jejunum and ileum recorded in experiments as in tests shown on Fig. 6.

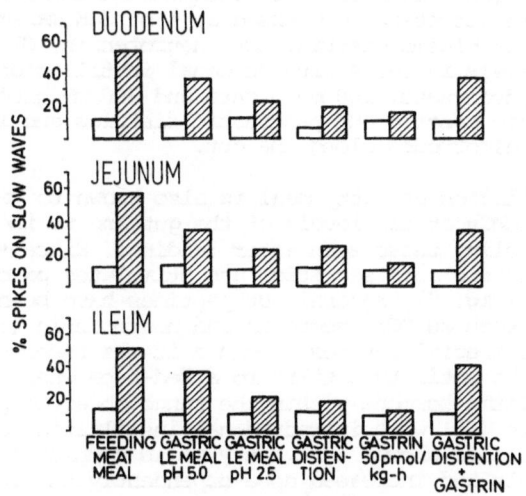

FIGURE 8   Per cent of spikes on slow waves recorded in the duodenum , jejunum and ileum in experiments as in tests shown on Fig. 6.

caused by the gut distention and CCK release by intestinal LE meal had
additive effects on the motility pattern and probably contributed to
the transformation of fasted to fed type pattern observed after intestinal perfusion with protein digestion products (Figs 9-11).

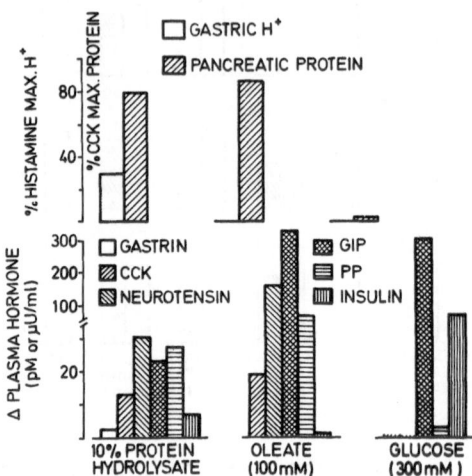

FIGURE 9   Gastric H$^+$ (expressed as % of histamine maximum) and pancreatic protein secretion (expressed as % of CCK maximum) and an
increment in plasma gastrin, CCK, neurotensin, GIP, PP and
insulin levels in tests with duodenal instillation of 10%
protein hydrolysate, 100 mM oleate and 300 mM glucose in dogs
with chronic gastric and pancreatic fistulas and implanted
monopolar electrodes along the gut.

Intestinal instillation of fatty meal is also known to cause prolonged abolition of MMCs at all levels of the gut and to increase
spike activity resembling those seen after feeding. Since fat in the
gut also inhibits gastric acid secretion and stimulates pancreatic bicarbonate secretion (Fig. 9), several gut peptides have been proposed
to mediate effects, such as CCK, secretin and neurotensin (59). The
latter peptide is of special interest because it was reported to block
MMCs and to change the motility pattern to a fed-type when infused at
a dose increasing plasma hormone within the range observed postprandially (59). Our results (60) with intraduodenal instillation of 20% intralipid or 100 mM oleate showed that fatty meals completely abolish
MMCs at all gut levels and increased dose-dependently the intestinal
spike activity. They also caused dose-dependent rise in plasma neurotensin level. Exogenous neurotensin at higher doses (0.6-2.5 µg/kg-hr)
mimicked the action of fat on intestinal motility. However, at lower
doses (0.15-0.6 µg/kg-hr), raising plasma hormone to the levels recorded after fatty meal, neurotensin decreased the occurrence of MMC, mainly in the proximal but not in the distal portion of the gut. Single
intravenous bolus injection of neurotensin at low doses induced in some animals the premature activity front of MMC in the jejunum and ileum

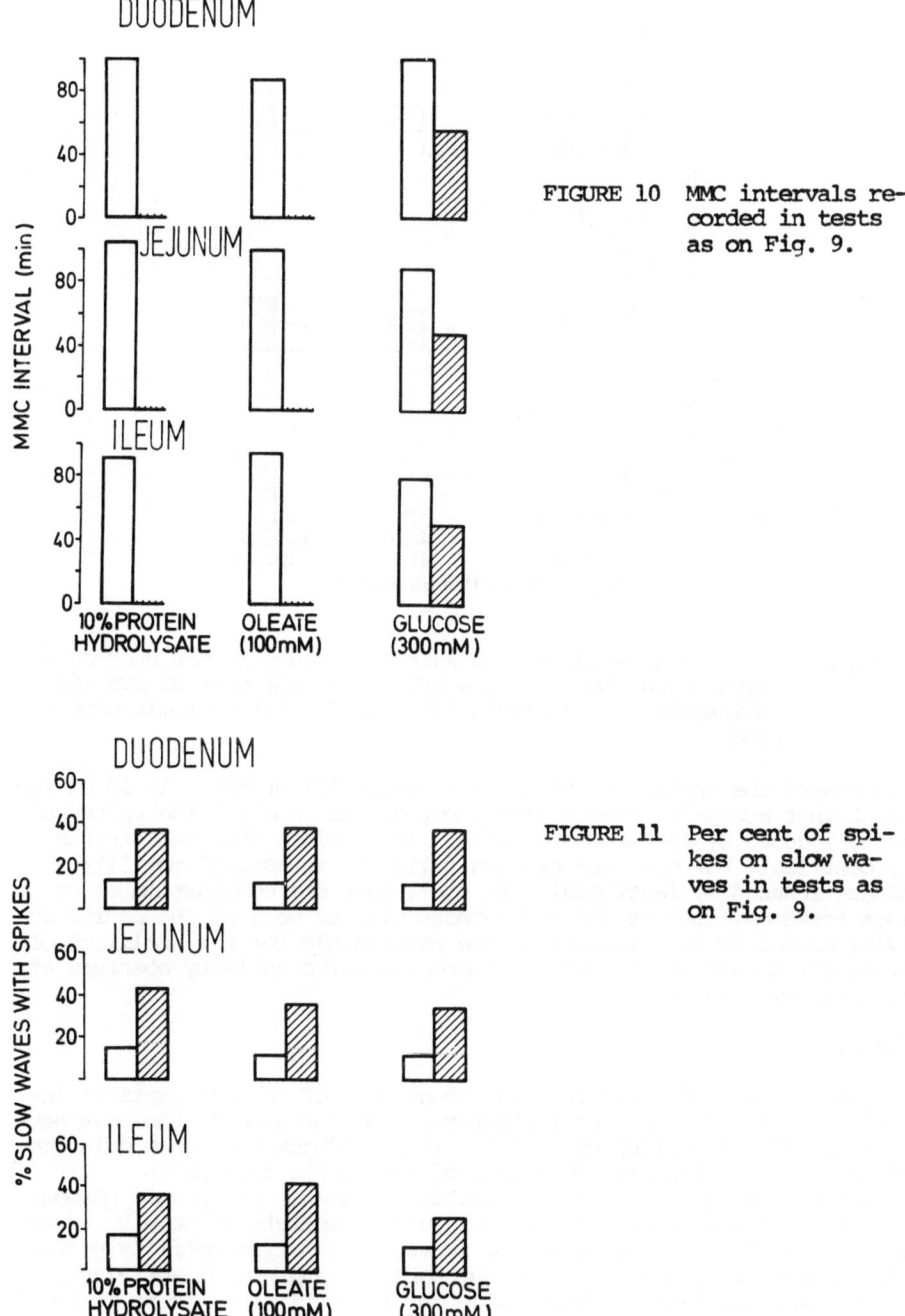

FIGURE 10   MMC intervals recorded in tests as on Fig. 9.

FIGURE 11   Per cent of spikes on slow waves in tests as on Fig. 9.

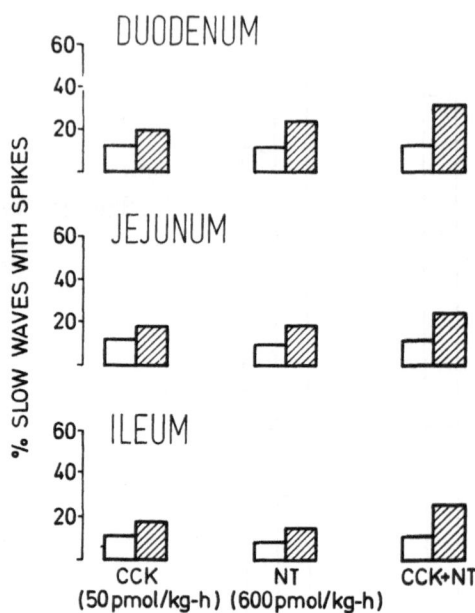

FIGURE 12   Per cent slow waves with spikes recorded in the duodenum,
jejunum and ileum in dogs after i.v. infusion of CCK (50
pmol/kg-hr), neurotensin (600 pmol/kg-hr) or their combination.

and delayed the appearance of the next phase III of MMC. It is of interest that atropine reduced inpart but did not abolish the spike activity induced by fat or neurotensin. We conclude that neurotensin
may contribute but does not explain fully the intestinal motility
changes induced by fatty meal. It seems that the combination of various hormones, such as CCK and neurotensin. as well as the neural activity caused by gut distention, are responsible for the abolition of
MMC at all levels of the gut and increased spike activity observed after fatty meal in the gut

SUMMARY

It appears that under fasting conditions none of the gut peptides including motilin serve as an initiator of MMC but some of them may serve as positive (motilin) or negative (PP) feedback factors modulating
both motor and secretory components of MMC in the foregut.
    Postprandially, in spite of dramatic changes in the plasma hormone
profile, again, none of gut hormones acting separately seems to be responsible for the transformation of fasted to fed-type motility pattern
but probably the combination of gut hormones and neural activity caused by gut distention is responsible for the motility pattern in fed
state.

REFERENCES

1. Dockray, G.B. (1979). Comparative biochemistry and physiology of gut hormones. Annu. Rev. Physiol. 41, 83-95
2. Erspamer, V., Melchiorri, P., Broccardo, M., Erspamer, G.F., Falaschi, P., Improta, G., Negri, L., and Renda, T. (1981). The brain-gut-skin triangle: New peptides. Peptides 2 (Suppl. 2) 7-16
3. Suchanek, G., and Kreil, G. (1977). Translation of melittin messenger RNA in vitro yields a product terminating with glutaminylglycine rather than with glutaminamide. Proc. Natl. Acad. Sci. U.S.A. 74, 975-978
4. Solcia, E., Capella, C., Buffa, R., Usellini, L., Fiocca, R., and Sessa, F. (1981) Endocrine cells of the digestive system. In: Johnson, L.R. (ed.). Physiology of the Gastrointestinal Tract vol. 1 pp. 39-58. (New York: Raven Press)
5. Jessen, K.R., Polak, J.M., Van Noorden, Bloom, S.R., and Burnstock, G. (1980). Peptide-containing neurones connect the two ganglionated plexuses of the enteric nervous system. Nature (Lond.). 283: 391-393
6. Lee, K.Y., Chey, W.Y., Tai, H.H., and Yajima, H. (1978). Radio-immunoassay of motilin. Validation and studies on the relationship between plasma motilin and interdigestive myoelectric activity of the duodenum of dog. Am. J. Dig. Dis. 23, 789-795
7. Janssens, J., Hellemans, J., Adrian, T.E., Bloom, S.R., Peeters, T.L., Christofides, N., and Vantrappen, G.R. (1982). Pancreatic polypeptide is not involved in the regulation of the migrating motor complex in man. Regulatory Peptides 3, 41-49
8. Peeters, T.L., Janssens, J., Vantrappen, G.R. (1983). Somatostatin and the interdigestive migrating motor complex in man. Regulatory Peptides 5, 209-217
9. Chey, W.Y., and Lee, K.Y. (1980). Motilin. Clinics in Gastroenterology 9, (3), 645-656
10. Lee, K.Y., Kim, M.S., and Chey, W.Y. (1980). Effects of a meal and gut hormones on plasma motilin and duodenal motility in dog. Am. J. Physiol. 238, G280-G283
11. Walsh, J.H. (1981) Gastrointestinal hormones and peptides. In: Johnson, L.R. (ed.). Physiology of the Gastrointestinal Tract vol. 1. pp. 59-144 (New York: Raven Press)
12. Creutzfeldt, W., Ebert, R., Nauck, M., Stöckmann, F. (1983). Disturbances of the entero-insular axis. Scand. J. Gastroent. 18 (Suppl. 82), 111-119
13. Go, V.L.W., and Miller, L.J. (1983). The role of gastrointestinal hormones in the control of postprandial and interdigestive gastrointestinal function. Scand. J. Gastroent. 18 (Suppl. 82), 135-142
14. Grossman, M.I. (1977). Physiological effects of gastrointestinal hormones. Fed. Proc. 36, 1930
15. Konturek, S.J., Thor, P., Krol, R., Dembinski, A., and Schally, A.V. (1980) Influence of methionine-enkephalin and morphine on myoelectric activity of small bowel. Am. J. Physiol. 238: G384-G389
16. Erckenbrecht, J., Caspary, J., Körner, M.M., Berges, W., and Wienbeck, J. (1982). The inhibiting effect of pentagastrin on interdigestive small bowel motility is antagonized by proglumide. Gastroenterology 82, 1050
17. Chey, W.Y., Kim, M.S., Lee, K.Y., and Chang, T.M. (1979). Effect

of rabbit antisecretin serum on postprandial pancreatic secretion in dogs. Gastroenterology 77, 1268-1275

18. Lee, K.Y., Chang, T.M., and Chey, W.Y. (1983) Effect of rabbit antimotilin serum on myoelectric activity and plasma motilin concentration in dog. Am. J. Physiol. (in press)

19. Sundler, F., Hakanson, R., Leander, S. (1980). Peptidergic nervous systems in the gut. Clinics in Gastroenterology 9 (3), 517-544

20. Boldyreff, W.N. (1905). Le travail periodique de l'appareil digestif endehors de la digestion. Arch. Des. Sci. Biol. 11, 1-157

21. Szurszewski, J.H. (1969). A migrating electric complex of the canine small intestine. Am. J. Physiol. 217, 1757-1763

22. Vantrappen, G.R., Janssens, J., Hellemans, J., and Ghoos, Y. (1977). The interdigestive motor complex of normal subjects and patients with bacterial overgrowth of the small intestine. J. Clin. Invest. 59, 1158-1166

23. Carlson, G.M., Bedi, B.S., and Code, C.F. (1972). Mechanism of propagation of intestinal interdigestive myoelectric complex. Am. J. Physiol. 222, 1027-1030

24. Code, C.F., and Marlett, J.A. (1975). The interdigestive myoelectric complex of the stomach and small bowel of dogs. J. Physiol. (Lond.) 246, 298-309

25. Schlegel, J.F., and Code, C.F. (1975). The gastric peristalsis of the interdigestive housekeeper. In: Vantrappen, G. (ed.). Proceedings of the Fifth International Symposium on Gastrointestinal Motility pp. 321-328. (Herentals: Typoff Press)

26. Weisbrodt, N.W., Copeland, E.M., Thor, P.J. (1976). The myoelectric activity of the small intestine of the dog during total parenteral nutrition. Proc. Soc. Exp. Biol. Med. 153, 121-124

27. Bueno, L., and Ruckebusch, Y. (1978). Migrating myoelectric complexes: disruption, enhancement and disorganisation. In: Duthie, H. (ed.). Gastrointestinal Motility in Health and Disease pp.83-91. (Lancaster: MTP, Press)

28. Boldyreff, W. (1911). Einige neue Seiten der Tätigkeit des Pancreas. Ergeb. der Physiol. 11, 121-217

29. Hoelzel, F. (1925). The relation between the secretory and motor activity in the fasting stomach (man). Am. J. Physiol. 73, 463-469

30. Vantrappen, G.R., Peeters, T.L., and Janssens, J. (1979). The secretory component of the interdigestive migrating motor complex in man. Scand. J. Gastroent. 14, 663-667

31. Kaene, F.B., DiMagno, E.P., Dozois, R.R., and Go, V.L.W. (1980). Relationship among canine interdigestive exocrine pancreatic and biliary flow, duodenal motor activity, plasma-pancreatic polypeptide and motilin. Gastroenterology 78, 310-316

32. Kaene, F.B., DiMagno, E.P., and Malagelada, J.R. (1981). Duodenogastric reflux in humans: Its relationship to fasting antroduodenal motility and gastric, pancreatic and biliary secretion. Gastroenterology 81, 726-731

33. Brown, J.C., Mutt, V., and Dryburgh, J.R. (1971). The further purification of motilin, a gastric motor activity stimulating polypeptide from the mucosa of the small intestine in hogs. Can. J. Physiol. Pharmacol. 48, 339-405

34. Itoh, Z., Honda, R., Hiwatashi, K., Takeuchi, S., Aizawa, I., Takayanagi, R., and Conch, E.F. (1976). Motilin-induced mechanical activity in the canine alimentary tract. Scand. J. Gastroent. 11 (Suppl. 39) 93-110

35. Wingate, D.L., Ruppin, H., Green, W.E.R., Thompson, H.H., Domsch-ke, W., Wunsch, E., Demling, L., and Ritchie, H.D. (1976). Motilin-induced electrical activity in the canine gastrointestinal tract. Scand. J. Gastroent. 11 (Suppl. 39), 111-118

36. Konturek, S.J., Dembinski, A., Krol, R., and Wünsch, E. (1976). Effect of motilin on gastric and pancreatic secretion in dogs. Scand. J. Gastroent. 11, 57-60

37. Itoh, Z., Takeuchi, S., Aizawa, I., Mori, K., Taminato, T., Sei-no, Y., Imura, H., and Yanaihara, N. (1978). Changes in plasma moti-lin concentration and gastrointestinal contractile activity in con-scious dogs. Am. J. Dig. Dis. 23, 929-935

38. Hall, K.E., Diamant, W.E., El-Sharkaway, T.Y., and Greenberg, G.R. (1953). Effects of pancreatic polypeptide on canine migrating motor complex and plasma motilin. Am. J. Physiol. 245, G178-G185

39. Wingate, D.L. (1983) The small intestine. In: Christensen, J., and Wingate, D.L. (ed). A Guide to Gastrointestinal Motility. pp. 128-156. (Bristol: Wright. PSG)

40. Sarna, S., Stoddard, C., Belbeck, L., and McWade, D. (1981). Intrinsic nervous control of migrating myoelectric complexes. Am. J. Physiol. 241, G16-G23

41. Thor, P., Krol, R., Konturek, S.J., Coy, D.H., and Schally, A.V. (1978). Effect of somatostatin on myoelectric activity of small bo-wel. Am. J. Physiol. 235, E249-254

42. Thor, P.J., Sendur, R., and Konturek, S.J. (1982). Influence of substance P on myoelectric activity of the small bowel. Am. J. Physiol. 243, G493-496

43. Sarna, S., Condon, R.E., and Cowles, W. (1983). Morphine versus motilin in the initiation of migrating myoelectric complexes. Am. J. Physiol. 245, G217-G220

44. Poitras, P., Steinbach, J.H., Van Deventer, G., Code, C.F., and Walsh, J.H. (1980). Motilin-independent ectopic fronts of the inter-digestive myoelectric complex in dogs. Am. J. Physiol. 239, G215-G220

45. Lorber, S.H., Komarov, S.A., and Shay, H. (1950). Effect of sham-feeding on gastric motor activity of the dog. Am. J. Physiol. 162, 447-451

46. Preshaw, R.M., and Knauf, R.S. (1966). The effect of sham-fee-ding on the secretion and motility of canine duodenal pouches. Gast-roenterology 51, 193-199

47. Steinbach, J.H., and Code, C.F. (1980). Increase in the period of the interdigestive myoelectric complex (IDMEC) with anticipation of feeding. In: Christensen, J. (ed.). Gastrointestinal Motility. pp. 247-252. (New York: Raven Press)

48. Defilippi, C., and Valenzuela, E. (1981). Sham-feeding disrupts the interdigestive motility complex in man. Scand. J. Gastroent. 16, 977-979

49. Peeters, T.L., Vantrappen, G., and Janssens, J. (1983). Sham-feeding amplifies the secretory component of interdigestive activity. Gastroenterology 84, 1272

50. Thor, P., Sendur, R., Konturek, S.J. (1982). Effect of sham-feeding and muscarinic receptors on myoelectric activity of the small intestine in the dog. Gastroenterology 82, 1197

51. Weisbrodt, N.W., Copeland, E.M., Thor, P., Mukhopadhyay, A.K., and Johnson, L.R. (1976). Nervous and humoral factors which influ-ence the fasted patterns of intestinal myoelectric activity. In: Vantrappen, G. (ed.). Proceedings of the 5th International Symposium

on Gastrointestinal Motility pp. 82-87.   (Herentals: Typoff Press)

52. Chang, J.C., Danchel, J., Sara, P., Angel, F., Bouchet, P., Lambert, A., and Grenier, J.F. (1978). Specific effects of different food components on intestinal motility. Eur. Surg. Res. 10, 425-432

53. Weisbrodt, N.W., Moore, E., Kearley, R., Copeland, E.M., and Johnson, L.R. (1974). Effects of pentagstrin on the myoelectric activity of the small intestine. Am. J. Physiol. 227, 425-429

54. Mukhopadhyay, A.K., Thor, P., Copeland, E.M., Johnson, L.R., and Weisbrodt, N.W. (1977). Effect of cholecystokinin on myoelectric activity of small intestine of the dog. Am. J. Physiol. 2321, E 44-E47

55. Mukhopadhyay, A.K., Johnson, L.R., Copeland, E.M., and Weisbrodt, N. (1975). Effect of secretin on electric activity of small intestine. Am. J. Physiol. 229, 484-488

56. Bueno, L., and Ruckebusch, M. (1976). Insulin and jejunal electrical activity in dogs and sheep. Am. J. Physiol. 230, 1539-1544

57. Thomes, P.A., Schang, J.C., Kelly, K.A., and Go, V.L.W. (1980). Can endogenous gastrin inhibit canine interdigestive gastric motility. Gastroenterology 78, 716-721

58. Wingate, D.L., Pearce, P.A., Hutton, M., and Thompson, H.H. (1978). Quantitative comparison of the effects of cholecystokinin, secretin and pentagastrin on gastrointestinal myoelectric activity in the conscious dog. Gut 19, 593-601

59. Thor, K., Rosell, S., Rokaeus, A., and Kager, L. (1982). (Glu^4)-Neurotensin changes the motility pattern of the duodenum and proximal jejunum from a fasting-type to a fed-type. Gastroenterology 83, 569-574

60. Thor, P.J., Konturek, J.W., Sendur, R., and Konturek, S.J. Comparison of neurotensin and fat on myoelectric activity pattern of the small bowel (in this issue)